AF167586

Communications
in Computer and Information Science   **2546**

Series Editors

Gang Li, *School of Information Technology, Deakin University, Burwood, VIC, Australia*
Joaquim Filipe, *Polytechnic Institute of Setúbal, Setúbal, Portugal*
Zhiwei Xu, *Chinese Academy of Sciences, Beijing, China*

Rationale

The CCIS series is devoted to the publication of proceedings of computer science conferences. Its aim is to efficiently disseminate original research results in informatics in printed and electronic form. While the focus is on publication of peer-reviewed full papers presenting mature work, inclusion of reviewed short papers reporting on work in progress is welcome, too. Besides globally relevant meetings with internationally representative program committees guaranteeing a strict peer-reviewing and paper selection process, conferences run by societies or of high regional or national relevance are also considered for publication.

Topics

The topical scope of CCIS spans the entire spectrum of informatics ranging from foundational topics in the theory of computing to information and communications science and technology and a broad variety of interdisciplinary application fields.

Information for Volume Editors and Authors

Publication in CCIS is free of charge. No royalties are paid, however, we offer registered conference participants temporary free access to the online version of the conference proceedings on SpringerLink (http://link.springer.com) by means of an http referrer from the conference website and/or a number of complimentary printed copies, as specified in the official acceptance email of the event.

CCIS proceedings can be published in time for distribution at conferences or as post-proceedings, and delivered in the form of printed books and/or electronically as USBs and/or e-content licenses for accessing proceedings at SpringerLink. Furthermore, CCIS proceedings are included in the CCIS electronic book series hosted in the SpringerLink digital library at http://link.springer.com/bookseries/7899. Conferences publishing in CCIS are allowed to use Online Conference Service (OCS) for managing the whole proceedings lifecycle (from submission and reviewing to preparing for publication) free of charge.

Publication process

The language of publication is exclusively English. Authors publishing in CCIS have to sign the Springer CCIS copyright transfer form, however, they are free to use their material published in CCIS for substantially changed, more elaborate subsequent publications elsewhere. For the preparation of the camera-ready papers/files, authors have to strictly adhere to the Springer CCIS Authors' Instructions and are strongly encouraged to use the CCIS LaTeX style files or templates.

Abstracting/Indexing

CCIS is abstracted/indexed in DBLP, Google Scholar, EI-Compendex, Mathematical Reviews, SCImago, Scopus. CCIS volumes are also submitted for the inclusion in ISI Proceedings.

How to start

To start the evaluation of your proposal for inclusion in the CCIS series, please send an e-mail to ccis@springer.com

Maria Pedro Guarino · Kazuhiro Hotta ·
Malik Yousef · Hui Liu · Giovanni Saggio ·
Hannes Schlieter · Ana Fred · Hugo Gamboa
Editors

Biomedical Engineering Systems and Technologies

17th International Joint Conference, BIOSTEC 2024
Rome, Italy, February 21–23, 2024
Revised Selected Papers

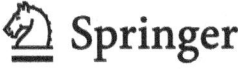 Springer

Editors
Maria Pedro Guarino
Polytechnic University of Leiria
Leiria, Portugal

Kazuhiro Hotta
Meijo University
Nagoya, Japan

Malik Yousef
Zefat Academic College
Dabburiya, Israel

Hui Liu
University of Bremen
Bremen, Germany

Giovanni Saggio
University of Rome Tor Vergata
Rome, Italy

Hannes Schlieter
Technische Universität Dresden
Dresden, Germany

Ana Fred
Instituto de Telecomunicações and Instituto
Superior Técnico
Lisbon, Portugal

Hugo Gamboa
Nova University of Lisbon
Lisbon, Portugal

ISSN 1865-0929   ISSN 1865-0937 (electronic)
Communications in Computer and Information Science
ISBN 978-3-031-96898-3   ISBN 978-3-031-96899-0 (eBook)
https://doi.org/10.1007/978-3-031-96899-0

This Springer imprint is published by the registered company Springer Nature Switzerland AG
The registered company address is: Gewerbestrasse 11, 6330 Cham, Switzerland

If disposing of this product, please recycle the paper.

Preface

The present book includes extended and revised versions of a set of selected papers from the 17th International Joint Conference on Biomedical Engineering Systems and Technologies (BIOSTEC 2024), held in Rome, Italy, from 21–23 February.

The purpose of BIOSTEC is to bring together researchers, professionals and practitioners, including engineers, biologists, health workers and informatics/computer scientists, interested in both theoretical advances and concrete applications of information systems, artificial intelligence, signal processing, electronics and other engineering tools in knowledge areas related to biology and medicine.

BIOSTEC 2024 received 242 paper submissions from 43 countries, of which 26 (11%) are included in this book.

The papers were selected by the event chairs and their selection was based on a number of criteria that included the classifications and comments provided by the program committee members, the session chairs' assessment and also the program chairs' global view of all papers included in the technical program. The authors of selected papers were then invited to submit revised and extended versions of their papers having at least one-third innovative material. The papers selected to be included in this book contribute to the understanding of relevant trends of current research on Biomedical Engineering Systems and Technologies, including: Assistive Technologies, Diagnostic Devices, Human-Machine Interaction in Healthcare IT, Medical Artificial Intelligence, Wearable and Mobile Devices, Health Monitoring Devices, Medical Informatics, Medical Signal Acquisition, Analysis and Processing, Cognitive Informatics and Biosensors, application of modelling frameworks, algorithmic concepts, computational methods, and information technologies to address challenging problems in Bioinformatics and Biomedical research.

We would like to thank all the authors for their contributions and also the reviewers who helped to ensure the quality of this publication.

February 2024

Maria Pedro Guarino
Kazuhiro Hotta
Malik Yousef
Hui Liu
Giovanni Saggio
Hannes Schlieter
Ana Fred
Hugo Gamboa

Organization

Conference Co-chairs

BIOSTEC

Ana Fred   Instituto de Telecomunicações and Instituto Superior Técnico (University of Lisbon), Portugal

Hugo Gamboa   Nova University of Lisbon, Portugal

Program Co-chairs

Biodevices

Maria Pedro Guarino   Polytechnic University of Leiria, Portugal

Bioimaging

Kazuhiro Hotta   Meijo University, Japan

Bioinformatics

Malik Yousef   Zefat Academic College, Israel

Biosignals

Hui Liu   University of Bremen, Germany

Giovanni Saggio   University of Rome Tor Vergata, Italy

HEALTHINF

Hannes Schlieter   Technische Universität Dresden, Germany

Program Committee

Biodevices

Carlos Abreu	Instituto Politécnico de Viana do Castelo, Portugal
Pedro Alpuim	International Iberian Nanotechnology Laboratory, Portugal
Manish Arora	Indian Institute of Science, India
Antonio Jesus Banegas-Luna	Universidad Católica San Antonio de Murcia, Spain
Steve Beeby	University of Southampton, UK
Gabriele Candiani	Polytechnic University of Milan, Italy
Vanessa Cardoso	University of Minho, Portugal
Eric Chappel	Debiotech SA, Switzerland
Mostafa Charmi	University of Zanjan, Iran
Cheng-Hsin Chuang	National Sun Yat-sen University, Taiwan
Youngjae Chun	University of Pittsburgh, USA
Alberto Cliquet Jr.	University of São Paulo & University of Campinas, Brazil
Willy Colier	Artinis Medical Systems, Netherlands
Maria Evelina Fantacci	University of Pisa and INFN, Italy
Mireya Fernández Chimeno	Universitat Politècnica de Catalunya, Spain
Rui Fonseca-Pinto	Polytechnic University of Leiria, Portugal
Gionata Fragomeni	University of Magna Graecia, Italy
Ugo Galvanetto	University of Padua, Italy
Miguel García Gonzalez	Universitat Politècnica de Catalunya, Spain
Javier Garcia-Casado	Universitat Politècnica de València, Spain
Gianluca Gatti	University of Calabria, Italy
Alessio Gizzi	Campus Bio-Medico University of Rome, Italy
Weihua Guan	Penn State University, USA
Evin Gultepe	Independent Researcher, USA
Ivan Ivanov	Technical University of Sofia, Bulgaria
Liudi Jiang	University of Southampton, UK
Yaroslav Korpan	Institute of Molecular Biology and Genetics, NAS of Ukraine, Ukraine
Dean Krusienski	Virginia Commonwealth University, USA
Hiroshi Kumagai	Kitasato University, Japan
Nicola Francesco Lopomo	Politecnico di Milano, Italy
Luyao Lu	George Washington University, USA
Ana Isabel Martins	Universidade de Aveiro, Portugal
Enzo Mastinu	Scuola Superiore Sant'Anna, Italy
Sabina Merlo	University of Pavia, Italy

Simona Miclaus	Nicolae Bălcescu Land Forces Academy, Romania
Ana Moita	Universidade de Lisboa, Portugal
Pedro Morouço	Polytechnic University of Leiria, Portugal
Robert Newcomb	University of Maryland, College Park, USA
Abraham Otero	Universidad San Pablo CEU, Spain
Zafer Ziya Öztürk	Gebze University of Technology, Turkey
Ji-Ho Park	Independent Researcher, South Korea
Onur Parlak	Karolinska Institute, Sweden
Helena Pereira	Coimbra Institute for Biomedical Imaging and Translational Research, Portugal
Gary Pickrell	Virginia Tech, USA
Rafael Pinheiro	Instituto Politécnico de Leiria, Portugal
Alexandre Rossi	Centro Brasileiro de Pesquisas Físicas, Brazil
Wim Rutten	University of Twente, Netherlands
Amir Sanati Nezhad	Independent Researcher, Canada
Wongwit Senavongse	Srinakharinwirot University, Thailand
Revati Shriram	Cummins College of Engineering for Women, India
Niall Tait	Carleton University, Canada
Tong-Boon Tang	Universiti Teknologi PETRONAS, Malaysia
Angel A. J. Torriero	Deakin University, Australia
John Tudor	University of Southampton, UK
Duarte Valério	Instituto Superior Técnico - Universidade de Lisboa, Portugal
Júlio Viana	University of Minho, Portugal
Nuno Vieira Lopes	Polytechnic of Leiria, Portugal
Roman Viter	University of Latvia, Latvia

Program Committee

Bioimaging

Peter Balazs	University of Szeged, Hungary
Richard Bayford	Middlesex University London, UK
Alpan Bek	Middle East Technical University, Turkey
Udo Birk	FH Graubünden, Switzerland
Fabio Augusto Cappabianco	Federal University of São Paulo, Brazil
Heang-Ping Chan	University of Michigan, USA
Mostafa Charmi	University of Zanjan, Iran
Giorgio De Nunzio	Università del Salento, Italy

João Batista Florindo	University of Campinas, Brazil
Dimitris Gorpas	Technical University of Munich, Germany
Tzung-Pei Hong	National University of Kaohsiung, Taiwan
Yuankai Huo	Vanderbilt University, USA
Turgay Ibrikci	Adana Alparslan Türkeş Science and Technology University, Turkey
Mohamed Esmail Karar	Menoufia University, Egypt
Algimantas Krisciukaitis	Lithuanian University of Health Sciences, Lithuania
Tengfei Li	University of North Carolina Chapel Hil, USA
Hongen Liao	Tsinghua University, China
Yingliang Ma	University of East Anglia, UK
Vaidotas Marozas	Kaunas University of Technology, Lithuania
Michal Mikl	Masaryk University, Czech Republic
Tim Nattkemper	Independent Researcher, Germany
Kalman Palagyi	University of Szeged, Hungary
Vadim Perez	Instituto Mexicano del Seguro Social, Mexico
Ivan Miguel Pires	Universidade de Aveiro, Portugal
Harikumar Rajaguru	Bannari Amman Institute of Technology, India
Oscar Ruiz-Salguero	Universidad EAFIT, Colombia
Hassan S. Salehi	California State University, USA
Gregory Sharp	Massachusetts General Hospital, USA
Jon Sporring	University of Copenhagen, Denmark
Arkadiusz Tomczyk	Lodz University of Technology, Poland
Carlos Travieso-González	Universidad de Las Palmas de Gran Canaria, Spain
Benjamin Tsui	Johns Hopkins University, USA

Additional Reviewers

Bioimaging

Darius Jegelevicius	Kaunas University of Technology, Lithuania

Program Committee

Bioinformatics

Heba Afify	Cairo University, Egypt
Tatsuya Akutsu	Kyoto University, Japan
Kazim Yalcin Arga	Marmara University, Turkey
Endre Barta	University of Debrecen, Hungary
Payam Behzadi	Shahr-e-Qods Branch, Islamic Azad University, Iran
Shifra Ben-Dor	Weizmann Institute of Science, Israel
Gilles Bernot	Université Côte d'Azur, France
Vannier Brigitte	University of Poitiers, France
Juan Caballero Pérez	Autonomous University of Queretaro, Mexico
Jean-Paul Comet	Université Côte d'Azur, France
Keith Crandall	George Washington University, USA
Thomas Dandekar	University of Würzburg, Germany
Riccardo Dondi	University of Bergamo, Italy
Maria Evelina Fantacci	University of Pisa and INFN, Italy
Stephen P. Ficklin	Washington State University, USA
Jean Fred Fontaine	Central Institute for Decision Support Systems in Crop Protection (ZEPP), Germany
Dmitrij Frishman	Technical University of Munich, Germany
Pascale Gaudet	Swiss Institute of Bioinformatics, Switzerland
Giorgio Giurato	University of Salerno, Italy
Alexandra Graf	FH Campus Wien - University of Applied Sciences, Austria
Junguk Hur	University of North Dakota School of Medicine and Health Sciences, USA
Mukesh Jain	Jawaharlal Nehru University, India
Giuseppe Jurman	Fondazione Bruno Kessler, Italy
Noam Kaplan	Technion Israel Institute of Technology, Israel
Andrzej Kloczkowski	Ohio State University, USA
Ivan Kulakovskiy	IPR RAS, Russian Federation
Yinglei Lai	George Washington University, USA
Man-Kee Lam	Universiti Teknologi PETRONAS, Malaysia
Lars Malmström	University of Zurich, Switzerland
Vincenzo Manca	University of Verona, Italy
Michal Marczyk	Silesian University of Technology, Poland
Enzo Martegani	University of Milano-Bicocca, Italy
Giancarlo Mauri	Università di Milano Bicocca, Italy
Paolo Milazzo	Università di Pisa, Italy

Jason Miller	Shepherd University, USA
Chilukuri Mohan	Syracuse University, USA
José Molina	Universidad Carlos III de Madrid, Spain
Shinichi Morishita	University of Tokyo, Japan
Brendan Mumey	Montana State University, USA
Pilib Ó Broin	University of Galway, Ireland
Theodore Perkins	Ottawa Hospital Research Institute, Canada
Graziano Pesole	University of Bari, Italy
Ovidiu Radulescu	University of Montpellier, France
Jagath Rajapakse	Nanyang Technological University, Singapore
Javier Reina-Tosina	University of Seville, Spain
Laura Roa	University of Seville, Spain
Vincent Rodin	UBO, LabSTICC/CNRS, France
Massimo La Rosa	National Research Council of Italy, Italy
Ulrich Rückert	Bielefeld University, Germany
Rovshan Sadygov	University of Texas Medical Branch, USA
J. Cristian Salgado	University of Chile, Chile
Andrew Schumann	University of Information Technology and Management in Rzeszow, Poland
Karel Sedlar	Brno University of Technology, Czech Republic
João Setubal	Universidade de São Paulo, Brazil
Jianting Sheng	Houston Methodist Research Institute, USA
Tiratha Raj Singh	Jaypee University of Information Technology, India
Sylvain Soliman	Inria Saclay, France
Martin Swain	Aberystwyth University, UK
Peter Sykacek	University of Natural Resources and Life Sciences, Vienna, Austria
Y-H. Taguchi	Chuo University, Japan
Giorgio Valentini	University of Milan, Italy
Nicola Vitulo	University of Verona, Italy

Additional Reviewers

Bioinformatics

Artem Kasianov	IITP RAS, Russian Federation
Isabella Mendolia	CNR-ICAR, Italy

Program Committee

Biosignals

Daniel Abasolo	University of Surrey, UK
Vahid Abolghasemi	University of Essex, UK
Siti Anom Ahmad	Putra Malaysia University, Malaysia
Eda Akman Aydin	Gazi University, Turkey
Raul Alcaraz	University of Castilla-La Mancha, Spain
Robert Allen	University of Southampton, UK
Óscar Barquero-Pérez	Rey Juan Carlos University, Spain
Eberhard Beck	Brandenburg University of Applied Sciences, Germany
Martin Bogdan	Universität Leipzig, Germany
Susana Brás	IEETA, LASI, Universidade de Aveiro, Portugal
Maria Claudia Castro	Centro Universitário FEI, Brazil
Ioanna Chouvarda	Aristotle University of Thessaloniki, Greece
Adam Czajka	University of Notre Dame, USA
Petr Dolezel	University of Pardubice, Czech Republic
Omar Farooq	Aligarh Muslim University, India
Marcos Faundez	Escola Universitaria Politecnica de Mataro - Tecnocampus, Spain
Dimitris Filos	Aristotle University of Thessaloniki, Greece
Javier Garcia-Casado	Universitat Politècnica de València, Spain
Carlos Gómez	University of Valladolid, Spain
Pedro Gómez Vilda	Independent Researcher, Spain
Rebeca Goya-Esteban	Rey Juan Carlos University, Spain
Teddy Surya Gunawan	International Islamic University Malaysia, Malaysia
David Halliday	University of York, UK
Dimitrios Hatzinakos	University of Toronto, Canada
Richard Hendriks	TU Delft, Netherlands
Thomas Hinze	Friedrich Schiller University Jena, Germany
Roberto Hornero	University of Valladolid, Spain
Aisyah Hartini Jahidin	Universiti Malaya, Malaysia
Irena Jekova	Bulgarian Academy of Sciences, Bulgaria
Aleksandar Jeremic	McMaster University, Canada
Akos Jobbagy	Budapest University of Technology and Economics, Hungary
Gordana Jovanovic Dolecek	INAOE, Mexico
Natalya Kizilova	Warsaw University of Technology, Poland
Krzysztof Kulpa	Independent Researcher, Poland

Lenka Lhotska	Czech Technical University in Prague, Czech Republic
Maria Lindén	Mälardalen University, Sweden
Mai Mabrouk	Nile University, Egypt
Luca Mainardi	Politecnico di Milano, Italy
Tomasz Marciniak	Politechnika Poznańska, Poland
Ahmet Mert	Bursa Technical University, Turkey
Fernando Monteiro	Polytechnic Institute of Bragança, Portugal
Mihaela Morega	University Politehnica of Bucharest, Romania
Minoru Nakayama	Institute of Science Tokyo, Japan
António Neves	University of Aveiro, Portugal
Joanna Isabelle Olszewska	University of the West of Scotland, UK
Rui Pedro Paiva	University of Coimbra, Portugal
Aleksander Paterno	Santa Catarina State University, Brazil
Riccardo Pernice	University of Palermo, Italy
Vitor Pires	Escola Superior de Tecnologia de Setúbal - Instituto Politécnico de Setúbal, Portugal
Fabienne Poree	Université de Rennes, France
Piotr Porwik	University of Silesia in Katowice, Poland
Shitala Prasad	I2R, A*Star Singapore, Singapore
Krothapalli Sreenivasa Rao	Indian Institute of Technology Kharagpur, India
José Joaquín Rieta	Universidad Politécnica de Valencia, Spain
Heather Ruskin	Dublin City University, Ireland
Goutam Saha	Indian Institute of Technology Kharagpur, India
Andrews Samraj	Mahendra Engineering College, India
Emanuele Schiavi	Universidad Rey Juan Carlos, Spain
Fabio Schneider	Federal University of Technology - Paraná, Brazil
Reinhard Schneider	Fachhochschule Vorarlberg, Austria
Zdenek Smekal	Brno University of Technology, Czech Republic
H. C. So	City University of Hong Kong, China
Jordi Solé-Casals	University of Vic - Central University of Catalonia, Spain
Iickho Song	Korea Advanced Institute of Science and Technology, South Korea
António Teixeira	University of Aveiro, Portugal
Carlos Thomaz	Centro Universitário FEI, Brazil
Hua-Nong Ting	University of Malaya, Malaysia
Alessandro Tognetti	University of Pisa, Italy
Carlos Travieso-González	Universidad de Las Palmas de Gran Canaria, Spain
Ursula van Rienen	University of Rostock, Germany
Aleksandra Vuckovic	University of Glasgow, UK

| Yuanyuan Wang | Fudan University, China |
| Rafal Zdunek | Politechnika Wrocławska, Poland |

Additional Reviewers

Biosignals

| Revathi Appali | University of Rostock, Germany |
| Ana Rocha | IEETA, University of Aveiro/LASI, Portugal |

Program Committee

HEALTHINF

Samina Abidi	Independent Researcher, Canada
Lucienne Abrahams	University of the Witwatersrand, Johannesburg, South Africa
Carlos Abreu	Instituto Politécnico de Viana do Castelo, Portugal
Ashir Ahmed	Kyushu University, Japan
Amin Aminifar	Heidelberg University, Germany
Luca Anselma	Università degli Studi di Torino, Italy
Shunxing Bao	Vanderbilt University, USA
Payam Behzadi	Shahr-e-Qods Branch, Islamic Azad University, Iran
José Alberto Benítez-Andrades	Universidad de León, Spain
Sorana Bolboaca	Iuliu Hațieganu University of Medicine and Pharmacy, Cluj-Napoca, Romania
Silvia Bonfanti	University of Bergamo, Italy
Alessio Bottrighi	Università del Piemonte Orientale, Italy
Andrew Boyd	University of Illinois Chicago, USA
Frederico Branco	University of Trás-os-Montes e Alto Douro, Portugal
Klaus Brinker	Hamm-Lippstadt University of Applied Sciences, Germany
Andrea Campagner	University of Milano-Bicocca, Italy
Manuel Campos-Martinez	University of Murcia, Spain
Prodromos Chatzoglou	Democritus University of Thrace, Greece
Davide Ciucci	Università degli Studi di Milano-Bicocca, Italy
Malcolm Clarke	Ondokuz Mayıs University, Turkey

Stefania Montani   Piemonte Orientale University, Italy
Roman Moucek   University of West Bohemia, Czech Republic
Hajar Mozaffar   University of Edinburgh, UK
Raymond Ng   University of British Columbia, Canada
Anne Ngu   Texas State University-San Marcos, USA
Kazunori Nozaki   Osaka University Dental Hospital, Japan
Takashi Obi   Tokyo Institute of Technology, Japan
Nelson Pacheco da Rocha   University of Aveiro, Portugal
Alessandro Pagano   University of Bari, Italy
Rui Pedro Paiva   University of Coimbra, Portugal
Petros Papapanagiotou   Independent Researcher, UK
Antonio Piccinno   University of Bari, Italy
Ivan Miguel Pires   Universidade de Aveiro, Portugal
Hardy Pundt   Harz University of Applied Sciences, Germany
Reza Rabiei   Shahid Beheshti University of Medical Sciences,
                                    Iran
Mahmudur Rahman   Morgan State University, USA
Murugesan Raju   University of Missouri, USA
Arkalgud Ramaprasad   University of Illinois Chicago, USA
Khaled Rasheed   University of Georgia, USA
Grzegorz Redlarski   Gdańsk University of Technology, Poland
Alejandro Rodríguez González   Universidad Politécnica de Madrid, Spain
Cristian Rotariu   Grigore T. Popa University of Medicine and
                                    Pharmacy, Romania
Stefan Rüping   Fraunhofer IAIS, Germany
Ovidio Salvetti   National Research Council of Italy - CNR, Italy
André Santanchè   University of Campinas, Brazil
Rishi Kanth Saripalle   Illinois State University, USA
Akio Sashima   AIST, Japan
Bettina Schnor   Potsdam University, Germany
Moushumi Sharmin   Western Washington University, USA
Revati Shriram   Cummins College of Engineering for Women,
                                    India
Geraldo Silva Junior   University of Fortaleza, Brazil
Carla Simone   University of Milano-Bicocca, Italy
Åsa Smedberg   Stockholm University, Sweden
Luca Spalazzi   Università Politecnica delle Marche, Italy
Zoran Stevic   University of Belgrade, Serbia
Manel Taboada   Autonomous University of Barcelona, Spain
Jorge Tavares   Universidade Nova de Lisboa, Portugal
Francesco Tiezzi   University of Camerino, Italy
Alberto Trombetta   Università degli Studi dell'Insubria, Italy

Yi-Ju Tseng	National Yang Ming Chiao Tung University, Taiwan
Lauri Tuovinen	University of Oulu, Finland
Mohy Uddin	King Abdullah International Medical Research Center, Saudi Arabia
Gary Ushaw	Newcastle University, UK
Ricardo Vardasca	ISLA Santarém, Portugal
Andrei Vasilateanu	Politehnica University of Bucharest, Romania
Francisco Veredas	Universidad de Málaga, Spain
Gennaro Vessio	University of Bari, Italy
Abdullah Wahbeh	Slippery Rock University, USA
Chien-Chih Wang	Ming Chi University of Technology, Taiwan
Dimitrios Zarakovitis	University of the Peloponnese, Greece
Dimitrios Zikos	Central Michigan University, USA

Additional Reviewers

HEALTHINF

Nuran Aydin	Independent Researcher, USA
Pier Felice Balestrucci	Università di Torino, Italy
Chariklia Chatzaki	Hellenic Mediterranean University, Greece

Invited Speakers

BIOSTEC

Norbert Noury	University of Lyon, France
Anna Maria M. Bianchi	Politecnico di Milano, Italy
Robert Turner	Max Planck Institute for Human Cognitive and Brain Sciences, Germany
Juan C. Augusto	Middlesex University London, UK

Contents

Bioinformatics Models, Methods and Algorithms

Bio-inspired Systems and Signal Processing

Health Informatics

Biomedical Electronics and Devices

A Sensitive Method to Rapidly Identify GBS

Zhi-Rui Xie[1,2], Yang Chen[2,3], Yu-Ying Hou[3], Bei-Bei Lin[3], Long-Teng Xie[4], and Yao-Gen Shu[2,3,4](✉)

[1] Postgraduate Training Base Alliance of Wenzhou Medical University, Wenzhou 325000, Zhejiang, China
[2] Wenzhou Institute, University of Chinese Academy of Sciences, Wenzhou 325024, Zhejiang, China
shuyaogen@ucas.ac.cn
[3] Oujiang Laboratory (Zhejiang Lab for Regenerative Medicine, Vision and Brain Health), Wenzhou 325024, Zhejiang, China
[4] Joint Research Center on Medicine, Xiangshan Hospital of Wenzhou Medical University, Ningbo 315700, Zhejiang, China

Abstract. Group B streptococcus (GBS) is a leading cause of invasive neonatal infections and a significant pathogen in immunocompromised adults. Screening pregnant women for GBS colonization can determine whether the pregnant woman needs antibiotic prophylaxis. Therefore, it is crucial to determine the GBS colonization status of pregnant women efficiently and quickly. Here, we set up a point-of-care testing (POCT) according to specific absorption spectroscopy method based on chromogenic culture media to replace the traditional visual identification of GBS. It first converts the bioinformatics (pigment concentration) into light absorption intensity, then transforms the latter into a electrical signal value, and finally computes the electrical signal value into the variable value we defined. In this way, we established a quantitative relationship between the variable value and the GBS concentration, which greatly improved the sensitivity of GBS detection and shortened the identification time of GBS colonization from the traditional 48 h to our POCT's 6 h as expected.

Keywords: GBS · Chromogenic culture media · POCT

1 Introduction

Group B streptococcus (GBS) is a Gram-positive encapsulated bacterium belonging to the group Streptococcus agalactiae that is an asymptomatic colonizer of the digestive and genitourinary tracts of healthy human adults. However, it can cause severe invasive infections in neonates and immunocompromised adult patients. In 1960s, GBS was identified into a leading cause of life-threatening neonatal infections [1,2].

In neonatology, two clinical syndromes are distinguished: one is called early-onset disease (EOD), in which GBS infection occurs within the first week of

M. P. Guarino et al. (Eds.): BIOSTEC 2024, CCIS 2546, pp. 3–12, 2026.
https://doi.org/10.1007/978-3-031-96899-0_1

life (particularly within the first 24 h); and the other is called late-onset disease (LOD), in which GBS infection presents after 7 to 90 days postpartum. EOD is caused by vertical transmission, either via ascending infection from the genital tract or infection during delivery. Numerous studies have shown that up to 30% of pregnant women worldwide are infected with GBS, and vertical transmission occurs in approximately 50% of infected mothers. Approximately 1% of infected neonates will develop EOD, which may be related to rupture of membranes, as the fetus cannot be infected unless it is exposed to GBS. Bacteremia without a focus of infection is the most common clinical syndrome, followed by pneumonia and meningitis. Even today, the mortality rate of EOD is estimated to be as high as 2% to 10%, with a higher mortality rate in premature infants [3].

Most EOD are caused by neonatal exposure to GBS during delivery; therefore, intrapartum antibiotic prophylaxis (IAP) for GBS carriers prevents vertical transmission in the vast majority of cases, and its widespread use has resulted in significant reductions in the incidence of EOD. However, LOD is most likely acquired through breast milk, nosocomial or community sources. Prematurity is the main risk factor for LOD, and bacteremia without a focus of infection is the most common presentation. LOD has a low mortality rate, but meningitis and subsequent sequelae are more frequently associated with LOD [4].

GBS can also causes significant maternal morbidity, including bacteremia, endometritis, chorioamnionitis, and postpartum wound infection. GBS urinary tract infections are associated with miscarriage, premature delivery, and low birth weight neonates. Although GBS rarely causes disease in healthy adults, it is responsible for serious infections in patients with diabetes, the elderly, nursing home residents, and other immunocompromised individuals. The successful administration of IAP and treatment of severe GBS infections rely on the effective and reliable detection of GBS in clinical specimens [5].

In recent years, the use of chromogenic culture media for the detection of GBS has increased rapidly. These culture media contain enzyme substrates linked to indoxyl chromogens, and the target microorganisms have a specific enzyme system that can metabolize the substrate, thereby releasing the chromogen. Subsequently, in an aerobic environment, the indoxyl molecules oxidize and dimerize to form a indigoid dye that precipitates within the colony, producing a typical bright contrast color [6]. Therefore, the magnitude of the color contrast is positively correlated with the concentration of GBS. However, traditional visual identification usually requires at least 48 h of bacterial culture to determine whether GBS is colonized. Thus, clinical diagnosis urgently needs a rapid and sensitive GBS quantitative detection technology.

2   Materials and Methods

2.1   A POCT Based on the Specific Absorption Spectrum of Chromogen

We developed a POCT (a point-of-care testing [7]) based on the specific absorption spectrum of chromogen, which first converts bioinformatics (pigment con-

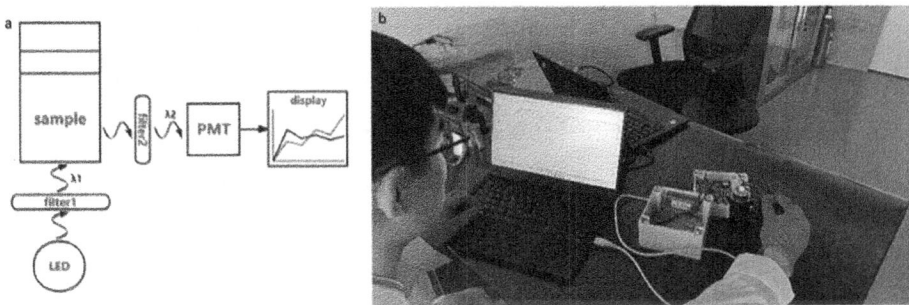

Fig. 1. a: Working principle of POCT. LED is the source of excited light. A beam of parallel excitation light with a wavelength of λ_1 is filtered out from filter 1 and incident on the sample in a direction perpendicular to the bottom of the tube. As a result, the irradiated sample emits another light (λ_2), which is the so-called emission light, but part of the λ_2 light will be absorbed by the indoxyl chromogen, and the rest of emission light will eventually be detected by PMT (photomultiplier tube) through filter 2. The absolute value of the time trajectory of the λ_2 light intensity is directly displayed in Fig. 2. **b:** The first genaration of POCT in experiment [8].

centration) into light absorption intensity, then transforms the latter into a digital electrical signal, and finally computes the electrical signal into the value of the variable we defined, thereby establishing a quantitative relationship between the variable and the GBS concentration, which meets the clinical demand for highly sensitive, rapid, and quantitative GBS detection.

Figure 1 shows the detection mechanism of the POCT device. A beam of parallel excitation light with a wavelength of λ_1 is filtered through filter 1 and then incident to the sample perpendicular to the bottom of the tube. As a result, the irradiated sample emits another beam of light (λ_2), which is the so-called emission light, but part of the λ_2 light will be absorbed by indoxyl chromogen, and the rest of emission light will eventually pass through filter 2 and be detected by the PMT (photomultiplier tube). The trajectory of the absolute detection value of the emission light intensity over time is shown in Fig. 2.

2.2   Definition of the Normalized Intensity of Absorbed Light ρ_j

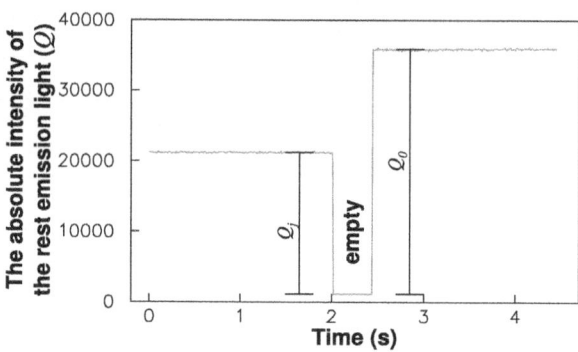

Fig. 2. Time trajectory of λ_2 light intensity and definition of absorption intensity $Q_0 - Q_j$.

The measured absolute intensity of the emitted light (Q_j) is equal to the value of higher platform minus the background noise (corresponding to the value of the lower platform (empty)). Therefore, the absorbed light intensity of the sample is $Q_0 - Q_j$, as shown in Fig. 2, where Q_0 is assumed to be the value without any indoxyl chromogens in the chromogenic media, such as sample "0" in Fig. 3a.

In order to quantitatively measure the concentration of GBS, we denominate the measurable variable ρ_j as the normalized intensity of the absorbed light of sample "j", which can be defined as

$$\rho_j \equiv 1 - \frac{Q_j}{Q_0}, \tag{1}$$

as shown in Fig. 3.

The amount of light λ_2 absorbed is proportional to the concentration of indoxyl chromogen, which in turn is positively correlated with the concentration of GBS. Therefore, the measurable amount of light λ_2 absorbed is also proportional to the concentration of GBS, that is, the concentration of GBS (c) can be quantitatively detected by the normalized intensity of absorbed light λ_2 (ρ_j) as defined by Eq. (1).

2.3   Preparation of Diluted Samples and Sensitivity Measurement

To determine the sensitivity of POCT, we performed a quantitative dilution experiment. Wenzhou Bacet Medical Instrument Co., Ltd. provided two tubes of 1.2 mL culture media, one contains a higher concentration of indoxyl chromogen, labeled as "5", and the other containing no chromogen, labeled as "0". Figure 3a shows the diluted samples, in which the culture media is uniformly mixed with different concentration of the chromogens, and corresponding measured absolute light intensity. The preparation and measurement are carried out simultaneously as follows:

1. We measured the intensity of the emission light from tube "0", and the platform "0" in Fig. 3a (the first higher platform from right) is the time trajectory of its measurement;
2. A 5 μL of samples "5" is injected into tube "0", the new sample is labeled as "1", and the time trajectory of the measured emission intensity is shown in platform "1" in Fig. 3a(the second higher platform from right) ;
3. Another 5 μL of samples "5" is injected into tube "1" again, the new sample is labeled as "2", and the time trajectory of the measured emission intensity is shown in platform "2" in Fig. 3a(the third higher platform from right);
4. A 10 μL of samples "5" is injected into tube "2", the new sample is labeled as "3", and the time trajectory of the measured emission intensity is shown in platform "3" in Fig. 3a(the fourth higher platform from right);
5. A 20 μL of samples "5" is injected into tube "3", the new sample is labeled as "4", and the time trajectory of the measured emission intensity is shown in platform "4" in Fig. 3a(the fifth higher platform from right);
6. Finally, we measured the emission intensity of tube "5", and the platform "5" (the sixth higher platform from right) in Fig. 3a is its measured time trajectory.

The normalized chromogen concentrations of sample "0~5"(relative to the sample "5"), c, are approximately 0, 4.15×10^{-3}, 8.26×10^{-3}, 1.64×10^{-2}, 3.23×10^{-2}, and 1.00 respectively.

In order to make the indoxyl chromogens uniformly distributed in the culture media, we use a vortexer to mix the culture media before each measurement.

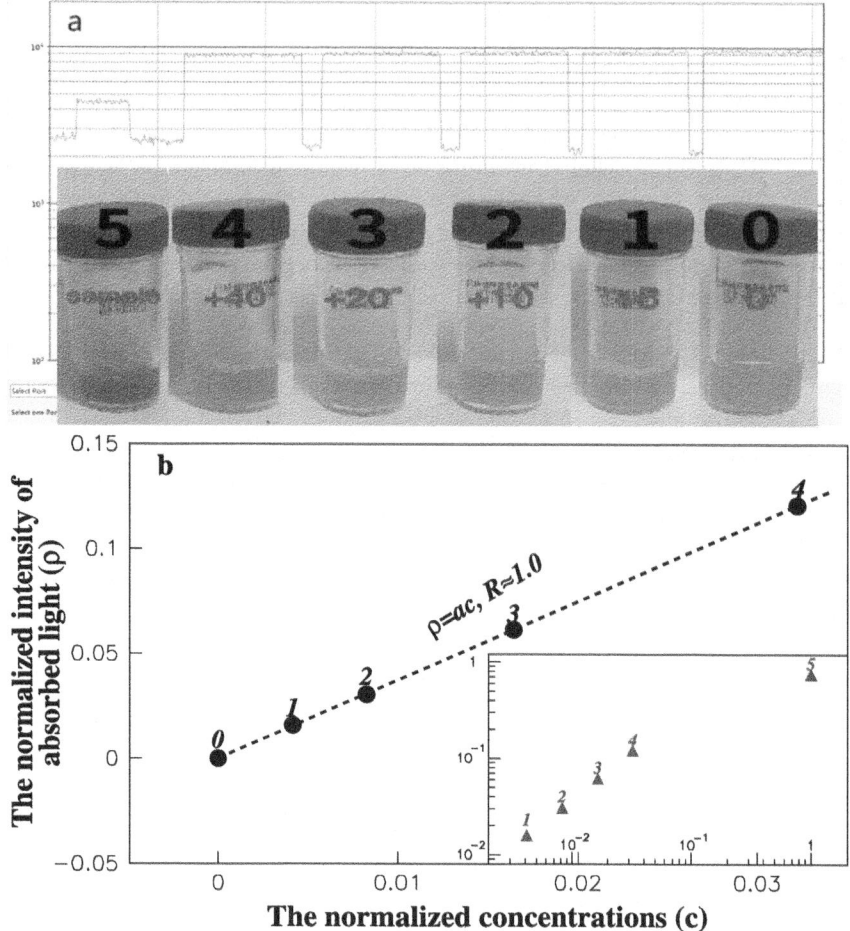

Fig. 3. a: Absolute light intensity (logarithmic scale) versus time of diluted samples measured by our POCT. From *right* to *left*, each higher platform corresponds to the value of samples "0","1","2","3","4" and "5" (**The inserted panel**) respectively, while the lower platform is the background value, so the absolute light intensity is the higher one minus the lower one. The normalized intensity of the absorbed light of sample j, ρ_j, can be defined by Eq. (1). **b:** ρ vs normalized concentrations of samples (c), which is almost linear ($\rho = ac$, where $a \approx 3.75$, is the fitted constant) at lower concentrations with regression coefficient($R \approx 1.0$). **The inserted panel** shows that the ρ_5/ρ_1 is close to 10^2, which means that our POCT is much more sensitive than the traditional visual detection [8].

2.4 Preparation of Clinical Samples and Measurement of Variable Values

For clinical samples, a challenging question arises: How long does the sample need to be cultured for our POCT to determine whether GBS is colonized?

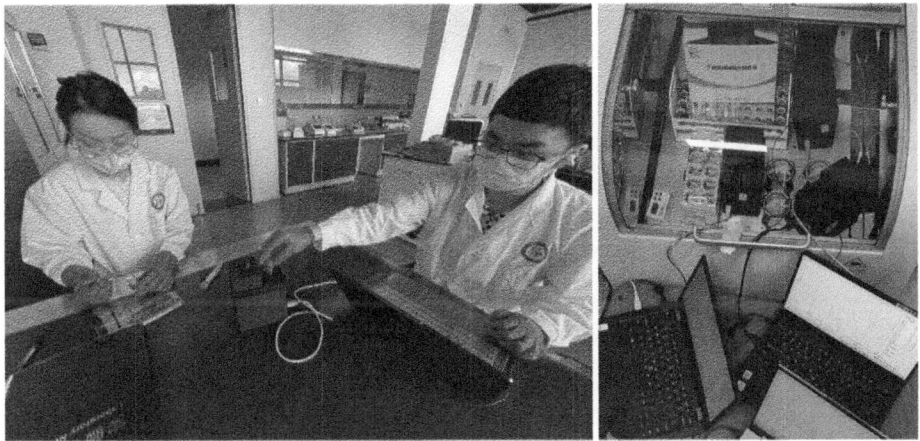

Fig. 4. left: Preparation of clinical samples. The black box at the centre of the panel is the second generation of our POCT. **right:** Online measurement in a constant incubator at 35 °C for 12 h. It was taken every 30 min automatically.

We performed online quantitative measurements of clinical samples in a 35 °C constant temperature incubator, as shown in Fig. 4. Wenzhou Bacet Medical Instrument Co., Ltd. provided 10 tubes of 1.2 mL culture media, and the Second Affiliated Hospital of Wenzhou Medical University supplied 7 clinical swab samples.

The experiment was conducted in two batches, the first batch enabled 4 POCTs corresponding to 4 clinical samples being cultured; the second batch enabled 3 POCTs corresponding to the remaining 3 clinical samples being cultured, as shown in Fig. 4. Online measurements were automatically performed every 30 min, as shown in Fig. 5. The labels "1", "2" and "3" of the second batch of samples were replaced by "5","6" and "7" in statistical results, respectively.

It should be pointed out that during the online measurement process, the pigment diffused very slowly in the media by itself, without any help of external mixing, which may be the main reason for the large fluctuations of data.

3   Results

In the dilution experiment (Sect. 2.3), the relationship between the normalized intensity of absorbed light (ρ) and the normalized concentrations of the samples (c) is almost linear at lower concentrations($\rho = ac$, where $a \approx 3.75$ is the fitted constant), and the regression coefficient($R \approx 1.0$). The values of samples "1" $\sim$ "4" are significantly higher than "$\rho_0 (\equiv 0)$", which means that the sensitivity of our method is much higher than that of the traditional visual identification method, as shown in Fig. 3. The huge quantitative difference between samples "1" and "5" further confirms the advanced nature of our POCT. With the help of our POCT, the time for identification GBS colonization can be greatly shortened.

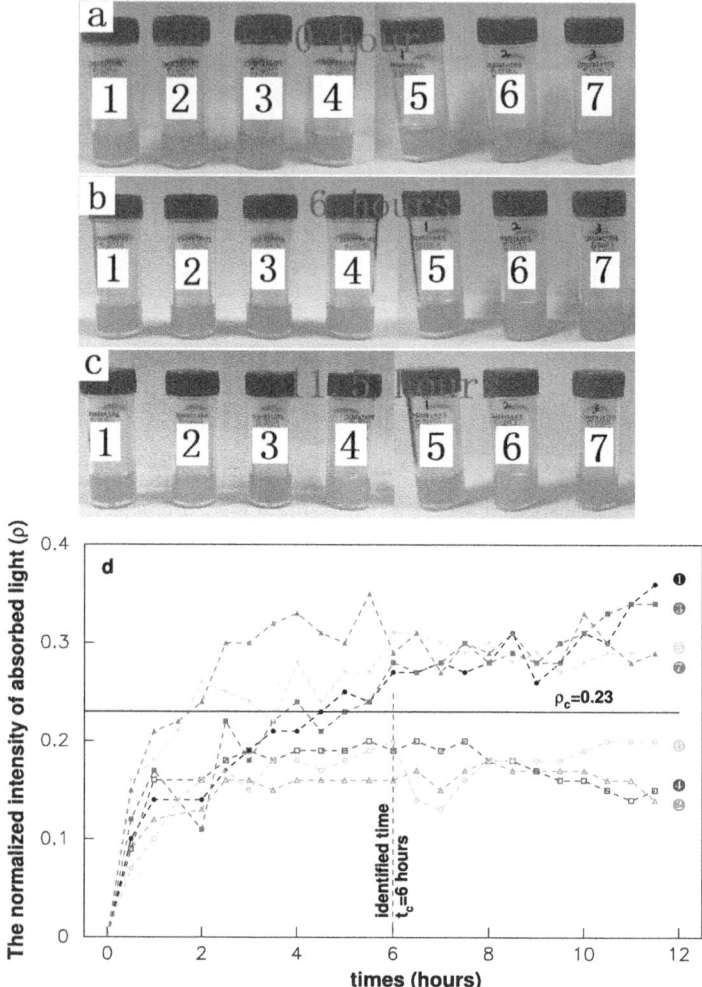

Fig. 5. **a/b/c:** The color display of different clinical samples after 0/6/11.5 h of culture respectively. They look like identical except the "1" and "3" in **c**. **d:** The relationship between the normalized intensity of absorbed light ρ and the culture time t. After 6 h of culture, the clinical samples were divided into two groups, the group with higher ρ is positive, while that with lower ρ is negative. In negative group, the trajectory of ρ seemed to be consistent with expectations, a straight line parallel to the time coordinate. There is a threshold of ρ ($\rho_c = 0.23$) that can be used to identify whether the GBS colonize. We denominate t_c (= 6 h) as the identification time in the clinical trials, which means that the traditional visual identification time of 48 h can be shortened to our identification time of 6 h. Although all ρ time trajectories fluctuate greatly, the positive/negative bifurcation at 6 h is obvious.

In the clinical trial (Sect. 2.4), the relationship between the normalized intensity of absorbed light (ρ) and the culture time (t) shows that at 6 h, the trajectory has a clear bifurcation, and the threshold of $\rho(\rho_c = 0.23)$ can be used to identify whether the sample is positive or negative. The traditional visual identification of culture tubes and our POCT measurement identification can be performed simultaneously. As predicted by the dilution experiment, our quantitative method can significantly shorten the positive identification time from the traditional 48 h to 6 h.

4   Conclusions and Discussion

The sensitivity of screening methods based on the culture identification of maternal carriage of GBS depends on the timing of specimen collection, the source of the specimen, and the culture technique used by the microbiology laboratory. Chromogenic culture media is a good alternative for the identification of GBS carrier status among near-term pregnant women. Decreasing identification time of GBS colonization and improving sensitivity is the original motivation for our development of POCT. As shown in Fig. 3, traditional visual identification is difficult to determine whether samples $1 \sim 4$ are colonized by GBS. However, our POCT achieves highly sensitivity and rapid detection of GBS and provides a competitive advantage for chromogenic culture methods. In Fig. 3a, the time traces of each platform show a high difference (this difference is not obvious visually because we use a logarithmic coordinate), indicating that our POCT is more sensitive than traditional visual detection.

The prediction results in the dilution experiment with perfect data as shown in Fig. 3 have been verified in clinical experiment. Although all ρ time trajectories fluctuate greatly, the positive/negative bifurcation at 6 h is obvious. Therefore, the clinical samples were divided into two groups according to their values of ρ, the higher ρ group is positive, while the lower ρ one is negative. As expected, the ρ in negative group remains constant, while that in positive group increase exponentially as:

$$\rho(t) = \alpha(2^{t/\tau} - 1), \tag{2}$$

where α is a constant, τ is the time for GBS to double in number after each generation through binary fission. Eq. (2) can be used to fit the positive time trajectories in Fig. 5. Then, if there are enough positive time trajectories, we can get the significant τ and α.

We denominate t_c ($= 6$ h) as the identification time in clinical trials and use a threshold of ρ ($\rho_c = 0.23$) to identify whether the GBS colonize. So far, we have gotten a simple two-step rapid identification method:

1. When the culture media temperature reaches 35 °C, for example, after 30 min of culture, the first measurement is performed to obtain the value of Q_0;
2. When the culture time t exceeds the identification time t_c, the second measurement is performed to obtain the value of $Q(t)$.

The normalized intensity of absorbed light at time t,

$$\rho(t > t_c) = 1 - \frac{Q(t)}{Q_0} \begin{cases} > \rho_c \text{ , positive} \\ < \rho_c \text{ , negative} \end{cases} \tag{3}$$

Therefore, the traditional visual identification time of 48 h can be shortened to our identification time of 6 h.

It should be pointed out that the diffusion of indoxyl chromogens in the culture media is very slow due to over damped, and it is very difficulty for the indoxyl chromogens to uniformly distributed in the culture media at all time in online experiment because there is no longer external vortexer to be engaged to mix the media as in diluted experiment, which may be the main reason for the large fluctuations in clinical experiment data. Therefore, the time trajectory of the online measurement is not as perfectly smooth as the curve of the dilution experiment.

It must also be pointed out that the quantitative relationship between the threshold of ρ (ρ_c) and the number of GBS has not been established. We will work hard to found the relationship and fit the α and τ with a large number of clinical swab samples.

Acknowledgements. The authors thank the Second Affiliated Hospital of Wenzhou Medical University and Wenzhou Bacet Medical Instrument Co., Ltd. for their supplying of samples and chromogenic media respectively, and the financial supports by Wenzhou Institute of UCAS (WIUCASQD2020009 and WIUCASICTP2022), Joint Research Center on Medicine of Xiangshan Hospital(XSZD2024004), the Discipline Cluster for Oncology of Wenzhou Medical University (z1-2023005), and Oujiang Laboratory (Zhejiang Lab for Regenerative Medicine, Vision and Brain Health) (OJQDJQ2022001).

Disclosure of Interests. The authors have no competing interests to declare that are relevant to the content of this article.

References

1. Hood, M., Janney, A., Dameron, G.: Am. J. Obstet. Gynecol. **82**, 809–818 (1961)
2. Rosa-Fraile, M., Spellerberg, B.: J. Clin. Microbiol. **55**, 2590–2598 (2017)
3. Edwards, M.S., Nizet, V., Baker, C.J.: Group B Streptococcal Infections: Remington and Klein's Infectious Diseases of the Fetus and Newborn Infant. Elsevier Saunders, Philadelphia (2016)
4. Verani, J.R., McGee, L., Schrag, S.J.: MMWR Recomm. Report **59**(RR-10), 1–36 (2010)
5. Edwards, M.S., Baker, C.J.: Clin. Infect. Dis. **41**, 839–847 (2005)
6. Orenga, S., James, A.L., Manafi, M., Perry, J.D., Pincus, D.H.: J. Microbiol. Methods **79**, 139–155 (2009)
7. Shu, Y.G., Chen, Y.: A trace analysis of GBS and its POCT. China patent **202211273343**, 6 (2022)
8. Chen, Y., Xie, Z. R., Shu, Y. G.:A POCT to rapid detect GBS with highly sensitivity. https://doi.org/10.5220/0012287600003657. Paper published under CC license (CC BY-NC-ND 4.0), In Proceedings of the 17th International Joint Conference on Biomedical Engineering Systems and Technologies (BIOSTEC 2024) - Volume 1, pp. 91–94. ISBN: 978-989-758-688-0; ISSN: 2184-4305

Low-Cost Flexible Sensor Glove for Measuring Functional Finger Range of Motion in Daily Activities

Shival Indermun[1,2(✉)] ⓘ and Taahirah Mangera[2] ⓘ

[1] Mechanical and Mechatronic Department, Stellenbosch University,
Western Cape, South Africa
s.indermun@gmail.com
[2] School of Mechanical, Aeronautical and Industrial Engineering, University of Witwatersrand,
Johannesburg, South Africa

Abstract. Hand impairments caused by conditions such as strokes and radial nerve palsy significantly impact the quality of life for many individuals, particularly in developing regions with limited access to rehabilitation services. Accurate measurement of the range of motion (ROM) of the hand is crucial for effective therapy and recovery monitoring. Traditional methods using goniometers are often cumbersome and dependent on the patient's ability to maintain static positions. This study utilizes a low-cost flexible sensor glove designed to measure the minimum range of ROM required to perform activities of daily living (ADLs). The prototype, developed using readily available flex sensors, was tested on 40 participants performing 11 ADLs. The investigation resulted in a ROM of 39.88°–69.42°, 18.92°–78.1°, and 13.42°–60.15° for the metacarpophalangeal (MCP), proximal interphalangeal (PIP) and interphalangeal joints (IP), respectively. These ranges indicate the necessary ROM for an individual to maintain functional independence based on the chosen ADLs. While the glove measurements were compared to those in previous studies, variations in measurement techniques, participant numbers and the selected ADLs influenced the variations observed in the results.

Keywords: Flex sensors · Prototype · Functional range of motion · Activities of daily living

1 Introduction

Various diseases and disorders can impair hand function, with cerebrovascular accidents (strokes) being particularly common. The incidence of stroke is increasing in developing countries [18] and is a leading cause of disability in South Africa [12], accounting for approximately 2–3% [12] of the total health services expenditure.

In addition to strokes, conditions such as radial nerve palsy also significantly affect hand function. Radial nerve palsy, which impairs wrist and finger extension, can result from physical injuries or infections and is prevalent among laborers due to repetitive arm use [14].

M. P. Guarino et al. (Eds.): BIOSTEC 2024, CCIS 2546, pp. 13–22, 2026.
https://doi.org/10.1007/978-3-031-96899-0_2

Many stroke patients in South Africa reside in rural areas, where access to therapy clinics is challenging due to distance [11]. Lower-income households spend a significant portion of their income on public transport [16], further increasing the cost of ongoing rehabilitation. High patient turnover in therapy clinics [3] often results in long waiting times, limiting the duration and quality of consultation and treatment. These issues are exacerbated by limited resources and opportunities for hand occupational therapy in South Africa, a challenge likely shared by other developing countries. Therefore, accessible treatment methods are crucial for these regions.

Effective rehabilitation is essential for stimulating recovery from hand impairments. Accurate assessment of hand impairment levels is a prerequisite for developing effective therapeutic methods. Measuring the range of motion (ROM) of the hand can help quantify impairment, monitor recovery, and potentially diagnose both neurological and hand-specific disorders. Hart et al. [5] found that patients with hand impairments who underwent rehabilitative therapy perceived improvements in their functional abilities and health. Quantifying hand ROM can validate observed improvements in therapy.

Traditionally, hand ROM measurement relies on goniometers. These devices have been used in numerous studies [1,6,8] to assess the static ROM of patients during activities of daily living (ADLs). However, the accuracy and reliability of goniometers depend on the patient's ability to maintain a static gesture, which can be tedious and time-consuming, affecting performance.

Recent advancements have introduced data gloves to address the limitations of goniometers and enhance the measurement of finger ROM. Lin et al. [10] developed a modular data glove system utilizing inertial measurement units (IMUs), ensuring precise capture of hand kinematics and improving the glove's flexibility and maintainability. Hazman et al. [7] followed with an IMU-based glove, demonstrating high accuracy and robustness in finger joint measurements. Connolly et al. [2] employed a neural network to improve data glove accuracy and usability, especially for individuals with limited joint mobility, eliminating the need for complex calibration procedures.

Moreover, modern methods for measuring finger ROM have increasingly incorporated smartphones to enhance accuracy and convenience. Miyake et al. [13] demonstrated the reliability of a smartphone application that utilizes the device's accelerometer to measure finger ROM, significantly reducing measurement time compared to traditional goniometers. Theile et al. [17] corroborated these findings, showing that a smartphone goniometer app provides measurements as reliable as traditional methods, with added portability and potential for patient self-measurement. Additionally, Zhao et al. [19] validated the use of smartphone photography for measuring finger ROM, demonstrating that contracture measurements obtained via smartphone photography were comparable to those taken using traditional goniometry, with potential applications in telemedicine.

Our previous work [9] developed a low-cost flexible sensor glove capable of measuring dynamic ROM. The aim of the study was to develop the prototype and evaluate the effectiveness of the glove in measuring finger ROM. Building on the positive results, the current study aims to use the glove to measure the static positions of candidates performing ADLs. Determining the minimum ROM required for finger joints to perform ADLs can provide crucial insights into therapy decisions and evaluating treatment outcomes. This information can assist therapists in tailoring rehabilitation programs to meet the specific needs of patients, ensuring more effective and targeted treatments. By understanding the functional ROM necessary for daily activities, therapists can better monitor progress and make informed adjustments to therapy plans, ultimately improving patient outcomes.

2   Materials and Methods

The current study was divided into two sections: (1) flexible sensor glove prototype and (2) candidate testing.

2.1   Flexible Sensor Glove Prototype

The flexible sensor glove prototype was developed in a prior study [9], where emphasis was placed on evaluating the glove's accuracy and performance in measuring dynamic finger range of motion. The prototype can be seen in Fig. 1.

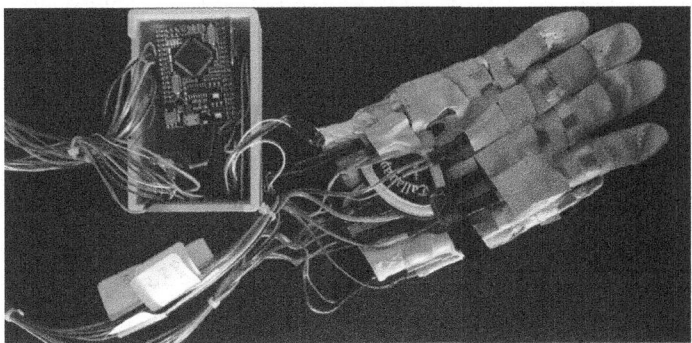

Fig. 1. Flexible sensor glove prototype.

The development of the glove, was focused on cost-effectiveness and sensor availability in South Africa and resulted in the selection of flex sensors (Sparkfun Electronics, USA). A flex sensor, shown in Fig. 2, is a device that quantifies bending by measuring changes in electrical resistance. Composed of a thin, flexible material embedded with conductive particles, the sensor's resistance increases as it bends due to the changing distance between particles.

The flex sensor analysis focused on evaluating the performance and reliability of the flex sensors used in the glove. Key aspects of the analysis included:

– **Signal Stability:** Sensors were tested for signal consistency using a voltage divider configuration with an Arduino Uno. A rig was used to keep the sensors straight, ensuring stable readings with minor fluctuations. The sensors displayed consistent resistance readings with less than 1% variance, indicating minimal signal drift.

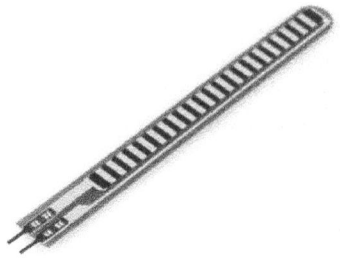

Fig. 2. Flex sensor (Sparkfun, USA).

- **Anatomical Variations:** To account for differences in hand sizes and joint locations, sensors were tested at various bend locations and radii. Bending sensors at offsets of 20, 30, and 40 mm from the base showed repeatable results with less than 2.2% variance. Tests with different bend radii (5, 10, and 12 mm) revealed that curvature had a greater impact on resistance than bend location, with up to 3.7% variance.
- **Repeatability:** The sensors produced repeatable results with deviations under 4%. A calibration phase was introduced to further minimize deviations and account for signal drift, ensuring accurate measurements of finger joint movements.

The results provided consistent and reliable data across different conditions, confirming their suitability for accurately capturing the range of motion in finger joints and supporting the prototype development.

In the glove design, flexible sleeves were initially placed on the proximal interphalangeal (PIP) joints, located in the middle section of the finger, providing reasonable comfort. However, extending the sleeves to both the PIP and metacarpophalangeal (MCP) joints, situated at the knuckle, increased resistance to motion and potentially caused discomfort or harm to hand-impaired users. The design of the glove underwent several iterations, ultimately resulting in attaching the sensors to a golf glove using medical tape. This approach aimed to maximize comfort, as alternative attachment methods introduced greater physical resistance across the joints.

The final circuit design of the glove involved a compact microcontroller (similar to Arduino MEGA) connected to ten flex sensors. The sensors were configured to measure the changes in resistance as the sensors bent. To determine the bend angle, a calibration was implemented.

The calibration procedure involved two phases to ensure accurate measurements of finger joint movements. Initially, the user placed their hand flat on a surface, and the sensor readings were recorded as the 0° reference. Following this, the user made a fist, and the sensor readings were recorded as the 90° reference. These two sets of data were then used to map the sensor resistances to corresponding angles. Visual cues using LEDs were provided during the calibration process to ensure accurate and consistent data collection. The validation of the glove involved measuring each finger joint at angles of 30°, 45°, and 60° using a goniometer. The results demonstrated an average Root Mean Square Error (RMSE) of 5.2° for the right hand and 4.8° for the left hand. After applying a correction factor to account for signal drift and physical slack in the glove,the results indicated an overall accuracy of $\pm 5°$, which are consistent with tests performed be [15].

To account for physical slack in the glove and signal drift, a correction factor was calculated from the differences between these calibration readings and subsequent measurements.

2.2   Candidate Testing

The initial study emphasized the dynamic ROM and demonstrated the glove's effectiveness as a measurement tool for potential diagnostic and rehabilitation applications. Building on these promising results, the current research aims to evaluate the glove's ability to measure static ROM while performing a subset of activities of daily living (ADLs) in order to determine the minimum ROM required to perform these activities.

Study Participants. A total of 40 healthy participants were recruited. Similar to the the preliminary study [9] participation was completely voluntary with the recorded data to remain disclosed through the use of number profiling. Additionally, participants only performed the set of activities with their dominant hand. In contrast to the previous study, left-handed candidates were present. This study was authorized and approved from the Human Research Ethics Committee (Medical) at the University of Witwatersrand. Both the principle investigator and each participant signed a declaration of consent before each test session.

Activities of Daily Living. The selection of activities was based on the International Classification of Functioning, Disability, and Health (ICF), which provides a framework for measuring health and disability levels. Following the categories used by [4], the activities included communication, mobility, self-care, and domestic life.

The test subjects for the current phase, were tasked to complete 11 activities, under ICF categories, shown in Table 1. The number of activities were reduced from the previous study to decrease the duration of testing for convenience of the prospective participants, given the lengthy testing that occurred.

Each participant performed a set of activities using both hands. Prior to testing, participants were briefed on the study, assessed for glove fit, and completed a questionnaire to determine hand dominance and any relevant medical history. The principal investigator ensured the flexible sensors were correctly positioned and secured before beginning calibration. During calibration, participants placed their hands flat on a desk to record the $0°$ position, then made a fist to record the $90°$ position. These data points were used to map sensor resistances to corresponding angles.

Participants were then directed to perform specific activities. After observing the initial performance, the activities were repeated while the device recorded the data. Upon completion, participants evaluated the glove's comfort and provided overall feedback on the study. This process ensured accurate and consistent data collection on the static ROM during various daily activities.

Table 1. Activities measured in each ICF category.

ICF Category	Action
Self-care	Brushing teeth
	Holding a cup
	Cutting with a knife
	Eating with a fork
Mobility	Holding a ball
	Holding a key
Technology and Communication	Holding a phone
	Holding a pen
Domestic	Holding a spray can
	Holding a cloth

3   Results and Discussion

3.1   ROM

All 40 candidates successfully completed the evaluation across 11 activities of daily living. As previously noted, the duration of each activity was shortened to facilitate the testing process and ensure participant convenience. Figure 3 illustrates the average, minimum, and maximum range of motion (ROM) for all joints, aggregated across all 40 participants.

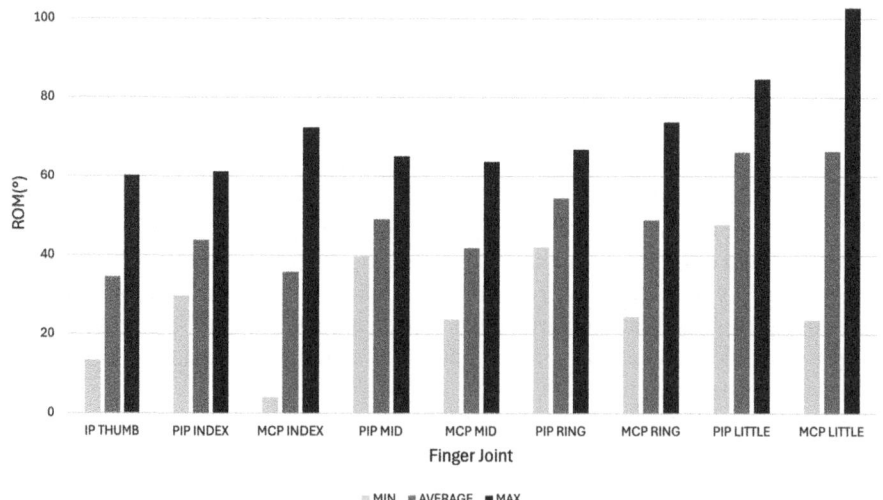

Fig. 3. Average, minimum and maximum ROM for all joints.

The little finger exhibited the highest ROM during the static tests. When gripping smaller objects, the little finger was often fully flexed, as it did not significantly contribute to the static hold (e.g., gripping a pen). Given that the tests involved holding objects of varying sizes, the little finger demonstrated the greatest variation in ROM.

The interphalangeal (IP) joint of the thumb showed considerable fluctuations in some candidates. This variability may be attributed to a connection problem within the circuit. Notably, these fluctuations were observed in only four candidates. Consequently, the thumb ROM data from these participants were excluded from the results. Despite this, the glove prototype produced consistent results with the remaining 36 candidates, yielding a success rate of 92%. The results of individual activities are not as significant, as the static phase of the study focused on a collective range of data that indicates the required ROM to perform all given activities.

3.2 Comparisons with Previous Work

Table 2 outlines the required ROM necessary to perform the propsed ADLs. Comparisons were made with studies aimed at determining the functional ROM required for performing ADLs. All previous studies mentioned, utilized either electric or standard goniometers to measure the ROM during the activities.

Table 2. Comparison of Static Test Results ($^\circ$).

Previous Studies	MCP	PIP	IP
Hume et al. [8]	61	60	18
Bain et al. [1]	23–87	10–64	-
Hayashi et al. [6]	>70	-	-
Current Study			
Average	53.34	48.21	34.51
Max	69.42	78.10	60.15
Min	39.88	18.92	13.42

Hume et al. [8] conducted a study on the functional ROM of the hand, aiming to investigate this motion during 11 ADLs. They were one of the first studies to systematically determine the functional ROM of the hand while performing ADLs. They defined active range of motion as the participant's normal range of motion, while functional motion represented the movements required to perform specific activities. All activities were selected to allow participants to fully flex and extend their hands by grasping objects of varying sizes.

In comparison to the average ROM presented in our results, the MCP and PIP joints attained lower magnitudes of ROM. Specifically, the differences were evaluated as 20.9% and 11.1% for the MCP and PIP joints, respectively. The variation in results may be influenced by the different activities performed in the studies. The size of the objects used in the activities played a significant role in determining the amount of

ROM a participant could utilize; larger objects required less flexion within the joints, and vice versa. Additionally, it is important to note that the flexible sensor glove used had an accuracy of $\pm 5°$.

Similar to Hume, Bain et al. [1] sought to determine the functional ROM of finger joints in 10 candidates performing ADLs. Their analysis focused on the pre-grasp and grasp positions during each activity, based on the Sollerman hand grip function test, which includes a range of 20 ADLs. Both active and passive ROM were assessed to define the range within the full arc of motion for each joint, thereby establishing boundaries for the functional ROM tests.

The results obtained from Bain et al. [1] represent a range between the minimum and maximum degrees of motion. When comparing the MCP joints, the minimum ROM is higher in our results, while the maximum ROM is higher according to Bain's results. For the PIP joint, both the minimum and maximum boundaries were higher in our study. Similar to the findings of Hume et al. [8], these results are significantly influenced by the selection of activities.

Bain et al. utilized a broader range of activities (20), which may more accurately represent the full use of the hand. The statistical range for the MCP joints in Bain's study and the current investigation are $64°$ and $29.54°$, respectively. Thus, both the number and types of activities can affect the ROM. However, for the PIP joint, the statistical range was greater in the current study. This discrepancy may also be attributed to the number of participants tested, as the current study included 40 participants compared to the 10 tested in Bain's investigation.

In a different approach, Hayashi et al. [6] focused specifically on the MCP joints of the hand, while using an orthotic device to limit ROM. To be functional, the required ROM of the MCP joints had to be greater than $70°$. The tests involved limiting the participants' ROM using orthoses set at various angles. Consequently, these experiments were based on imposed restrictions, leading to the conclusion that $70°$ was the minimum required ROM to functionally perform the Jebsen Taylor and O'Connor dexterity tests.

Comparitively, the maximum ROM for the MCP joint in the current study was $69.42°$, which does not coincide with Hayashi's identified limit. However, it is important to note that Hayashi's experiments relied on restricting the ROM while performing activities, whereas the current study measured the ROM required for performing the activities without such restrictions. Another key difference is that the current study focused on measuring the ROM necessary for ADLs rather than specific hand dexterity tests. Therefore, it may not be necessary to have an MCP joint ROM greater than $70°$ to be functional in performing ADLs.

Beyond the selection of activities and the number of participants, direct comparison of the results remains challenging. Assessing the accuracy of the measuring devices is crucial. The goniometer used in the study had an accuracy of $\pm 1°$, compared to the $\pm 5°$ accuracy of the glove. Using a goniometer requires participants to maintain rigid gestures during measurements, whereas the glove allows for more natural positioning. There is no assurance that participants did not move their joints between physical measurements with the goniometer. In contrast, the glove enables instant measurements, allowing the therapist or investigator to choose the timing of each measurement.

4   Conclusions

The flexible sensor glove successfully recorded the static ROM of 40 candidates performing a subset of 11 activities of daily living (ADLs). The results were averaged for each joint of the hand, determining the maximum and minimum limits. The static tests yielded a ROM of 39.88°–69.42°, 18.92°–78.1°, and 13.42°–60.15° for the MCP, PIP, and IP joints, respectively. These ranges represent the required ROM for an individual to be functionally independent, based on the selected ADLs. Although the glove measurements were compared with previous studies, differences in measurement methods, the number of participants and the selection of ADLs had a significant influence on the disparity between the results.

Disclosure of Interests. The authors have no competing interests to declare that are relevant to the content of this article.

References

1. Bain, G., Polites, N., Higgs, B., et al.: The functional range of motion of the finger joints. J. Hand Surg. Eur. **40**(4), 406–411 (2015)
2. Connolly, J., Condell, J., Curran, K., Gardiner, P.: Improving data glove accuracy and usability using a neural network when measuring finger joint range of motion. Sensors **22**(6), 2228 (2022). https://doi.org/10.3390/s22062228
3. De Klerk, S., Badenhorst, E., Buttle, A., et al.: Occupation-based hand therapy in South Africa: challenges and opportunities. S. Afr. J. Occup. Ther. **46**(3), 10–15 (2016)
4. Gracia, V., Vergara, M., Sancho-Bru, J., et al.: Functional range of motion of the hand joints in activities of the international classification of functioning, disability and health. J. Hand Ther. **30**, 337–343 (2017)
5. Hart, D.L., Tepper, S.: Changes in health status for persons with wrist or hand impairments receiving occupational therapy or physical therapy. Am. J. Occup. Ther. **55**(1), 68–74 (2001)
6. Hayashi, H., Shimizu, H., Okumura, S., et al.: Necessary metacarpophalangeal joints range of motion to maintain hand function. Hong Kong J. Occup. Ther. **24**(2), 51–55 (2014)
7. Hazman, M.A.W., et al.: IMU sensor-based data glove for finger joint measurement. Indonesian J. Electr. Eng. Comput. Sci. **20**(1), 82–88 (2020). https://doi.org/10.11591/ijeecs.v20.i1.pp82-88
8. Hume, M., Gellman, H., McKellop, H., et al.: Functional range of motion of the joints of the hand. J. Hand. Surg. Am. **15**(2), 240–243 (1990)
9. Indermun, S., Mangera, T.: Prototyping a low-cost flexible sensor glove for diagnostics and rehabilitation. In: Proceedings of the 17th International Joint Conference on Biomedical Engineering Systems and Technologies - Volume 1: BIODEVICES, pp. 103–110. INSTICC, SciTePress (2024). https://doi.org/10.5220/0012314800003657
10. Lin, B.S., Lee, I.J., Chiang, P.Y., Huang, S.Y., Peng, C.W.: A modular data glove system for finger and hand motion capture based on inertial sensors. J. Med. Biol. Eng. **39**, 532–540 (2019). https://doi.org/10.1007/s40846-018-0434-6
11. Maredza, M., Bertram, M., Tollman, S.: Disease burden of stroke in rural South Africa: an estimate of incidence, mortality and disability adjusted life years. BMC Neurol. **15**(1), 54 (2015)

12. Maredza, M., Chola, L.: Economic burden of stroke in a rural South African setting. eNeu-rologicalSci **3**, 26–32 (2016)
13. Miyake, K., et al.: A new method measurement for finger range of motion using a smart-phone. J. Plast. Surg. Hand Surg. **54**(4), 207–214 (2020). https://doi.org/10.1080/2000656X.2020.1755296
14. Moodley, D.: Radial Nerve Injuries. Interview - Occupational Therapist at Charlotte Maxeke Johannesburg Academic Hospital, SA (2018)
15. Oess, N., Wanek, J., Curt, A.: Design and evaluation of a low-cost instrumented glove for hand function assessment. J. Neuroeng. Rehabil. **9**(1), 1–11 (2012)
16. StatsSA: Measuring household expenditure on public transport (2015). http://www.statssa.gov.za/?p=5943, http://www.statssa.gov.za/?p=5943. Accessed 28 Jan 2019
17. Theile, H., Walsh, S., Scougall, P., Ryan, D., Chopra, S.: Smartphone goniometer for reliable and convenient measurement of finger range of motion: a comparative study. Aust. J. Plastic Surg. **5**(2), 335 (2022). https://doi.org/10.34239/ajops.v5n2.335
18. Yan, L., Li, C., Chen, J., et al.: Prevention, management, and rehabilitation of stroke in low and middle-income countries. eNeurologicalSci **2**(8), 21–30 (2016)
19. Zhao, J.Z., Blazar, P.E., Mora, A.N., Earp, B.E.: Range of motion measurements of the fin-gers via smartphone photography. HAND **15**(5), 679–685 (2019). https://doi.org/10.1177/1558944718820955

EMG-Based Action Unit Recognition: Feature Engineering, Machine Learning, and Real-Time Classification

Hui Liu$^{(\boxtimes)}$ (ID), Abhinav Veldanda (ID), Rainer Koschke (ID), Tanja Schultz (ID), and Dennis Küster$^{(\boxtimes)}$ (ID)

Cognitive Systems Lab, University of Bremen, Bremen, Germany
{hui.liu,kuester}@uni-bremen.de

Abstract. This article is an extended version of the work originally presented at the BIODEVICES 2024 conference, which exclusively focuses on utilizing fEMG as the primary method for action unit recognition (AUR). Within the framework of this study, we employ a proprietary dataset of facial electromyography (fEMG) sensor data, which contains synchronized video modality data with fEMG recordings and output labels corresponding to appropriate AUs, to predict a subset of action units. Abundant feature engineering practice and machine learning experiments are conducted to study fEMG-based AUR.

Keywords: Action units · Electromyography · Facial action coding system · Facial expression · EMG · sEMG · fEMG · Pattern recognition · Machine learning

1 Background and Related Works

1.1 Facial Expression and Emotion

A significant part of human interaction is thought to rely on nonverbal and visual cues, many of which are conveyed through facial expressions [33]. This is evident in everyday situations such as phone conversations in which facial cues are absent, interactions with individuals wearing face masks [21], or engaging with others in virtual reality environments [57]. The human face has been shown to play a major role in nonverbal communication in general and in expressing emotions in particular. Apart from emotions, faces convey a multitude of social information, ranging from gender and ethnicity to health and social status [33]. Dating back to Charles Darwin's seminal work on the expression of emotions in man and animals [12], the role of the face in signaling emotional states has thus been in the spotlight of a long tradition of emotion researchers [33].

M. P. Guarino et al. (Eds.): BIOSTEC 2024, CCIS 2546, pp. 23–43, 2026.
https://doi.org/10.1007/978-3-031-96899-0_3

1.2   Facial Action Coding Systems (FACS), Action Units (AUs), and Action Unit Recognition (AUR)

Since the early 1970s, extensive research has been conducted on facial expression analysis. One of the most important contributions is the facial action coding system (FACS) designed by Paul Ekman and Wallace Friesen [17]. The system is based on previous research [30] categorizing facial structures [4] that are described by Duchenne [13].

FACS enables classifying all possible facial expressions into constituent action units (AUs) that reflect the activity of facial muscles that can be independently controlled. Compared to the discrete or so-called "basic emotions" [16], AU can essentially describe certain muscle activities rather than providing inferential labels [73]. Hence, accurate AU tracking lay the foundations for facial emotional expression research and three-dimensional emotion modeling [65]. FACS contains 44 AUs as a set of coding essentials [17].

Action unit recognition (AUR) represents a crucial area of research within facial expression analysis, focusing on automating the identification of specific AUs associated with emotions, expressions, and actions. This approach examines subtle facial changes such as wrinkling of the nose, raising eyebrow(s), or pulling the corners of the lips. Historically, AUR relied heavily on manual recognition by certified FACS experts, a process that was both costly and time-consuming, requiring hours to annotate one minute of video data [5, 73]. Recently, advances in automatic affect recognition tools have made facial activity analysis more cost-effective in various experimental research paradigms [37]. From early tools like the Computer Expression Recognition Toolbox [42] to contemporary open-source solutions such as OpenFace [2], researchers now have access to a wide array of software for automatic affect recognition based on external sensing technologies. Such kind of tools aimed to differentiate prototypical expressions associated with discrete emotional states like happiness, anger, or sadness, influenced by basic emotion theories (BETs) [14, 58]; More recently, there has been a growing focus on the reliable assessment and validation of facial AUs, which provide an objective measure independent of BET frameworks [37].

While some previous studies have evaluated their internal datasets without comparative analysis across different platforms [35], state-of-the-art research has prominently focused on machine learning (ML) models for video camera-based AUR challenges within facial expression recognition and analysis [73]. Furthermore, several studies have examined the performance of freely available pre-trained AUR systems like OpenFace [40, 54, 55]. Collectively, these studies underline the utility and reliability of camera-based AUR systems. Nevertheless, methodological and conceptual challenges persist, particularly concerning the heavy reliance on visual data in facial AUR. The academic community is currently focusing on the role that electromyography (EMG) and inertial sensors, such as accelerometers and gyroscopes, can play in the field of AUR [69].

1.3   Shortcomings of Camera-Based AUR

Rich machine learning models, including deep learning and even large language models, have been widely applied in the research of camera-based AUR [6]. The performance of camera-based AUR varies depending on various factors, such as specific datasets [73], specific AUs involved [54], and specific viewing angles [55]. Evaluations and challenges in cross-database studies for both discrete and AU-based affect recognition have focused primarily on a limited number of well-known databases consisting mostly of posed expressions [37,73]. Spontaneous facial expressions in natural environments, involving complex dynamics, are more subtle than those in controlled posture datasets [73]. They contain additional cues like head movements (for example, nodding) [73]. Spontaneous facial behavior also encompasses the simultaneous activation of multiple AUs, such as smiling with eyes and mouth, which can potentially result in numerous distinct expression combinations [73]. These factors raise concerns about classifier generalizability during application to newly collected, less standardized data. Furthermore, the presence of a camera can sometimes influence the phenomena being measured: for instance, awareness of being observed has been shown to diminish facial feedback effects previously thought to be robust and well established [56]. The challenges mentioned above underscore ongoing complexities in the field of camera-based AUR.

1.4 Exploring a New AUR Path Towards Biosignals: Using Electromyography (EMG)

Facial expression research continues to grapple with significant challenges, particularly in achieving consensus across various measures of emotion [33] and in contextualizing AUs within their physical and social settings [36]. Previous reviews have highlighted the surprising lack of agreement between physiological measures of emotion and subjective self-reports [53]. This phenomenon is also strongly reflected in research on other human behaviors, such as motivation drop during sports [72]. Further challenges include interindividual differences and the variability of facial expressions, head motion, and occlusions [4,32]. Moreover, traditional theories of emotion, which assume coordination among biosignals, cognitive, and behavioral components, have faced repeated empirical challenges regarding their strong concordance [31]. In response, novel machine learning approaches that integrate multiple modalities may offer more robust predictions compared to earlier psychological models, potentially shedding light on how different components of emotional responses interact.

The integration of easily accessible data, such as jointly recorded audiovisual emotional responses, has been a central objective in multimodal emotion recognition challenges for over a decade [62]. Recent applications of these approaches have shown promise across diverse fields, including the recognition of emotional engagement in individuals with dementia [64]. However, despite these advancements, facial electromyography (fEMG) has been notably absent from many of these approaches.

While current research on facial expressions primarily relies on video data supplemented occasionally by EMG, fEMG has long served as the definitive standard for highly precise recording of facial expressions in psychophysiological laboratories [19,70]. In particular, facial surface EMG can detect extremely subtle muscle activities, including muscle relaxation (e.g., of the eyebrows), beyond the perceptible range of the naked eye [33,39]. Currently, facial electromyography is often used in experimental studies examining subtle psychological effects on facial activity. E.g., recent work has leveraged facial EMG to examine to what extent social touch may modulate affective responses during affective image viewing [71]. Moreover, previous studies have highlighted the potential of fEMG not only in accurately detecting emotional facial expressions, but also in significantly enhancing human-computer interaction [1, 20]. Last but not least, EMG

Recent methodological work in this field has further aimed to identify the most suitable placement schema for facial EMG electrodes to allow for discriminating between patterns of Ekman's six discrete emotional expressions via high-resolution electromyography from up to 19 simultaneously recorded positions [23]. As there is no gold standard that could unambiguously identify emotions across individuals and contexts, there is now wide agreement among emotion researchers that different modalities and biosignals need to be investigated to more accurately assess emotional expressions and advance our understanding of emotions [38].

Beyond the technical challenges associated with the capture of high-quality and high-resolution fEMG signals of facial activity, a significant conceptual hurdle lies in interpreting facial muscle activity beyond the FACS-based categorization framework. Increasingly, studies have questioned the validity of concepts like Ekman's "basic emotions" [10, 11, 16, 58]. While acknowledging this ongoing debate, our current focus remains methodological. By demonstrating the feasibility of reliably automatically recognizing facial AUs from EMG data, our purpose is to contribute towards establishing a more sensitive and detailed measure of facial activity compared to conventional webcam-based approaches. In addition, up-to-date in-house work has affirmed the practicality, convenience, and effectiveness of EMG in human activity recognition (HAR) [25–27], providing a solid basis for AUR because research on facial expressions is also strongly related to HAR in scientific fields [45]. Such experiences also provide strong support for our collection, processing, and modeling of EMG data.

1.5   Contribution

This article is an extended version of the work originally presented at the conference [68], which aims to advance fEMG as the primary method for AUR beyond the current video-based approaches.

Within the framework of this work, we collected and analyzed a proprietary dataset of fEMG sensor data, which contains synchronized video modality data with fEMG recordings and output labels corresponding to appropriate AUs, to predict a subset of AUs. Abundant feature engineering practice and machine learning experiments are conducted to study EMG-based AUR.

To the best of our knowledge, though facial EMG has been a popular tool in psychological studies on **facial expressions** for many years, no existing work, except for our preliminary conference paper mentioned above, has yet been published on **AUR** that has exclusively relied on EMG data as its sole modality to model facial activity as AUs.

2 Equipment and Data Acquisition

2.1 Biosignal Aquisition Device, EMG Sensors, and Sensor Positions

High-quality sensory observations applicable to recognizing users' activities and behaviors are inseparable from sensors' sophisticated design and appropriate application [44]. The *biosignalsplux* Research Kits[1] were applied as a biosignal acquisition toolkit due to their proven reliability in previous in-house research similar to the data collection requirements of this work, which yields two big datasets [46,52] and validates two open-source time-series processing codebanks [3,18] for the academic community.

We used two channels among the eight sockets to record two-dimensional 2,000 Hz, 16-bit EMG signals, and the time alignment of both channels was automatically ensured throughout the recording sessions. Given that fEMG signals typically range from 15 to 500 Hz [7], a sampling frequency of 2,000 Hz ensures an accurate representation of the signal.

The fEMG setup utilized a bipolar configuration with two channels covering the frontalis and corrugator supercili facial muscles. These sensor positions adhered to guidelines from the Society for Psychophysiological Research [19], with slight adjustments based on extensive pre-testing to minimize crosstalk and optimize electrode placement for our slightly larger electrodes compared to standard guidelines, as demonstrated by Fig. 1.

2.2 Hardware, Software Implementation, and Annotation

Our recording setup included a computer for demonstration of stimuli, a webcam for recording video, and the fEMG recording system introduced in Sect. 2.1.

An acquisition software tool with an interactive graphical user interface (GUI) was implemented, as shown in the screenshot of Fig. 2, where the synchronization between the imitated actions and the fEMG sensor data was achieved using the lab streaming layer (LSL) protocol. Alongside fEMG data, video data of the participant captured by the laptop's built-in webcam was recorded. The timestamps of the video stream, facilitated by the LSL, allowed precise annotation, alignment, and extraction of relevant fEMG signals for subsequent processing and analysis.

2.3 AU Classes, Data Acquisition Procedure, and Dataset

During each recording trial, the participant was instructed to mimic facial expressions presented in stimulus videos via the custom GUI (see Fig. 1). These stimulus videos were sourced from the MPI Video Database [34], recognized for accurately depicting AU activations as verified by FACS coders.

Four AUs were selected to be mimicked during data collection. Additionally, we captured fEMG data of neutral (baseline) expressions, which is subsequently referred to as "AU0."

---

[1] www.pluxbiosignals.com, accessed August 12, 2024.

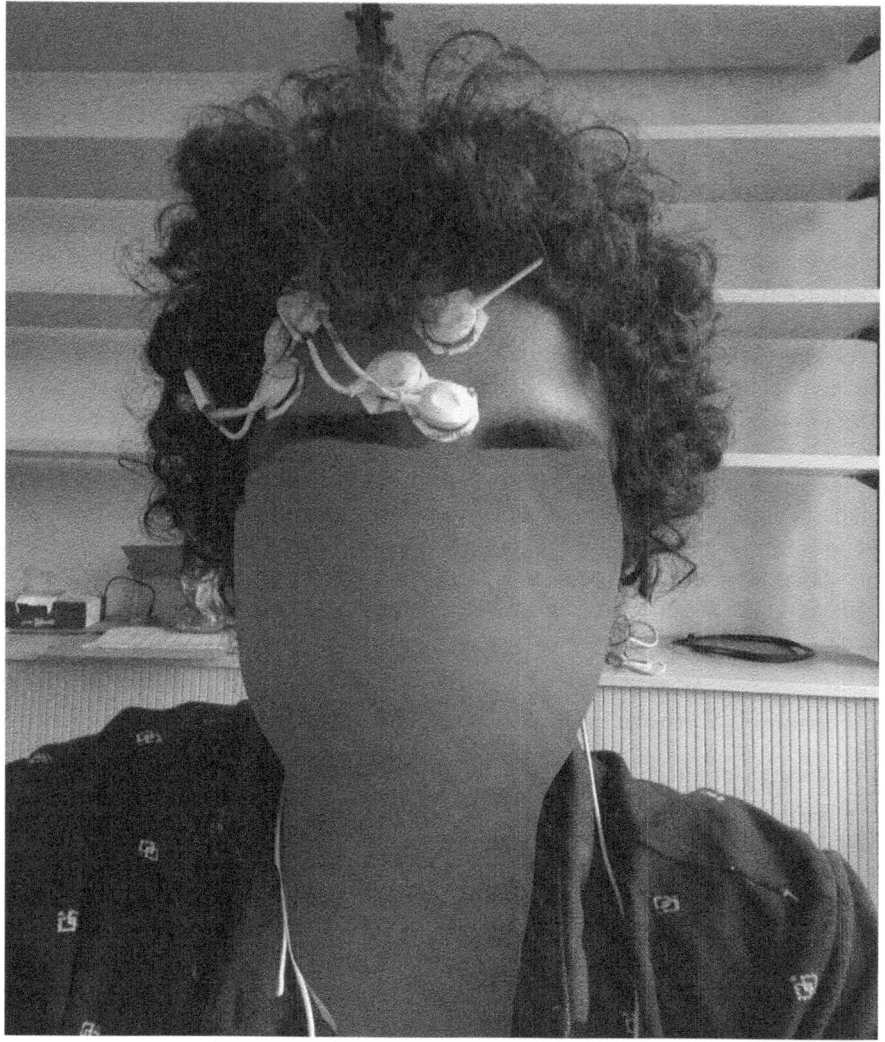

Fig. 1. The positions of the bipoloar fEMG sensors [68].

- AU1: Inner Brow Raiser
- AU2: Outer Brow Raiser
- AU4: Brow Lowerer
- AU9: Nose Wrinkler
- AU0: Neutral Expression

Participants were instructed to exhibit maximum intensity (apex) expressions, and to maintain each expression for at least five seconds while simultaneous fEMG data was recorded.

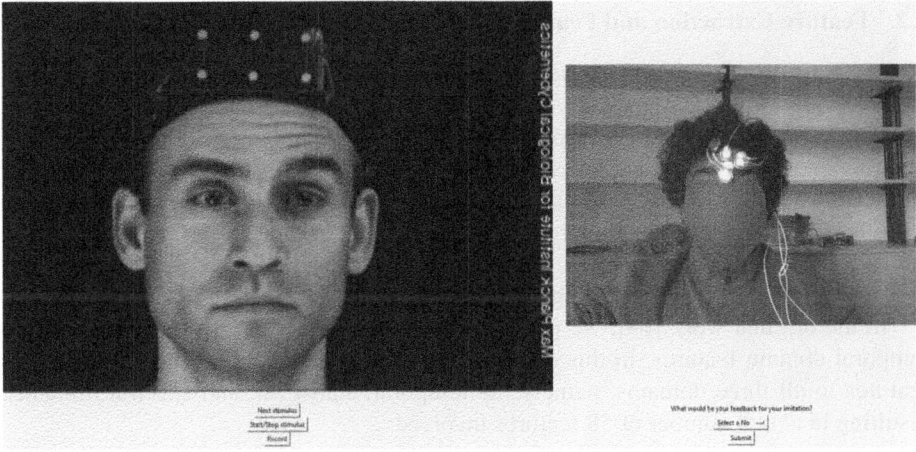

Fig. 2. GUI implemented for recording trials [68].

The proof-of-concept event recorded data from one male subject across four sessions, each consisting of 25 recording trials, totaling a trial count of 100. On average, each trial provided approximately 2.12 ± 0.8 min of data in all sessions, accumulating a dataset comprising a total of 3.53-h, which is considered sufficient for pilot experiments.

3 Feature Engineering and Classifiers

3.1 Applying Raw EMG Data and Windowing

Raw EMG data is typically interfered by a substantial amount of electrical noise, which should be removed prior to amplification [66]. Conventionally, the remaining noise, such as the 50/60 Hz low-frequency noise, and artifacts, can be removed via filtering before further processing and statistical analyses [19, 66].

Recent work, however, has attempted to view these types of noise from a different perspective. Within the field of ML based on biomedical/physiological signals, artificial intelligence (AI) algorithms may better explain low-frequency noise than filters that may filter out useful information. In addition, the device and sensors applied in the acquisition event (see Sect. 2.1) are claimed to be endowed with essential anti-noise functionalities, which ensures a strong signal-to-noise ratio (SNR)[2]. Some successful early or late stage work in the field of wearable biosignal-based human behavior research [49–51] has further suggested running feature extractors directly on raw EMG that were acquired from the same devices and sensors as in this work. We therefore decided to adopt this approach also the current experiments.

The raw EMG data was first segmented into windows of a specified length with a pre-defined overlap percentage.

---

[2] https://www.pluxbiosignals.com/products/electromyography-emg, accessed on August 12, 2024.

3.2   Feature Extraction and Feature Space Reduction

Feature extraction is a necessary step in machine learning algorithms. Generally speaking, deep algorithms automatically learn features through raw inputs, while high-level feature design in the field of human behavior research, although more efficient and interpretable, is targeted at a specific research direction and does not have universal applicability [24, 28]. This work aims to verify whether AUR can be achieved using only the EMG modality for the proof-of-concept; thus, the data collected is not sufficient for the above two approaches. We therefore adopted handcrafted feature extraction and applied it to various lightweight ML models.

In the original work [68], we performed experiments using the 16 most common temporal domain features. In this extension article, we expand the selection range of features to all three domains, namely the temporal, statistical, and spectral domains, resulting in a total number of 58 features involved:

- Temporal features
  - Absolute energy
  - Area under the curve (AUC)
  - Autocorrelation
  - Centroid
  - Entropy
  - Mean absolute difference (MAD)
  - Median difference
  - Negative turning points
  - Neighborhood peaks
  - Peak to peak distance
  - Positive turning points
  - Signal distance
  - Slope
  - Sum absolute difference (SAD)
  - Total energy
  - Zero crossing rate
- Statistical features
  - Empirical cumulative distribution function (ECDF)
  - ECDF Percentile
  - ECDF Percentile Count
  - Histogram
  - Interquartile range
  - Kurtosis
  - Max
  - Mean
  - Mean absolute deviation
  - Median
  - Median absolute deviation
  - Min
  - Root mean square
  - Skewness

- Standard deviation
- Variance
- Spectral features
  - Fast Fourier transform (FFT) mean coefficient
  - Fundamental frequency
  - Human range energy
  - Linear predictive cepstral coefficient (LPCC)
  - Mel-Frequency Cepstral Coefficients (MFCC)
  - Max power spectrum
  - Maximum frequency
  - Median frequency
  - Power bandwidth
  - Spectral centroid
  - Spectral decrease
  - Spectral distance
  - Spectral entropy
  - Spectral kurtosis
  - Spectral positive turning points
  - Spectral roll-off
  - Spectral roll-on
  - Spectral skewness
  - Spectral slope
  - Spectral spread
  - Spectral variation
  - Wavelet absolute mean
  - Wavelet energy
  - Wavelet entropy
  - Wavelet standard deviation
  - Wavelet variance

Physiological signals are a set of time series, from which existing open-source resources can easily extract various features to form feature vectors. We used the Time Series Feature Extraction Library (TSFEL) [3] that has been widely applied and validated in various research fields, not only due to its ease of use and wide inclusion, but also because it has been reported to compute features the fastest among peer codebanks [29], laying the foundation for future research in real-time systems and interactivity. In the field of human behavioral study based on physiological signals, real-time systems have high requirements for computational efficiency. Most of the features applied in this work are considered fast to compute according to the previous literature [43,61]. Besides, TSFEL provides some unique features that do not exist in other libraries, such as negative turning points, whose effectiveness has been validated in previous research [48].

Two conventional feature dimensionality reduction approaches, namely linear discriminant analysis (LDA) [25,26,47] and principal component analysis (PCA) with a conventional 95% variance retained, have been applied after feature extraction.

In addition to feature extraction and space reduction, feature engineering in time series can also involve other research topics such as feature stacking, aiming at further improving recognition rates by preserving temporal information, which is an important research task for future work.

3.3   Machine Learning (ML) and Deep Learning (DL) Models

As a proof-of-concept, we examined four widely-used lightweight ML models:

– Random forest (RF)
– Support vector machine (SVM)
– Gaussian naïve Bayes (GNB)
– k-nearest neighbors (k-NN)

The input sources of the four lightweight models mentioned above are the handcrafted features extracted as detailed in Sect. 3.2. All models are trained on the default hyperparameters provided by the *scikit-learn* library [59].

In order to further enrich the experimental results, we also introduced temporal convolutional networks (TCN) as a reference, although we initially believed that such a deep model was not suitable for our small-scale datasets at present. The TCN classifier takes the raw windowed data instead of handcrafted features as input. The input and output lengths of the TCN module are identical, where the output is flattened and fed into a single neural network with the same number of output nodes and categories, and then *softmax* activation is performed for prediction. It can be expected that after further enriching the dataset and tuning the model parameters, TCN may play a pivotal role. However, it is not in the scope of this article.

4   Experimental Results and Analysis

4.1   Cross-Validation Recognition Results

As one of the four sessions will be used as a separate test set to validate the results (see Sect. 4.3), we conducted multiple five-fold cross-validation experiments with stratified sampling using three of the acquired data sessions as our ML materials. All three combinations of temporal, spectral, and statistical domain features were tested, along with dimensionality reduction using LDA and PCA. The results of applying the whole 58 features are omitted because their results are inferior to those of the three individual domains. The results of the 400-ms window with 20% overlap configuration are selected to demonstrate its stable and outperforming statistics (see Table 1), which provides essential parameter suggestions for similar research.

We can observe that different feature domains yield similar accuracy. Nevertheless, the choice of features can impact real-time tracking due to computational efficiency, and temporal features are understandably faster to compute. Furthermore, the TCN's performance improves significantly with increased training data sessions, which aligns with the general understanding of deep learning. Among all models tested, the RF classifier exhibited the highest and most stable performance.

4.2   Experiments on Separate Muscles

Given the high performance observed in the cross-validation results applying both EMG channels (see Sect. 4.1), we sought to assess how our models would work when trained solely on individual EMG channels with different muscles.

Table 1. Feature domain-related accuracies for the results accumulated from five-fold cross-validation using combinations of different sessions of data with linear discriminant analysis (LDA) and principal component analysis (PCA).

Domain	Model	LDA			PCA		
		Session 1	Ses. 1&2	Ses. 1–3	Session 1	Ses. 1–2	Ses. 1–3
Temporal	RF	0.99	0.99	0.99	0.99	0.98	0.98
	SVM	0.95	0.95	0.96	0.95	0.95	0.96
	GNB	0.99	0.98	0.97	0.99	0.97	0.97
	k-NN	0.98	0.98	0.98	0.98	0.97	0.98
	TCN	0.77	0.80	0.76	0.69	0.67	0.91
Statistical	RF	0.99	0.98	0.97	0.99	0.98	0.97
	SVM	0.91	0.93	0.90	0.91	0.93	0.90
	GNB	0.99	0.97	0.95	0.99	0.97	0.95
	k-NN	0.96	0.93	0.91	0.96	0.93	0.91
	TCN	0.90	0.79	0.90	0.70	0.77	0.88
Spectral	RF	0.99	0.97	0.97	0.99	0.98	0.97
	SVM	0.99	0.97	0.96	0.99	0.97	0.96
	GNB	0.98	0.96	0.95	0.98	0.96	0.95
	k-NN	0.99	0.97	0.96	0.99	0.97	0.96
	TCN	0.85	0.85	0.78	0.73	0.79	0.80

We conducted cross-validation studies using the same training data, focusing on individual channels from our dataset to analyze the impact of varying the number of channels on the model performance, presented in Table 2.

Table 2. Feature domain-related accuracies for the results on individual EMG channels accumulated from five-fold cross-validation using combinations of different sessions of data with linear discriminant analysis (LDA) and principal component analysis (PCA).

Domain	Model	LDA		PCA	
		Frontalis	Corrugator	Frontalis	Conrugator
Temporal	RF	0.97	0.91	0.89	0.91
	SVM	0.75	0.83	0.77	0.87
	GNB	0.88	0.84	0.78	0.83
	k-NN	0.89	0.89	0.80	0.86
	TCN	0.28	0.37	0.29	0.29
Statistical	RF	0.84	0.89	0.84	0.89
	SVM	0.51	0.84	0.51	0.84
	GNB	0.74	0.85	0.74	0.85
	k-NN	0.64	0.85	0.64	0.85
	TCN	0.30	0.29	0.20	0.29
Spectral	RF	0.89	0.90	0.89	0.90
	SVM	0.76	0.70	0.76	0.70
	GNB	0.78	0.86	0.78	0.86
	k-NN	0.82	0.77	0.82	0.77
	TCN	0.20	0.29	0.20	0.20

As expected, noticeable decreases can be observed in model performance on individual channels. Interestingly, there was no clear discernible pattern indicating that one channel consistently outperformed others in terms of temporal and spectral features. For instance, by using temporal features, RF exhibited better performance with frontalis data, while SVM showed superior results with corrugator data; but when spectral features were applied, the situation reverses. In contrast, in the case of spectral features, Corrugator often outperformed Frontalis. Another finding to summarize is that when using statistical features, corrugator generally has better capability to distinguish AUs than frontalis, while their abilities are fuzzy regarding the other two feature domains.

In particular, TCN demonstrated the most significant decline in performance, suggesting a potential need for multichannel feature combinations to effectively classify AUs. In general, individual-channel experiments highlight the importance of leveraging multiple channels for robust AUR proposed in this work.

4.3   Results on the Separate Test Set

While validation scores provide insights into how models perform on data distributions similar to those used during training, we aimed to assess their performance on completely unseen datasets. Specifically, we aimed to examine session-independent data. In the absence of large datasets, such a procedure can be regarded as a pseudo-black-box verification to test the robustness of the classifiers.

We trained the five ML models and further evaluated their accuracy metrics on the remaining separate test set that had been withheld from the outset. The results are depicted in Fig. 3, which is selected from multiple experiments relevant to different feature domains. Overall, the evidence suggests that the trained models achieved excellent scores on the test set.

4.4   Joint Study of Window Length and Overlap Rate Using Temporal Domain Features

The temporal domain feature set has been proven to perform the best on the entire dataset. Applying the current best-performing RF classier, we conducted a series of experiments on window length and overlap rate, with the former ranging from 150 ms to 500 ms, increasing by 50 ms, and the latter ranging from 10% to 50%, increasing by 10%. The experimental results, as documented in Table 3, indicate that the recognition accuracy of all parameter pairs are very close. From the perspective of real-time application, longer window length and smaller overlap are clearly more advantageous in reducing the system's computational consumption and response delay. The current offline models on the recorded data can achieve the most effective computation at the cost of sacrificing about 1% accuracy.

5   From Offline Towards Read-Time

RF has been selected as the foundational model for the next stage of study, a preliminary real-time system, due to its excellent performance in offline experiments (see

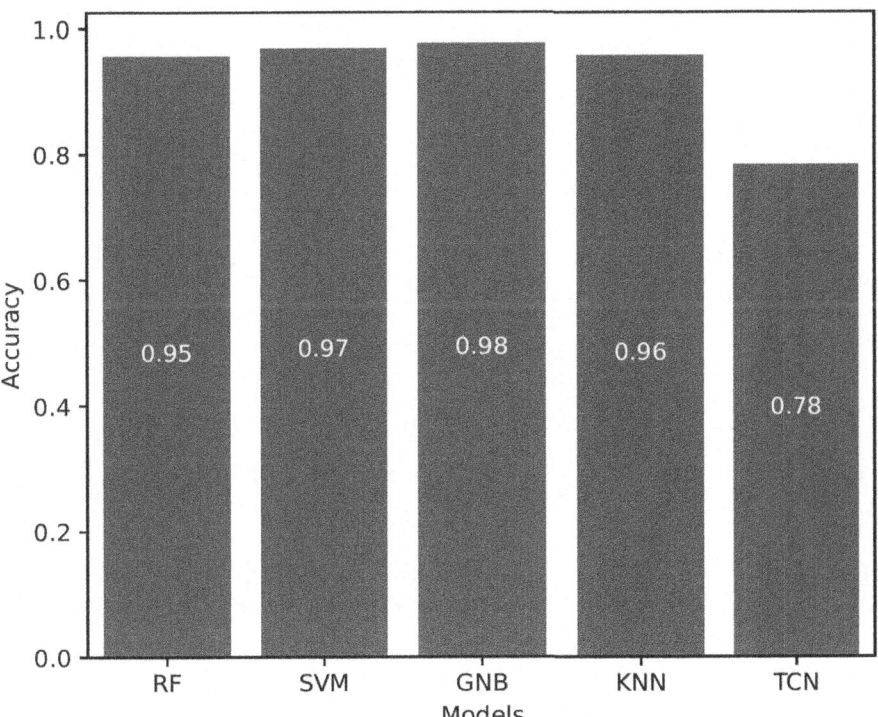

Fig. 3. Recognition results on the pseudo-black-box test set with the setup of 400-ms window length, 20% overlap, and temporal domain features (adapted from [68]).

Table 3. Recognition accuracies with five-fold cross-validation on joint experiments of window length and overlap rate using random forest classifier and temporal domain features [68].

	Overlap Rate				
Window length	10%	20%	30%	40%	50%
150 ms	0.97	0.97	0.97	0.97	0.97
200 ms	0.97	0.98	0.98	0.98	0.98
250 ms	0.98	0.98	0.98	0.98	0.98
300 ms	0.98	0.98	0.98	0.98	0.98
350 ms	0.98	0.98	0.98	0.98	0.99
400 ms	0.99	0.98	0.98	0.98	0.98
450 ms	0.98	0.98	0.98	0.98	0.98
500 ms	0.98	0.98	0.98	0.98	0.98

Sect. 4.1). In real-time tracking, participants are required to execute the same stimulus model, but the predictions happen in real-time. After accumulating EMG signals that meet a window length, the feature extractor starts to work on the collected samples.

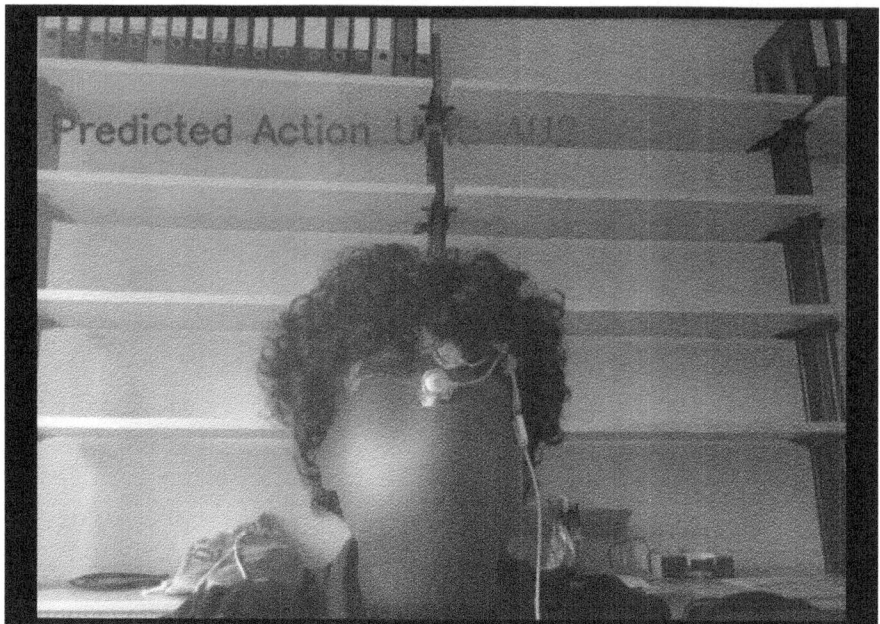

Fig. 4. A Screenshot of the pilot real-time EMG-based action unit recognition system [68].

Subsequently, the trained RF model receives input of features, classifies the results, and displays the AU class on the screen (see Fig. 4). It is satisfactory that the classifier can recognize participants' facial AUs with unremarkable delay and remarkable accuracy. This supports our hypothesis that EMG signals can be used solely to predict AUs. The preliminary offline research and real-time validation illuminate this research direction, with gratifying results.

6   Evaluation, Discussion, and Comparison

In our study, we focus on recording EMG data from two specific muscle sites: frontalis and corrugator supercili, to monitor eyebrow activity and distinguish between four different AUs: AU1, AU2, AU4, and AU9. Although we did not directly record from the levator labii (nose wrinkler) muscle site, we anticipated that sufficient signals could still be detected from nearby sites to reliably classify AU9. Our results demonstrated successful and robust classification, even when using single-channel EMG data. Previous research has highlighted challenges related to crosstalk between neighboring muscles [8,67]; however, our models effectively utilized these data to identify the targeted AUs.

Our validation results indicated that all lightweight learning models performed well, irrespective of features domains or dimensionality reduction technique. Given the limited data size, the TCN, a deep learning-based model, exhibited unstable performance, as anticipated. Despite this instability, TCN showed promising results comparable to those of lightweight ML models. Future research could explore whether TCN-based models can achieve more stable and improved results with larger EMG datasets and sufficient parameter tunings.

To our knowledge, there have been few or even no previous studies aimed at using EMG data alone for AUR. [60] trained models on the fusion of computer vision and EMG data, while [20] used EMG data only to predict prototypical facial expressions. Similarly, [22] developed a wearable device that can detect smiles and frowns based on two electrode pairs. Some works relied on independent video data [2] or used other biosignal modalities like electroencephalography (EEG) [41]. A recent method utilized earbud inertial measurement unit (IMU) [69] to detect and recognize various AUs using TCN. However, despite obtaining promising results in a subject-dependent study, ear-mounted IMU sensors may be disadvantageous in terms of detecting more subtle natu-ralistic facial activity, the presence of movement artifacts like head movements, or inter-ference from the sound waves produced by the earbud. The sound waves may excite the IMUs and the earable device [69].

7   Conclusions and Outlook

This article introduces a novel approach to the recognition of upper-face action units using electromyography data, as evidenced by the successful training of subject-dependent models in this initial case study. Based on the original conference paper, we further investigated feature engineering and machine learning modeling in detail. Our findings also suggest the potential for classifying new AUs using more distally placed electrodes in future applications, such as virtual reality (VR). Additionally, experiments indicate that deep learning models like temporal convolutional networks warrant further exploration in this domain, while underscoring the challenges associated with using fewer channels. Overall, this research contributes to the evolving field of EMG-based AUR recognition and sets the stage for future investigations.

We envision our EMG approach as complementary to the development of earable devices based on IMU, which face distinct sources of noise and practical constraints. EMG sensors, requiring direct contact with the skin, offer robustness against artifacts from head movements or sound waves generated by earable devices. Conversely, ear-buds may be less susceptible to electrical interference from other devices, while EMG excels in detecting subtle facial expressions. Given the complexities of multimodal emotion recognition in natural settings [37], we advocate for a hybrid system incor-porating both IMUs and a select number of EMG sensors to achieve robust and precise AUR performance. Nevertheless, refining EMG-based AUR to ensure versatility and reliability remains an ongoing challenge.

Despite achieving successful AUR in this pilot study, our current models are con-strained to subject-specific data collected near traditional recording sites for upper-face action units. As highlighted in previous research, the control of facial muscles is intri-cate [9], influenced by anatomical variations [15], and variable in signal strength across muscle sites [63]. To address these complexities, our future efforts will focus on devel-oping subject-independent models to assess the consistency of muscle activity patterns. Moving forward, we aim to extend our EMG-based AUR approach to include lower face AUs and explore the feasibility of distal electrode placements through multi-subject studies.

References

1. Facial expression recognition using surface electromyography. https://www.semanticscholar.org/paper/Facial-Expression-Recognition-using-Surface-Schultz/7370f7109318a0ed91ae8a87371bb01d774e6
2. Baltrusaitis, T., Zadeh, A., Lim, Y.C., Morency, L.P.: OpenFace 2.0: facial behavior analysis toolkit. In: 2018 13th IEEE International Conference on Automatic Face & Gesture Recognition (FG 2018), pp. 59–66. IEEE, Xi'an (2018). https://doi.org/10.1109/FG.2018.00019, https://ieeexplore.ieee.org/document/8373812/
3. Barandas, M., et al.: TSFEL: time series feature extraction library. SoftwareX **11**, 100456 (2020). https://doi.org/10.1016/j.softx.2020.100456, https://www.sciencedirect.com/science/article/pii/S2352711020300017
4. Barrett, L.F., Adolphs, R., Marsella, S., Martinez, A.M., Pollak, S.D.: Emotional expressions reconsidered: challenges to inferring emotion from human facial movements. Psychol. Sci. Public Interest: J. Am. Psychol. Soc. **20**(1), 1–68 (2019). https://doi.org/10.1177/1529100619832930, https://journals.sagepub.com/doi/abs/10.1177/1529100619832930
5. Bartlett, M.S., Littlewort, G.C., Frank, M.G., Lainscsek, C., Fasel, I.R., Movellan, J.R.: Automatic recognition of facial actions in spontaneous expressions. J. Multimed. **1**(6), 22–35 (2006). https://doi.org/10.4304/jmm.1.6.22-35, http://ojs.academypublisher.com/index.php/jmm/article/view/2125
6. Bian, Y., Küster, D., Liu, H., Krumhuber, E.G.: Understanding naturalistic facial expressions with deep learning and multimodal large language models. Sensors **24**(1) (2024). https://doi.org/10.3390/s24010126, https://www.mdpi.com/1424-8220/24/1/126
7. Boxtel, A.: Optimal signal bandwidth for the recording of surface EMG activity of facial, jaw, oral, and neck muscles. Psychophysiology **38**(1), 22–34 (2001). https://doi.org/10.1111/1469-8986.3810022, https://onlinelibrary.wiley.com/doi/10.1111/1469-8986.3810022
8. van Boxtel, A., Boelhouwer, A., Bos, A.: Optimal EMG signal bandwidth and interelectrode distance for the recording of acoustic, electrocutaneous, and photic blink reflexes. Psychophysiology **35**(6), 690–697 (1998). https://doi.org/10.1111/1469-8986.3560690, https://onlinelibrary.wiley.com/doi/abs/10.1111/1469-8986.3560690
9. Cattaneo, L., Pavesi, G.: The facial motor system. Neuroscience & Biobehav. Rev. **38**, 135–159 (2014). https://doi.org/10.1016/j.neubiorev.2013.11.002, https://linkinghub.elsevier.com/retrieve/pii/S0149763413002674
10. Crivelli, C., Fridlund, A.J.: Facial displays are tools for social influence. Trends Cogn. Sci. **22**(5), 388–399 (2018). https://doi.org/10.1016/j.tics.2018.02.006, https://www.cell.com/trends/cognitive-sciences/abstract/S1364-6613(18)30029-9, publisher: Elsevier
11. Crivelli, C., Fridlund, A.J.: Inside-out: from basic emotions theory to the behavioral ecology view. J. Nonverbal Behav. **43**(2), 161–194 (2019). https://doi.org/10.1007/s10919-019-00294-2
12. Darwin, C.: The Expression of the Emotions in Man and Animals. Oxford University Press, New York, 1998 ed. edn. (1872)
13. Duchenne, G.B., Cuthbertson, R.A.: The mechanism of human facial expression. Studies in emotion and social interaction, Cambridge University Press ; Editions de la Maison des Sciences de l'Homme, Cambridge [England] ; New York: Paris (1990)
14. Dupré, D., Krumhuber, E.G., Küster, D., McKeown, G.J.: A performance comparison of eight commercially available automatic classifiers for facial affect recognition. PLoS ONE **15**(4), e0231968 (2020). https://doi.org/10.1371/journal.pone.0231968, https://journals.plos.org/plosone/article?id=10.1371/journal.pone.0231968, publisher: Public Library of Science
15. D'Andrea, E., Barbaix, E.: Anatomic research on the perioral muscles, functional matrix of the maxillary and mandibular bones. Surg. Radiol. Anat. **28**(3), 261–266 (2006). https://doi.org/10.1007/s00276-006-0095-y, http://link.springer.com/10.1007/s00276-006-0095-y

16. Ekman, P.: Basic emotions. In: Handbook of Cognition and Emotion, pp. 45–60. Wiley, Hoboken (1999). https://doi.org/10.1002/0470013494.ch3

17. Ekman, P., Friesen, W.V., Hager, J.C.: Facial Action Coding System: The Manual. Research Nexus, Salt Lake City, Utah (2002)

18. Folgado, D., et al.: TSSEARCH: time series subsequence search library. SoftwareX **18**, 101049 (2022). https://doi.org/10.1016/j.softx.2022.101049, https://www.sciencedirect.com/science/article/pii/S2352711022000425

19. Fridlund, A.J., Cacioppo, J.T.: Guidelines for human electromyographic research. Psychophysiology **23**(5), 567–589 (1986). https://doi.org/10.1111/j.1469-8986.1986.tb00676.x, https://onlinelibrary.wiley.com/doi/10.1111/j.1469-8986.1986.tb00676.x

20. Gibert, G., Pruzinec, M., Schultz, T., Stevens, C.: Enhancement of human computer interaction with facial electromyographic sensors. In: Proceedings of the 21st Annual Conference of the Australian Computer-Human Interaction Special Interest Group: Design: Open 24/7, pp. 421–424. ACM, Melbourne Australia (2009). https://doi.org/10.1145/1738826.1738914

21. Giovanelli, E., Valzolgher, C., Gessa, E., Todeschini, M., Pavani, F.: Unmasking the difficulty of listening to talkers with masks: lessons from the Covid-19 pandemic. I-Perception **12**(2), 2041669521998393 (2021). https://doi.org/10.1177/2041669521998393

22. Gruebler, A., Suzuki, K.: Design of a wearable device for reading positive expressions from facial EMG signals. IEEE Trans. Affect. Comput. **5**(3), 227–237 (2014). https://doi.org/10.1109/TAFFC.2014.2313557, https://ieeexplore.ieee.org/document/6778017

23. Guntinas-Lichius, O., et al.: High-resolution surface electromyographic activities of facial muscles during the six basic emotional expressions in healthy adults: a prospective observational study **13**(1) (1921). https://doi.org/10.1038/s41598-023-45779-9, https://www.nature.com/articles/s41598-023-45779-9

24. Hartmann, Y., Liu, H., Lahrberg, S., Schultz, T.: Interpretable high-level features for human activity recognition. In: Proceedings of the 15th International Joint Conference on Biomedical Engineering Systems and Technologies (BIOSTEC 2022) - Volume 4: BIOSIGNALS, pp. 40–49 (2022). https://doi.org/10.5220/0010840500003123, https://www.scitepress.org/Link.aspx?doi=10.5220/0010840500003123

25. Hartmann, Y., Liu, H., Schultz, T.: Feature space reduction for multimodal human activity recognition. In: Proceedings of the 13th International Joint Conference on Biomedical Engineering Systems and Technologies (BIOSTEC 2020) - Volume 4: BIOSIGNALS, pp. 135–140 (2020). https://doi.org/10.5220/0008851401350140

26. Hartmann, Y., Liu, H., Schultz, T.: Feature space reduction for human activity recognition based on multi-channel biosignals. In: Proceedings of the 14th International Joint Conference on Biomedical Engineering Systems and Technologies (BIOSTEC 2021) - Volume 4: BIOSIGNALS, pp. 215–222. INSTICC, SCITEPRESS - Science and Technology Publications (2021). https://doi.org/10.5220/0010260802150222, https://www.scitepress.org/Link.aspx?doi=10.5220/0010260802150222

27. Hartmann, Y., Liu, H., Schultz, T.: Interactive and interpretable online human activity recognition. In: PERCOM 2022 - 20th IEEE International Conference on Pervasive Computing and Communications Workshops and other Affiliated Events (PerCom Workshops), pp. 109–111 (2022). https://doi.org/10.1109/PerComWorkshops53856.2022.9767207, https://ieeexplore.ieee.org/document/9767207

28. Hartmann, Y., Liu, H., Schultz, T.: High-level features for human activity recognition and modeling. In: Roque, A.C.A., Gracanin, D., Lorenz, R., Tsanas, A., Bier, N., Fred, A., Gamboa, H. (eds.) Biomedical Engineering Systems and Technologies, pp. 141–163. Springer Nature Switzerland, Cham (2023). https://doi.org/10.1007/978-3-031-38854-5_8

29. Henderson, T., Fulcher, B.D.: An empirical evaluation of time-series feature sets. In: 2021 International Conference on Data Mining Workshops (ICDMW), pp. 1032–

1038 (2021). https://doi.org/10.1109/ICDMW53433.2021.00134, https://ieeexplore.ieee.org/abstract/document/9679937

30. Hjortsjö, C.H.: Man's Face and Mimic Language. Studentlitteratur, Lund, Sweden (1969)
31. Hollenstein, T., Lanteigne, D.: Models and methods of emotional concordance. Biol. Psychol. **98**, 1–5 (2014). https://doi.org/10.1016/j.biopsycho.2013.12.012, http://linkinghub.elsevier.com/retrieve/pii/S0301051113002597
32. Huang, X., Zhao, G., Zheng, W., Pietikäinen, M.: Towards a dynamic expression recognition system under facial occlusion. Pattern Recogn. Lett. **33**(16), 2181–2191 (2012). https://doi.org/10.1016/j.patrec.2012.07.015, https://linkinghub.elsevier.com/retrieve/pii/S0167865512002371
33. Kappas, A., Krumhuber, E., Küster, D.: Facial behavior, pp. 131–165 (2013). https://doi.org/10.1515/9783110238150.131
34. Kleiner, M., Wallraven, C., Breidt, M., Cunningham, D.W., Bülthoff, H.H.: Multi-viewpoint video capture for facial perception research. In: Workshop on Modelling and Motion Capture Techniques for Virtual Environments (CAPTECH 2004). Geneva, Switzerland (2004). http://www.kyb.tuebingen.mpg.de/fileadmin/user_upload/files/publications/pdf3058.pdf
35. Krumhuber, E.G., Küster, D., Namba, S., Skora, L.: Human and machine validation of 14 databases of dynamic facial expressions. Behav. Res. Methods **53**(2), 686–701 (2021). https://doi.org/10.3758/s13428-020-01443-y, https://link.springer.com/10.3758/s13428-020-01443-y
36. Kuester, D., Kappas, A.: Measuring emotions in individuals and internet communities. In: Benski, T., Fisher, E. (eds.) Internet and emotions, pp. 48–62. Routledge (2013)
37. Küster, D., Krumhuber, E.G., Steinert, L., Ahuja, A., Baker, M., Schultz, T.: Opportunities and challenges for using automatic human affect analysis in consumer research. Front. Neurosci. **14**, 400 (2020)
38. Küster, D., Kappas, A.: Measuring Emotions Online: Expression and Physiology. In: Holyst, J.A. (ed.) Cyberemotions, pp. 71–93 (2016). https://doi.org/10.1007/978-3-319-43639-5_5
39. Larsen, J.T., Norris, C.J., Cacioppo, J.T.: Effects of positive and negative affect on electromyographic activity over zygomaticus major and corrugator supercilii. Psychophysiology **40**(5), 776–785 (2003). https://doi.org/10.1111/1469-8986.00078, https://onlinelibrary.wiley.com/doi/abs/10.1111/1469-8986.00078
40. Lewinski, P., den Uyl, T.M., Butler, C.: Automated facial coding: validation of basic emotions and FACS AUs in FaceReader. J. Neurosci. Psychol. Econ. **7**(4), 227–236 (2014). https://doi.org/10.1037/npe0000028, http://doi.apa.org/getdoi.cfm?doi=10.1037/npe0000028
41. Li, X., Zhang, X., Yang, H., Duan, W., Dai, W., Yin, L.: An EEG-based multi-modal emotion database with both posed and authentic facial actions for emotion analysis. In: 2020 15th IEEE International Conference on Automatic Face and Gesture Recognition (FG 2020), pp. 336–343. IEEE, Buenos Aires, Argentina (2020). https://doi.org/10.1109/FG47880.2020.00050, https://ieeexplore.ieee.org/document/9320173/
42. Littlewort, G., Whitehill, J., Wu, T., Fasel, I., Frank, M., Movellan, J., Bartlett, M.: The computer expression recognition toolbox (CERT). In: 2011 IEEE International Conference on Automatic Face & Gesture Recognition (FG), pp. 298–305 (2011). https://doi.org/10.1109/FG.2011.5771414
43. Liu, H.: Biosignal processing and activity modeling for multimodal human activity recognition. Ph.D. thesis, University of Bremen (2021). https://doi.org/10.26092/elib/1219, https://www.csl.uni-bremen.de/cms/images/documents/publications/Liu2021Diss.pdf
44. Liu, H., Gamboa, H., Schultz, T. (eds.): Sensors for human activity recognition. MDPI (2023). https://doi.org/10.3390/books978-3-0365-7555-1, https://www.mdpi.com/books/reprint/7447-sensors-for-human-activity-recognition

45. Liu, H., Gamboa, H., Schultz, T.: Human activity recognition, monitoring, and analysis facil-itated by novel and widespread applications of sensors. Sensors **24**(16) (2024). https://doi.org/10.3390/s24165250, https://www.mdpi.com/1424-8220/24/16/5250

46. Liu, H., Hartmann, Y., Schultz, T.: CSL-SHARE: a multimodal wearable sensor-based human activity dataset. Front. Comput. Sci. **3**, 90 (2021). https://doi.org/10.3389/fcomp.2021.759136, https://www.frontiersin.org/journals/computer-science/articles/10.3389/fcomp.2021.759136

47. Liu, H., Hartmann, Y., Schultz, T.: Motion units: generalized sequence modeling of human activities for sensor-based activity recognition. In: 29th European Signal Processing Con-ference (EUSIPCO 2021). IEEE (2021). https://doi.org/10.23919/EUSIPCO54536.2021.9616298, https://ieeexplore.ieee.org/document/9616298

48. Liu, H., Jiang, K., Gamboa, H., Xue, T., Schultz, T.: Bell shape embodying zhongyong: The pitch histogram of traditional chinese anhemitonic pentatonic folk songs. Appl. Sci. **12**(16) (2022). https://doi.org/10.3390/app12168343, https://www.mdpi.com/2076-3417/12/16/8343

49. Liu, H., Schultz, T.: ASK: a framework for data acquisition and activity recognition. In: Proceedings of the 11th International Joint Conference on Biomedical Engineering Systems and Technologies (BIOSTEC 2018) - Volume 3: BIOSIGNALS, pp. 262–268. INSTICC, SciTePress (2018). https://doi.org/10.5220/0006732902620268, https://www.scitepress.org/Link.aspx?doi=10.5220/0006732902620268

50. Liu, H., Schultz, T.: A wearable real-time human activity recognition system using biosen-sors integrated into a knee bandage. In: Proceedings of the 12th International Joint Confer-ence on Biomedical Engineering Systems and Technologies (BIOSTEC 2019) - Volume 1: BIODEVICES, pp. 47–55 (2019). https://doi.org/10.5220/0007398800470055, https://www.scitepress.org/Link.aspx?doi=10.5220/0007398800470055

51. Liu, H., Xue, T., Schultz, T.: On a real real-time wearable human activity recogni-tion system. In: Proceedings of the 16th International Joint Conference on Biomedi-cal Engineering Systems and Technologies (BIOSTEC 2023) - Volume 5: HEALTHINF: WHC, pp. 711–720. INSTICC, SCITEPRESS - Science and Technology Publications (2023). https://doi.org/10.5220/0011927700003414, https://www.scitepress.org/Link.aspx?doi=10.5220/0011927700003414

52. Liu, H., Zhang, S., Gamboa, H., Xue, T., Zhou, C., Schultz, T.: Taxonomy and real-time classification of artifacts during biosignal acquisition: a starter study and dataset of ECG. IEEE Sens. J. **24**(6), 9162–9171 (2024). https://doi.org/10.1109/JSEN.2024.3356651, https://ieeexplore.ieee.org/document/10415350

53. Mauss, I.B., Robinson, M.D.: Measures of emotion: a review. Cognit. Emotion **23**(2), 209–237 (2009). https://doi.org/10.1080/02699930802204677, http://www.tandfonline.com/doi/abs/10.1080/02699930802204677

54. Namba, S., Sato, W., Osumi, M., Shimokawa, K.: Assessing automated facial action unit detection systems for analyzing cross-domain facial expression databases. Sensors **21**(12), 4222 (2021). https://doi.org/10.3390/s21124222, https://www.mdpi.com/1424-8220/21/12/4222

55. Namba, S., Sato, W., Yoshikawa, S.: Viewpoint robustness of automated facial action unit detection systems. Appl. Sci. **11**(23), 11171 (2021). https://doi.org/10.3390/app112311171, https://www.mdpi.com/2076-3417/11/23/11171

56. Noah, T., Schul, Y., Mayo, R.: When both the original study and its failed replica-tion are correct: feeling observed eliminates the facial-feedback effect. J. Pers. Soc. Psychol. **114**(5), 657–664 (2018). https://doi.org/10.1037/pspa0000121, http://doi.apa.org/getdoi.cfm?doi=10.1037/pspa0000121

57. Oh Kruzic, C., Kruzic, D., Herrera, F., Bailenson, J.: Facial expressions contribute more than body movements to conversational outcomes in avatar-mediated virtual environments. Sci. Rep. **10**(1), 20626 (2020). https://doi.org/10.1038/s41598-020-76672-4, https://www.nature.com/articles/s41598-020-76672-4

58. Ortony, A.: Are All "Basic emotions" emotions? A problem for the (basic) emotions construct. Perspect. Psychol. Sci. **17**(1), 41–61 (2022). https://doi.org/10.1177/1745691620985415, http://journals.sagepub.com/doi/10.1177/1745691620985415

59. Pedregosa, F., et al.: Scikit-learn: machine learning in Python. J. Mach. Learn. Res. **12**, 2825–2830 (2011)

60. Perusquia-Hernandez, M., Dollack, F., Tan, C.K., Namba, S., Ayabe-Kanamura, S., Suzuki, K.: Smile action unit detection from distal wearable electromyography and computer vision. In: 2021 16th IEEE International Conference on Automatic Face and Gesture Recognition (FG 2021), pp. 1–8. IEEE, Jodhpur, India (2021). https://doi.org/10.1109/FG52635.2021.9667047, https://ieeexplore.ieee.org/document/9667047/

61. Rodrigues, J., Liu, H., Folgado, D., Belo, D., Schultz, T., Gamboa, H.: Feature-based information retrieval of multimodal biosignals with a self-similarity matrix: focus on automatic segmentation. Biosensors **12**(12) (2022). https://doi.org/10.3390/bios12121182, https://www.mdpi.com/2079-6374/12/12/1182

62. Schuller, B., Valster, M., Eyben, F., Cowie, R., Pantic, M.: AVEC 2012: the continuous audio/visual emotion challenge. In: Proceedings of the 14th ACM international conference on Multimodal interaction, pp. 449–456. ICMI 2012, Association for Computing Machinery, New York, NY, USA (2012). https://doi.org/10.1145/2388676.2388776

63. Schultz, T., et al.: Towards restoration of articulatory movements: Functional electrical stimulation of orofacial muscles. In: 2019 41st Annual International Conference of the IEEE Engineering in Medicine and Biology Society (EMBC), pp. 3111–3114 (2019). https://doi.org/10.1109/EMBC.2019.8857670, https://ieeexplore.ieee.org/abstract/document/8857670

64. Steinert, L., Putze, F., Küster, D., Schultz, T.: Audio-visual recognition of emotional engagement of people with dementia. In: Interspeech, pp. 1024–1028 (2021)

65. van der Struijk, S., Huang, H.H., Mirzaei, M.S., Nishida, T.: FACSvatar: an open source modular framework for real-time FACS based facial animation. In: Proceedings of the 18th International Conference on Intelligent Virtual Agents, pp. 159–164. IVA 2018, Association for Computing Machinery, New York, NY, USA (2018). https://doi.org/10.1145/3267851.3267918, https://dl.acm.org/doi/10.1145/3267851.3267918

66. Tassinary, L.G., Cacioppo, J.T., Vanman, E.J.: The Skeletomotor system: surface electromyography. In: Cacioppo, J.T., Tassinary, L.G., Berntson, G. (eds.) Handbook of Psychophysiology, pp. 267–300. Cambridge University Press, Cambridge, 3 edn. (2007). https://doi.org/10.1017/CBO9780511546396.012, http://ebooks.cambridge.org/ref/id/CBO9780511546396A020

67. Van Boxtel, A., Jessurun, M.: Amplitude and bilateral coherency of facial and jaw-elevator EMG activity as an index of effort during a two-choice serial reaction task. Psychophysiology **30**(6), 589–604 (1993). https://doi.org/10.1111/j.1469-8986.1993.tb02085.x, https://onlinelibrary.wiley.com/doi/abs/10.1111/j.1469-8986.1993.tb02085.x

68. Veldanda, A., Liu, H., Koschke, R., Schultz, T., Küster, D.: Can electromyography alone reveal facial action units? A pilot EMG-based action unit recognition study with real-time validation. In: Proceedings of the 17th International Joint Conference on Biomedical Engineering Systems and Technologies (BIOSTEC 2024) - Volume 1: BIODEVICES. pp. 142–151. INSTICC, SCITEPRESS - Science and Technology Publications (2024). https://doi.org/10.5220/0012399100003657, https://www.scitepress.org/Link.aspx?doi=10.5220/0012399100003657

69. Verma, D., Bhalla, S., Sahnan, D., Shukla, J., Parnami, A.: ExpressEar: sensing fine-grained facial expressions with earables. Proc. ACM Interact. Mob. Wearable Ubiquitous Technol. **5**(3), 1–28 (2021). https://doi.org/10.1145/3478085, https://dl.acm.org/doi/10.1145/3478085

70. Wingenbach, T.S.H.: Facial EMG – Investigating the interplay of facial muscles and emotions. In: Boggio, P.S., Wingenbach, T.S.H., da Silveira Coêlho, M.L., Comfort, W.E., Murrins Marques, L., Alves, M.V.C. (eds.) Social and Affective Neuroscience of Everyday Human Interaction: From Theory to Methodology, pp. 283–300. Springer International Publishing, Cham (2023). https://doi.org/10.1007/978-3-031-08651-9_17

71. Wingenbach, T.S.H., Ribeiro, B., Nakao, C., Boggio, P.S.: Modulation of facial muscle responses by another person's presence and affiliative touch during affective image viewing **38**(1), 59–70 (2024). https://doi.org/10.1080/02699931.2023.2258588, https://www.tandfonline.com/doi/full/10.1080/02699931.2023.2258588

72. Zhang, S., Kolensnikov, S., Rennspieß, T., Porzel, R., Schultz, T., Liu, H.: Really can't hold on anymore? Physiological indicators versus self-reported motivation drop during jogging. In: Proceedings of the 17th International Joint Conference on Biomedical Engineering Systems and Technologies (BIOSTEC 2024) - Volume 1: BIOSIGNALS, pp. 821–831. INSTICC, SCITEPRESS - Science and Technology Publications (2024). https://doi.org/10.5220/0012577300003657, https://www.scitepress.org/Link.aspx?doi=10.5220/0012577300003657

73. Zhi, R., Liu, M., Zhang, D.: A comprehensive survey on automatic facial action unit analysis. Vis. Comput. **36**(5), 1067–1093 (2020). https://doi.org/10.1007/s00371-019-01707-5

RehabVisual: A Platform for Visual Stimulation Applied to Patients with Multiple Sclerosis

Margarida Henriques[1](✉) ⓘD, Maria Irene Mendes[3], Ana Martins[3], Carla Quintão[1,2] ⓘD, and Cláudia Quaresma[1,2] ⓘD

[1] Physics Department, NOVA School of Science and Technology - FCT NOVA, Universidade Nova de Lisboa, 2829-516 Caparica, Portugal
m1.henriques@campus.fct.unl.pt
[2] LIBPhys-UNL, Physics Department, NOVA School of Science and Technology - FCT NOVA, Universidade Nova de Lisboa, 2829-516 Caparica, Portugal
[3] Neurology Department, Hospital Garcia de Orta, 2805-267 Almada, Portugal

Abstract. Multiple Sclerosis (MS), which is the most prevalent immune-mediated inflammatory demyelinating disease affecting the Central Nervous System (CNS), has an estimated global incidence of 2,8 million individuals. Although its symptomatology is highly varied and unpredictable, depending on the lesions' location in the CNS, visual impairments are among the most common manifestations. However, conventional methods for assessing and rehabilitating visuomotor competences are not sufficient to deliver objective assessments or personalized therapies. To address this gap, RehabVisual was adapted and its usability for MS patients was assessed. RehabVisual, developed in previous studies, aims to objectively assess visuomotor skills through an integrated low-cost eye tracking system. Before clinical application, a normative base was established using 50 healthy individuals for later comparison. The experimental group comprised 25 MS patients with and without confirmed visuomotor alterations. The protocol involved viewing three visual stimuli for later calculation of the mean Euclidean distance between the gaze and stimulus positions using the eye tracking system, for further assessment of the patients' performance in tracking the stimulus. The current paper aims to detail the results obtained, revealing relevant results that had not yet been addressed. It was possible to confirm diagnosed visual impairments, and to assess the usability of the RehabVisual platform for monitoring and rehabilitation purposes.

Keywords: Multiple sclerosis · Visuomotor skills · Eye tracker

1 Introduction

Multiple Sclerosis (MS) is the most prevalent immune-mediated inflammatory demyelinating disease affecting the Central Nervous System (CNS), with an estimated incidence of 2.9 million individuals worldwide, according to the Multiple Sclerosis International Federation [1].

In MS, the immune system mistakenly attacks the protective covering of nerve fibers, called myelin. This causes inflammation and attracts more immune cells to the

M. P. Guarino et al. (Eds.): BIOSTEC 2024, CCIS 2546, pp. 44–62, 2026.
https://doi.org/10.1007/978-3-031-96899-0_4

affected area, which further damages the myelin and nerve fibers. Since myelin helps the efficient transmission of electrical signals between the brain and the rest of the body, when it is damaged or destroyed (demyelination), the signals can become slower, distorted, or completely blocked [11]. As any region of the CNS may be affected, the MS symptoms are very variable and unpredictable, depending from one person to another and in the same person over time. However, visual impairments are often the first indication of the disease and are among its most prevalent symptoms [2].

Nevertheless, clinical tools to objectively assess ocular motor dysfunction are lacking. Currently, assessments are mainly based on bedside visual examinations and observations by experienced professionals. Consequently, these impairments may often be overlooked or undervalued by clinicians. In this sense, conducting a detailed and quantitative evaluation of eye movement function holds considerable promise for enhancing patient care, particularly for healthcare professionals focused on monitoring disease progression and rehabilitating visual function [10].

To address this need, eye tracking systems have been included in several studies in order to quantitatively assess eye movements. In 2003, Frohman et al. [6] compared the accuracy of quantitative infrared oculography to the clinical detection of internuclear ophthalmoplegia (INO). INO results from damage to the Medial Longitudinal Fasciculus in the brain, which plays a critical role in coordinating eye movements, particularly the conjugate movement of both eyes. It is distinguished by the limitation or slowing of the adducting ipsilateral eye relative to the abducting eye, often accompanied by abducting nystagmus in the contralateral eye. The referred study suggested that INO may be overlooked on clinical examination, and the use of a quantitative system provides greater precision in the diagnostic confirmation.

Considering this, the RehabVisual platform was applied to MS patients at the Hospital Garcia de Orta to assess its usability for these individuals [7], after the Ethics Committee's approval of the experimental protocol's execution. RehabVisual is a web-based platform designed to stimulate visuomotor skills and includes an integrated eye tracking system. In this context, three different stimuli were used to evaluate the presence of common visual impairments in MS patients, and the eye tracking system enabled the assessment of their eye movement function.

The present paper aims to compare the results obtained from the MS patients with those obtained from the healthy volunteers in the control group through a more detailed analysis.

2   Materials and Methods

The current chapter details the materials used in this work, namely the RehabVisual platform, covered in Sect. 2.1, along with its integrated eye tracking system. Additionally, the data acquisition methodology is described, including the samples characterization in Sect. 2.2, and the experimental protocol in Sect. 2.3.

2.1   RehabVisual Platform

RehabVisual is a computer application designed to stimulate visuomotor skills through the presentation of various stimuli on a computer screen. Its integrated eye tracking system enables objective monitoring and analysis of eye movements, enhancing the understanding of patients' needs and facilitating the design of individualized rehabilitation plans.

In the Department of Physical Medicine and Rehabilitation at Hospital Dona Estefânia, it was identified that there was a lack of methodology for assessing and intervening in visuomotor skills in infants up to 18 months old with developmental abnormalities. Consequently, in collaboration with physicians and occupational therapists, the RehabVisual platform was developed to address this problem [8].

The application aimed to provide individualized and specific treatment to meet the needs of these children and monitor their therapeutic progress. Therefore, two sections were designed: one for assessment and another for intervention [8].

- **Assessment Section:** This consists of a database to record all relevant clinical information of the patients, including their clinical records and ophthalmological, behavioral, and functional assessments. These data facilitate long-term monitoring and enable the possibility of conducting prospective longitudinal studies in the future.
- **Intervention Section:** This includes various protocols with different stimuli tailored to the visuomotor function of each patient (differing in form, dimension, color, contrast, movement, and presentation distance), allowing the utilization of an appropriate set of stimuli for specific patients.

Following an initial behavioral assessment of the infants, therapists select the most appropriate stimuli available on the platform based on the outcomes of this assessment. The videos presented in subsequent sessions depend on the results of the previous sessions. Hence, the platform allows a global and integrated evaluation and intervention, addressing both assessment and rehabilitation aspects [8].

An eye tracking system was developed to integrate the platform and quantitatively assess visual impairments [3]. Additionally, the platform was adapted to include the adult population, particularly post-stroke patients [9]. RehabVisual has been tested on these patients, and the eye tracker has been improved and validated [4,5].

The computer application was developed using HTML, PHP, CSS, and JS, while SQL was used to create the database. It includes eight different pages: homepage, users, clinical record, general ophthalmological assessment, neuropsychological assessment, behavioral assessment, functional assessment, and intervention program. Figure 1 demonstrates the homepage of the RehabVisual application, with the available menus visible on the left side. Additionally, it allows access to four different profiles with different permissions within the platform: administrator, physician/technician, occupational therapist, and caregiver.

Recently, RehabVisual was tested on individuals diagnosed with Multiple Sclerosis [7]. As the neuropsychology assessment is typically carried out on these patients, a new area was added to the platform (currently included in the menus available on the left side of Fig. 1). It includes information about whether or not the patient has executive alterations and allows the addition of observations considered relevant by the healthcare professional. Executive alterations refer to cognitive difficulties or dysfunctions related to the executive system which are diagnosed by a neuropsychologist and are relevant in

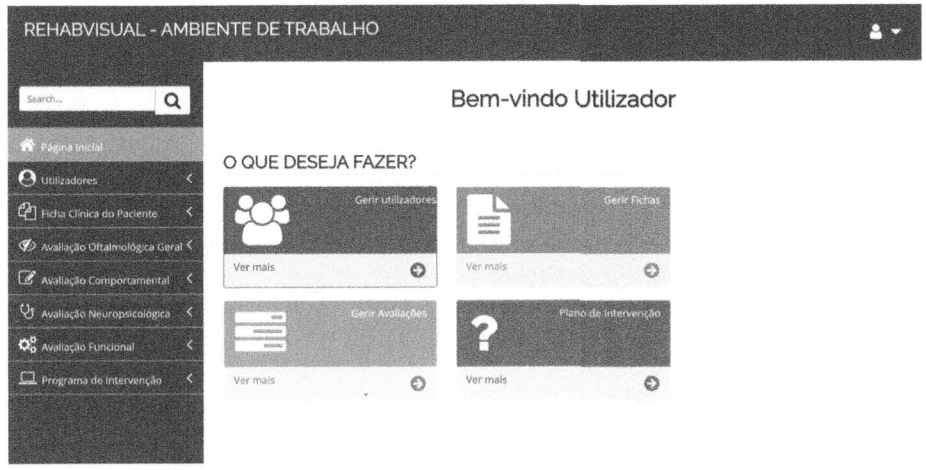

Fig. 1. Homepage of RehabVisual, with the available menus on the left side.

evaluating the progression of the pathology, hence the integration of this assessment in the platform.

The functional assessment includes the protocol developed particularly for MS patients, addressed in Sect. 2.3. The intervention section was not changed nor applied in this work, since the present research focused on the possibility of confirming and monitoring diagnosed visual alterations with the utilization of RehabVisual on MS patients [7].

Eye Tracking System. The eye tracking system was developed using Matlab R2017a software and operates offline, only requiring prior recording of the participants' face during stimulus observation.

The process is semi-automated, starting with the selection of the video to be analyzed, i.e. a recording of the participant's face while visualizing a specific stimulus. Subsequently, the user defines the tolerance value for each eye, from 0 to 1, which will be used as an argument in the grayconnected() function, responsible for the image binarization. After the manual selection of the position of each eye and a reference point (usually the nose) in the first frame, the image processing initiates by converting the image into grayscale and identifying the darkest point (lowest intensity), which is presumed to belong to the pupil. Using this pixel as a basis, the image segmentation technique defines the approved range of similar intensity values based on the inserted tolerance values, hence achieving the iris segmentation. This tolerance values depend on the image's lighting conditions, as well as the individual's eye color (e.g. blue eyes normally require a higher tolerance value than brown eyes).

The eye detection is attained through the iris detection by the imfindcircles() function, which is programmed to identify black circles within a binary image and store their positions and radii in matrices. After these steps, the system automatically analyses the whole recording, processing every frame and storing the circles with a radius ranging from 80% to 120% of the radius of the previous frame's circle. These values are converted into screen positions (in pixels) through a calibration system for later comparison with the coordinates of the stimulus's position throughout the video shown to the participant.

These two distinct positions - coordinates of the participant's gaze and the stimulus in the screen - are used to calculate the mean Euclidean distance between them for each eye. This metric showed a promising result in the previous study that validated the present eye tracking system [5], hence its utilization in the current research. To analyze the results, four graphs are also generated, one for each eye and for each direction (vertical and horizontal), representing the overlay of the stimulus positions with the gaze's direction of each eye (both in pixels) as a function of the video frame number.

2.2   Samples Characterization

The experimental protocol was employed in two distinct samples: a control group, constituted by healthy individuals, and an experimental group with MS patients monitored at the HGO [7].

It is important to mention that the Ethics Committee of both the HGO and the NOVA School of Science and Technology (where the control group samples were collected) reviewed the experimental protocol and approved its execution in their facilities.

Control Group. The control group consists of 50 volunteers, who willingly agreed to collaborate in the present study by providing their free consent. To be included in this sample, the individuals had to have a minimum of 18 years of age and could not have a known pathology that might influence ocular movements in any way. The group was constituted by 38 (76%) females and 12 (24%) males, with ages ranging from 19 to 63 years old and a mean of 30,3 ± 13,3 years. The mean age for the females is 32,7 ± 14,4 years, while for the males is 22,5 ± 1,6 years.

Multiple Sclerosis Group. The experimental group included 25 individuals diagnosed with MS, who provided free informed consent before taking part on the present study. Patients with a recent history of MS relapse (less than six months) or a physical handicap that affected the execution of the experimental protocol were excluded. This sample is constituted by 18 females (72%) and 7 males (28%), with ages also raging from 19 to 63 years old, although with a mean of 41,8 ± 11,7 years. The mean age for the female cohort is 41,2 ± 11,5, while for the male cohort is 43,3 ± 12,9 years. Additional information was also collected from the participants, namely their MS subtype and whether they had had a diagnosis of internuclear ophthalmoplegia, optic neuropathy or alterations of the executive system. 22 (88%) of the individuals are diagnosed with Relapsing-remitting MS, while the other 3 (12%) are diagnosed with Secondary Progressive MS. 9 patients (36%) had already been diagnosed with internuclear ophthalmoplegia, 9 patients (36%) with optic neuropathy, and 12 (48%) with executive alterations.

2.3   Experimental Protocol

All participants were informed about the purpose and protocol of the study and subsequently signed the informed consent form. They were then asked to watch three different videos in a specific order, with intervals in between, while resting their head on a support. An external camera recorded their face during this process. To minimize movement of the reference point, participants were instructed to keep their head still throughout the recordings. If participants wore glasses, they were asked to remove them to prevent interference with the eye tracker. In such cases, it was ensured that stimulus recognition was not affected.

This experimental protocol was identical for both the control and experimental groups and was designed in collaboration with the Neurology team of Hospital Garcia de Orta (HGO).

Below are the descriptions of the experimental setup and the stimuli presented in the experimental protocol.

Experimental Setup. Although the data acquisition site was different for each group, the experimental setup was the same, with their conditions as equal as possible in order to obtain more reliable and comparable results. The following equipment was used: a laptop, Acer Aspire E15; a head support, with a chin- and a forehead-rest; an external camera, Logitech C920 HD PRO Webcam, which a 78° field of view and a recording resolution of 1920×1080 pixels (full HD) at 30 frames per second; and an external monitor (22''), with a resolution of 1680×1050 pixels at 60 Hz. The positioning of the equipment was chosen empirically and is represented in Fig. 2.

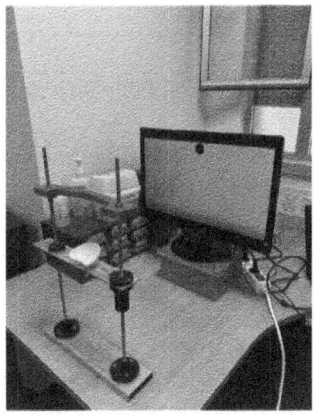

Fig. 2. Experimental setup.

The monitor and camera were arranged at a height of approximately 20 cm to correspond with eye level, and positioned about 60 cm away from the participant, ensuring the stimuli were comfortably visible within the subject's field of vision. Figure 3 represents the first frame of a recording, captured by the webcam.

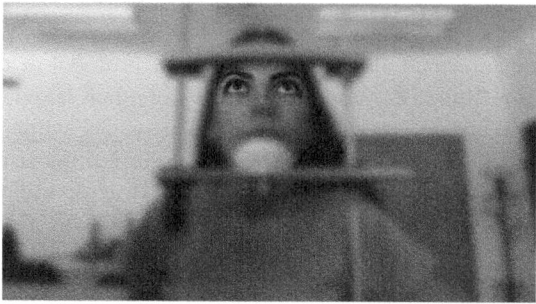

Fig. 3. Image of the webcam during the experimental protocol.

Stimuli. The three different videos were designed and planned in collaboration with the Neurology Service of the HGO. The shape of the stimulus was always the same, a black circle with a red center in a white background (Fig. 4, on the left), presenting a high contrast and a diameter of approximately 2 cm when displayed in the monitor.

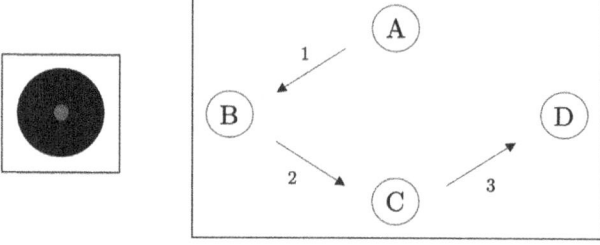

Fig. 4. Visual stimulus (on the left) and calibration path scheme (on the right).

What differed from one video to another is the trajectory followed by the stimulus, with increasing complexity. However, all three videos started with a 15-s (450 frames) calibration, according to the scheme detailed on the right side of Fig. 4), where the stimulus covers the maximum and minimum vertical and horizontal values on the screen, hence allowing a correspondence between these values and the maximum and minimum amplitude of the eyes' movements.

The first video was included to assess the presence of nystagmus by evaluating the ability of the participant to maintain a steady gaze at a fixed point. It has a duration of 28 s, in which, after the calibration, the stimulus moves to the center of the screen and remains static for 10 s, as it is schematized on the left side of Fig. 5.

In the second video, with a total duration of 41 s, the stimulus follows the trajectory schematized on the right side of Fig. 5, presenting vertical and horizontal movements after the calibration. Its goal was to evaluate if the participant could achieve a smooth pursuit of the stimulus, which could indicate the presence or absence of saccadic intrusions.

Finally, the third stimulus aimed to assess the participant's visual field and visual attention by following a more complex trajectory, including a continuous movement along the screen edges and an intermittent movement afterwards. Considering the scheme presented in Fig. 6, the stimulus primarily follows the sequence B-D-H-F-E-B-H-I-A-G-C (which includes the calibration sequence). Posteriorly, the stimulus disappears and reappears in another area, where it remains static for 3 s, hence describing the above mentioned intermittent movement, following the sequence E-A-I-D-F-B-G-C-H.

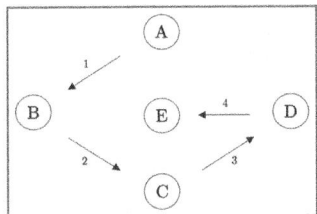 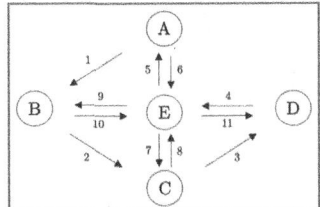

Fig. 5. Schemes of the first (left) and second (right) stimuli.

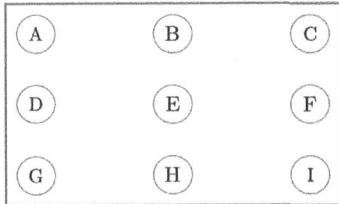

Fig. 6. Screen locations of the stimulus's trajectory for the third video.

Figure 7 represents the graphs generated by the eye tracking system for the more complex stimulus, the third one. In these, the stimulus's screen position in pixels is represented as a function of the video frame number with the red line.

As it was mentioned before, the graphs are separated in the two directions (horizontal on the left, and vertical on the right). The slope alterations up to frame 450 correspond to the initial above mentioned calibration, where the stimulus performs diagonal movements. Additionally, horizontal lines represent unchanged coordinates in the respective axis. The diagonal movements along the screen edges are represented by changes in the values of both coordinates, hence the slope alterations in both graphs at the same frame. Additionally, the intermittent movement is evident by the abrupt lines, as the coordinate in both axes is null when the stimulus disappears.

3   Results and Discussion

As previously mentioned, the metric used to quantify the capacity to adequately follow the stimulus was the mean Euclidean distance between the stimulus and gaze positions, automatically calculated by the eye tracking system. This metric was calculated for the first two videos for each subject to establish a reference value for later comparison with the experimental group. The third video was analyzed separately.

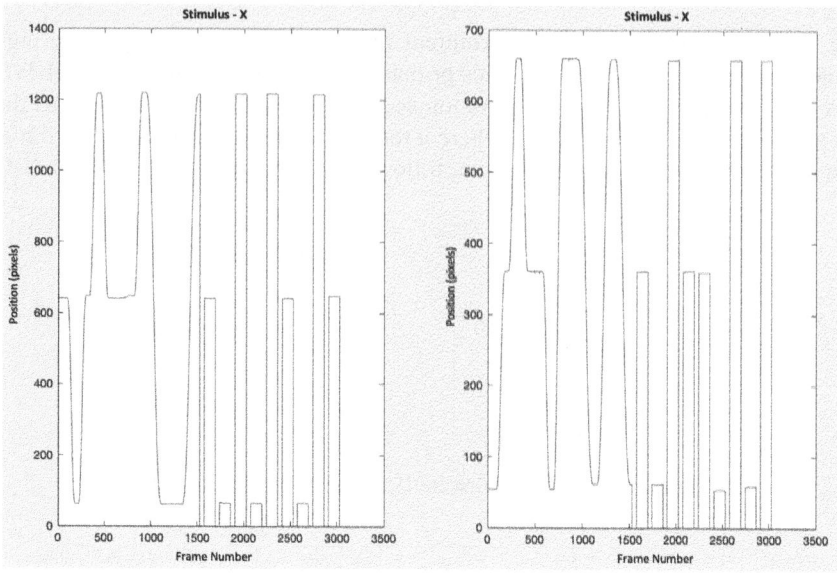

Fig. 7. Position in pixels of the third stimulus as a function of the frame number (x coordinates on the left and y coordinated on the right).

Following the approach of the previous study that validated the eye tracking system [5], and given that the control group was able to follow the stimulus without difficulties, a reference threshold was established to distinguish the success and failure of stimulus tracking for the experimental group. The approximate values of the maximum mean Euclidean distances between the gaze and stimulus positions were used to establish this threshold.

To complement this analysis, the graphs generated by the eye tracker were also observed to assess the continuity of the participants' eye movements.

In the current chapter, the results are presented separately for the three videos, encompassing the findings for both the control and experimental groups.

3.1   First Stimulus

Table 1 summarizes the mean Euclidean distances between the gaze and the stimulus positions (in pixels) for both groups. The maximum value obtained for the control group was 125 pixels, hence it was established a threshold at 130 pixels, following the methodology mentioned above. In this sense, a mean Euclidean distance between the gaze and the stimulus positions above this established value was considered an indicator of difficulties in tracking the stimulus, and the respective graphs were analyzed.

Upon initial examination, we can conclude that the mean Euclidean distances values are higher for the experimental group. This result was anticipated, since the latest sample includes individuals with diagnosed visual impairments that were expected to demonstrate difficulties in following the stimulus only with eye movements.

Figure 8 depicts the graphs generated by the eye tracking system for one participant of the normative base, corresponding to the visualization of the first stimulus. The mean

Table 1. Descriptive statistics of the mean Euclidean distance between the stimulus and the gaze positions (in pixels) for the first stimulus and for both groups, considering both eyes.

Mean Euclidean distances (pixels)	Control Group		Experimental Group	
	Right Eye	Left Eye	Right Eye	Left Eye
Maximum	125	119	336	346
Minimun	49	44	58	48
Mean	84	89	113	128
Standard Deviation	20	18	57	73

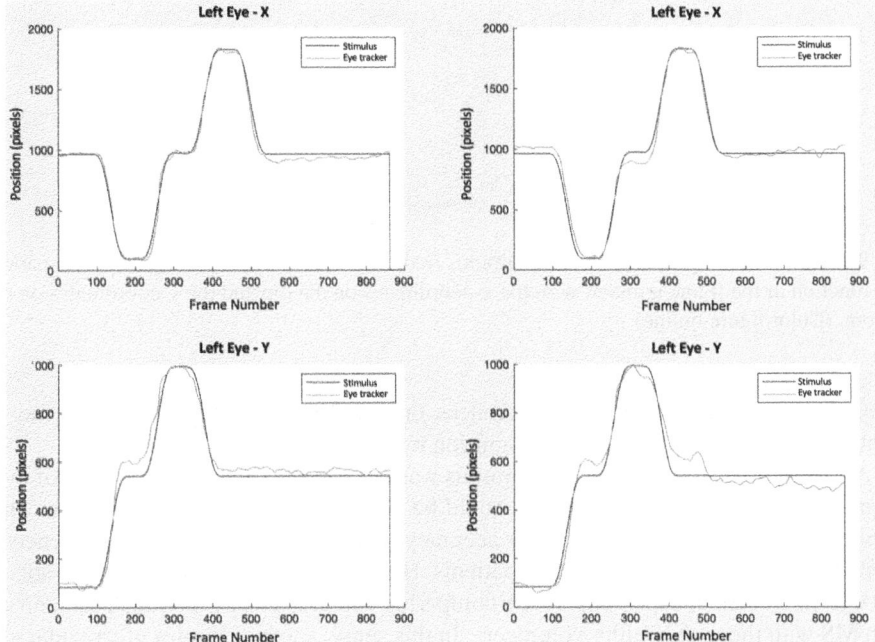

Fig. 8. Graphs of the coordinates of the first stimulus (red) and the participant's gaze (green) as a function of the frame number. On the left side, the x positions (top) and y positions (bottom) are presented for the left eye, and on the right side, the x positions (top) and y positions (bottom) are presented for the right eye (Color figure online).

Euclidean distances between the gaze and the stimulus positions were 59 ± 26 pixels for the right eye and 44 ± 27 pixels for the left eye.

As evident from the observation, the green line is noisier than the red one, which represents the theoretical values. Additionally, the estimation of the y-coordinate (vertical movement) of the eye position appears less accurate than the x-coordinate (horizontal movement). This phenomenon was expected and observed across all three videos, as previously demonstrated in Fonseca et al. (2022). This discrepancy might be attributed

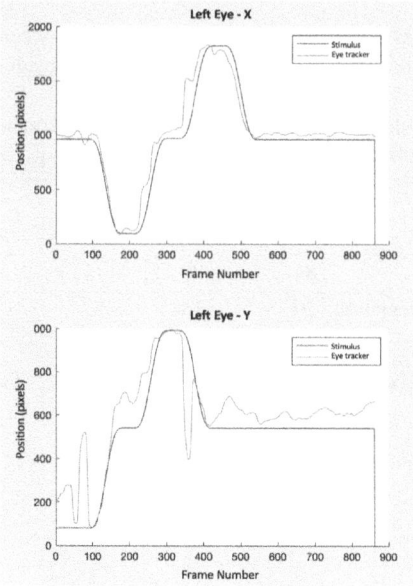

Fig. 9. Coordinates in pixels of the first stimulus (red) and the left eye's gaze (green) of a patient as a function of the frame number, with the x-coordinates on the top and the y-coordinates on the bottom. (Color figure online)

to eye morphology, particularly differences in eyelid opening during vertical movements, which can complicate iris recognition by the eye tracking system.

As mentioned above, the initial stimulus was intended to assess the presence of nystagmus, but no definitive conclusions could be drawn about this visual alteration. This ambiguity might be attributed to a low accuracy of the eye tracker or a low incidence or intensity of nystagmus in the studied patients. However, it was possible to detect abnormal eye movements, especially when comparing the graphs of individuals diagnosed with MS with those of healthy volunteers. In this sense, some examples of irregular eye movements are illustrated.

Figure 9 shows the left eye movements of one of the patients while visualizing the first stimulus. This patient is a 28-year-old female diagnosed with Relapsing-remitting Multiple Sclerosis and executive alterations. The mean Euclidean distances between the stimulus and the gaze positions were 134 ± 113 pixels for the left eye and 159 ± 96 pixels for the right eye.

Although the mean Euclidean distances were higher than the established threshold, as this patient had no diagnosed visual alterations, it was expected that they did not experience difficulties during the execution of the experimental protocol. However, when analyzing these graphs and the respective recording, it is clear that the patient did not follow the stimulus's continuous movement. This is particularly evident in the interval between frames 200 and 450 of the x-coordinates graph, where the green line is very irregular and does not match the linearity of the red line. These abrupt movements may indicate the presence of saccadic intrusions.

Figure 10 corresponds to the right eye movements of another patient, a 49-year-old female diagnosed with Relapsing-Remitting Multiple Sclerosis with an unknown presence of executive alterations, while visualizing the first stimulus. The mean Euclidean distances between the stimulus and the gaze positions were 98 ± 71 pixels for the right eye and 121 ± 58 pixels for the left eye.

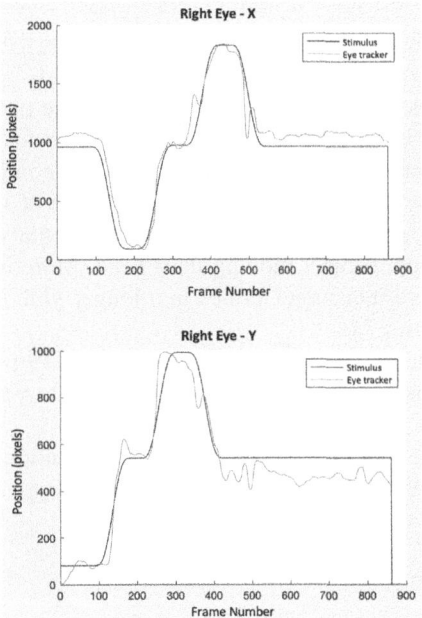

Fig. 10. Coordinates in pixels of the first stimulus (red) and the right eye's gaze (green) of a patient as a function of the frame number, with the x-coordinates on the top and the y-coordinates on the bottom. (Color figure online)

As we can observe, these graphs are very different from the ones obtained for the healthy individual (Fig. 8). Similarly to the previous patient, there are some peaks that indicate that the stimulus tracking was not continuous, mainly visible between frames 300 and 550 in the x coordinates graph. Additionally, we can see that the slope of the green line was higher than the slope of the red line, especially visible between frames 100 and 200 and 250 and 300 in the y coordinates graph, which indicate that the patient anticipated the stimulus movement, not being able to accompany its slow dislocation.

It is also important to mention that the mean Euclidean distances between the gaze and the stimulus positions for this case were below the defined threshold, even though there are evident visual alterations demonstrated by the graphs generated by the eye tracking system.

3.2 Second Stimulus

Table 2 summarizes the results obtained for both groups regarding the visualization of the second stimulus. As it was expected, the obtained values are greater for the second

Table 2. Descriptive statistics of the mean Euclidean distance between the stimulus and the gaze positions (in pixels) for the second stimulus and for both groups, considering both eyes.

Mean Euclidean distances (pixels)	Control Group		Experimental Group	
	Right Eye	Left Eye	Right Eye	Left Eye
Maximum	137	149	367	457
Minimun	53	61	81	72
Mean	109	116	159	171
Standard Deviation	23	27	68	90

video within both groups. This result may be related to the participants' performance, as well as to the eye tracking system. A longer video demands a longer attention span and can lead to visual fatigue, therefore resulting in a more imprecise tracking. On the other hand, a longer time interval implies a higher chance of situations where the eye is not correctly detected, namely due to blinking or momentary changes in brightness, and a higher chance of the subject moving their head. Moreover, an initial imprecise calibration results in more inaccurate values in a longer video, thus leading to higher mean Euclidean distances.

The maximum mean Euclidean distance calculated was 149 pixels. In this sense, and following the above mentioned methodology, the threshold was defined at 150 pixels for the second video.

Figure 11 depicts the graphs representing the visualization of the second stimulus by one of the participants of the normative base. Accordingly, the red line represents

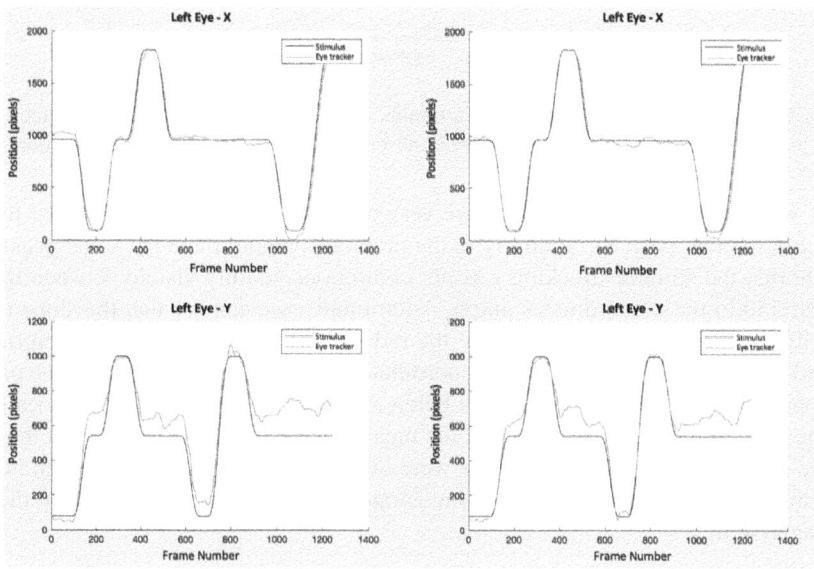

Fig. 11. Graphs of the coordinates of the second stimulus (red) and the participant's gaze (green) as a function of the frame number. On the left side, the x positions (top) and y positions (bottom) are presented for the left eye, and on the right side, the x positions (top) and y positions (bottom) are presented for the right eye. (Color figure online)

the screen position of the stimulus, and the green line represents the screen position of the gaze for each eye. The mean Euclidean distances between the gaze and the stimulus positions were 72 ± 54 pixels for the right eye and 104 ± 54 pixels for the left eye.

By observation, we can conclude that the participant was able to continuously follow the stimulus, as there are no evident delays or anticipations. However, the y coordinate estimation is considerably less accurate.

Below are some examples of graphs obtained for MS patients included in the experimental group that demonstrated visual alterations when following the stimulus in the second video.

Figure 12 corresponds to one patient, a 24-year-old female diagnosed with Relapsing-remitting Multiple Sclerosis and confirmed executive alterations. The mean Euclidean distances calculated were 121 ± 121 pixels for the right eye and 143 ± 135 pixels for the left eye.

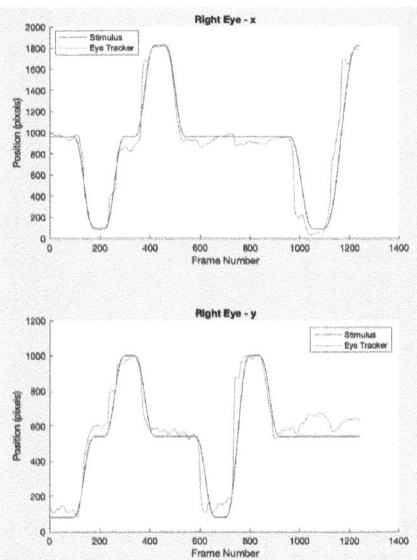

Fig. 12. Coordinates in pixels of the second stimulus (red) and the right eye's gaze (green) of a patient as a function of the frame number, with the x-coordinates on the top and the y-coordinates on the bottom. (Color figure online)

When comparing these graphs with those obtained from the healthy volunteer in the normative base (Fig. 11), it is evident that this patient had difficulties in following the continuous movement of the stimulus. The "jumps" observed in the green line, particularly around frames 240, 275, and 1005 (mainly visible in the x-coordinate graph), may indicate the presence of saccadic intrusions, similar to the example observed in the previous section. Additionally, the y-coordinate graph shows a greater slope of the green line compared to the red one, suggesting that the patient anticipated the stimulus, unable to wait for its movement. This phenomenon may be attributed to executive alterations, which can affect the ability of an individual to strictly follow the experimental protocol.

Figure 13 shows the left eye movements of another patient while visualizing the second stimulus. This patient is a 36-year-old female diagnosed with Relapsing-Remitting Multiple Sclerosis with an unknown presence of executive alterations. The mean Euclidean distances between the stimulus and the gaze positions were 93 ± 75 pixels for the right eye and 95 ± 79 pixels for the left eye.

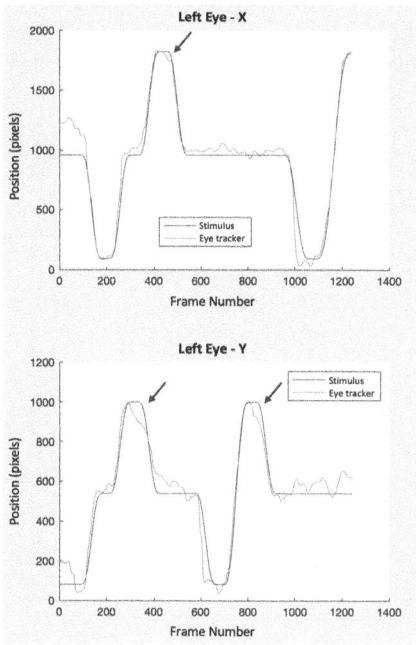

Fig. 13. Coordinates in pixels of the second stimulus (red) and the left eye's gaze (green) of a patient as a function of the frame number, with the x-coordinates on the top and the y-coordinates on the bottom. (Color figure online)

This case is particularly relevant as the graphs generated by the eye tracking system revealed abnormal movements that were almost imperceptible to the human eye. After analyzing the recording of this patient visualizing the second video, some minimal abnormal movements were observed. However, with the eye tracking system analysis, we were able to quantify and objectively observe these uncommon alterations. These movements are marked with arrows in Fig. 13, where the green line, after reaching its maximum value, decreases in amplitude.

Through the analysis of these graphs, it can be assumed that this specific patient experiences greater difficulty in maintaining gaze in the signaled extreme positions. This information is crucial for designing an individualized rehabilitation plan tailored to this patient's needs.

Regarding the metric used to identify difficulties in following the stimulus, both patients referred in this section showed values of mean Euclidean distances between the gaze and the stimulus positions below the defined threshold. However, it was possible to identify visual alteration in both cases, which indicates that the metric in question may not be suitable for the intended analysis. In this sense, it is always beneficial to analyze the graphs obtained through the eye tracking system.

3.3 Third Stimulus

In the previous study conducted by Fonseca et al. (2022), where the RehabVisual platform was applied to post-stroke patients, this video was used. Two participants experienced a notable difficulty in locating the stimulus once it reappeared on the screen, particularly in the affected area of the visual field. This phenomenon was associated with the presence of neglect (neurological disorder associated with loss of awareness of one side of the visual field due to brain damage) as a symptom in this type of patients, being a consequence that frequently follows a Stroke, and was captured by the eye tracking system, which demonstrated relevant results because it could have been easily overlooked by the patient and by the physician.

In MS, the visual field may be affected due to the inflammation of the optic nerve. However, at the time of the acquisition, none of the patients was in this situation, so none of them exhibited a loss of the visual field, and therefore, no new results were expected in comparison to the outcomes obtained with the two previous stimuli. This hypothesis was corroborated, as the patients did not encounter difficulties that had not already been identified with the initial videos, nor did they experience difficulties in locating the stimulus during intermittent movement.

Figure 14 represents the visualization of the third stimulus by one healthy volunteer.

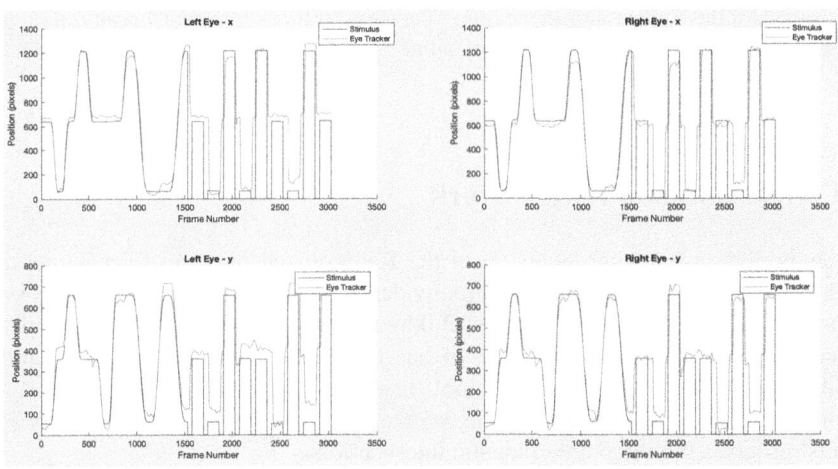

Fig. 14. Graphs of the coordinates of the third stimulus (red) and the participant's gaze (green) as a function of the frame number. On the left side, the x positions (top) and y positions (bottom) are presented for the left eye, and on the right side, the x positions (top) and y positions (bottom) are presented for the right eye. (Color figure online)

Figure 15 presents the graphs obtained through the eye tracker for one patient who exhibited visuomotor alterations at the first two stimuli.

By observation, it is clear that this patient exhibits visual alterations during the first part of the video, where the stimulus follows a continuous movement. However, this result was already observed during the first video . In this sense, and in accordance with the above mentioned, the third stimulus did not provide us with new information about the disabilities present in the studied population of. MS patients, as none of the individuals of the experimental group showed difficulties in locating the stimulus during the intermittent movement.

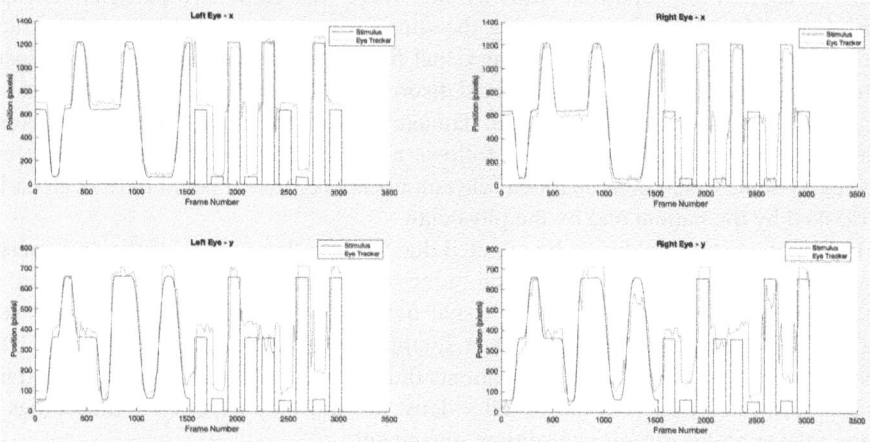

Fig. 15. Graphs of the coordinates of the third stimulus (red) and the gaze of a patient (green) as a function of the frame number. On the left side, the x positions (top) and y positions (bottom) are presented for the left eye, and on the right side, the x positions (top) and y positions (bottom) are presented for the right eye. (Color figure online)

4   Conclusions and Future Work

This study demonstrates the potential of the RehabVisual platform for patients diagnosed with Multiple Sclerosis (MS). Initially developed to assist healthcare professionals in the visuomotor rehabilitation of children with developmental delays and later applied to post-stroke patients, this tool has been adapted to include MS patients. In addition to serving as an auxiliary tool for diagnosing visuomotor impairments, it aims to aid in rehabilitation by providing standardized yet individualized monitoring of patients' progress throughout therapeutic interventions.

The main objective of the present work was to continue the analysis of the application of RehabVisual on individuals with Multiple Sclerosis, previously started in another study [7].

The integrated eye tracking system generates four distinct graphs: one for each eye and for each direction (vertical and horizontal), representing the overlay of the stimulus positions with the gaze's direction of each eye (both in pixels) as a function of the video frame number. Additionally, the mean Euclidean distance between the participant's gaze and the stimulus positions was automatically calculated. This metric, validated in a previous study [5], was considered in the current paper. However, the results showed that the mean Euclidean distance may be a limitation, as it did not serve as an indicator of difficulties in following the stimulus as expected. To address this obstacle, the graphs generated by the eye tracking system were also analyzed to assess the presence of abnormal eye movements.

The inclusion of individuals with diagnosed executive alterations in the experimental group complicated the analysis of the results. These alterations may affect the capability of strictly following the experimental protocol, such as maintaining the head immobile throughout the visualization of the three videos, which undoubtedly affects the generated graphs.

Regarding limitations, it is also relevant to mention that the analysis of the recordings by the eye tracking system is a very time-consuming process. This fact was considered when analyzing the recordings of the patients visualizing the third video, as the computational time needed to process the videos was greater than 20 min. Therefore, it is important to improve the performance of the eye tracking system, not only to decrease the computational time but also to enhance the accuracy of the coordinates estimation of the gaze.

In summary, the results obtained confirmed the presence of visual alterations in several individuals, mainly through a qualitative analysis of the graphs obtained through the eye tracking system. This objective identification of individualized difficulties allows systematic and standardized monitoring of patients and facilitates the design of tailored rehabilitation plans. Thus, the application of the RehabVisual platform on patients with Multiple Sclerosis has demonstrated high potential, both in monitoring and therapeutic intervention.

Acknowledgments. This research was supported by Fundação para a Ciência e a Tecnologia through research grants UIDB/FIS/04559/2020 and UIDP/FIS/04559/2020 (LIBPhys).

Disclosure of Interests. The authors have no competing interests to declare that are relevant to the content of this article.

References

1. New prevalence and incidence data now available in the atlas of MS - MS international federation. https://www.msif.org/news/2023/08/21/new-prevalence-and-incidence-data-now-available-in-the-atlas-of-ms/
2. Costello, F.: Vision disturbances in multiple sclerosis. Seminars Neurol. **36**, 185–195 (2016). https://doi.org/10.1055/S-0036-1579692/ID/JR0072-19/BIB
3. Dias, P.: Actualização e validação da plataforma RehabVisual: Ferramenta para estimulação das competências visuomotoras. Master's thesis, NOVA School of Science and Technology (2019)

4. Ferreira, A., et al.: Rehabvisual: application on subjects with stroke. IFIP Adv. Inf. Commun. Technol. **577**, 355–365 (2020). https://doi.org/10.1007/978-3-030-45124-0_34/COVER

5. Fonseca, P.: Validação da plataforma RehabVisual: Ferramenta para estimulação das competências visuomotoras - Aplicação a doentes com AVC. Master's thesis, NOVA School of Science and Technology (2022)

6. Frohman, T.C., et al.: Accuracy of clinical detection of INO in MS: corroboration with quantitative infrared oculography. Neurology **61**, 848–850 (2003). https://doi.org/10.1212/01.WNL.0000085863.54218.72

7. Henriques., M., Mendes., M., Martins., A., Quintão., C., Quaresma., C.: Rehabvisual: adapting and testing the visuomotor skills stimulation platform on patients with multiple sclerosis. In: Proceedings of the 17th International Joint Conference on Biomedical Engineering Systems and Technologies - BIODEVICES, pp. 164–171. INSTICC, SciTePress (2024). https://doi.org/10.5220/0012463700003657

8. Machado., R., Ferreira., A., Quintão., C., Quaresma., C.: Rehabvisual: Development of an application to stimulate visuomotor skills. In: Proceedings of the 11th International Joint Conference on Biomedical Engineering Systems and Technologies (BIOSTEC 2018) - BIODEVICES, pp. 173–178. INSTICC, SciTePress (2018). https://doi.org/10.5220/0006597001730178

9. Monteiro, M.: Adaptação da plataforma RehabVisual: ferramenta para estimulação das competências visuomotoras para a população adulta. Master's thesis, NOVA School of Science and Technology (2022)

10. Sheehy, C.K., Beaudry-Richard, A., Bensinger, E., Theis, J., Green, A.J.: Methods to assess ocular motor dysfunction in multiple sclerosis. J. Neuro-Ophthalmol. **38**, 488–493 (2018). https://doi.org/10.1097/WNO.0000000000000734

11. Thompson, A.J., Baranzini, S.E., Geurts, J., Hemmer, B., Ciccarelli, O.: Multiple sclerosis. The Lancet **391**, 1622–1636 (2018). https://doi.org/10.1016/S0140-6736(18)30481-1

Design and Numerical Optimization of a Lab-on-a-Chip Device for Blood Cells' Analysis

Ahmed Fadlelmoula[1], Vítor Carvalho[2,3]([envelope]), Graça Minas[1,4], and Susana O. Catarino[1,4]

[1] Center for MicroElectromechanical Systems (CMEMS-UMinho), University of Minho, 4800-058 Guimaraes, Portugal
[2] 2Ai, School of Technology, IPCA, 4750-810 Barcelos, Portugal
vcarvalho@ipca.pt
[3] Algoritmi Research Center, University of Minho, 4800-058 Guimaraes, Portugal
[4] LABBELS–Associate Laboratory, University of Minho, 4800-058 Guimaraes, Portugal

Abstract. The blood circulation carries valuable information about the human body's functioning. Thus, there is a continuous need for novel, accurate, and fast techniques to analyse blood samples. The objective of this research is to design, numerically simulate and optimize a low-cost microfluidic lab-on-a-chip device, which, in the future, can be used to quickly help the diagnosis of different diseases, by using a single drop of blood from a patient. The designed microdevice includes two fluid inlets, an outlet, a serpentine area for achieving a fully developed continuous flow, as well as a detection chamber able for optical measurements. The numerical model of the designed microdevice was computed in COMSOL Multiphysics, taking into account the flow and tracing of microparticles that mimic blood cells. In order to reach the optimal lab-on-a-chip geometry, i.e., achieving a high and stable number of particles in the detection chamber during the entire microfluidic assay, the inlet velocities, the channel width, and the diameter of the detection chamber were individually optimized. A mesh study was also performed to improve the accuracy of the results, aiming the lowest computational effort. From the obtained results, it was observed that a lab-on-a-chip geometry with a 1 mm channel width and a 3 mm detection chamber radius, with fluid inlet velocities, for both particles and buffer fluid, of 1 mm/s, was the one with the most interesting results for the intended application, with a relatively constant number of particles flowing through the detection chamber (more than 2000 particles, on average, for the selected inlet conditions).

Keywords: COMSOL Multiphysics · Lab-on-a-Chip · Microfluidics · Numerical simulation · Particle tracing

1 Introduction

Blood presents valuable data about the functioning of the whole body. Every minute, the entire blood volume circulates throughout the body, delivering oxygen and nutrients to the cells and transporting products and analytes from and toward all different tissues.

M. P. Guarino et al. (Eds.): BIOSTEC 2024, CCIS 2546, pp. 63–80, 2026.
https://doi.org/10.1007/978-3-031-96899-0_5

As a result, blood harbors a massive amount of physiological information about the functioning of all tissues and organs in the body [1]. Consequently, blood sampling and analysis are of prime interest for medical and science applications, holding a key role in diagnosing several physiologic and pathologic conditions, both localized and systemic. However, for clinical and scientific applications, besides blood biology, it is also necessary to understand the diagnosis technologies involved [2]. Blood diagnosis knowledge has always evolved in parallel with the general knowledge of biology, and several breakthroughs were facilitated by technological advances. Numerous devices and techniques have been reported and used to analyze blood cells with good sensitivity, detecting the presence and alterations in the platelets, and white and red blood cells [3]. Microfluidics has demonstrated an enormous potential in filling the continuous need for fast and precise techniques for blood analysis. However, designing a customized microfluidic platform, and gaining a better understanding of its operation and the underlying physics and mechanics still pose significant technical challenges, including flow control, achieving flow development, and avoiding microchannel clogging, among others. Experimental approaches, although expensive and laborious, have been commonly used for the development of microfluidic devices since they are accurate and evidence-based methods [4].

Numerical approaches, on the other hand, are recognized as reliable complementary methodologies, aiming for a reduction of cost, time, and effort, while being relatively accurate [5]. So, this work aims to design, simulate, and optimize a low-cost polymeric lab-on-a-chip (LOC) device, which can be used to quickly evaluate and analyze blood cells using optical methods (for instance, through spectrophotometry or Fourier-transform infrared spectroscopy). This article presents the numerical modeling and the simulation study of an optimized microchannel geometry for the intended application. Therefore, it simulates the flow of a fluid (representing plasma) filled with microparticles, mimicking flowing blood cells. A complementary buffer fluid (mimicking dextran or phosphate buffered saline, commonly used in experimental assays) also circulates in the microchannel, helping to control the fluid velocity and avoiding clogging or cells' deposition in the substrate. The microdevice will comprise a serpentine region, for a longer transit time, achieving a fully developed flow [6] and a circular detection chamber, where the optical measurements will occur. In this region, the number of particles/cells (mimicking different hematocrit values) should be as high and steady as possible during the entire duration of the assays.

In a previous study [7], the authors proposed the basis geometry for the LOC device to be developed and performed a preliminary numerical analysis. Herein, following those initial results, the authors significantly improved the computational numerical method and compared how the microchannel fills with cells/particles, over time, for different dimensions of the channel and for different flow conditions, and when different concentrations of cells (mimicking different hematocrit values) are introduced in the microfluidic inlet.

This paper is organized into 4 sections: Sect. 2 presents the numerical methods; Sect. 3 presents the obtained results and discussion; and, Sect. 4 presents the main conclusions of this work, as well as suggestions for further developments.

2 Implementation of the Numerical Methods

This section describes the implementation of the finite element numerical methods in COMSOL Multiphysics, aiming at the simulation of the designed microdevice.

2.1 2D Geometry Model

Figure 1 shows the initially proposed lab-on-a-chip geometry and dimensions, which will be optimized, according to the computational results that will be presented and discussed in Sect. 3.

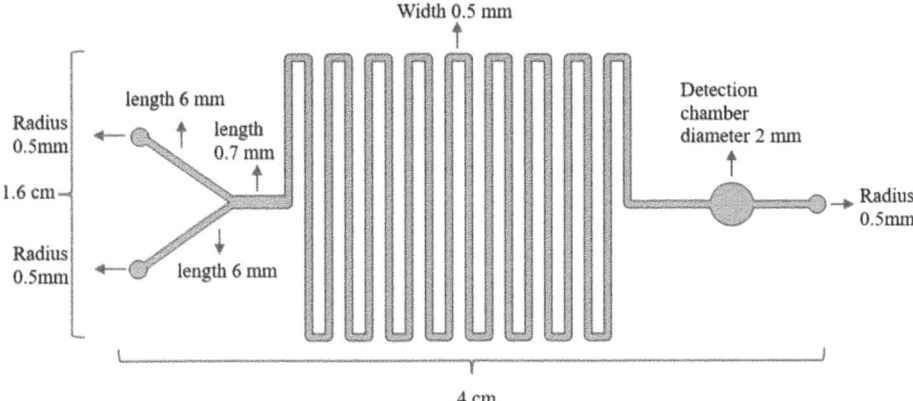

Fig. 1. Schematics of the lab-on-a-chip initial design, before optimization. Reprinted from [7], ScitePress, under a Creative Commons Attribution (CC BY-NC-ND 4.0) license.

Overall, and as observed in Fig. 1, the total chip length is 4 cm, the height is 1.6 cm, and there are 2 inlets and one outlet, all of them with a 0.5 mm radius (so, when fabricated, tube connectors can fit properly in the experimental assays). The serpentine includes 9 turns; each turn width is 0.5 mm, while, in this first version, the circular detection chamber has a 2 mm diameter. Relatively to the domains' materials and properties, the microchannel walls are constituted by polydimethylsiloxane (PDMS) while, in the interior of the device, water will be flowing at room temperature (1000 kg/m^3 density and 0.001 Pa·s viscosity) [8].

2.2 Governing Equations

The COMSOL Multiphysics Laminar Flow interface was used to compute the velocity and pressure fields for the flow of a single-phase fluid in the laminar flow regime. Equations (1) and (2) present the fluid flow governing equations:

$$P\left(\frac{\delta u}{\delta t} + \nabla uu\right) = -\nabla p + \nabla.\tau \qquad (1)$$

$$\tau = \eta(\nabla u + \nabla u\mathrm{T}) = 2\eta D \tag{2}$$

where ∇ represents the gradient operator, u is the velocity vector, t is the time, p is the pressure, τ represents the Newtonian extra stress tensor, η is the dynamic viscosity and D is the symmetric rate of strain tensor.

Besides the laminar flow, particle tracing for the fluid flow was used as a numerical method for computing the paths and migration of individual particles by solving their equations of motion over time. The particle traceability is examined under different conditions, to reach the maximum number of particles that will pass through the detection chamber. Equation (3) presents the particle tracing governing equation:

$$Ft = d(mpv)dt \tag{3}$$

where Ft, mp, and v are, respectively, the total force, the particle mass, and the particle velocity. Particles moving through a fluid are subjected to a force, known as drag force, which acts in the direction of the fluid's motion relative to the object. Equation (4) presents the Stokes' law equation, which allows the determination of the drag force (FD).

$$FD = 6\pi.\mu.rp.us \tag{4}$$

where rp is the radius of the particle and us is the velocity of the fluid relative to the sphere, also called slip velocity.

2.3 Boundary and Initial Conditions

To implement the numerical model, the following boundary and initial conditions were considered:

Laminar Flow: The default boundary condition in laminar flow is a non-slip wall ($u = 0$), which means viscous effects at the wall are negligible and the fluid velocity at the wall is zero. Two different inlets were considered in the microchannel (Inlet 1, for the fluid with particles, and Inlet 2, for the complementary buffer fluid). Both are independently described by fluid velocities, that range from 1 to 8 mm/s. At the outlet, a zero-pressure boundary is set to ensure the outflow. Regarding the numerical initial conditions, both initial velocity and pressure were set to zero.

Particle Tracing for Fluid Flow: The default wall boundary condition in particle tracing was assumed as a slipping particle wall, which means particles reflect from the wall, such that the particle momentum is conserved. Regarding the inlet of particles, these were released on both inlets, since the beginning of the assay (time = 0 s), and also at time steps of 0.1 s, for a total duration of 15 s.

At each 0.1 s release, 50 or 200 particles entered the microchannel, according to the simulations. The number of particles was selected to represent the number of blood cells in a diluted whole blood sample flowing in the channel, with two different hematocrit values. In these simulations, all the particles have a 5 μm diameter and a 1050 kg/m³ density, representing the size and density of red blood cells.

2.4 Mesh

After defining the numerical model, the geometry was meshed, aiming for its computational solution. To reach the best type of mesh, aiming for optimized results, regarding accuracy, with the lowest computational cost, a mesh study was performed. For that, simulations of the fluid flow were performed in three different regions of the microdevice, and the maximum fluid velocity was evaluated in each of those regions, as represented in Fig. 2. Velocity 1 represents the maximum velocity in the serpentine, where the fluid reaches a fully developed flow, Velocity 2 represents the maximum velocity at the entrance of the channel, immediately following the junction of the inlets, and Velocity 3 represents the maximum velocity in the detection chamber.

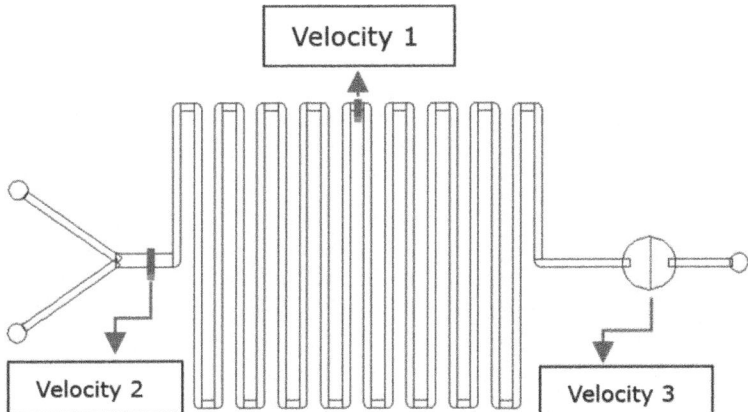

Fig. 2. Schematic of the three regions where the maximum velocity was evaluated for, during the mesh study simulations. Reprinted from [7], ScitePress, under a Creative Commons Attribution (CC BY-NC-ND 4.0) license.

After computing the model for 9 different meshes (predefined at COMSOL Multiphysics, version 5.3), with different number of elements, the maximum velocity was evaluated in each of the 3 sections. Figure 3 shows the maximum velocity, at each of the three regions (Velocity 1, Velocity 2, and Velocity 3), for all the simulated meshes elements. Reprinted from [7], ScitePress, under a Creative Commons Attribution (CC BY-NC-ND 4.0) license.

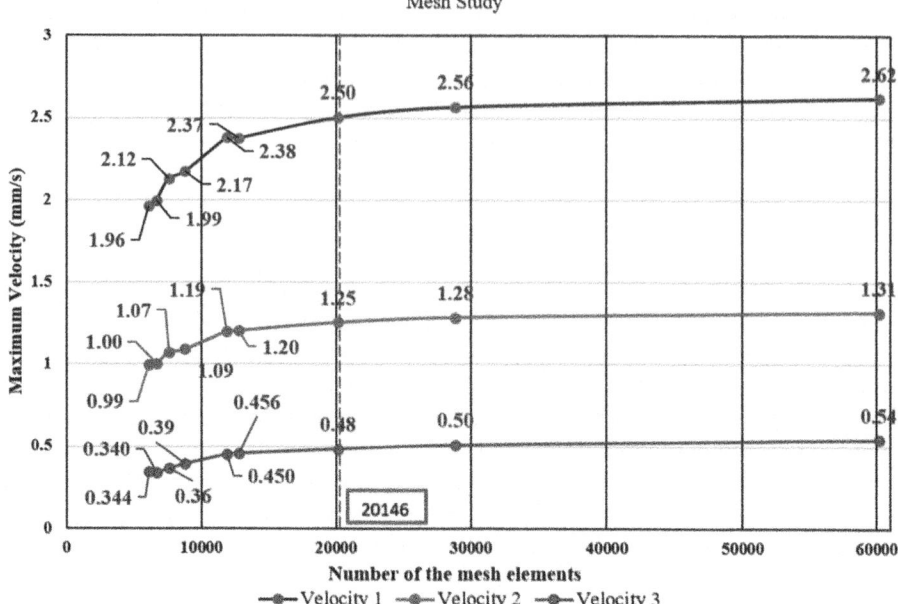

Fig. 3. Maximum velocity (mm/s) in the microchannel as a function of the number of mesh

From the presented plot, it can be observed that, above the 20146 mesh elements, even if the number of elements is increased (obviously with higher computational efforts since the number of calculus points increases significantly), there is no significant variation or improvement in the maximum velocity in any of the considered regions. As it reaches a plateau, it will be considered as the ideal mesh for this model, as the mesh results converged, allowing to achieve accurate results, without an excessive computational cost (both regarding time and memory). To correspond to the ideal number of mesh elements, a predefined "Finer" mesh was selected in COMSOL Multiphysics. This mesh, with 20146 triangular elements (9351 of them mesh vertices), achieved the best results in terms of velocity stability and computational time. This mesh has a minimum element quality of 0.5016 (0–1 scale) and an average element quality of 0.8256, and it is represented in Fig. 4. It is clear that there is a higher density of mesh elements in the serpentine curves and in the inlets and in the outlet of the channel, corresponding to the regions with maximum computational requirements.

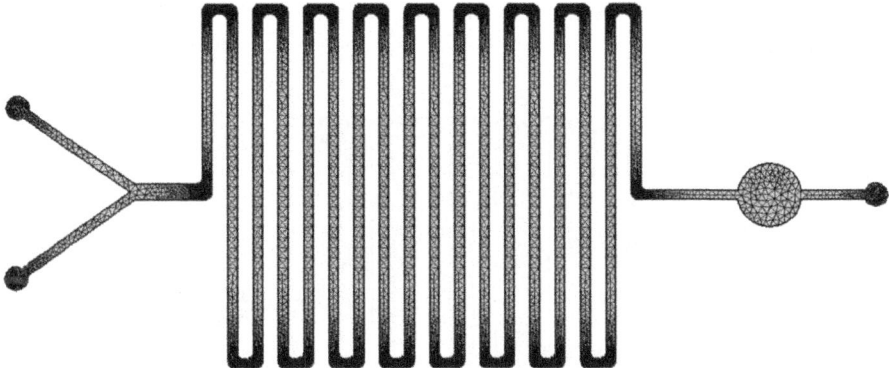

Fig. 4. Representation of the 2D mesh. Reprinted from [7], ScitePress, under a Creative Commons Attribution (CC BY-NC-ND 4.0) license.

2.5 Solver

The laminar flow, as a steady-state condition, was simulated using a stationary solver. For this simulation, a Parallel Direct Sparse Solver Interface (PARDISO) fully coupled algorithm was considered, with a 0.001 relative tolerance. The particle tracing was simulated considering a time-dependent solver, for a total duration of 120 s, with 0.1 s time steps, and 1e−5 relative tolerance. In this simulation, an iterative Jacobi preconditioned Generalized Minimal Residual Method (GMRES) algorithm was implemented.

3 Results and Discussion

The simulated results, using COMSOL Multiphysics, were achieved considering the effect of the fluid flow (velocity and pressure profile along the lab-on-a-chip) and the particle's migration in the detection chamber. For achieving a high and stable number of particles in the detection chamber during the entire microfluidic assay, the inlet velocities, the channel width, and the diameter of the detection chamber were individually optimized, outputting the best LOC geometry. The layout geometry described in Fig. 1 was used for the initial simulations, considering initially inlet velocities of 1 mm/s. Figure 5 shows the plot of the stationary fluids' velocity magnitude, which is the flow field applied to the particles, during their migration along the microdevice. Analyzing Fig. 6, which represents the velocity profile through a half-width cut of one of the simulated detection chambers, it can be concluded that the velocity in the near wall region decreases, being 0 at the wall, and being maximum at the center of the detection chamber, which is in agreement with the typical laminar flow profile.

Surface: Velocity magnitude (m/s)

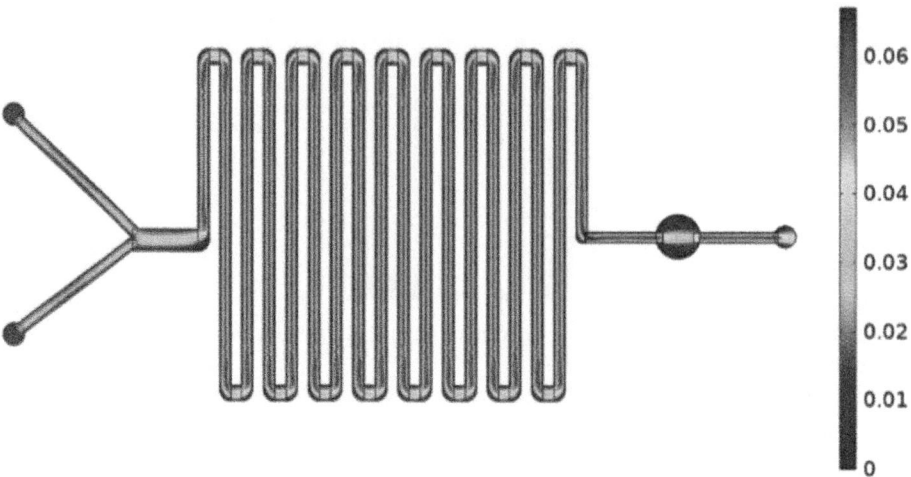

Fig. 5. Stationary velocity magnitude (mm/s) in the microdevice represented in Fig. 1. Reprinted from [7], ScitePress, under a Creative Commons Attribution (CC BY-NC-ND 4.0) license.

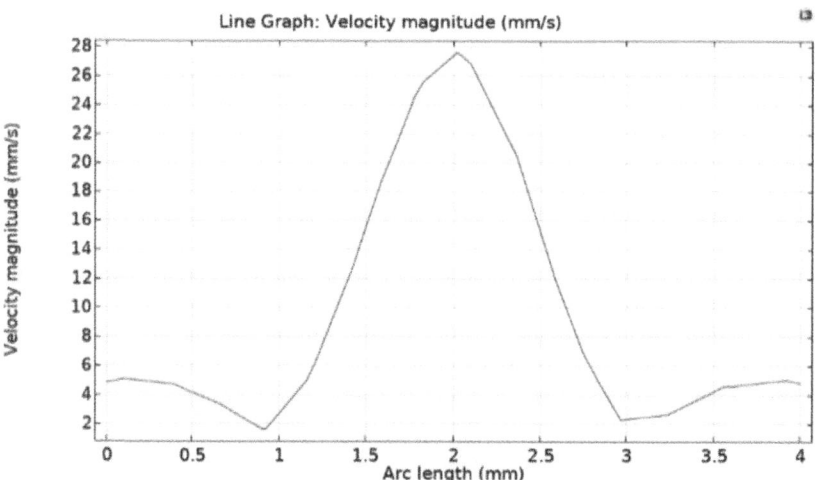

Fig. 6. Example of a cross-section plot of the stationary velocity magnitude (mm/s), at the detection chamber half-width, in the microchannel represented in Fig. 1. Reprinted from [7], ScitePress, under a Creative Commons Attribution (CC BY-NC-ND 4.0) license.

Moreover, Fig. 7 shows that the obtained pressure varies along the LOC channels from the highest at the beginning of the microdevice (around 600 Pa), decreasing gradually until the end of the microdevice, which forces the fluid to naturally exit the microchannel. Figure 8 shows an example of the particle migration inside the microdevice, at t = 25 s, where the color bar on the right-hand side represents the particles' velocity in the microdevice and, as it can be seen, the velocity profile at the center of the detection chamber, with maximum around 28 mm/s, is in complete agreement with the velocity magnitude (Fig. 5), showing that the velocity field is the biggest responsible for the dragging force that leads the particles' migration. It is also possible to observe that, as the fluid flow develops, the particles, which start by moving next to the microchannel walls, in the first serpentine's turns, slowly adjust their position and move towards the center of the microchannel, as observable in the last turns of the serpentine, where the flow is fully developed and stable. As an example, Fig. 9 shows the total number of particles passing in the detection chamber over time, considering 200 particles entering the channel, every 0.1 s. A total simulation time of 60 s was considered to present the complete variation in the number of particles, from the time needed for the first particles reach the chamber until the last ones leave the chamber to the outlet.

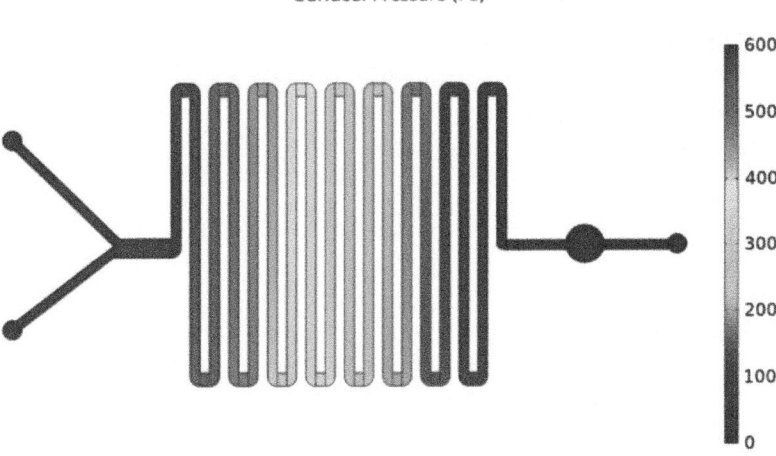

Fig. 7. Pressure distribution along the microdevice represented in Fig. 1. Reprinted from [7], ScitePress, under a Creative Commons Attribution (CC BY-NC-ND 4.0) license.

Then, following an initial characterization of the flows in the microchannel, it was performed the device optimization, regarding its dimensions and operation velocities. As the results presented above show a fully developed flow in the serpentine, with the particle migration tending to the center of the microchannel, there was no need to optimize the number of turns of the serpentine. It is important to note that, in all tables and plots presented below, the average and standard deviation values were calculated based on the number of particles in the chamber when they reached a relatively stable plateau (a 10% tolerance was considered). This means that when the chamber was filling or starting to empty (in the plot above, Fig. 9, it would be before 25 s and after 38 s), not being filled with particles anymore, those time steps were not included in the estimation of the particles' number.

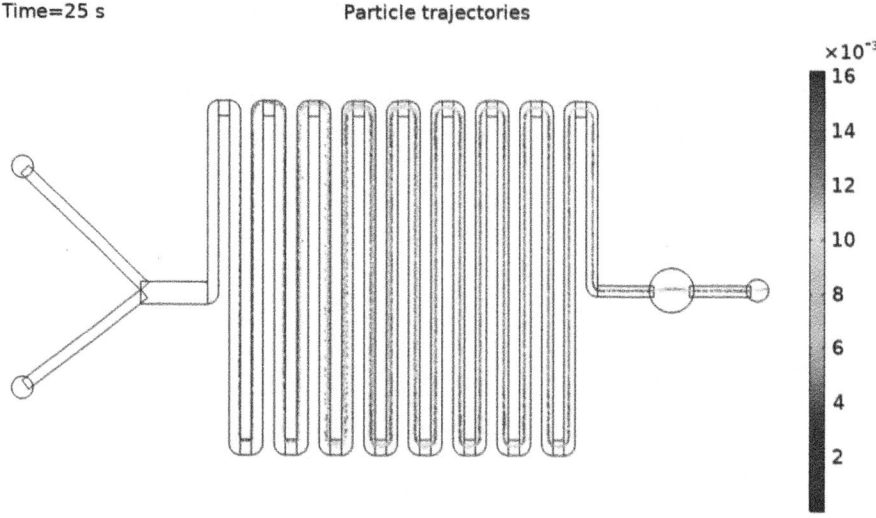

Fig. 8. Example of the particles' migration inside the microdevice, at t = 25 s. The color bar on the right-hand side represents the instantaneous particles' velocity (m/s).

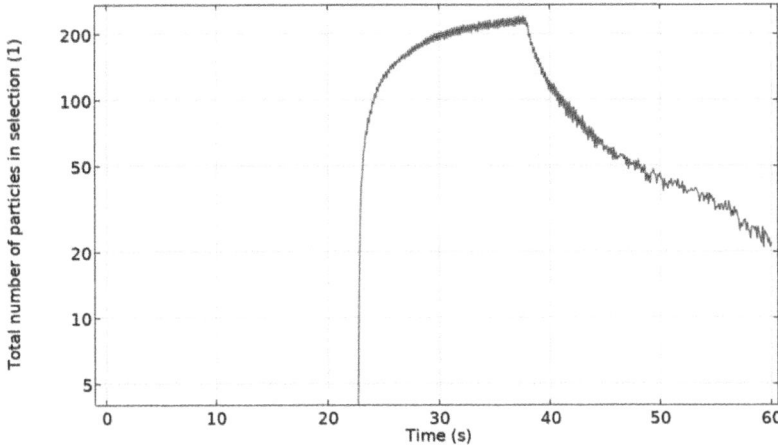

Fig. 9. Total number of particles passing in the detection chamber over time, considering 200 particles entering the channel every 0.1 s, and a total flowing time of 60 s to present the complete variation in the number of particles.

The first layout geometry optimization was performed by fixing the channel width and the detection chamber radius and changing the inlet velocity of the fluid with particles – inlet 1 (keeping the buffer velocity – inlet 2 - constant). The channels' width was kept at 0.5 mm and the detection chamber radius at 1 mm. The velocity was changed from 1 to 8 mm/s, in 1 mm/s steps. Figure 10 shows the average and the standard deviation of the number of particles that passed through the detection chamber, during the entire simulation. It is observed that the number of particles in the channel detection area is, as expected, directly proportional to the particles' concentration in the inlet (50 or 200 particles every 0.1 s). The results show that modifying the inlet velocity, from 1 to 8 mm/s, has a significant effect on the number of particles crossing the detection chamber, as increasing the velocity decreases the time the particles spend in the detection region. Thus, the 1 mm/s velocity leads to the highest number of particles simultaneously in the detection chamber (for 200 particles in the entrance, more than 180 particles at each time, with a standard deviation of less than 10), and it was selected for the next optimization steps.

A)

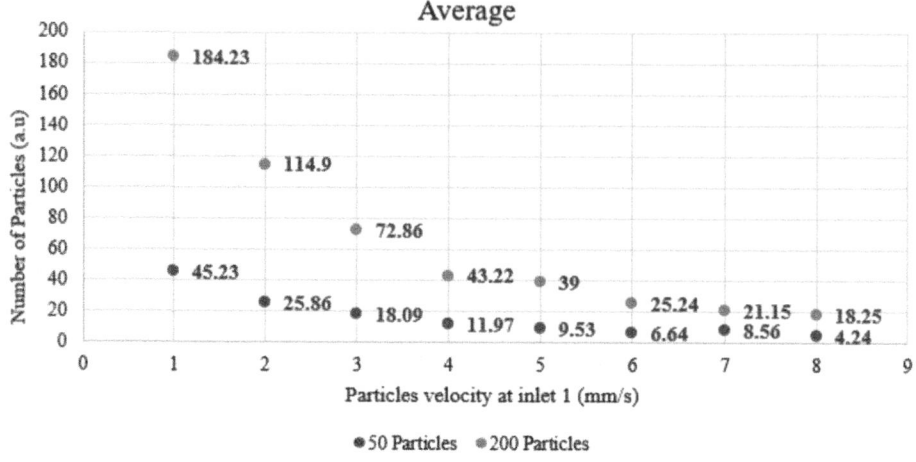

B)

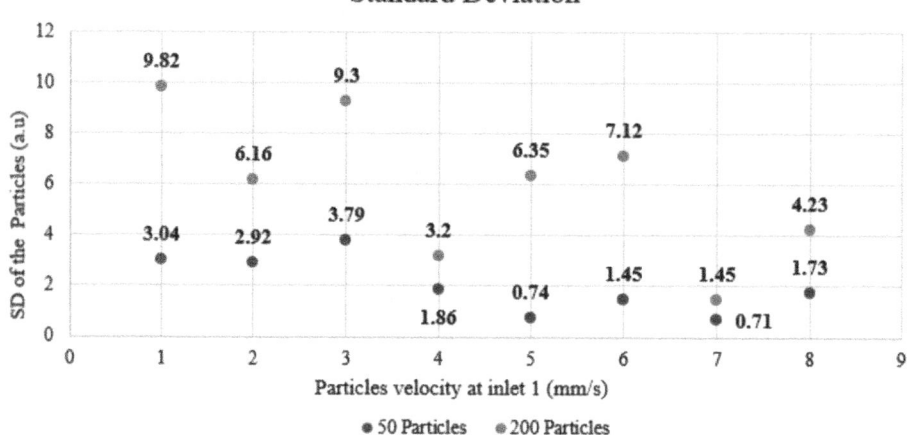

Fig. 10. Number of particles passing through the detection chamber, for different inlet 1 velocities, considering 50 and 200 particles entering the channel at each 0.1 s: A) average; B) standard deviation.

In the second optimization phase, the 0.5 mm channel width and the 1 mm/s inlet velocities were fixed, and the detection chamber radius was changed from 1 to 3 mm, in steps of 0.5 mm. Figure 11 shows the average and the standard deviation of the number of particles that passed through the detection chamber, during the duration of the simulation. The results show that increasing the radius of the detection chamber leads to a significant increase in the average number of particles in that area (up to more than 1300 particles, with a standard deviation below 60). Thus, a 3 mm radius, with a resulting average number of particles around 1323.04 (for 200 particles in the entrance), was selected for the next optimization steps.

A)

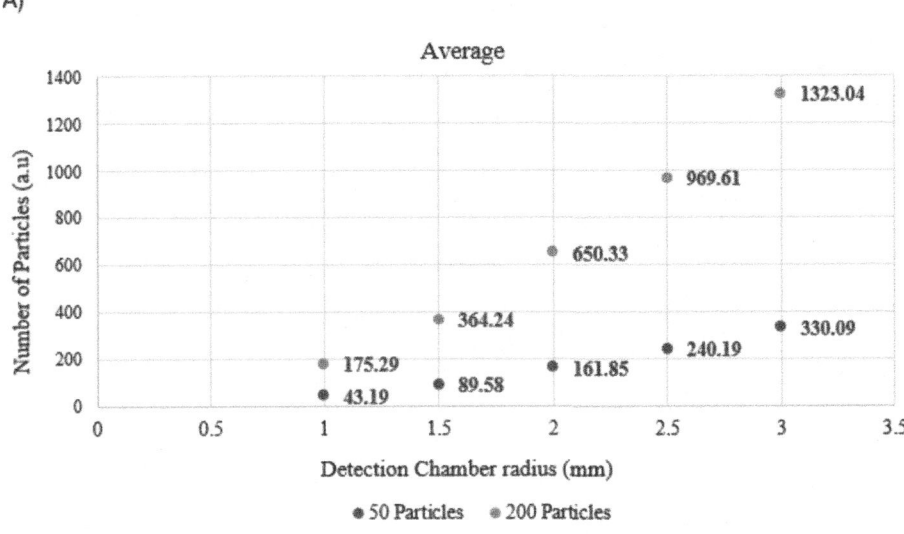

B)

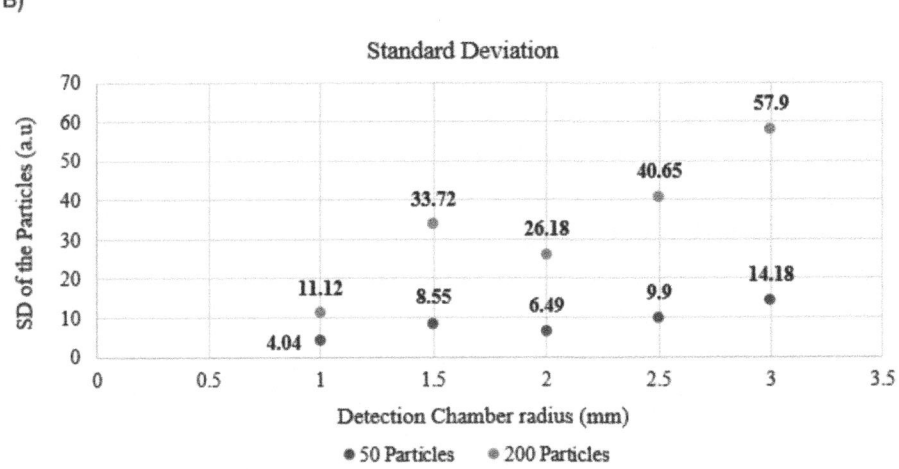

Fig. 11. Number of particles passing through the detection chamber, for different detection chamber radius, considering 50 and 200 particles entering the channel at every 0.1 s: A) average; B) standard deviation.

In the third optimization phase, the inlet velocities, of 1 mm/s, and the detection chamber radius, of 3 mm, were fixed, and the width of the channel was varied from 0.5 to 1 mm in 0.1 mm steps. Figure 12 shows the average and the standard deviation of the number of particles that passed through the detection chamber during the duration of the assay. The results show that an increase in the channel's width implies more fluid volume in the microchannel at each time, and also leads to an increase in the total number of particles in the detection chamber. From the average and the standard deviation, an adequate channel width, combining a high and stable number of particles in the chamber is 1 mm (more than 2150 particles simultaneously in the chamber, with a standard deviation of around 70).

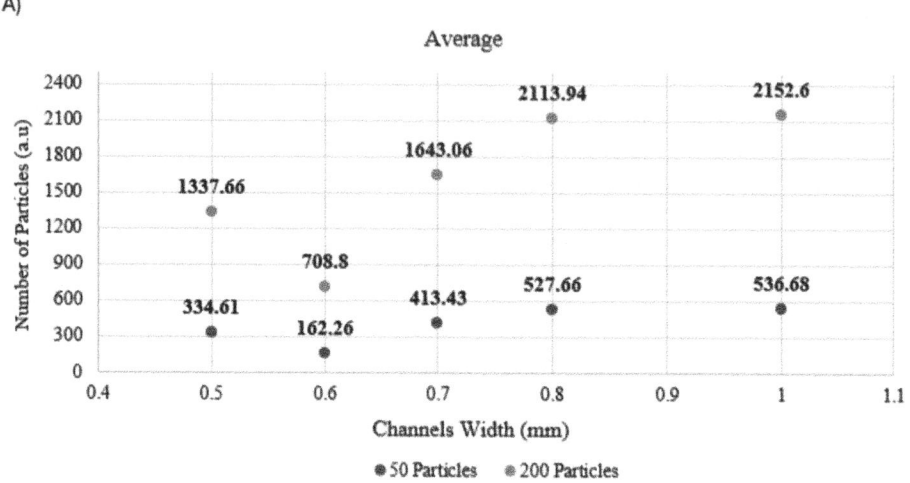

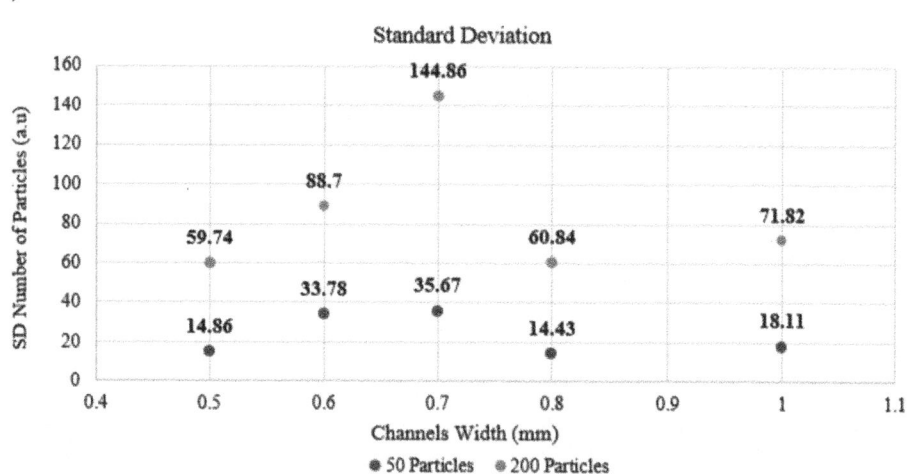

Fig. 12. Number of particles passing through the detection chamber, for different channel widths, considering 50 and 200 particles entering the channel at every 0.1 s: A) average; B) standard deviation.

Following the optimization of the dimensions, it was studied the effect of the buffer velocity in the resultant number of particles in the detection chamber. Figure 13 shows the number of particles (average and standard deviation) that passed through the detection chamber for different velocities at the inlet 2 (buffer fluid velocity), maintaining the previously optimized parameters (3 mm detection chamber radius, 1 mm channel width, and 1 mm/s inlet 1 velocity). It was observed that, for the studied geometry and inlet conditions, the inlet 2 velocity (buffer) affects the number of particles passing through the detection chamber, as higher velocities lead to a lower simultaneous number of particles in the detection chamber. It is a similar behavior to the one observed for inlet 1 velocity, as higher velocities lead to a lower time of the particles in the microchannel. Thus, the 1 mm/s velocity in inlet 2 allowed for the highest number of particles and, consequently, it was the selected velocity for the optimized version of the LOC device.

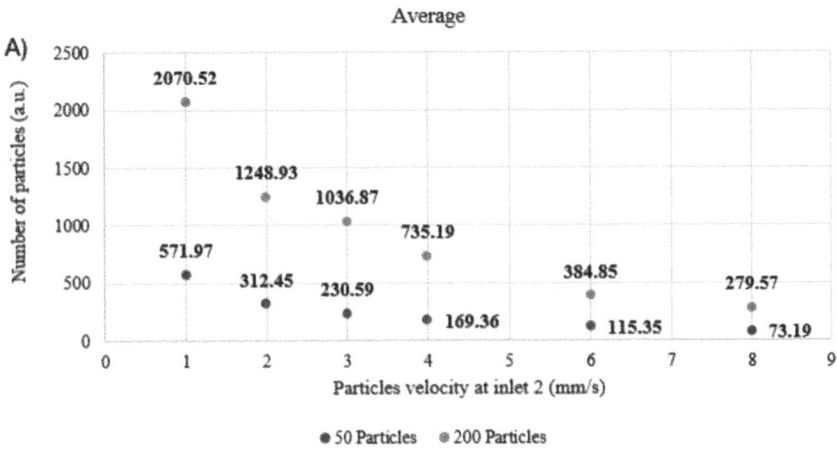

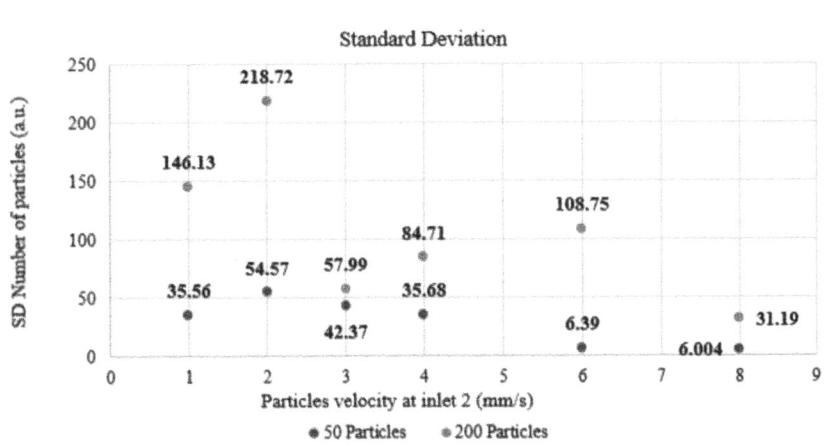

Fig. 13. Number of particles that passed through the detection chamber, for different inlet 2 velocities, considering 50 and 200 particles entering the channel at every 0.1 s: A) average; B) standard deviation.

Considering all the previously presented results, Fig. 14 presents the optimized design of the LOC device and its dimensions: 1 mm channel width, detection chamber radius of 3 mm, and inlet velocities of 1 mm/s, at both inlets 1 and 2. For those conditions, Fig. 15 shows the instantaneous number of particles simultaneously passing through the detection chamber, for the optimized parameters.

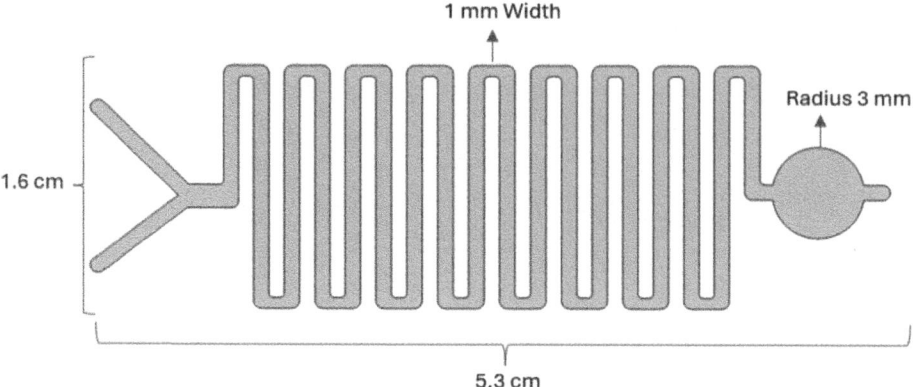

Fig. 14. Schematic representation of the optimized design of the lab-on-a-chip. The total chip length is 5.3 cm, the total width is 1.6 cm, and there are 2 inlets and an outlet, both with a 0.5 mm radius (for tube fitting after fabrication). There are 9 serpentine turns, each with a 1 mm width, and the circular detection chamber has a 3 mm radius.

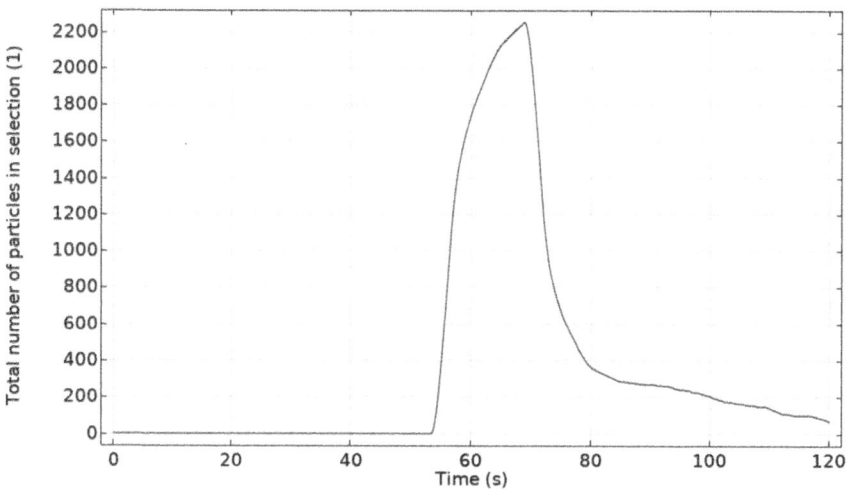

Fig. 15. Total number of particles passing in the detection chamber over time, considering 200 particles entering the channel every 0.1 s, and a total simulation time of 120 s, to present the complete variation in the number of particles, so we can observe the maximum variation within the detection chamber. In this example, the average number of particles simultaneously in the chamber, with a 10% tolerance, is 2070.52 and the standard deviation is 146.13.

It is important to notice that, after fabrication of the designed microchannels, and in experimental assays, the inlet of particles/cells in the microchannel is typically constant and controlled by a pumping system, so, instead of a short time plateau with a maximum number of cells, as observed in these computational assays, the number of cells will be stable, from the moment the first cells reach the detection chamber (and until the pumping syringe is shut down). In these simulations, that behavior was mimicked, but limited to a shorter time to assure the saving of computational resources (both time and memory consumption related).

4   Conclusion and Future Work

This work presented the design, numerical simulation and optimization of the dimensions and operating velocities of a LOC device for blood analysis. The numerical model was computed, using COMSOL Multiphysics software, taking into account the flow and microparticles (to mimic the blood cells) tracing. Regarding the flow, the pressure along the LOC reached the maximum value at the inlet and decreased gradually until reached the minimum in the outlet. The stationary velocity followed the laminar flow profile, and reached the maximum value in the serpentine channels, followed by the center of the detection chamber. It was observed that increasing the channel width and the chamber radius led to a significant increase in the total number of particles in the detection chamber. Oppositely, increasing the velocities at the inlets led to a decrease in the total number of particles at the detection region. Thus, the obtained results showed that the ideal LOC design comprises a 1 mm channel width, a detection chamber radius of 3 mm, and inlet velocities of 1 mm/s, achieving a maximum total number of more than 2000 particles flowing in the detection chamber at the same time (see Figs. 13 A and 15). Further works will consolidate the physical implementation of the simulated LOC model and their testing, examining the velocity, pressure, and particle flow inside the chip, and performing design updates if required. 3D simulations will allow to assess the effect of the microchannel thickness in velocity and particles' tracing, taking into account that this dimension, corresponding to the optical path, will be key in optical measurements (as targeted in this application). Numerical simulations will include the effect of other blood cells with different sizes (such as white blood cells and platelets), before advancing for the fabrication (through soft-lithography and replica molding) and experimental characterization of the optimized device, with samples at different hematocrit values and under different flow rates.

Acknowledgments. This work was supported by the project PTDC/EEI-EEE/2846/2021 (https:// doi.org/10.54499/PTDC/EEI-EEE/2846/2021), funded by national funds (OE), within the scope of the Scientific Research and Technological Development Projects (IC&DT) program in all scientific domains (PTDC), through the Foundation for Science and Technology, I.P. (FCT, I.P), and by the R&D Unit Project Scope: UIDB/04436/2020, UIDB/05549/2020 and UIDP/05549/2020 funded by the Foundation for Science and Technology, I.P. (FCT). This study has also been funded by a grant 2023 from the European Society of Clinical Microbiology and Infectious Diseases (Europäische Gesellschaft für klinische Mikrobiologie und Infektionskrankheiten) (ESCMID) to CATARINO. A.F. thanks the FCT for his 2023.03312.BD PhD grant. S.O.C. thanks the FCT for her 2020. 00215.CEECIND contract funding (DOI: https://doi.org/10.54499/2020.00215.CEECIND/ CP1600/CT0009). The authors declare no conflicts of interest.

References

1. Kouzehkanan, Z.M., et al.: A large dataset of white blood cells containing cell locations and types, along with segmented nuclei and cytoplasm. Sci. Rep. **12** (2022)
2. Balogh, E.P., Miller, B.T., Ball, J.R.: Improving diagnosis in health care. In Improving Diagnosis in Health Care. National Academies Press (2016). https://doi.org/10.17226/21794
3. Rohde, T., Martinez, R.: Equipment and energy usage in a large teaching hospital in Norway. J. Healthc. Eng. **6** (2015)
4. Fadlelmoula, A., Pinho, D., Carvalho, V.H., Catarino, S.O. Minas, G.: Fourier Transform Infrared (FTIR) spectroscopy to analyse human blood over the last 20 years: a review towards lab-on-a-chip devices. Micromachines **13** (2022). https://doi.org/10.3390/mi13020187
5. Nagarajan, S., Stella, L., Lawton, L.A., Irvine, J.T.S., Robertson, P.K.J.: Mixing regime simulation and cellulose particle tracing in a stacked frame photocatalytic reactor. Chem. Eng. J. **313**, 301–308 (2017)
6. Catarino, S.O. et al.: Blood cells separation and sorting techniques of passive microfluidic devices: From fabrication to applications. Micromachines **10** (2019). https://doi.org/10.3390/mi10090593
7. Fadlelmoula, A., Carvalho, V., Catarino, S., Minas, G.: Numerical Modelling and Simulation of a Lab-on-a-Chip for Blood Cells' Optical Analysis, pp. 185–190. Scitepress (2024). https://doi.org/10.5220/0012571900003657
8. Norouzi, N., Bhakta, H.C. Grover, W.H.: Sorting cells by their density. PLoS One **12** (2017)

Cardiorespiratory and Bicep Muscle Responses to Assembly Line Work Volume

Dania Furk, Luís Silva(✉), Mariana Dias, Phillip Probst, and Hugo Gamboa

Laboratório de Instrumentação, Engenharia Biomédica e Física da Radiação (LIBPhys-UNL), Departamento de Física, Faculdade de Ciências e Tecnologia, FCT, Universidade Nova de Lisboa, 2829-516 Caparica, Portugal
lmd.silva@fct.unl.pt

Abstract. Automobile assembly workers routinely engage in repetitive tasks with varying workload volumes, dictated by their specific workstation assignments. Such occupational activities, especially with inadequate recovery (return to the body's resting condition), can lead to the development of cardiovascular and musculoskeletal disorders. However, the adoption of biosignal-monitoring-based strategies to mitigate these risks remains limited. This study aims to examine the Electromyogram (EMG), Electrocardiogram (ECG), and Respiratory Inductance Plethysmography (RIP) data to comprehend the evolution of both muscular and cardiorespiratory load for different workstations. Sixteen male operators (age = 38 ± 8 years; BMI = $25 \pm 3 \, \text{kg/m}^2$) from three workstations (H_1, H_2, and H_3) with work cycle durations of 1, 3, and 5 min, respectively, volunteered for the study. The results indicated that distinct workload volumes led to unique cardiovascular patterns, identified through heart rate variability (HRV), as well as respiratory frequency, variability, and coordination over the monitored period. Significant differences were observed in the biceps' load between recording moments for H_3 and H_2, in terms of median frequency and amplitude, respectively. Simultaneous monitoring of these biosignals offers the potential for a more comprehensive and individualized risk assessment of assembly-line tasks.

Keywords: Cardiovascular · Respiratory · Muscle load · Workload · Occupational health

1 Introduction

Musculoskeletal disorders are the most common occupational-related health problem in the EU [1], and account for the largest percentage of global compensation costs for work-related diseases, followed by heart and circulatory diseases [2]. In the EU, machine operators and assemblers, work for an average of 39.7 h per week [3].

During most of that time, they are exposed to numerous occupational risk factors such as repetitive movements, awkward postures, static positioning, and forceful exertions [4]. These types of activity have been shown to have serious consequences on worker's health.

M. P. Guarino et al. (Eds.): BIOSTEC 2024, CCIS 2546, pp. 81–102, 2026.
https://doi.org/10.1007/978-3-031-96899-0_6

Low-intensity assembly line-like occupational tasks have been associated with high rates of musculoskeletal injuries [5]. Surface Electromyography (sEMG) has been an often used tool to quantify localized muscular fatigue and can be used as a biomarker for cumulative exposure to repetitive work [6].

This type of occupation has also been shown to negatively influence cardiovascular health due to insufficient recovery of the cardiac system, leading to continuous stimulation of the inflammatory response of the body, which can increase the risk for cardiac diseases or encourage their aggravation. [7].

Specifically, assembly line jobs have previously been linked with high blood pressure, [8], atherosclerosis [9], a well-known cardiovascular risk factor, increased mortality [10] and long-term sickness absence [11].

The monitoring of respiration frequency is used to assess effort in sports [12] and has shown its usefulness in the identification of cognitive load, environmental stress, and other relevant factors in occupational settings [13].

Current occupational risk quantification tools consider different body parts and key indicators of biomechanical load, where an expert fills in a predefined scoring sheet by watching workers perform their tasks. Some of the most common scoring sheets are the job strain index, OCRA (Occupational Repetitive Action), the EAWS (European Assembly Worksheet), and the revised NIOSH (National Institute for Occupational Safety and Health) equation [14]. These risk quantification tools, besides establishing work practice guidelines, do for example recommend that the demands put on workers should not surpass 30% of their aerobic capacity in an 8-hour continuous shift [15].

The incorporation of this risk information into workplace management has shown positive outcomes such as a reduction in work-related disorders, workers' compensation costs, absenteeism, and increased productivity [16, 17]. The previously mentioned tools present multiple shortcomings as they focus only on the biomechanical aspect of work not accounting for other factors such as individual differences and physiological load. Furthermore, these rely mainly on observational methods that are time consuming and do not provide sufficient resolution for smaller anatomical structures [18], while also not regarding internal adaptations to the assessed work tasks [19]. Finally, most of these tools are only employed after complaints from workers have been filed or symptoms have been reported, showing that these are also not being effective prevention measures. [20].

The use of wearables allows direct measurement of motion and activity of biosignals in real-time, providing a means of more individual-specific planning and interventions in real occupational settings [16, 21]. Former work that included sEMG analysis in similar contexts, not only focused on fatigue manifestation but also measured kinematic variables through IMU units. Monaco et al. [22] studied three workers at an automobile assembly line, while performing the same task. They found that the Erector Spinae Lumbar Region and the Multifidus muscles were highly activated, having mean values of amplitude between 10–20% MVC, something confirmed by the kinematic data, suggesting a significant load at the spine level. Bosch et al. [23] simulated assembly-line tasks with two intensities while monitoring the trapezius fatigue. Median frequency decreased for both tasks, while amplitude remained constant. The decrease in frequency progressed differently depending on the intensity of the task. The same author also investigated the influence of work-pace on workload and fatigue, but did not find significant differences between both [24].

Previous studies on real assembly lines have put their main focus on cardiovascular response rather than respiratory, when looking at overall physical load. Lundberg et al. [25] measured self-reports of work characteristics and of perceived physical load, accompanied by the evaluation of objective measures: HR (Heart Rate), blood pressure, catecholamines, and cortisol, finding that perceived stress was associated with neuroendocrine response and that during work both HR and blood pressure were significantly increased. With the aim of studying the impact of minimization of non-productive time during work activities (rationalization), to complement biomechanical exposure, Palmerud et al. [26] quantified job exposure based on HR monitoring by extracting the Reserve Heart Rate k(RHR) of the workers, where the they found that mean HR decreased. In [27], they measured mechanical exposures of car disassembly tasks to compare with what was seen in assembly studies. This mechanical exposure included cardiovascular load, which was revealed to be higher in disassembly than in assembly tasks. The modeling of ideal working time based on energy expenditure of assembly-line workers was also developed, based on moderate workload tasks [28]. The energy expenditure was computed based on HR measurements of workers, with smart watches, from three different assembly lines. They found that the most significant variables to model this time were the calories spent by the workers and the operation time.

Research has also been conducted on the effect of this kind of work on cardiorespiratory adaptations. Nardolillo et al. simulated assembly line tasks and extracted Heart Rate Variability (HRV) from HR of participants, measured with a wearable device. The participants included individuals who were either currently employed in the sector or a related field, as well as students of varying ages and genders. It was concluded that there were no significant differences in frequency domain metrics between stages of work, but there were marked differences in some of the time metrics Mean RRi (intervals between consecutive heartbeats), Standard Deviation (SD) of Normal to Normal RRi intervals, and RRi Triangular Index) between some of the trials [29].

In our previous work, Respiratory Inductance Plethysmography (RIP), ECG and EMG were monitored in simulated repetitive tasks under a fatigue-inducing protocol, where thoraco-abdominal coordination, local muscle load [30] and HRV [31] parameters were analyzed. In these studies, results showed a decrease in correlation and Phase Synchrony (PS) between the respiratory movements of the chest and abdominal walls, and an increase in the normalized amplitude for the bicep brachii from the Baseline to Fatigue trials. Also, it was found a decrease in HRV between trials.

As shown above, current research on assembly lines focuses on exploring either RHR (Relative Heart Rate) or EMG amplitude and median frequency, separately, as a measure of job exposure. The main goal was to predict or analyze the effects of interventions made on the line organization, using unimodal acquisition methods. In cases where a multimodal approach was employed, the acquisitions were carried not carried out in real work contexts (i.e., factory settings) but in simulated work environments (i.e., lab settings).

This study aimed to search for differences in muscular and cardiorespiratory load adaptation linked to specific work volumes. We monitored workers' muscle, heart and respiratory signals, EMG, ECG, and RIP, respectively, on a real assembly line during their regular work.

This work is part of the OPERATOR 4.0 project (Zenithwings, Fraunhofer AICOS, LIBPhys-UNL, Volkswagen Autoeuropa, NST Apparel Lda, FPCEUP, Controlconsul, Universidade do Minho, Institute for Medical Engineering and Science at MIT, 2020), which has the support of MIT Portugal.

The remaining sections of this document are organized as follows: in Sect. 2 the materials and methods used are described, including a brief description of the study sample, the followed data acquisition protocol, and adopted statistical analysis. In Sect. 4 the results are presented, in Sect. 5 their discussion, and in Sect. 6 the drawn conclusions and the proposed future work.

2　Materials and Methods

To characterize cardiovascular, respiratory and local muscle load responses to work volume, the corresponding biosignals of assembly line operators were monitored on the field, during real occupational activities.

2.1　Participants

Data collected from 16 subjects on the assembly workstations were analyzed (age: 38 ± 8 yrs; body mass index: 25 ± 3 kg.m^2; physical activity: 220 ± 135 min per week).

The included participants were part of three assembly process workstations, 8 from H_3, 4 from H_2, and 4 from H_1. All were right-handed male workers on automotive assembly lines, rotating between workstations.

2.2　Workstations

In this factory, the manufacturing of vehicles relies on multiple processes. This study focused only on the activities carried out in the final stage of production as they are based on manual handling: the assembly and alignment of the last parts to be mounted on the car. The tasks performed at the studied workstations are specified:

- H1: setting of tail lights and pre-fitting alignments. The mean cycle time each tasks was 3 min
- H2: alignments of side doors, rear and front end. The mean cycle time of each task was 5 min
- H3: final stages of assembly, including mounting of rearview mirror, cowl top, boot panel, and trunk symbol. The mean cycle time of each task was 1 min.

In Fig. 1 the dominant positions in which workers perform each of the activities mentioned above are shown.

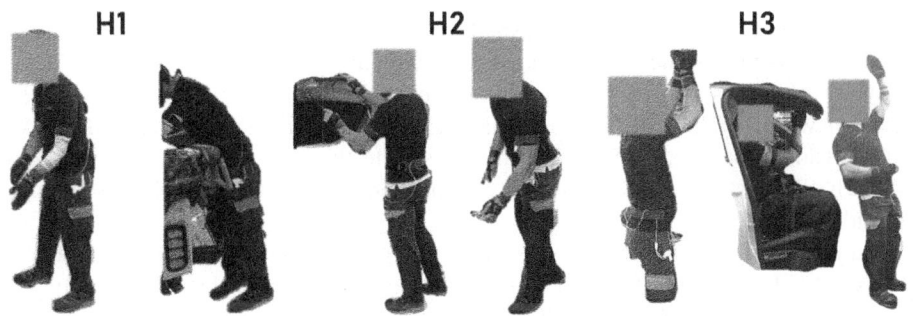

Fig. 1. Main positions in each workstation from [32].

2.3   Sensor Setup

The followed protocol comprised the measurement of ECG, RIP, EMG and ACC signals. The sensor placement started with cleaning the skin areas where electrodes were to be attached, to optimize skin-electrode conductivity. The cleaning process included hair removal, abrasion, and alcohol cleaning.

Firstly, three disposable Ag/AgCl adhesive electrodes (Ambu®), attached to each electrode cable of the ECG sensor (PLUX WIRELESS BIOSIGNALS S.A.), were placed in a configuration to minimize artifacts of arm and chest movements. On the left side of the sternum, the positive was positioned at the level of the manubrium, and the negative was put on the superior part of the sternum's body. The ground electrode was placed on the left anterior superior iliac spine.

Subsequently, the RIP signals were monitored with two inductive sensors (PLUX WIRELESS BIOSIGNALS S.A.) attached to two elastic belts: one over the chest passing below the armpit and the other band at the umbilicus level [30,33], they were adjusted to the anatomy of the participant.

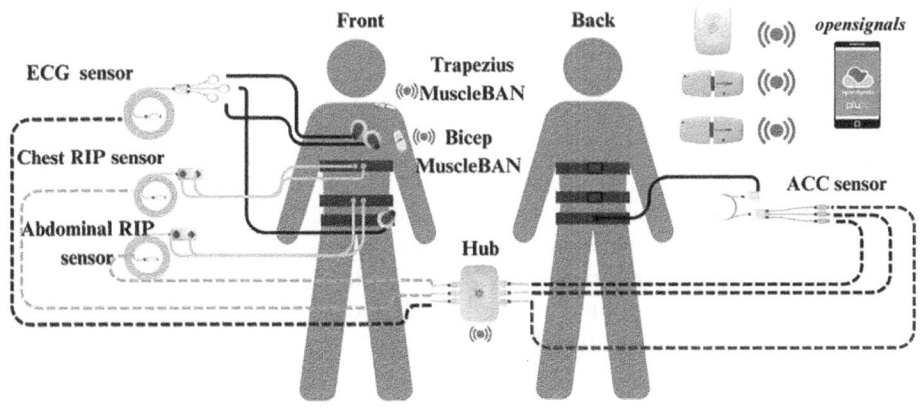

Fig. 2. Sensor setup for biosignal collection from [32].

A triaxial ACC (PLUX WIRELESS BIOSIGNALS S.A.) was also used and was placed on the center of the lower back, secured with an elastic belt.

These three sensors with an acquisition rate of 350 Hz, were all connected to the 8-channel wireless Hub, PLUX Biosignals (PLUX WIRELESS BIOSIGNALS SA), which streamed the data from each of the sensors to the *opensignals*, (PLUX WIRE-LESS BIOSIGNALS S.A.) software, to a smartphone (Xiaomi Redmi Note 9, running Android 10).

The EMG of the dominant side bicep was also captured with a MuscleBAN, (PLUX WIRELESS BIOSIGNALS S.A.) device, at a rate of 1000 Hz and transmitted to *opensignals*, (PLUX WIRELESS BIOSIGNALS S.A.). The bicep brachii was chosen to be monitored as it is the main muscle involved in the tasks (arm flexion and extension).

The ACC data from the lower back and bicep were acquired for device synchronization and signal segmentation since the tasks involve mainly repetitive arm movements.

A scheme of the sensor configuration is shown in Fig. 2.

2.4   Data Collection

All subjects read and signed the informed consent. The study was conducted in accordance with the Declaration of Helsinki, and the protocol was approved by the Ethics Committee of the University of Porto. The participants were asked personal information (age, height, physical activity habits and dominant hand). After this, their body mass was measured with a digital scale.

Next, all devices for biosignal monitoring were mounted as detailed in Sect. 2.3 and the volunteers placed the mobile phone in their uniform pockets. Before data collection, the Maximum Voluntary Contraction (MVC) test was performed for the bicep brachii. Subjects were asked to place their arms next to their trunk with the forearms positioned at a 90° angle to the upper arm, thus being both parallel to each other and the ground. They were asked to gradually exert force against the researcher's hands, which was offering resistance in the subjects' wrist region. Verbal encouragement was given to achieve maximum force from the subjects. This test was repeated 2 times. At the beginning of the data collection, volunteers were asked to perform 10 jumps for data synchronization purposes. Their activity was monitored for about 50 min of normal work. During the data collection, a video of the first 4–5 cycles of the performed task was recorded.

2.5   Data Cleaning

During the carried-out acquisitions, some data loss was experienced as in some cases issues with the wireless connection appeared. This left us with 16 subjects to analyse in terms of the cardiorespiratory sensors and 14 of those same subjects for the bicep sensors. The data collected from the trapezius suffered to much data loss, and we were not able to include it in this analysis.

2.6   Signal Processing

Electrocardiography. The preprocessing for the ECG focuses on the detection of the R-peaks, requiring the suppression of other waveforms. To achieve this, a Maximum

Overlap Discrete Wavelet Transform (MODWT) was used to filter the ECG signal, taking into account its non-stationary nature [34,35]. The optimal wavelet for each subject was determined by maximizing the signal energy to the signal Shannon entropy ratio [36], with the db2 wavelet emerging as the most effective. The ECG time series were decomposed into six wavelet levels and the signal was reconstructed using level 4 coefficients (10.94–21.88 Hz) through the inverse wavelet transform.

An R-peak detection algorithm based on the Shannon energy envelope [37] was then applied to the filtered signals. The amplitude of the signal was first normalized by the signal's maximum value, then the Shannon energy and envelope were calculated using a moving root mean square with a window of 70 samples. This process enhanced the R-peaks, which were then detected using the findpeaks function of Scipy [38], with a minimum distance of 120 samples and a minimum height of 0.15.

Several features commonly used in previous studies to assess cardiovascular load in occupational settings, were extracted from the detected R-peaks to quantify both heart rate variability (HRV) and HR based indicators. HRV metrics were:

– Standard Deviation of consecutive RR peak intervals (SDRRi);
– Root Mean Square of consecutive RR peak intervals (RMSSD);
– Poincaré plot standard deviation perpendicular to the line of identity (SD1);
– Poincaré plot standard deviation along the line of identity (SD2).

The extracted HR based metrics were:

– Relative heart rate (RHR);
– Cardiovascular load (CVL);
– Cardiovascular strain (CVS).

The metrics based on HR rely on the calculation of age-adjusted maximum HR (HR_{max} = 208–0.7 × age) [39].

Respiratory Inductance Plethysmography. The respiratory signals from the chest and abdomen were first submitted to a finite impulse response bandpass filter of 0.15 to 0.45 Hz [30]. Subsequently, Masked Sift Empirical Mode Decomposition (EMD) was used on the signals, leading to their breakdown into Intrinsic Mode Functions (IMFs) [40]. The signals were then reconstructed using IMF-4, as it resulted in the clearest respiratory pattern.

Using a zero-crossing detection algorithm, the respiratory rate (RR) in breaths per minute was extracted from the filtered signals [41]. Additionally, the rib-cage percentage (RC%), which is the Rib Cage's (RC) contribution to tidal volume as a percentage of the combined RC and Abdominal (ABD) volume variation [42], was computed. With a moving window of 400 samples, the full cross-correlation between the RC and ABD signals was determined [43]. Finally, by applying the Hilbert Transform to both RC and ABD signals and subtracting their imaginary parts (phase), PS was obtained [30].

Electromyography. The first step to process the EMG signals was filtering with a 4th order band-pass of 10 Hz to 500 Hz [30]. The signals were then downsampled to 350 Hz for synchronization with the data collected with the hub device and work cycle detection.

Smoothing using a moving root mean square with a window of 70 samples, was also applied. This process was followed for both MVC and activity monitoring recordings.

From the EMG signals recorded during workers' activities, normalized amplitude by the MVC test and median frequency were extracted, as they can quantify the local muscle load [44]. The former was obtained by first rectifying the EMG, and the activity EMGs' values were divided by the maximum value found in the MVC. The latter was computed with Welch's modified periodogram.

Accelerometer. To remove noise from the ACC data collected from the triaxial ACC placed at the center of the lower back and the ACCs in the MuscleBAN device, a band-pass filter with cut-off frequencies set at 0.1 Hz and 10 Hz was applied [30,45]. Subsequently, the signals were smoothened using a 0.2-second window.

2.7 Signal Segmentation

Signal Synchronization. The first step to identify the work-cycles was to synchronize the signals acquired from the multiple devices. This was accomplished by first matching the sampling frequencies of the signals, i.e.,dowmsampling the data collected from the hubs from 1000 Hz to 350 Hz. Next they were aligned through the computation of the full cross-correlation between the ACC signals of the two devices.

Self-similarity Matrix. Since this study was conducted on an actual automobile assembly line, there were unexpected occurrences like line stops, bathroom breaks, and tasks performed with additional or altered movements. Despite these interruptions, the monitored activities are expected to follow a repeating pattern, since they are typically executed with specific movements in a set order. As the video recordings only covered the begining of each collection, the cycles were identified by applying the Self-Similarity Matrix (SSM) and the signals were segmented accordingly. Using the available videos, it was possible to compare the resulting segmentation with the observable work cycles. This method has been successfully applied in segmenting time series, human activity recognition, biosignal segmentation [46], and work-cycle anomaly and pattern detection [47]. This process consisted of three main steps, represented in Fig. 3:

1. Signal selection and Downsampling: the accelerometer signals from the three devices (back, biceps) were visually inspected, and the axis (x,y,z) with the most cyclical pattern was chosen. Next, this signal was downsampled to the frame rate of the video camera.
2. Synchronization: the signals were synchronized with the videos, by identification of the last jump.
3. SSM and Signal Segmentation: features were extracted from the signals (peak to peak distance, absolute energy, mean, standard deviation, autocorrelation, traveled distance, kurtosis, and skewness of the signal), building the feature vector. These were computed with a specific window (w) and overlap (o) to each workstation. H1: $w \in [50, 120]$ samples, $o = 5\%$; $H2 : w \in [100, 150]$ samples, $o \in [1, 5]\%$; H3: $w \in [25, 40]$, $o \in [5, 10]\%$, creating the feature matrix, were the rows are the features and the columns are the windows. The dot product between the z-normalized matrix and

its transpose gave us the SSM matrix. From this matrix the self-similarity function was calculated by the colum-wise sum of the features. This makes the parts of the signal with similar structures evident and makes it possible to detect anomalies and cycles. Finally the first detected cycles were compared with the available annotations from the video [48].

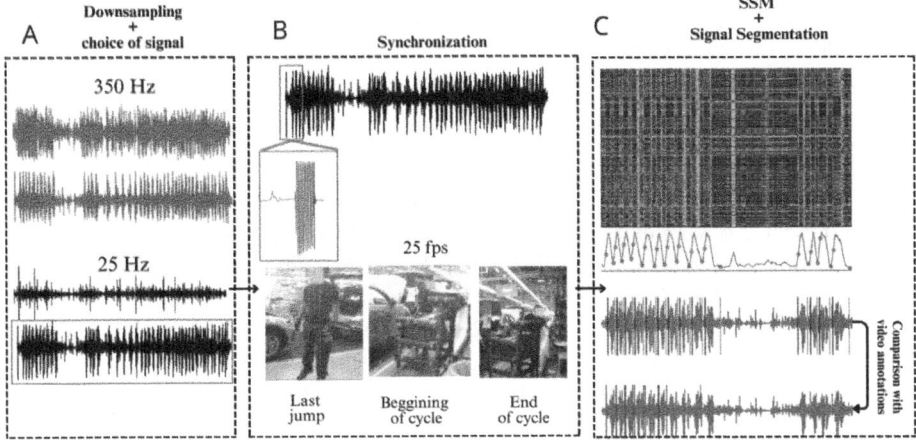

Fig. 3. Data segmentation process from [48].

2.8 Data Normalization

In some cases, there were unexpected assembly line stops, such as the example given in Fig. 3. This led us to exclude those recordings from the analysis, to guarantee that only comparable data were used. All the signals were cut from the first to the last detected work cycles. This cut of data left the 16 cardiorespiratory recordings with 40 min each, and the 14 available EMG recordings with 50 min each. They have different lengths, since one of the 2 subjects that did not have EMG data available performed less time of actual work.

3 Statistical Analysis

3.1 Cardiorespiratory Analysis

To evaluate how the work volume affects the cardiorespiratory response during acquisition, signals were studied at two time points: the first 10 min and the last 10 min. Cardiac and respiratory indicators described in the Sect. 2.6, were extracted at each of these time periods.

A Mixed ANOVA was used for the statistical analysis, considering two factors: the workstation and the phase (first and last 10 min) at which the metrics were extracted. To perform a more robust test, the features from the 16 subjects were oversampled to 24 subjects, to balance the minority workstations through cluster-based oversampling, specifically using the SMOTE (Synthetic Minority Over-sampling Technique) algorithm [49].

To ensure the reliability of the results, 500 simulations were performed by changing the random seed of the oversampler, and the p-value was determined using the harmonic mean combined p-value method, suitable for dependent tests [50].

The obtained p-values were corrected for violations of normality and equality of variance principles using the Yeo-Johnson power transform [51] and the Welch correction, respectively. The level of significance was set at 5%, and indicators below this threshold were further analyzed using the Tukey post-hoc test.

3.2   EMG Analysis

To study the evolution of the biceps' responses to work volume, EMG indicators detailed in Sect. 2.6 were extracted from the identified work cycles. To be able to compare the workstations and their muscle load evolution throughout the data collection, the total duration was divided into four equal segments, that will be mentioned as Moments of work, Moment 1 (M1), Moment 2 (M2), Moment 3 (M3) and Moment 4 (M4), as illustrated in Fig. 4-A. For each of these segments, the indicators described in Sect. 2.6 were extracted from each identified work cycle within that segment (Fig. 4-B). Finally, the mean of these subsegments was calculated. These four averaged segment values were then used for the formal analysis (Fig. 4-C). As EMG data should be analyzed with complementary data [52], such as inertial measurements (which was used to identify the work-cycles), our approach allows us to extract meaningful insights into fast changes in muscular activity, that would be smoothed in longer windows.

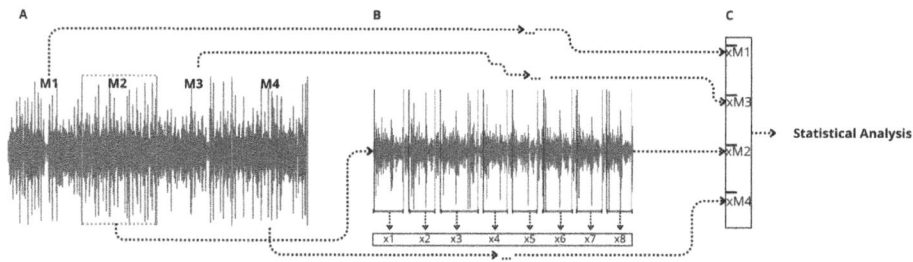

Fig. 4. EMG feature extraction process. A- Division into 4 equal segments, the Moments (M1, M2, M3 and M4). B- Extraction of feature X from the nth work-cycle and computation of the mean value from all work-cycles in that Moment. C- All mean values of feature x for each Moment are computed, and are used in the statistical analysis.

A repeated measures ANOVA with the workstation as a between factor was the chosen statistical test. Again, the sample size was increased in the same way as described in Sect. 3.1 to increase the robustness of the test. When the assumption of sphericity was violated the Greenhouse-Geisser correction was applied. The significance level was set at 5%, and the post hoc chosen was the Bonferroni test.

4   Results

4.1   Cardiovascular Response

The results of the mixed test showed that H_3 had an evident decrease in SDRRi, SD of RHR, coefficient of variation of HR, and SD2. The H_2 workstation had a significant decrease in HR over time. The values of the extracted ECG metrics of station H_1 were generally smaller and remained constant throughout the recording.

The results of the mixed ANOVA simulation statistics of the cardiac indicators are presented in Table 1 where the p-value of each interaction is shown, and significant results are presented with an *.

The post-hoc tests are presented in Fig. 5.

Table 1. Mixed ANOVA results for the cardiovascular metrics. From [32].

Variables	p_g	p_{ph}	p_{int}
HR	0.432	0.006*	0.043*
Max HR	0.486	0.097	0.038*
SDRRi	0.530	0.018*	0.009*
CV HR	0.273	0.001*	0.017*
RHR	0.229	<0.001*	0.021*
SD RHR	0.274	<0.001*	0.030*
CV RHR	0.071	0.563	0.007*
CVS	0.051	0.008*	0.094
CVL	0.027*	0.006*	0.058
CVL range	0.075	0.198	0.040*
SD2	0.502	0.015*	0.008*

HR- Heart Rate; SDRRi- Standard deviation of consecutive RR intervals; RHR- Relative Heart Rate; CVS- Cardiovascular Strain; CVL- Cardiovascular Load; SD2- Poincaré plot standard deviation along the line of identity; Max- Maximum; Min-Minimum; SD Standard Deviation; CV- Coefficient of Variation; p_g- harmonic mean combined p-value for the between factor; p_{ph}- harmonic mean combined p-value for the within factor; p_{int}- harmonic mean combined p-value for the interaction; * significant result at a confidence level of 5%.

Table 2. Mixed ANOVA results for the respiratory metrics. From [32].

Variables	p_g	p_{ph}	p_{int}
Max RC	0.534	0.033*	<0.001*
Min RC	0.891	0.533	<0.001*
SD RC	0.391	0.491	0.013*
ABD	0.190	0.468	<0.001*
Max ABD	0.697	<0.001*	<0.001*
SD ABD	0.539	0.008*	0.077
Correlation	0.022*	<0.001*	0.013*
PS	0.022*	<0.001*	0.015*

RC- Ribcage; ABD- Abdominal; PS- Phase synchrony; p_g- harmonic mean combined p-value for the between factor; p_{ph}- harmonic mean combined p-value for the within factor; p_{int}- harmonic mean combined p-value for the interaction; Max- Maximum; Min-Minimum; SD Standard Deviation; * significant result at a confidence level of 5%.

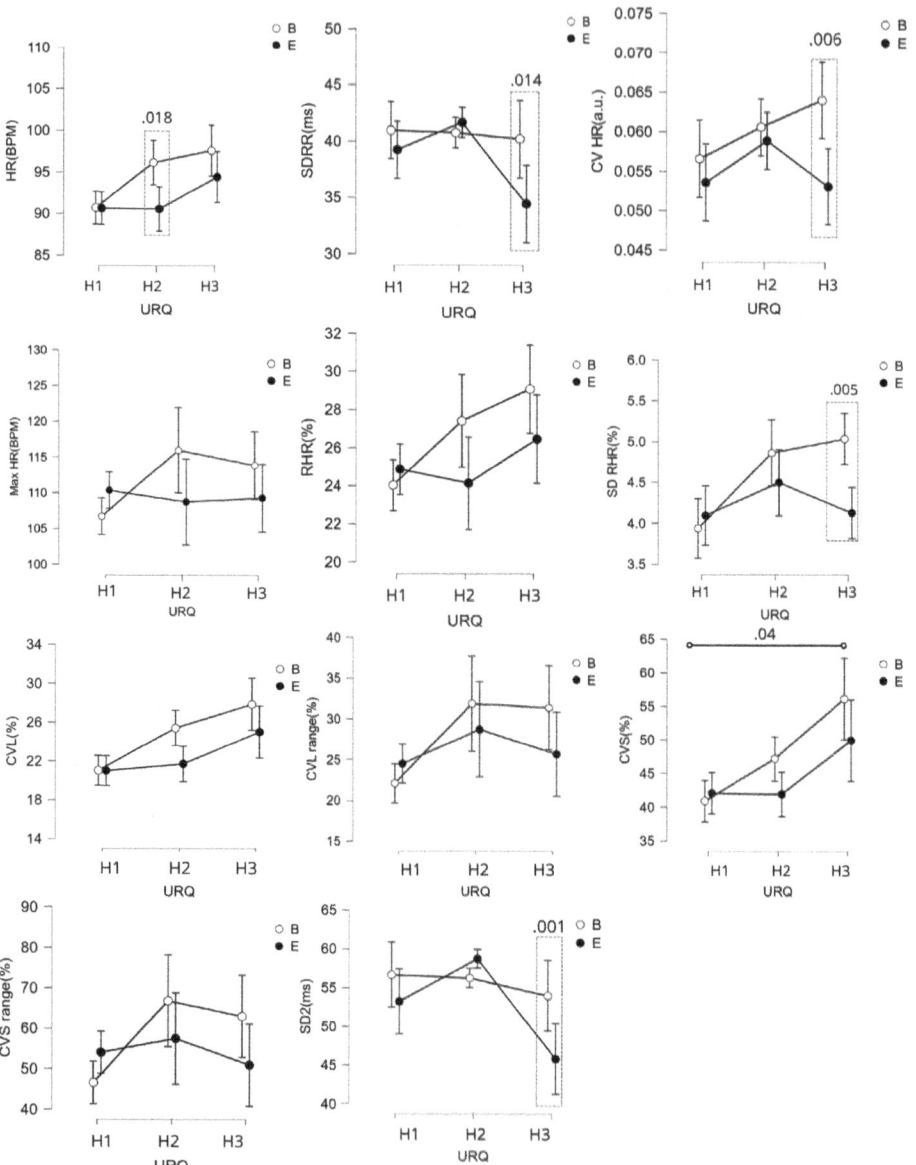

Fig. 5. Descriptive plots with Tukey test results for the significant cardiac variables. URQ: Workstation; B: Beginning; E: Ending. The dashed line box represents a significant result in the within factor. The solid line on top of the plot represents significant differences in the between factors, with markers on its tips: B-circle; E-solid circle. From [32].

4.2 Respiratory Response

The statistical analysis revealed that the mean and maximum ABD RR increased significantly, and so did its SD for the H_2 workstation. Significant reduction in respiratory correlation and PS was observed for H_2 and H_1 stations, respectively. In contrast, H_3 subjects maintained the PS between both RC and ABD wall motions from the first and last 10 min, having the highest mean values of this metric within the assembly line.

The results from the Mixed ANOVA simulation tests of respiratory indicators are presented in Table 2.

The post-hoc results are presented in Fig. 6.

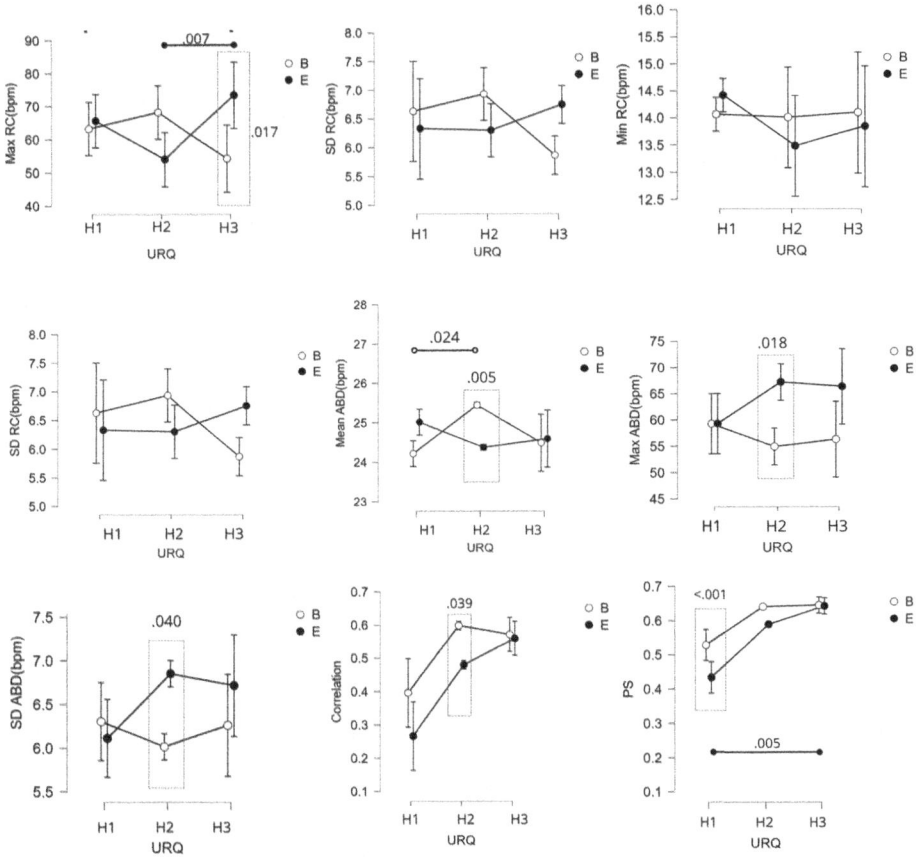

Fig. 6. Descriptive plots with Tukey test results for the significant respiratory variables. URQ: Workstation; H1- medium cycle station; H2- long cycle station; H3- short cycle station; B: Beginning; E: Ending. The dashed line box represents a significant result in the within factor. The solid line on top of the plot represents significant differences in the between factors, with markers on its tips: B-circle; E-solid circle. From [32].

4.3 Muscular Response

The results of the bicep's response showed that there were significant differences between moments of work within the workstations (M*URQ) in both relative amplitude ($p_M = 0.018$, $p_{M*URQ} = 0.001$) and median frequency ($p_M = 0.034$, $p_{M*URQ} = 0.044$). Between workstations there were not significant differences, neither for amplitude ($p_{URQ} = 0.154$) or for median frequency ($p_{URQ} = 0.777$). These values were obtained with the Greenhouse-Geisser sphericity correction. The Bonferroni post-hocs are represented in Fig. 7. These revealed that there was a significant reduction of median frequency from M1 to M3 ($p = 0.046$) and from M1 to M4 ($p = 0.022$) for the H3 workstation. In terms of normalized amplitude, only the H2 workstation presented significant reductions from M1 to M2 ($p = 0.002$), from M1 to M3 ($p < 0.001$) and from M1 to M4 ($p < 0.001$).

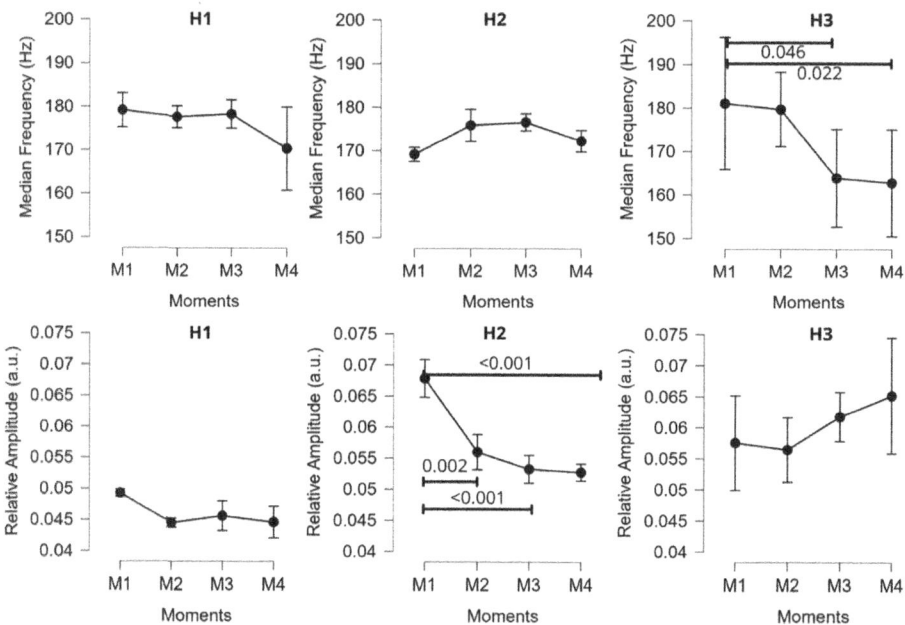

Fig. 7. Descriptive plots with Bonferroni test results for the significant muscular variables. H1- medium cycle station; H2- long cycle station; H3- short cycle station; M1- first moment; M2: second moment; M3: third moment; M4: fourth moment; The solid line on top of the plot represents significant differences between the repeated measures.

5 Discussion

This research aimed to better understand muscular and cardiorespiratory adaptations to repetitive work. From the monitorization of EMG, ECG, and RIP data throughout the performance of tasks with different work volumes, we searched for acute physiological changes. For the cardiorespiratory variables, two factors were considered: the phase of work (beginning and ending) and the workstation. For the EMG the more immediate changes in muscular load were investigated, considering the moment of the monitored activity (M1, M2, M3 and M4) and the workstation.

In the realm of cardiovascular indicators, HR serves as a marker of cardiovascular stress [53,54], while HRV provides valuable insight into autonomic regulation in response to various stimuli [55]. The influence of the parasympathetic nervous system on HR is more pronounced than that of the sympathetic nervous system at rest and during moderate exercise, resulting in increased variability of inter-beat intervals [56]. A reduction in HRV parameters has been associated with fatigue and work-related stress, as well as responses to the intensity and duration of physical activity [57–59].

Examining the cardiovascular stress indicators in Table 1 and the HRV trends in Fig. 5, it appears that tasks at the H_3 workstation place a greater demand on the cardiovascular system in terms of both stress and regulatory mechanisms. This increased demand is likely due to the higher frequency of repetitive movements at this workstation, which has been associated with greater metabolic, cardiac, and perceived stress [60]. In addition, many tasks at the H_3 workstation involve overhead movements, which have been shown to increase HR and blood pressure in similar activities [61]. Carvalho et al. [31] have also shown a significant decrease in HRV parameters in simulated assembly line tasks that included a fatigue inducing protocol.

In terms of respiratory adaptations, respiratory frequency is used as an indicator of physical workload [62]. Thoraco-abdominal asynchrony, defined as the uncoordinated movements of the thoracic (RC) and abdominal (ABD) walls and expressed in phase angle, is used to measure respiratory muscle workload [63].

From the observed workstations, the H_2's ABD respiratory variables present the most distinct evolution from the initial to the final 10 min, as shown in Fig. 6. The substancial drop in H2's ABD and RC correlation combined with the drop in mean ABD respiratory rate, increase in maximal ABD respiratory rate, while RC parameters did not change suggests a chaotic movement of the abdominal muscles, as confirmed by Table 2. The tasks performed in H2 involve the exertion of the upper-arms force to align the doors and front-end, hence, a possible explanation for these results is the fact that the inspiratory thoracic muscles are exerting less force for breathing, leaving ABD expiration muscles and the diaphragm to compensate [64].

The decline in phase synchrony was evident in H_1 and in correlation in the H_2 workstation. This result is consistent with the findings from Silva et al., where PS and correlation decreased between baseline and fatigue trials in a simulated repetitive task [30]. The H_3 subjects maintained the synchrony between ABD and RC wall motions throughout the analyzed time, suggesting different adaptation mechanisms inherent to this station compared to the others.

Concerning the EMG analysis, amplitude and median frequency serve as indicators of muscle fatigue. In a fatigued state, the amplitude of the signal increases while the median frequency decreases [65].

As illustrated in Fig. 2, the median frequency of H3 exhibited a notable decline throughout the observation period, indicating the potential for fatigue in the biceps muscle. This result also indicates that the biceps muscle is most utilized in this workstation, as evidenced by the increasing relative amplitude. For low-intensity tasks ($<20\%$ MVC), in [23] a significant decrease in median frequency and maintenance of amplitude were also found in the trapezius muscle EMG recording during simulated manual assembly work. This result is reasonable since a simultaneous increase of amplitude and decrease of median frequency has not been consistently seen in dynamic, longer, and realistic assembly line tasks [66].

Workstation H2 demonstrated notable fluctuations in relative amplitude, with a decline observed over moments. This suggests that the biceps were less active as the tasks progressed. In contrast to H3, H2 does not include movements above the head. In this workstation, bending positions and applying downward force are predominant, with the potential recruitment and compensation through other muscle activity, or motor compensation strategies, being present. A similar outcome was reported in [30], where an elevated activity of the biceps was observed during the second fatigue trial compared to the third. This phenomenon is attributed to the engagement of shoulder musculature and the implementation of alternative movements to mitigate localized fatigue. Kinematic and muscular adaptations to sustained task execution have been found in cyclic lifting tasks [67] and in fatiguing upper-limb work with different tasks [68].

At the H1 workstation, the relative amplitude remains relatively constant, and the median frequency tends to decrease at the last moment. However, this decrease was not statistically significant, and the increase of standard deviation points to the variability of compensation strategies among the subjects. Previous studies on repetitive work have also found that biomechanical compensation is very individual specific, resulting in high subject inter-variability [68,69].

These parameters can be easily monitored with different wearable applications. This information could be used to leverage task rotation, by identifying which tasks are harder for the individual employee. This type of approach has already been used in the construction sector to quantify task demands [70]. Also, muscular patterns and compensation mechanisms could be analysed to create a more individual specific risk score, such as the one suggested in [22]. Another possible application is the monitoring and prevention of health problems of the operators. For instance, the identification of a parameter that is above or under recommended limits, where an alert could be sent to the worker and supervisor that they need a break. This has already been applied in Tsai, but in the construction industry [57].

When considering all the analysed biosignals, worktation H3 seams to have the most straining effect on subjects both in cardiovascular and bicep loads. This makes these workers exposed to increased inflammation and subject to possible bicep fatigue. Only the respiratory response did not have a visible effect. This may be due to the contamination of the RC respiration patterns with arm movements. The RIP belt measures the changes in volume that it surrounds. As workers in this station perform most of the tasks with their arms above head with hyperflextion and abduction movements, these volume changes might not solely represent breathing.

These results indicate that workers should not perform tasks of the H3 station for long periods. As mentioned in Sect. 1, the reduction of HRV without sufficient recovery time puts these workers through increased inflammation which then elevates the risk for developing a disease. Also, the reduction in median frequency of the biceps muscle activity points to possible muscle fatigue, leaving them at increased risk of musculoskeletal disorders. They need to rotate to other workstations, take longer breaks or have earlier shift changes.

In this study some limitations are pointed out. First, the work experience of the volunteers was guaranteed to be at least one year at the factory, but how many years of that experience was in that workstation was not known. The years of experience in a certain task may influence physiological adaptations. As this study was carried out in a real factory, researchers were subject to the worker's availability, and not all recordings were taken in the same conditions. Some were taken in the morning and others in the afternoon, some after their break and others had already been working. In the future it should be interesting to understand the influence this has on physiological measurements.

6   Conclusions and Future Work

Cardiorespiratory and bicep responses to different work volumes were studied using ECG, RIP and EMG signals monitoring during a period of the shift of multiple operators.

The analysis of the evolution of the chosen cardiac and respiratory indicators showed contrasts among tasks with distinct work volumes, where cardiac load was higher in the H_3 workstation and respiratory difficulty appeared to be higher in the H_1 and H_2 workstations, revealing distinct strategies of adaptation depending on work-volume. In terms of local muscle load, H_3 has the most evident bicep activation, with a possible manifestation of muscle fatigue.

The results of this study further prove the powerful information contained in biosignals to understand underlying physiological mechanisms and the advantage of ubiquitous monitoring for the development of more comprehensive risk quantification tools and possibly lead to early detection of work-related health issues.

Increasing acquisition time should be considered in the following studies, to capture long-term adaptations of these biological phenomena, monitoring of different muscles could also shed more light on motor strategies and increasing the sample size to allow the association between biosignals.

The integration of muscular and cardiorespiratory responses offers a more holistic view of the occupational demands placed on workers, addressing the full spectrum of physical stressors encountered in the manufacturing sector. By examining both cardiovascular and muscular responses, we can better understand the cumulative impact of repetitive and strenuous tasks on the body, leading to more effective interventions and ergonomic improvements at the workplace.

Acknowledgements. This work was supported by Project OPERATOR (NORTE01-0247-FEDER-045910), co-financed by the European Regional Development Fund through the North Portugal Regional Operational Program and Lisbon Regional Operational Program and by the Portuguese Foundation for Science and Technology, under the MIT Portugal Program. M. Dias and P. Probst were supported by the doctoral Grants SFRH/BD/151375/2021 and

RT/BD/152843/2021, respectively, financed by the Portuguese Foundation for Science and Technology (FCT), and with funds from the State Budget, under the MIT Portugal Program.

Disclosure of Interests. The authors have no competing interests to declare that are relevant to the content of this article.

References

1. de Kok, J., et al.: Work-related musculoskeletal disorders: Prevalence, costs and demographics in the eu. Technical report, European Agency for Safety and Health at Work (EU-OSHA) (2019). https://osha.europa.eu/en/publications/msds-facts-and-figures-overview-prevalence-costs-and-demographics-msds-europe
2. (ILO), I.L.O.: Global trends on occupational accidents and diseases. Technical report. International Labour Organization (ILO) (2008). https://webapps.ilo.org/legacy/english/osh/en/story_content/external_files/fs_st_1-ILO_5_en.pdf
3. Eurostat: Hours of work - Annual Statistics (2023). https://ec.europa.eu/eurostat/statistics-explained/index.php?title=Hours_of_work_-_annual_statistics&oldid=565451#How_does_the_average_usual_working_week_vary_across_economic_activities_and_occupations.3F
4. Niu, S.: Ergonomics and occupational safety and health: An ILO perspective. Appl. Ergon. 41(6), 744–753 (2010). https://doi.org/10.1016/j.apergo.2010.03.004. https://www.sciencedirect.com/science/article/pii/S0003687010000499
5. Aarås, A., Westgaard, R.: Further studies of postural load and musculo-skeletal injuries of workers at an electro-mechanical assembly plant. Appl. Ergon. 18(3), 211–219 (1987). https://doi.org/10.1016/0003-6870(87)90006-8. https://www.sciencedirect.com/science/article/pii/0003687087900068
6. Nussbaum, M.A.: Static and dynamic myoelectric measures of shoulder muscle fatigue during intermittent dynamic exertions of low to moderate intensity. Eur. J. Appl. Physiol. 85, 299–309 (2001)
7. Geurts, S.A., Sonnentag, S.: Recovery as an explanatory mechanism in the relation between acute stress reactions and chronic health impairment. Scand. J. Work Environ. Health 482–492 (2006)
8. Pickering, T.G., et al.: Environmental influences on blood pressure and the role of job strain. Journal of hypertension. Suppl. Off. J. Int. Soc. Hypertens. 14(5), S179–85 (1996). http://europepmc.org/abstract/MED/9120676
9. Krause, N., et al.: Occupational physical activity, energy expenditure and 11-year progression of carotid atherosclerosis. Scand. J. Work Environ. Health 6, 405–424 (2007). https://doi.org/10.5271/sjweh.1171. https://www.sjweh.fi/show_abstract.php?abstract_id=1171
10. Krause, N., Arah, O.A., Kauhanen, J.: Physical activity and 22-year all-cause and coronary heart disease mortality. Am. J. Ind. Med. 60(11), 976–990 (2017). https://doi.org/10.1002/ajim.22756. https://onlinelibrary.wiley.com/doi/abs/10.1002/ajim.22756
11. Holtermann, A., Hansen, J.V., Burr, H., Søgaard, K., Sjøgaard, G.: The health paradox of occupational and leisure-time physical activity. Br. J. Sports Med. 46(4), 291–295 (2012). https://doi.org/10.1136/bjsm.2010.079582. https://bjsm.bmj.com/content/46/4/291
12. Nicolò, A., Massaroni, C., Passfield, L.: Respiratory frequency during exercise: the neglected physiological measure. Front. Physiol. 8, 922 (2017). https://doi.org/10.3389/fphys.2017.00922
13. Massaroni, C., Nicolò, A., Lo Presti, D., Sacchetti, M., Silvestri, S., Schena, E.: Contact-based methods for measuring respiratory rate. Sensors 19(4), 908 (2019). https://doi.org/10.3390/s19040908

14. Andreas, G.W.J., Johanssons, E.: Observational methods for assessing ergonomic risks for work-related musculoskeletal disorders: a scoping review. Revista Ciencias de la Salud **16**, 8–38 (2018). http://www.scielo.org.co/scielo.php?script=sci_arttext&pid=S1692-72732018000400008&nrm=iso

15. NIOSH: Work Practices Guide for Manual Lifting. No. 81-122 in DHHS (NIOSH) publication, U.S. Department of Health and Human Services, Public Health Service, Centers for Disease Control, National Institute for Occupational Safety and Health, Division of Biomedical and Behavioral Science (1981). https://books.google.pt/books?id=uoY3OpylFTwC

16. Goggins, R.W., Spielholz, P., Nothstein, G.L.: Estimating the effectiveness of ergonomics interventions through case studies: implications for predictive cost-benefit analysis. J. Safety Res. **39**(3), 339–344 (2008). https://doi.org/10.1016/j.jsr.2007.12.006. https://www.sciencedirect.com/science/article/pii/S0022437508000480

17. Baraldi, E.C., Kaminski, P.C.: Ergonomic planned supply in an automotive assembly line. Hum. Fact. Ergon. Manuf. Serv. Ind. **21**(1), 104–119 (2011). https://doi.org/10.1002/hfm.20228. https://onlinelibrary.wiley.com/doi/abs/10.1002/hfm.20228

18. Takala, E.P., et al.: Systematic evaluation of observational methods assessing biomechanical exposures at work. Scand. J. Work Environ. Health **1**, 3–24 (2010). https://doi.org/10.5271/sjweh.2876. https://www.sjweh.fi/show_abstract.php?abstract_id=2876

19. van der Beek, A.J., Frings-Dresen, M.H.: Assessment of mechanical exposure in ergonomic epidemiology. Occup. Environ. Med. **55**(5), 291–299 (1998). https://doi.org/10.1136/oem.55.5.291. https://oem.bmj.com/content/55/5/291

20. Eliasson, K., Lind, C.M., Nyman, T.: Factors influencing ergonomists' use of observation-based risk-assessment. In: Work, pp. 93–106 (2019)

21. Romero, D., et al.: Towards an operator 4.0 typology: a human-centric perspective on the fourth industrial revolution technologies, pp. 29–31 (2016)

22. Monaco, M.G.L., et al.: Combined use of semg and inertial sensing to evaluate biomechanical overload in manufacturing: an on-the-field experience. Machines **11**(4) (2023). https://doi.org/10.3390/machines11040417. https://www.mdpi.com/2075-1702/11/4/417

23. Bosch, T., de Looze, M., Kingma, I., Visser, B., van Dieën, J.: Electromyographical manifestations of muscle fatigue during different levels of simulated light manual assembly work. J. Electromyogr. Kinesiol. **19**(4), e246–e256 (2009). https://doi.org/10.1016/j.jelekin.2008.04.014. https://www.sciencedirect.com/science/article/pii/S1050641108000758

24. Bosch, T., Mathiassen, S., Visser, B., Looze, M., Van Dieen, J.: The effect of work pace on workload, motor variability and fatigue during simulated light assembly work. Ergonomics **54**, 154–68 (2011). https://doi.org/10.1080/00140139.2010.538723

25. Lundberg, U., Granqvist, M., Hanssonand, T., Magnusson, M., Wallin, L.: Psychological and physiological stress responses during repetitive work at an assembly line. Work Stress **3**(2), 143–153 (1989). https://doi.org/10.1080/02678378908256940

26. Palmerud, G., Forsman, M., Neumann, W.P., Winkel, J.: Mechanical exposure implications of rationalization: a comparison of two flow strategies in a Swedish manufacturing plant. Appl. Ergon. **43**(6), 1110–1121 (2012). https://doi.org/10.1016/j.apergo.2012.04.001. https://www.sciencedirect.com/science/article/pii/S0003687012000518

27. Kazmierczak, K., Mathiassen, S.E., Forsman, M., Winkel, J.: An integrated analysis of ergonomics and time consumption in Swedish 'craft-type' car disassembly. Appl. Ergon. **36**(3), 263–273 (2005). https://doi.org/10.1016/j.apergo.2005.01.010. https://www.sciencedirect.com/science/article/pii/S0003687005000372

28. Ayabar, A., De la Riva, J., Sanchez, J., Balderrama, C.: Regression model to estimate standard time through energy consumption of workers in manual assembly lines under moderate workload. J. Ind. Eng. **2015** (2015). https://doi.org/10.1155/2015/382673

29. Nardolillo, A.M., Baghdadi, A., Cavuoto, L.A.: Heart rate variability during a simulated assembly task. Influence Age Gend. **61**, 1853–1857 (2017). https://doi.org/10.1177/1541931213601943
30. Silva, L., et al.: Respiratory inductance plethysmography to assess fatigability during repetitive work. Sensors **22** (2022). https://doi.org/10.3390/s22114247
31. Carvalho, D., et al.: Cardiovascular Reactivity (CVR) during repetitive work in the presence of fatigue. In: Ahram, T., Karwowski, W., Bucchianico, P.D., Taiar, R., Casarotto, L., Costa, P. (eds.) Intelligent Human Systems Integration (IHSI 2023): Integrating People and Intelligent Systems, vol. 69. AHFE Open Access, AHFE International (2023). https://doi.org/10.54941/ahfe1002833
32. Furk, D., Silva, L., Dias, M., Probst, P., Gamboa, H.: Cardiorespiratory adaptations to work volume on an automobile assembly line. In: Proceedings of the 17th International Joint Conference on Biomedical Engineering Systems and Technologies, vol. 1, pp. 71–81 (2024https://doi.org/10.5220/0012587800003657
33. Gastinger, S., Donnelly, A., Dumond, R., Prioux, J.: A review of the evidence for the use of ventilation as a surrogate measure of energy expenditure. JPEN. J. Parent. Enteral Nutr. **38** (2014). https://doi.org/10.1177/0148607114530432
34. Hessnielsen, N., Wickerhauser, M.: Wavelets and time-frequency analysis. Proc. IEEE **84**, 523–540 (1996). https://doi.org/10.1109/5.488698
35. Chen, C.C., Tsui, F.R.: Comparing different wavelet transforms on removing electrocardiogram baseline wanders and special trends. BMC Med. Inf. Decis. Mak. **20** (2020). https://doi.org/10.1186/s12911-020-01349-x
36. He, H., Tan, Y., Wang, Y.: Optimal base wavelet selection for ECG noise reduction using a comprehensive entropy criterion. Entropy **17**(9), 6093–6109 (2015)
37. Xu, W., Du, F.: A robust qrs complex detection method based on shannon energy envelope and hilbert transform. J. Mech. Med. Biol. **22**(03), 2240013 (2022). https://doi.org/10.1142/S0219519422400139. https://doi.org/10.1142/S0219519422400139
38. Virtanen, P., et al.: Fundamental algorithms for scientific computing in python. Nat. Methods **17**, 261–272 (2020). https://doi.org/10.1038/s41592-019-0686-2. https://rdcu.be/b08Wh
39. Tanaka, H., Monahan, K.D., Seals, D.R.: Age-predicted maximal heart rate revisited. J. Am. Coll. Cardiol. **37**(1), 153–156 (2001). https://doi.org/10.1016/S0735-1097(00)01054-8. https://www.sciencedirect.com/science/article/pii/S0735109700010548
40. Liu, S., Gao, R.X., John, D., Staudenmayer, J., Freedson, P.: Tissue artifact removal from respiratory signals based on empirical mode decomposition. Ann. Biomed. Eng. **41**, 1003–1015 (2013). https://doi.org/10.1007/s10439-013-0742-5
41. Rétory, Y., Niedzialkowski, P., de Picciotto, C., Bonay, M., Petitjean, M.: New respiratory inductive plethysmography (RIP) method for evaluating ventilatory adaptation during mild physical activities. PLoS ONE **11** (2016). https://api.semanticscholar.org/CorpusID:4684787
42. Ryan, L., Rahman, T., Strang, A., Heinle, R., Shaffer, T.H.: Diagnostic differences in respiratory breathing patterns and work of breathing indices in children with Duchenne muscular dystrophy. PLoS ONE **15** (2020). https://doi.org/10.1371/journal.pone.0226980
43. Makowski, D., et al.: NeuroKit2: a python toolbox for neurophysiological signal processing. Behav. Res. Methods **53**(4), 1689–1696 (2021). https://doi.org/10.3758/s13428-020-01516-y
44. Tuček, D., Dombeková, B.: Local muscular load measurement with the help of a datalogger. Acta Polytech. Hung **14**, 215–234 (2017)
45. Lester, J., Hannaford, B., Borriello, G.: "Are You with Me?" – using accelerometers to determine if two devices are carried by the same person, vol. 3001, pp. 33–50 (2004). https://doi.org/10.1007/978-3-540-24646-6_3

46. Rodrigues, J., Liu, H., Folgado, D., Belo, D., Schultz, T., Gamboa, H.: Feature-based information retrieval of multimodal biosignals with a self-similarity matrix: focus on automatic segmentation. Biosensors **12**(12) (2022). https://doi.org/10.3390/bios12121182. https://www.mdpi.com/2079-6374/12/12/1182
47. Santos, A., Rodrigues, J., Folgado, D., Santos, S., Fujão, C., Gamboa, H.: Self-similarity matrix of morphological features for motion data analysis in manufacturing scenarios, pp. 80–90 (2021). https://doi.org/10.5220/0010252800800090
48. Furk, D., Silva, L., Dias, M., Fujão, C., Probst, P., Liu, H., Gamboa, H.: Cardiorespiratory response to workload volume and ergonomic risk: Automotive assembly line operators' adaptations. Appl. Sci. **14**(9) (2024). https://doi.org/10.3390/app14093921. https://www.mdpi.com/2076-3417/14/9/3921
49. Chawla, N., Bowyer, K., Hall, L., Kegelmeyer, W.: SMOTE: synthetic minority oversampling technique. J. Artif. Intell. Res. (JAIR) **16**, 321–357 (2002). https://doi.org/10.1613/jair.953
50. Wilson, D.J.: The harmonic mean p-value for combining dependent tests. Proc. Natl. Acad. Sci. **116**(4), 1195–1200 (2019). https://doi.org/10.1073/pnas.1814092116. https://www.pnas.org/doi/abs/10.1073/pnas.1814092116
51. Yeo, I.K., Johnson, R.A.: A new family of power transformations to improve normality or symmetry. Biometrika **87**(4), 954–959 (2000). http://www.jstor.org/stable/2673623
52. Felici, F., Del Vecchio, A.: Surface electromyography: what limits its use in exercise and sport physiology? Front. Neurol. **11** (2020). https://doi.org/10.3389/fneur.2020.578504. https://www.frontiersin.org/journals/neurology/articles/10.3389/fneur.2020.578504
53. Samani, A., Holtermann, A., Søgaard, K., Holtermann, A., Madeleine, P.: Following ergonomics guidelines decreases physical and cardiovascular workload during cleaning tasks. Ergonomics **55**(3), 295–307 (2012). https://doi.org/10.1080/00140139.2011.640945. https://doi.org/10.1080/00140139.2011.640945, pMID: 22409167
54. Umer, W.: Sensors based physical exertion monitoring for construction tasks: Comparison between traditional physiological and heart rate variability based metrics. In: Proceedings of Joint CIB WO99 & TG59 Conference (2020)
55. Mccraty, R., Shaffer, F.: Heart rate variability: new perspectives on physiological mechanisms, assessment of self-regulatory capacity, and health risk. Glob. Adv. Health Med. **4**(1), 46–61 (2015). https://doi.org/10.7453/gahmj.2014.073. pMID: 25694852
56. Sammito, S., Thielmann, B., Seibt, R., Klussmann, A., Weippert, M., Böckelmann, I.: Guideline for the application of heart rate and heart rate variability in occupational medicine and occupational science. ASU Int. **2015**(06), 1–29 (2015)
57. Tsai, M.K.: Applying physiological status monitoring in improving construction safety management. KSCE J. Civil Eng. **21**, 2061–2066 (2017). https://doi.org/10.1007/s12205-016-0980-9
58. Tonello, L., Rodrigues, F., Souza, J., Campbell, C., Leicht, A., Boullosa, D.: The role of physical activity and heart rate variability for the control of work related stress. Front. Physiol. **5** (2014https://doi.org/10.3389/fphys.2014.00067. https://www.frontiersin.org/articles/10.3389/fphys.2014.00067
59. Brockmann, L., Hunt, K.J.: Heart rate variability changes with respect to time and exercise intensity during heart-rate-controlled steady-state treadmill running. Sci. Rep. **13**, 8515 (2023). https://doi.org/10.1038/s41598-023-35717-0
60. Mang, Z.A., et al.: The effect of repetition tempo on cardiovascular and metabolic stress when time under tension is matched during lower body exercise. Eur. J. Appl. Physiol. **122**(6), 1485–1495 (2022). https://doi.org/10.1007/s00421-022-04941-3
61. Astrand, I., Guharay, A., Wahren, J.: Circulatory responses to arm exercise with different arm positions. J. Appl. Physiol. **25**(5), 528–532 (1968). https://doi.org/10.1152/jappl.1968.25.5.528

62. Nicolò, A., Marcora, S.M., Bazzucchi, I., Sacchetti, M.: Differential control of respiratory frequency and tidal volume during high-intensity interval training. Exp. Physiol. **102**(8), 934–949 (2017)
63. Hammer, J., Newth, C.: Assessment of thoraco-abdominal asynchrony. Paediatr. Respir. Rev. **10**(2), 75–80 (2009). https://doi.org/10.1016/j.prrv.2009.02.004. https://www.sciencedirect.com/science/article/pii/S1526054209000190
64. Celli, B.R., Criner, G., Rassulo, J.: Ventilatory muscle recruitment during unsupported arm exercise in normal subjects. J. Appl. Physiol. **64**(5), 1936–1941 (1988). https://doi.org/10.1152/jappl.1988.64.5.1936
65. de Looze, M., Bosch, T., van Dieën, J.: Manifestations of shoulder fatigue in prolonged activities involving low-force contractions. In: Contemporary Sport, Leisure and Ergonomics, pp. 15–28 (2009)
66. de Looze, M., Bosch, T., van Dieën, J.H.: Manifestations of shoulder fatigue in prolonged activities involving low-force contractions. Ergonomics **52**(4), 428–437 (2009). https://doi.org/10.1080/00140130802707709
67. Bonato, P., et al.: Muscle fatigue and fatigue-related biomechanical changes during a cyclic lifting task. Spine **28**(16), 1810–1820 (2003)
68. McDonald, A.C., Mulla, D.M., Keir, P.J.: Muscular and kinematic adaptations to fatiguing repetitive upper extremity work. Appl. Ergon. **75**, 250–256 (2019). https://doi.org/10.1016/j.apergo.2018.11.001. https://www.sciencedirect.com/science/article/pii/S0003687018306008
69. Mulla, D.M., McDonald, A.C., Keir, P.J.: Joint moment trade-offs across the upper extremity and trunk during repetitive work. Appl. Ergon. **88**, 103142 (2020). https://doi.org/10.1016/j.apergo.2020.103142, https://www.sciencedirect.com/science/article/pii/S0003687020300995
70. Sadat-Mohammadi, M., Shakerian, S., Liu, Y., Asadi, S., Jebelli, H.: Non-invasive physical demand assessment using wearable respiration sensor and random forest classifier. J. Build. Eng. **44**, 103–279 (2021)

Towards the Development of Safer Biomedical Devices for ECG Acquisition: Using DPI for the Assessment of Electromagnetic Susceptibility

Tiago Nunes[1,3](✉)[iD], Hugo Plácido da Silva[1,2][iD], and Hugo Gamboa[1,3][iD]

[1] PLUX Wireless Biosignals, Lisbon, Portugal
tnunes@pluxbiosignals.com, hsilva@lx.it.pt
[2] Instituto de Telecomunicações, Lisbon, Portugal
[3] NOVA School of Science and Technology, Almada, Portugal
hgamboa@fct.unl.pt

Abstract. Ensuring reliability of electronic medical devices is becoming increasingly challenging. The number of incidents with devices intended for clinical usage associated with electromagnetic interference has been increasing over the years and this trend is expected to be maintained. Ensuring proper behaviour on a given device from an electromagnetic point of view can be very expensive given the equipment and facilities required to conduct standardised tests. However, this topic shall not be disregarded, as the smallest source of interference on a medical device can make the difference when a diagnosis is dependent on the readings of a device. This work exposes the issue related with EMI induced malfunction in medical devices and proposes a method for simple and affordable pre-assessment of electromagnetic susceptibility on a device for ECG acquisition. The setup created for this purpose is presented as well as the good practices that shall be taken into account for the development of the system. This is used to replicated two scenarios previously evaluated in an anechoic chamber. It is shown that it is possible to replicate certain conditions using this system leading to conclusions identical to those observed in the anechoic chamber.

Keywords: Biosignals · Electromagnetic · Interference · Immunity · Risk-based EMC · ECG

1 Introduction

In the course of the past years, the number of incidents with medical technology associated with Electromagnetic Interference (EMI) has seen an exponential increase. Such an incident occurs when two devices that coexist in the same environment interact with each other in an unwanted manner leading to undesired and unforeseen consequences (more or less severe). In this scenario, one device is

M. P. Guarino et al. (Eds.): BIOSTEC 2024, CCIS 2546, pp. 103–118, 2026.
https://doi.org/10.1007/978-3-031-96899-0_7

the victim and the other is the source. Part of the reason behind the increase in incidents with medical devices is the increase in availability of these devices to the masses, mostly in the shape of wearables (increasing the number of potential victims). In addition, the number of electronic devices capable of wireless communication in general has also augmented, doubling over the past five years. This number is expected to keep growing yearly in the near future, thus increasing the number of potential sources of EMI to medical devices [1–3].

Devices for ECG Acquisition

One of the most addressed signals in the context of wearables is the Electrocardiogram (ECG). The raising interest on the exploration of this signal comes in part from its wide range of applications in physical activity monitoring but also, and more importantly, monitoring of Cardiovascular Disease (CVD), the leading cause for deaths worldwide.

In fact, for more than 30 years, the number of deaths per year associated with CVDs has been greater than 12 millions and increasing every year, reaching 18 millions in 2019 with ischaemic heart disease being the leading condition, [4–8]. This comes with no surprise in a world with an increasingly older population, the most affected by these conditions [9].

Proper surveillance and early diagnosis is key in the outcome of a patient presenting a CVD. As we transition to an era of digital medicine and with the advent of wearable technology for constant monitoring of various physiological parameters, the range of products available for monitoring the heart activity is more diverse than ever.

Made possible by the non stopping advances in technology, everyday, more patients and practitioners adopt these technologies as a solution for continuous and remote monitoring of these and other conditions [10, 11]. With these devices, physicians are able to track the evolution of their patients relying on the signals acquired by the equipment in question.

All electronic devices are susceptible to some interference and, in some cases, these are undetected or cause minor consequences or disturbances to the application and end user. However, when the device in question has a medical function, where reliance on the information provided is key, it is of paramount importance that the well functioning of the device is ensured.

In this regard, some works have looked into these effects in devices for ECG acquisition in particular. For this biosignal the smallest deviation on the signal can be misinterpreted as a medical condition or, on the contrary, mask an existing one which, if left untreated, might have dramatic outcomes. The results showed that in various cases, an ECG signal may be misinterpreted as presenting a medical condition when in truth it was the result of an electronic device placed nearby [12].

Ensuring resilience to electromagnetic interference when developing a new device is essential to ensure it will operate safely when placed in the intended use environment. [13, 14]. This assurance is typically made via standardised tests performed in anechoic chambers. These are time and resources consuming specially when the test fails thus requiring more investment in correcting the product. In fact, one of the most common causes for Printed Circuit Board (PCB) redesign are Electromagnetic Compatibility (EMC) related issues identified only at the final stage of the development during the certification tests.

To avoid these situations, it is crucial that proper measures are taken early in the development of a new product so that potential weaknesses are identified as soon as possible allowing for its correction.

2 Direct Power Injection

The current small form factor of wearables that we commonly see available in the market is made possible thanks to the constant miniaturization of the components they are made of. This simple fact makes Integrated Circuits (IC) intrinsically less prone to be disturbed by EMI. However, as soon as they are placed on the PCB, an indispensable element in any electronic device, the traces that lead to it are able to pick up noise from the environment and conduct it to the pins of the component [15–17].

A typical embedded application relies on a microcontroller, a power source, communication module and in the case of medical technology, the biomedical sensor specifically design to acquire the signal of interest. Figure 1 illustrates the case of a device for Electromyography acquisition. For this purpose, and given the nature of biosignals, a series of filter and amplification stages are often require to acquire the signal while rejecting the unwanted artifacts.

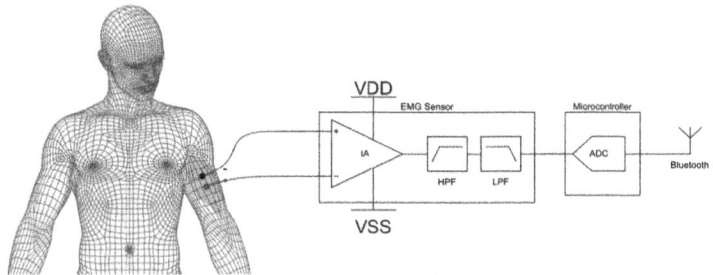

Fig. 1. Example of an acquisition device for Electromyography acquisition.

Each of these components, and the PCB that brings them together by the means of traces, is a potential victim to EMI which, if not dealt with from the very beginning of the development phase, might hinder the fulfilment of the desired function or fail in the certification tests.

As an alternative to testing in anechoic chambers, different studies have proposed the application of Direct Power Injection (DPI) to analyse the susceptibility of the various potential victims in an application such as the one mentioned above (Fig. 2).

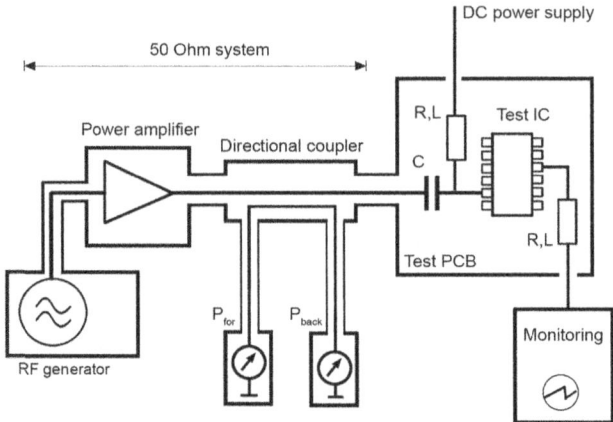

Fig. 2. Typical setup for DPI testing of ICs. Adapted from [18].

This method, established by the standard IEC62132-4 [19] is one of the most reproducible methods to evaluate a systems susceptibility to EMI. By injecting an interference on the Device Under Test (DUT) capacitively, it allows to characterize the immunity of a system to various Radio Frequency (RF) disturbances without the need for expensive facilities and/or equipment. Furthermore, it can be used throughout the development process and as soon as the first prototypes are ready, providing with information on the potential weaknesses of the device for them to be corrected as early as possible thus reducing time-to-market [20, 21].

Susceptibility of the Different Components

The potential of this method and the ease to implement it in a traditional laboratory has lead to the publication of multiple works demonstrating its ability to assess the susceptibility of various ICs, most of them used in the typical wearable device.

A study conducted by Dai et al. looked into the evaluation of conducted immunity of a microcontroller by exposing the component to a continuous-wave electromagnetic interference using DPI. It was possible to demonstrate the failure of the IC under particular conditions confirming the damage inflicted to it with an electron microscope [22].

Jian-fei et al. investigated the behaviour of an Low Dropout Voltage regulator (LDO) when exposed to given RF disturbances. They verified, both by simulation and using DPI, that this component, used in embedded applications to provide a stable voltage supply, was significantly affected by the disturbance injected as it led to an offset of the value at the output of the component [17].

Multiple works have looked into the effects of EMI on amplifiers. This component, essential in the design of sensors for biosignals, was tested using DPI to deliver an interfering signal on the ground plane and output pin of the device in various topologies and configurations, such as precision voltage references [16, 23–26].

From simple amplifiers to microcontrollers, all these components are commonly used in applications for biosignal acquisition. These and other works have demonstrated the potential in the use of DPI to assess the ability of a given device to sustain electromagnetic disturbances. While anechoic chambers might not be within reach to most Small and Medium Enterprises (SME)'s and researchers, DPI is a rather simple and easy technique that can and shall be applied during the development of an electronic device to evaluate its susceptibility to interference.

3   An Affordable Alternative

The solution hereinafter proposed is intended to evaluate the behaviour of an equipment for ECG monitoring in the presence of a disturbing signal while an acquisition is taking place. This solution uses the DPI method to inject a disturbance in the DUT capacitively and an ECG simulator to create the signal of interest.

Both signals are created using a arbitrary waveform generator, Analog Discovery 2, manufactured by Digilent. It is able to produce simple sinusoidal signals but also arbitrary signals with a 5 V amplitude and 14-bit resolution Digital to Analog Converter (DAC). Although dedicated software exists to operate the device, MATLAB 2023b is used via the toolbox provided by Digilent. This solution eases and simplifies the process of generating the signals required and sending them for the generator to synthesize them into single ended signals.

By nature, the ECG signal has very low amplitude ($\pm$ 1 mV) and requires high amplification gain on the sensor ($\pm$ 60 dB) [27]. For this reason, and since the generator is not capable of providing high resolution, low amplitude signals within the range of the ECG sensor, two independent PCBs were produced to accommodate both the signal of interest and the interference.

3.1   Considerations for PCB Design

When designing a PCB, there are good practices that can be employed to make sure it will be resilient to electromagnetic disturbances and, just as important, that it will not be a source of Electromagnetic Disturbance (EMD) for devices that might be present in the vicinity of the PCB being developed.

In a PCB, interference can be grouped in two categories: internal and external. The first is associated with signal degradation along the traces or transmission path due to crosstalk, for example, and leading to signal losses and reflections. As for the external issues, a PCB can be seen as a source of interference or a victim. In the first case, radiated emissions might occur associated with periodic signals or harmonics of clocks. In the case of susceptibility, it should not be disregarded that PCBs, independently of how small they might be, may be affected by EMD or RF disturbances as these can couple into input/output lines which in turn carry the interfering signal to the ICs they are connected to.

The probability of occurrence and severity of consequences of these are dependent of various parameters: the frequency, the amplitude, the duration (continuous or transient), the impedance (of both source and victim) and the dimensions of the emitting device. Most of these parameters can be tailored when designing a PCB. The length of traces and its inherent impedance, for example, is one of the most versatile and customizable feature of a PCB that can play a major role in determining its emission and susceptibility behaviour, as it they are directly related to transmission paths to RF signals [28].

However simple these guidelines might be, it is important to take them into consideration from an early stage of the development of any PCB in general. For the system here presented, the following considerations were particularly addressed:

Multilayer PCB. Once the schematics of the product being developed have been finalized, it is time to design the board itself. When doing so, many constraints (technical or by design) exist that force the engineer to compromise on some aspects in favour of others. Among these aspects, one of the first is the number of layers that the PCB will contain. In fact, even if on the outside most people only see the top and bottom of the PCB where the components are placed, most PCBs have in fact 4, 6, 8, 10 or more layers interconnected between them and with different purposes (Fig. 3).

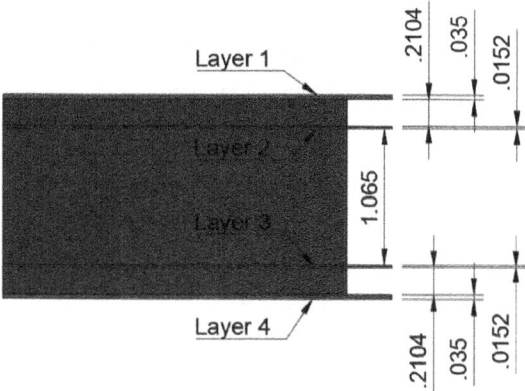

Fig. 3. Cross section of the PCB showing the different layers that compose it. All units are in millimeters. Adapted from [29].

The two PCBs used in this system use 4 layers instead of the simpler 2 layer PCB. With the compromise of slightly increase the complexity and potentially the cost, there are advantages in this configuration that justify the decision. Choosing a 4 layer PCB not only provides with more options to run the traces that connect the different components of the devices but also, and more importantly, provide more signal integrity by using ground and power planes effectively reducing crosstalk and EMI. The configuration employed for the PCB developed for this system is as follows:

- Layer 1 (or top layer) is where all the components are placed. Here, only small traces are connecting pins of different components to reduce potential antennas that could pick up noise from the environment. Those who are spaced far from each other are connected via an internal layer (Layer 3) protecting the longer traces with the surrounding planes.
- Layer 2 and 4 are ground planes. While in simple applications a trace connecting the ground pins might be sufficient, having Layer 2 as a ground plane provides a more stable reference plane to all the components placed on Layer 1, even in high frequencies [30]. Furthermore, having the two planes connected to each other with a dense network of vias, and in combination with via fencing on the boarder of the PCB, a Faraday cage is created protecting layer 3 from all interference presenting a wavelength greater than the distance between two vias [31].
- Layer 3 is used to route the signal traces connecting the different components on the top layer. In addition, it also provides a power plane to supply all the active components directly to the pin through a via.

Fencing and Via Spacing. As mentioned in Sect. 2, the decreasing size of IC used in current days has lead to smaller final products, more ergonomic and practical to use but also considerably more complex. In truth, as the components decrease in size, the problems associated with signal integrity and crosstalk increase. Therefore, it is important that the two ground planes used in this configuration have a good connection by the means of via spacing and via fencing to prevent signals from propagating within the PCB and out of it through the edges where it can propagate radially. Having two ground planes shielding high speed traces might not only protect them but also serve as a waveguide that can lead the radiated energy from the traces to the edges of the showing the different. This phenomenon constitutes one of the main sources of radiated interference from PCBs [31,32] (Fig. 4).

Power Supply Decoupling. Active components, such as the ones commonly found in wearable devices and mentioned above, rely on a stable power supply. Some of these devices rely on LDOs to achieve this goal but, as mentioned above (Sect. 2), these have been shown to be susceptible to EMI. Additional measures must be implemented to ensure that power lines supplying the different components are as stable as possible. For this, a common solution is to use decoupling capacitors to compensate fluctuation in the voltage level associated with high frequency noise. These shall be placed as close as possible to the power supply pins of each active component.

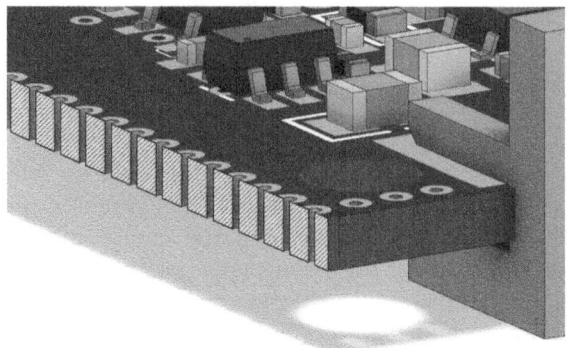

Fig. 4. Fencing used around the PCB's to prevent radially propagated electromagnetic emissions. Adapted from [29].

Coaxial Connections. In order to be able to predict and characterize the signals being used, these must arrive to the DUT as close to the signal generated as possible. The best way to protect them from external signal that could superpose is by using coaxial cables that shield the signal of interest between the source and the end connection. Just like traditional signal generator, the Analog Discovery 2 allows the use of BNC connections to output the signals. By placing an SMA connector on the PCB we are able to use a BNC to SMA cable to guide the signals of interest to the PCBs designed (Fig. 5).

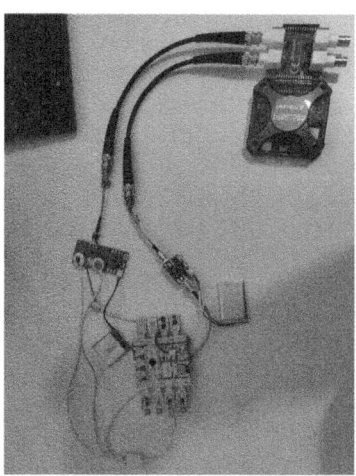

Fig. 5. System assembled with the signal generator connected to both PCBs via coaxial cables.

3.2   ECG Signal Simulator

The PCB created for the simulation of the ECG signal has three main goals: convert the single ended signal into a differential one, adapt the amplitude of the signal generated by the Analog Discovery 2 and create an interface for the electrode lead wires of the DUT to connect easily (Fig. 6).

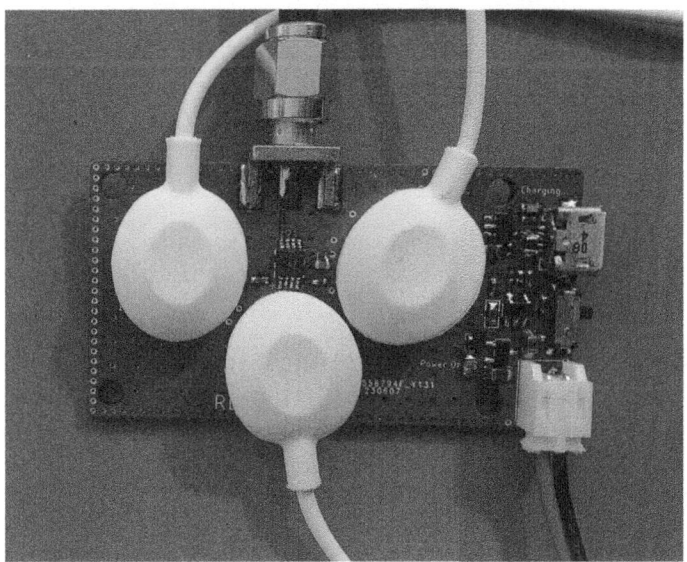

Fig. 6. PCB designed to convert and adapt a simulated single ended ECG signal into a differential one.

As mentioned above, the DAC of the generator has 14 bits resolution rending it capable of producing very high resolution signals. The ECG signal however, is a very low amplitude signal. The limitation of the DAC is the ability to generate small amplitude signals. In this case, only the least signifiant bits are used producing a low resolution, staircase like signal. In order to improve the resolution of the signal obtained, we create a high amplitude, high resolution signal using the full scale of the DAC and reduce the amplitude of the resulting signal using a voltage divider implemented on the showing the different. In addition, the ECG signal must be converted from single ended to differential for the ECG sensor to acquire it. For this purpose, a dedicate IC is used, the LTC6363. The two outputs of this device will be referenced to a voltage level provided by the acquisition device.

Finally, the PCB is fitted with three snap connectors mimicking the electrodes that would be placed on the body and to which the electrode lead wires can be easily connected to.

3.3   Direct Power Injection Board

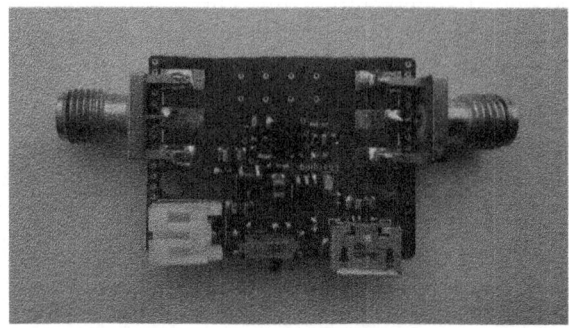

Fig. 7. PCB for direct power injection.

For the particular case of ECG acquisition, a dedicated board was designed to inject a disturbing signal using DPI. This PCB is at the interface of the signal generator and the DUT. In this application, the sensor being studied presents a very high gain to be able to amplify the ECG signal to a value that can be read by the microcontroller. If a high amplitude disturbance is injected in this port, the amplifier will easily saturate and no conclusions can be drawn from the tests (Fig. 7).

The PCB developed has the purpose of not only providing a stable and protected connection from the signal generator to the DUT using shielded cables and SMA connectors but also accommodate the signal, decreasing its amplitude with a voltage divider.

This system is intended to be used with various types of disturbances, not only simple continuous-wave signals. To be able to have complex signals correctly represented and with good resolution, the full scale of the DAC is used, similarly to the ECG signal generator.

4   Validation

The device chosen to validate the system here proposed is a BITalino (r)evolution board (PLUX Wireless Biosignals, Lisbon, Portugal). Given its small form factor and ability to be customized into wearable devices capable of ECG acquisition, it was a good candidate to verify its resilience to EMI while acquiring an ECG signal and transmitting it to a nearby computer via Bluetooth.

A particular weakness in the realm of biosignals is the susceptibility to the 50 Hz noise coming from the mains supply. In a real scenario this signal can couple capacitively to the human body and the electrode cables of the system. Here, the human body is not taken into account but the electrode cables might act as antenna and pick up noise from the environment completely masking both the signal of interest and, in this case the synthesized disturbances. To protect the system from this situation, a metallic enclosure is used. Even though it is not completely sealed, the biggest apertures were carefully planned to be small enough to prevent the 50 Hz noise from reaching to the components inside while allowing for the Bluetooth connection to remain established.

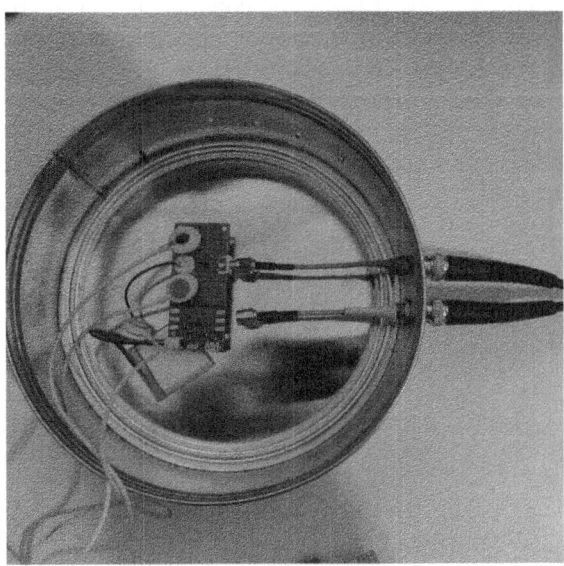

Fig. 8. Enclosure used to protect the setup. A lid (not present in this figure) completes the enclosure, protecting the system inside.

As illustrated by Fig. 8, the enclosure was fitted with BNC feedthroughs so that the shielded cables carrying the signals from the signal generator could easily connect to the box. On the inside, the feedthroughs were connected to SMA cables which in turn lead to the two PCBs. With this system in place, both signals are safely transferred from the signal generator to the two PCBs. From the PCB's, the ECG simulator is connected to the DUT using snap connectors and the disturbance is injected into the board using a probe to allow for testing of different points.

Test Cases

The test cases here reported have been previously presented in more detail in conference and aim to reproduce experiments conducted in an anechoic environment [29].

Test Case 1. The first test reproduced in with this system, aimed to reproduce a previous work by Bastian et al. [33] where the effects of small deviations on the modulating frequency used in standardised test procedures are investigating. This work targeted protocols such as the one proposed by IEC61000-4-3 where the interference is modulated by a 1 kHz sine wave AM at 80% depth [34]. In their work, Bastian et al. were able to demonstrate by changing modulating frequency in small increments that when this frequency matched the sampling frequency of the DUT, some failure modes might be missed. This test case aims to reproduce the same phenomenon and see if the same conclusions can be drawn. While the DUT is acquiring a simulated ECG signal, a high frequency signal modulated in amplitude at 80% depth with a carrier of 1 kHz is injected in the DUT. The live stream of the signal acquired shows no difference, however, when an increment of 0.1 kHz is made, the effects on the ECG signal are clearly visible. Figure 9 allows to see the moment where the increment was made and the effects it had on the signal of interest.

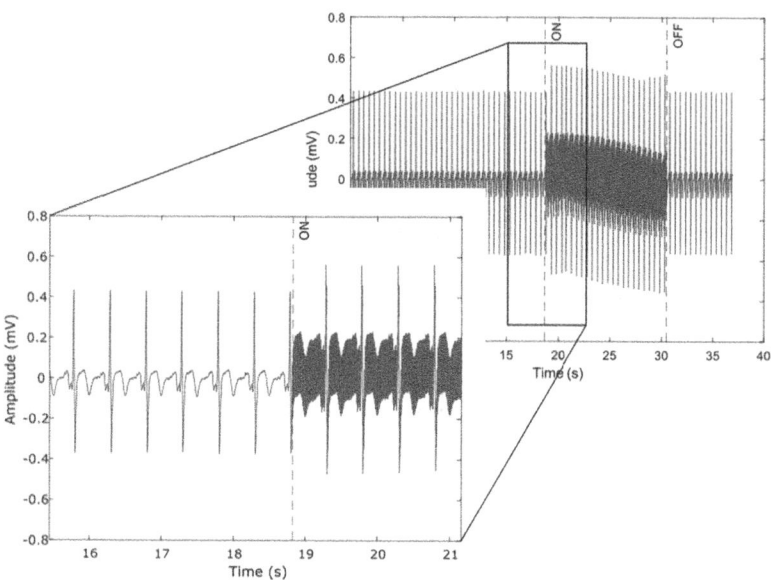

Fig. 9. Acquired ECG in the presence of a disturbance modulated at 1.1 kHz. Adapted from [29].

Test Case 2. In another case study, we tried to demonstrate the effects of having a low frequency AM modulation near a biosignals acquisition device. Once again, this has been attempted in anechoic environment using a 20 Hz AM modulation at 80% depth [35]. Similarly to the first case here presented, we inject an interference AM modulated by a 20 Hz signal at 80% depth. The interference was injected in the input pin of ECG sensor. With a passing band comprised between 0.5 Hz and 40 Hz the ECG sensor picks up the modulating signal rending which superposed to the signal of interest rending the latter unexploitable. Figure 10 shows the signal acquired where it is clear the moment where the interference was activated and deactivated.

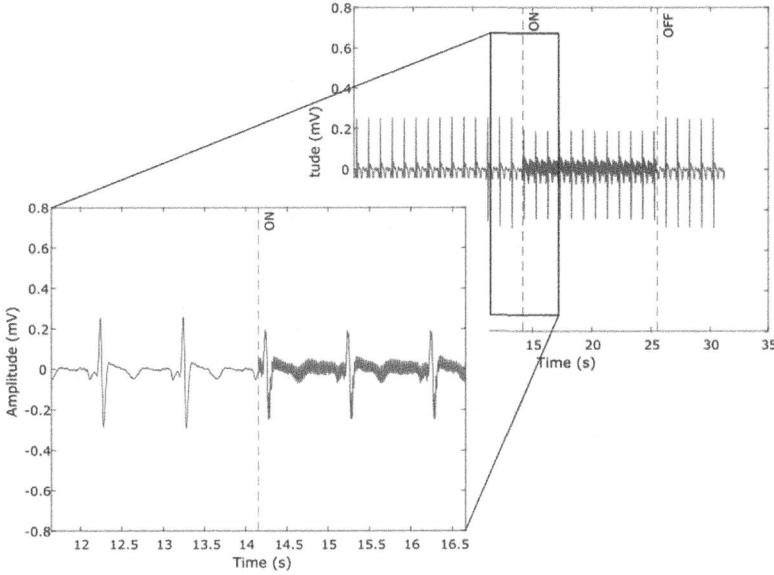

Fig. 10. Acquired ECG in the presence of a disturbance modulated at 20 Hz. Adapted from [29].

5   Conclusions

In a world where the number of incidents with medical devices associated with EMI is increasing every year and with a society increasingly relying on electrical medical equipment, it is of paramount importance that appropriate measures are taken when developing these devices. Common tests performed in anechoic environments are often out of reach for most SME's. This, however, should not be seen as an excuse not to conduct proper evaluation of a device throughout its development when other solutions exist using affordable equipment commonly found in most laboratories. DPI is a good example of a well established methodology for assessing a device's susceptibility to a wide range of interference using benchtop equipment within reach to most SME's, researchers or even students. The solution here presented demonstrates the possibility of reproducing some of the tests conducted in anechoic environment leading to the same conclusions.

Acknowledgements. The research leading to these results has received funding from the European Union's EU Framework Programme for Research and Innovation Horizon 2020 under Grant Agreement No. 955.816.

Disclosure of Interests. The authors have no competing interests to declare that are relevant to the content of this article.

References

1. Alaeldine, A., Perdriau, R., Ramdani, M., Levant, J.L., Drissi, M.: A direct power injection model for immunity prediction in integrated circuits. IEEE Trans. Electromagn. Compatibil. **50**(1), 52–62 (2008)
2. Sinha, S.: State of IoT 2023: Number of connected IoT devices growing 16% to 16.7 billion globally. Technical report (2023)
3. Vailshery, L.S.: IoT connected devices worldwide 2019–2030. Technical report (2023)
4. Celik, N., Manivannan, N., Strudwick, A., Balachandran, W.: Graphene-enabled electrodes for electrocardiogram monitoring. Nanomaterials (Basel) **6**(9), 156 (2016)
5. Yoo, J., Yan, L., Lee, S., Kim, H., Yoo, H.-J.: A wearable ECG acquisition system with compact planar-fashionable circuit board-based shirt. IEEE Trans. Inf Technol. Biomed. **13**(6), 897–902 (2009)
6. Osório, D.N., et al.: Comparison of different polymeric materials for mobile off-the-person ECG. In: Inácio, P.R.M., Duarte, A., Fazendeiro, P., Pombo, N. (eds.) HealthyIoT 2018. EICC, pp. 15–22. Springer, Cham (2020). https://doi.org/10.1007/978-3-030-30335-8_2
7. Ritchie, H., Roser, M.: Causes of death. Our World in Data (2018)
8. World Health Organization. The top 10 causes of death. Technical report (2020)
9. Rodgers, J.L., et al.: Cardiovascular risks associated with gender and aging. J. Cardiovasc. Dev. Dis. **6**(2), 19 (2019)
10. Lymberis, A., de Rossi, D.: Wearable EHealth Systems for Personalised Health Management: State of the Art and Future Challenges. IOS Press, Amsterdam (2004)
11. Kroll, R.R., et al.: Use of wearable devices for post-discharge monitoring of ICU patients: a feasibility study. J. Intensive Care **5**(1), 64 (2017)
12. Baranchuk, A., et al.: Electromagnetic interference of communication devices on ECG machines. Clin. Cardiol. **32**(10), 588–592 (2009)
13. Smuck, M., Odonkor, C.A., Wilt, J.K., Schmidt, N., Swiernik, M.A.: The emerging clinical role of wearables: factors for successful implementation in healthcare. NPJ Dig. Med. **4**(1), 1–8 (2021)
14. Lin, L., et al.: Wearable health devices in health care: narrative systematic review. JMIR Mhealth Uhealth **8**(11), e18907
15. Lavarda, A., Deutschmann, B.: Direct power injection (DPI) simulation framework and postprocessing. In: Proceedings of IEEE International Symposium on Electromagnetic Compatibility - EMC Europe, pp. 1248–1253 (2015)
16. Lavarda, A., Deutschmann, B., Haerle, D.: Enhancement of the DPI method for IC immunity characterization. In: Proceedings of International Workshop on the Electromagnetic Compatibility of Integrated Circuits (EMCCompo), pp. 178–183 (2017)
17. Wu, J., Sicard, E., Ndoye, A.C., Lafon, F., Li, J., Shen, R.: Investigation on DPI effects in a low dropout voltage regulator. In: Proceedings of the 8th Workshop on Electromagnetic Compatibility of Integrated Circuits, pp. 153–158 (2011)

18. Langer EMV - ICIM DPI, Measurement service IC Immunity Measurement Direct Power Injection (DPI) acc. IEC 62132-4. https://www.langer-emv.de/en/product/immunity/43/icim-dpi-measurement-service-ic-immunity-measurement-direct-power-injection-dpi-acc-iec-62132-4/864

19. IEC. IEC 62132-4:2006 Integrated circuits - Measurement of electromagnetic immunity 150 kHz to 1 GHz - Part 4: Direct RF power injection method (2006)

20. Pues, H., Pissoort, D.: Design of IEC 62132-4 compliant DPI test Boards that work up to 2 GHz. In: Proceedings of IEEE International Symposium on Electromagnetic Compatibility - EMC EUROPE 2012, pp. 1–4 (2012)

21. Miropolsky, S., Frei, S.: Comparability of RF immunity test methods for IC design purposes. In: Proceedings of the 8th Workshop on Electromagnetic Compatibility of Integrated Circuits, pp. 59–64 (2011)

22. Dai, S., Lu, X.J., Zhang, Y., Liu, L., Fang, W.: Electromagnetic conductive immunity of a microcontroller by direct power injection. In: Proceedings of International Conference on Integrated Circuits and Microsystems (ICICM), pp. 280–284 (2021)

23. Deutschmann, B., Winkler, G.: Characterizing the electromagnetic immunity of operational amplifiers based on EMIRR and DPI. In: Proceedings of International Symposium on Electromagnetic Compatibility – EMC Europe, pp. 1–4 (2023)

24. Richelli, A., Delaini, G., Grassi, M., Redouté, J.-M.: Susceptibility of operational amplifiers to conducted EMI injected through the ground plane into their output terminal. IEEE Trans. Reliab. **65**(3), 1369–1379 (2016)

25. Richelli, A., Colalongo, L., Kovacs-Vajna, Z.: EMI susceptibility of the output pin in CMOS amplifiers. Electronics **9**(2), 304 (2020)

26. Richelli, A., Colalongo, L., Toninelli, L., Rusu, I., Redouté, J.-M.: Measurements of EMI susceptibility of precision voltage references. In: Proceedings of International Workshop on the Electromagnetic Compatibility of Integrated Circuits (EMC-Compo), pp. 162–167 (2017)

27. Singh, Y.N., Singh, S.K., Ray, A.K.: Bioelectrical signals as emerging biometrics: issues and challenges. Int. Schol. Res. Notices **2012**(1), 712032 (2012)

28. Montrose, M.I.: Printed Circuit Board Design Techniques for EMC Compliance: A Handbook for Designers, 2 edn. IEEE Press Series on Electronics Technology. IEEE Press, Piscataway (2000)

29. Nunes, T., Da Silva, H.P., Gamboa, H.: Development of an affordable emc immunity assessment setup using direct power injection for biosignals instrumentation: application to ECG monitoring. In: Proceedings of the 17th International Joint Conference on Biomedical Engineering Systems and Technologies, Rome, Italy, pp. 82–87. SCITEPRESS - Science and Technology Publications (2024)

30. Armstrong, M.K.: PCB design techniques for lowest-cost EMC compliance. Part 1. Electron. Commun. Eng. J. **11**(4), 185–194 (1999)

31. Lindseth, W.: Effectiveness of PCB perimeter Via fencing: radially propagating EMC emissions reduction technique. In: Proceedings of IEEE International Symposium on Electromagnetic Compatibility - EMC Europe, pp. 627–632 (2016)

32. Suntives, A., Khajooeizadeh, A., Abhari, R.: Using via fences for crosstalk reduction in PCB circuits. In: Proceedings of IEEE International Symposium on Electromagnetic Compatibility, EMC Europe, vol. 1, pp. 34–37 (2006)

33. Bastian, G.G., Nunes, T.P., Quílez, M., Fernández-Chimeno, M., Silva, F.: Analysis of the effect of deviated modulating signal characteristics on the susceptibility of a small medical device. In: Proceedings of International Symposium on Electromagnetic Compatibility – EMC Europe 2023, pp. 1–6 (2023)
34. CENELEC. Medical Electrical Equipment—Part 1–2: General Requirements for Basic Safety and Essential Performance—Collateral Standard: Electromagnetic Disturbances—Requirements and Tests (2015)
35. Nunes, T.P., Quílez, M., Fernández-Chimeno, M., Silva, F., da Silva, H.P.: Stage-by-stage evaluation of a biomedical system regarding its electromagnetic susceptibility. In: Proceedings of International Symposium on Electromagnetic Compatibility – EMC Europe 2023, pp. 1–6 (2023)

Bioimaging

A Comparative Study of Deep Neural Network Architectures in Magnification Invariant Breast Cancer Histopathology Image Analysis

Pranav Jeevan$^{(\boxtimes)}$[iD], Nikhil Cherian Kurian[iD], and Amit Sethi[iD]

Department of Electrical Engineering, Indian Institute of Technology Bombay, Mumbai, India
{pranavjp.ee,nikhilkurian,asethi}@iitb.ac.in

Abstract. Deep Neural networks are prevalent in medical image analysis, yet their performance deteriorates when there is a mismatch between the magnification levels of training and testing images. This study evaluates the robustness of various deep learning architectures for breast cancer histopathological image classification under differing magnification scales. We compare CNN-based models like ResNet and MobileNet, self-attention-based Vision Transformers and Swin Transformers, and token-mixing models such as FNet, ConvMixer, MLP-Mixer, and WaveMix. Using the BreakHis dataset, which includes images at multiple magnification levels, we demonstrate that WaveMix achieves stable and high classification accuracy, regardless of magnification differences between training and testing data. Our findings underscore the importance of selecting robust deep learning architectures capable of handling domain shifts, such as magnification variation, to ensure reliable performance in histopathological image analysis. Additionally, we assess the classification performance using popular off-the-shelf, pre-trained computer vision backbones to identify suitable models for medical applications.

Keywords: Histopathology · Classification · Vision-transformer · Token-mixers · Generalization

1 Introduction

Computer-aided medical image analysis is becoming increasingly essential for diagnosing and treating various diseases [2,6]. Convolutional neural networks (CNNs) are the most frequently used deep learning models in this field [17]. These models have achieved near-human performance in analyzing medical images, including magnetic resonance imaging (MRI), computed tomography (CT), and histology images, when training and testing data come from the same sources [3,7]. However, their effectiveness can be compromised by factors such as variations in image quality, lighting conditions, and magnification scales. Specifically, differences in magnification scales between training and testing datasets can significantly impact the accuracy and robustness of deep learning models in medical image analysis [8]. Training a CNN on images at one magnification scale typically results in high performance at that scale, but this does not necessarily generalize to other scales [1]. This issue is particularly problematic in histology imaging, where magnification changes are common due to varying

M. P. Guarino et al. (Eds.): BIOSTEC 2024, CCIS 2546, pp. 121–133, 2026.
https://doi.org/10.1007/978-3-031-96899-0_8

sensors and lenses across different hospitals and datasets. Although augmenting input images with scale perturbations can marginally improve CNN performance, there is a pressing need to develop deep learning architectures that can inherently produce features invariant to scale changes. Such architectures must be capable of capturing crucial image features regardless of magnification variations to ensure reliable performance in clinical settings.

In this study, we assess the robustness of various popular deep learning architectures under conditions where the magnification of test data differs from the training data. We evaluate CNN-based models such as ResNet [10] and MobileNet [12], self-attention-based models including vision transformers (VIT) [5] and swin transformers [19], as well as token mixing models like Fourier-Net (FNet) [16], ConvMixer [27], Multi-Layer Perceptron-Mixer (MLP-Mixer) [26], and WaveMix [15]. Our experiments use the BreakHis [24] dataset, which contains breast cancer histopathological images at different magnification levels. By comparing the empirical performance of these models, we aim to identify the most robust architecture for histopathological image analysis when faced with magnification variations.

In the medical domain, deep learning practitioners commonly rely on popular machine learning libraries, such as TorchVision [22]. They often use off-the-shelf pre-trained models, which are then fine-tune on specific medical datasets. This approach is favored because medical machine learning practitioners typically have access to limited data, and using pre-trained networks has been shown to improve performance and accelerate convergence compared to training models from scratch. However, many practitioners tend to select models that have achieved the highest accuracy on the ImageNet dataset without considering the specific distribution of their medical data. This practice can be misleading, as the domain of natural images in ImageNet significantly differs from that of medical images, such as histology or radiology. This discrepancy highlights the need for careful model selection tailored to the unique characteristics of medical imaging datasets. To assist machine learning practitioners in selecting the most suitable pre-trained computer vision backbones, we have chosen some of the most commonly used lightweight machine learning backbones and provide an empirical comparison of their performance on the BreakHis Histopathology dataset. This comparison aims to offer a clearer understanding of which models are most effective for specific medical image classification tasks, helping practitioners make more informed decisions for their applications.

2   Experiments

2.1   Dataset

We used the BreakHis dataset [24], a well-known public resource of digital breast histopathology images, for our experiments. The BreakHis dataset has been extensively used in the development and evaluation of computer-aided diagnosis (CAD) systems for breast cancer [4]. It offers a challenging benchmark for CAD system development due to the significant variations in tissue appearances, making it an ideal choice for assessing the robustness and performance of different machine learning models.

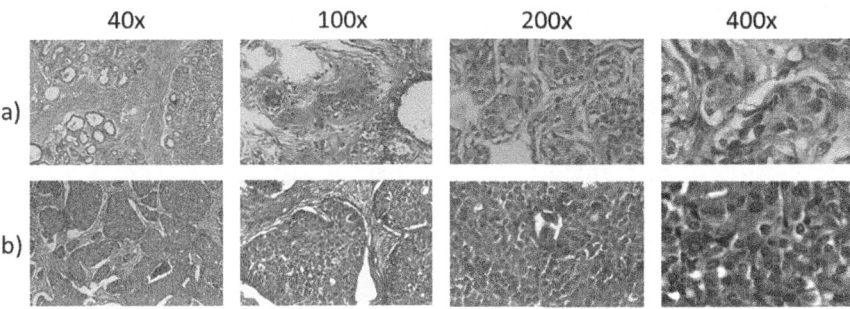

Fig. 1. BreakHis dataset contains images at four different magnifications: $40\times$, $100\times$, $200\times$, and $400\times$. The top row shows (a) benign images, and bottom row shows (b) malignant images at four different magnification levels [14].

The BreakHis dataset consists of 7,909 microscopy images of breast tissue biopsy specimens from 82 patients diagnosed with either benign or malignant breast tumors. These images, collected from four different institutions, are provided at four different magnification scales: $40\times$, $100\times$, $200\times$, and $400\times$, corresponding to objective lenses of $4\times$, $10\times$, $20\times$, and $40\times$, respectively, as illustrated in Fig. 1. This variety in magnification scales adds another layer of complexity and makes the dataset particularly useful for evaluating the performance of machine learning models in handling different magnifications.

In addition to the malignancy information for each image, the BreakHis dataset includes further annotations with clinical information such as the patient's age, the subtype of malignancy, and the type of biopsy performed. The dataset is slightly imbalanced, both in terms of the distribution of benign versus malignant cases and the distribution of different magnifications. Specifically, there are 5,429 malignant cases compared to only 2,480 benign cases. This imbalance adds another challenge for developing and evaluating robust machine learning models for histopathological image analysis.

As the BreakHis dataset contains multiple images at different magnification levels, it serves as a challenging and representative test bed for evaluating the robustness of deep learning architectures across various magnification scales. To assess this robustness, we will train several recently reported deep learning architectures on one magnification level of the BreakHis dataset and test these trained models across multiple held-out magnification levels. By observing the average test accuracy across different magnification levels, we can determine how well these deep learning architectures handle varying image magnifications during inference.

To compare the performance of the pre-trained backbones, we calculate the classification accuracy for each magnification level separately and then averaged the results across all four magnification levels. This approach allows us to identify which of the selected models could best handle histopathology images, providing a clearer understanding of their suitability for this application.

Table 1. Train-validation-test split of the BreakHis dataset in our experiments for each magnification [14].

Magnification	Train	Validation	Test
40×	1395	201	399
100×	1455	209	417
200×	1408	202	403
400×	1273	182	365

2.2 Models

CNNs and Vision Transformers. For the CNN-based models, we assessed the performance of ResNet-18, ResNet-34, and ResNet-50 from ResNet family [10], as well as MobileNetV3-small-0.50, MobileNetV3-small-0.75, and MobileNetV3-small-100 from the MobileNet series. In addition, we conducted experiments with ViT-Tiny, ViT-Small, and ViT-Base (each using a patch size of 16, as detailed in [5]), along with Swin-Tiny and Swin-Base (both utilizing a patch size of 4 and a window size of 7, see [19]).

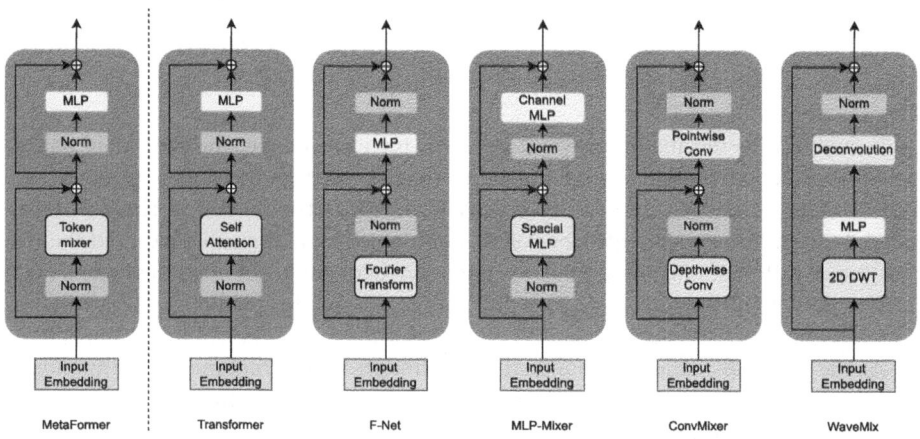

Fig. 2. Architectures of various token-mixers along with the general MetaFormer block where the token-mixing operation in different models is performed by different operations, such as spatial MLP, depth-wise convolution, self-attention, Fourier and wavelet transforms [14].

Token-Mixers. Token-mixers are a family of models that use an architecture similar to MetaFormer [29] as their fundamental block, as illustrated in Fig. 2. Transformer models can be considered token-mixing models that utilize self-attention for token-mixing. Other token-mixers employ different operations for token-mixing, such as Fourier transforms (FNet) [16], Wavelet transforms (WaveMix) [15], spatial-MLP (MLP-Mixer) [26], and depth-wise convolutions (ConvMixer) [27]. These token-mixing models have been shown to be more efficient in terms of parameters and computation compared to attention-based transformers [29].

FNet [16] was initially designed for natural language processing (NLP) tasks to handle 1D input sequences. It demonstrated impressive performance compared to transformer-based large language models in terms of parameter efficiency and speed. In our study, we used a modified version of FNet, known as 2D-FNet, which employs a 2D Fourier transform for spatial token-mixing instead of the 1D Fourier transform used in the original FNet. The 2D-FNet can process images in their 2D form without needing to convert them into sequences of patches or pixels, as is required in transformers and the original FNet. We conducted experiments by varying the embedding dimension and the number of layers to find the best model hyper-parameters.

WaveMix [15] employs the 2D-Discrete Wavelet Transform (2D-DWT) for token-mixing. This approach has demonstrated accuracy, efficiency, and robustness across various computer vision tasks, including image classification and semantic segmentation. In our experiments, we varied the embedding dimension, the number of layers, and the number of levels of 2D-DWT used in WaveMix to identify the model configuration that achieved the highest validation accuracy on the dataset.

ConvMixer [27] utilizes depth-wise convolutions for spatial token-mixing and point-wise convolutions for channel token-mixing. ConvMixer has demonstrated impressive parametric efficiency in image classification performance across various datasets. For our experiments, we used ConvMixer-1536/20, ConvMixer-768/32, and ConvMixer-1024/20 models available in the Timm model library [28].

MLP-Mixer [26] employs spatial MLP and channel MLP to mix spatial and channel tokens, respectively. In our experiments, we used MLP-Mixer-Small (with a patch size of 16) and MLP-Mixer-Base (also with a patch size of 16).

Pre-trained Torchvision Backbones. To compare the performance of pre-trained backbones on fine-tuning using histopathology images, we selected eleven of the most widely used backbones available in Torchvision [22] and Github. These models include WaveMix [15], ResNet-50 [10], ConvNeXt-Tiny [20], Swin-Transformer-Tiny [19], Swin-TransformerV2-Tiny [18], EfficientNet-V2 [25], DenseNet [13], MobileNet-V3 [11], RegNet [23], ResNeXt-50 [23], and ShuffleNetV2 [21]. We choose models less than 30 million parameters since most practitioners use lightweight models. These pre-trained backbones were initially trained for the classification of images in ImageNet-1k dataset.

2.3   Implementation Details

The dataset was partitioned into training, validation, and test sets in a 7:1:2 ratio for each magnification level, as shown in Table 1. Due to limited computational resources, the training process was capped at a maximum of 300 epochs. All experiments were conducted using a single 80 GB Nvidia A100 GPU, and all models were trained from scratch on the BreakHis dataset without any pre-trained weights. We utilized ResNet, MobileNet, Vision Transformer, Swin Transformer, ConvMixer, and MLP-Mixer models available in the Timm (PyTorch Image Models) library [28]. Since WaveMix and FNet were not available in the Timm library, they were implemented based on their original research papers. The Timm training script [28] with default hyper-parameter settings was used for all models. Cross-entropy loss was employed for training, and automatic mixed precision in PyTorch was used to enhance speed and memory efficiency.

For the experiments, the images were resized to 672×448. However, for transformer-based models and the MLP-Mixer, the images needed to be resized to 384×384 and 224×224, respectively. We trained models of varying sizes within the same architecture on the training set and evaluated their performance on the validation set to determine the optimal model size for the BreakHis dataset [24]. The model size that achieved the highest average validation performance across all magnifications was then used for evaluation on the test set.

For the task of measuring the fine-tuning performance of pre-trained backbones, all images were resized to 672×448 pixels. We used the implementation of these models available in the TorchVision library, utilizing the pre-trained ImageNet weights provided by TorchVision [22]. We reported the class-weighted accuracy of these pre-trained backbones for better comparison.

Table 2. Results (test accuracy) of cross-magnification classification performance of all CNNs, transformers and token-mixers on BreakHis [24] dataset [14].

CNNs

ResNet-34

Training Magnification	Testing Magnification				Average testing performance over all magnifications
	40×	100×	200×	400×	
40×	94.74	92.81	81.89	84.11	88.38
100×	88.72	95.20	90.32	90.69	91.23
200×	86.97	89.21	95.53	93.43	91.28
400×	78.20	85.61	87.10	96.44	86.84

MobileNetV3-Small 075

Training Magnification	Testing Magnification				Average testing performance over all magnifications
	40×	100×	200×	400×	
40×	92.48	91.13	84.62	82.19	87.60
100×	87.47	89.69	88.59	89.04	88.70
200×	86.97	89.21	94.54	90.96	90.42
400×	85.71	86.81	90.07	94.79	89.35

Transformers

ViT-S/16

Training Magnification	Testing Magnification				Average testing performance over all magnifications
	40×	100×	200×	400×	
40×	89.72	86.33	85.11	69.04	82.55
100×	86.72	88.73	87.84	89.86	88.29
200×	86.47	88.49	87.35	88.49	87.70
400×	86.22	87.29	87.59	90.69	87.95

Swin-B

Training Magnification	Testing Magnification				Average testing performance over all magnifications
	40×	100×	200×	400×	
40×	91.48	87.05	75.43	70.68	81.16
100×	88.22	88.49	90.57	86.85	88.53
200×	85.97	89.21	92.06	88.22	88.86
400×	87.97	88.01	89.83	91.78	89.40

Token-Mixers

ConvMixer-1024/20

Training Magnification	Testing Magnification				Average testing performance over all magnifications
	40×	100×	200×	400×	
40×	96.49	88.49	81.14	81.92	87.01
100×	89.22	96.40	90.07	85.75	90.36
200×	87.47	91.61	96.28	92.33	**91.92**
400×	85.46	88.73	90.57	95.62	90.09

MLP-Mixer-S/16

Training Magnification	Testing Magnification				Average testing performance over all magnifications
	40×	100×	200×	400×	
40×	91.98	80.58	78.16	81.10	82.95
100×	86.72	88.73	87.84	89.86	88.29
200×	88.47	88.49	94.29	91.78	90.76
400×	83.46	86.57	84.86	87.67	85.64

WaveMix-224/10

Training Magnification	Testing Magnification				Average testing performance over all magnifications
	40×	100×	200×	400×	
40×	95.99	93.77	87.10	90.68	**91.88**
100×	89.97	94.72	92.31	89.86	**91.72**
200×	87.97	89.69	94.79	93.70	91.54
400×	89.31	88.49	91.47	97.69	**91.74**

FNet-256/8

Training Magnification	Testing Magnification				Average testing performance over all magnifications
	40×	100×	200×	400×	
40×	94.50	85.10	83.90	84.90	87.10
100×	88.70	89.00	84.70	83.40	87.50
200×	86.70	87.10	89.30	88.50	87.90
400×	84.70	82.50	86.40	87.90	85.40

The maximum batch-size was set to 128. For larger models, we reduced the batch-size so that it can fit in the GPU. Top-1 accuracy on the test set of the best of three runs with random initialization is reported as a generalization metric based on prevailing protocols [9]. We also reported the class-weighted accuracy of token-mixers to compensate for dataset imbalance.

3 Results and Discussion

3.1 Magnification Invariance

The cross-magnification classification performance of the top-performing model variants, including CNN, transformer, and token-mixer models, is presented in Table 2. It is evident that WaveMix outperforms all other models in maintaining high performance across different testing magnifications. Notably, only ConvMixer, another token-mixer, managed to surpass WaveMix in performance at one magnification level ($200\times$). Furthermore, WaveMix demonstrates the most stable accuracy, never dropping below 87%. In contrast, other well-performing models like ConvMixer and ResNet-34 exhibit instability, with their accuracy dropping to 81% and 78%, respectively. We attribute WaveMix's superior performance to the 2D wavelet transform's capability to capture multi-scale features and effectively mix spatial token information. Additionally, the use of deconvolution layers contributes to the rapid expansion of the receptive field after each wavelet block. The residual connections within each block facilitate multiple levels of wavelet transform on the feature maps, further enhancing long-range token-mixing.

As demonstrated in Fig. 3, WaveMix achieves the highest overall performance in terms of average testing accuracy across all magnifications. Furthermore, our analysis reveals that token-mixer models (green), including MLP-Mixer and FNet, exhibit performance levels comparable to those of transformer-based models (red). Notably, CNN-based models (blue) surpass the performance of transformer models (Table 3).

Table 3. Comparison of computational requirements and throughput of all the models for image classification on the BreakHis dataset [14].

Model	InputResolution	#Params	GPU consumption for batch size of 64 (GB)	Throughput (img/s)	
				Train	Inference
ResNet-34	672×448	21.3 M	37.6	107	80
MobileNetV3-Small 075	672×448	1.0 M	9.1	87	100
ViT-S/16	384×384	21.7 M	17.4	106	101
Swin-B	384×384	86.7 M	52.5	75	82
ConvMixer-1024/20	672×448	23.5 M	53.6	53	83
MLP-Mixer-S/16	224×224	18.0 M	10.3	141	104
FNet-256/8	672×448	2.4 M	1254.4	2	13
WaveMix-224/10	672×448	10.6 M	70.2	72	81

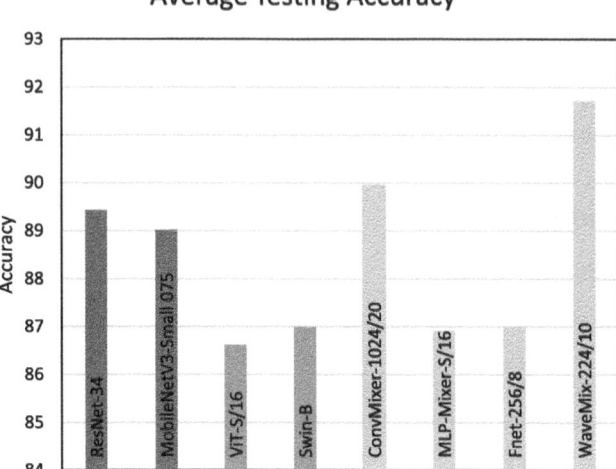

Fig. 3. Average of all test accuracy reported for various training magnifications for each of the models compared. [14]. (Color figure online)

Figure 4 presents the average test accuracy achieved when training and testing were conducted on the same magnifications. Our observations indicate that ConvMixer outperforms WaveMix under these conditions. Additionally, ResNet-34 demonstrates performance nearly on par with both WaveMix and ConvMixer. These results suggest that while other models exhibit strong performance when the magnifications of the training and test data are identical, they struggle to maintain this performance when there is a discrepancy in magnifications between the training and testing sets. In contrast, WaveMix shows a high degree of invariance to changes in magnification, consistently outperforming other CNN, transformer, and token-mixing models in such scenarios.

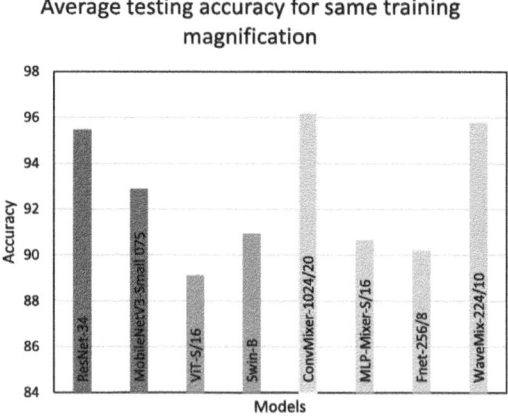

Fig. 4. Average test accuracy when training and testing was done on same magnification for each model [14].

To comprehensively evaluate the performance of all models on the BreakHis dataset, we also measure the class-weighted accuracy. This metric calculates accuracy for each class individually and then computes an overall accuracy using a weighted average, with weights based on the inverse of the class frequencies. Class-weighted accuracy is particularly valuable for imbalanced datasets, as it assigns greater importance to minority classes, which are often the primary focus in practical applications like cancer detection. Traditional accuracy metrics can be misleading on imbalanced datasets such as BreakHis, where malignant cases outnumber benign cases by more than 2:1. The class-weighted accuracy for all token-mixers is presented in Table 4, revealing similar trends to those observed in Table 2, with WaveMix outperforming all other token-mixers.

Table 4. Cross-magnification classification performance of token-mixer models on the BreakHis dataset, evaluated using class-weighted accuracy. This metric accounts for class imbalance by assigning weights based on the inverse proportion of samples in each class, providing a more accurate reflection of model performance across different classes [14].

Token-Mixers										
ConvMixer-1024/20					MLP-Mixer-S/16					
Training Magnification	Testing Magnification				Average testing performance over all magnifications	Training Magnification	Testing Magnification				Average testing performance over all magnifications
	$40\times$	$100\times$	$200\times$	$400\times$			$40\times$	$100\times$	$200\times$	$400\times$	
$40\times$	93.58	85.93	85.41	80.59	86.38	$40\times$	89.19	85.67	81.25	71.85	81.99
$100\times$	86.89	90.35	86.38	79.12	85.69	$100\times$	82.16	85.11	87.84	86.77	85.47
$200\times$	88.35	90.75	96.32	91.76	**91.80**	$200\times$	83.39	84.27	92.94	89.68	87.57
$400\times$	81.32	81.69	83.2	96.21	85.61	$400\times$	83.46	83.57	84.86	86.57	84.62
WaveMix-224/10						F-Net-256/8					
Training Magnification	Testing Magnification				Average testing performance over all magnifications	Training Magnification	Testing Magnification				Average testing performance over all magnifications
	$40\times$	$100\times$	$200\times$	$400\times$			$40\times$	$100\times$	$200\times$	$400\times$	
$40\times$	91.03	90.70	83.00	81.23	**86.49**	$40\times$	85.61	84.11	83.50	79.66	83.22
$100\times$	93.59	96.48	90.20	85.23	**91.38**	$100\times$	83.36	84.79	83.25	82.36	83.44
$200\times$	85.78	90.94	98.51	90.37	91.40	$200\times$	82.31	84.43	86.99	86.03	84.94
$400\times$	82.33	84.95	85.81	96.87	**87.49**	$400\times$	71.33	75.40	82.36	83.33	78.10

FNet exhibited the highest GPU RAM consumption, utilizing 4 to 8 times more memory compared to other architectures. In the BreakHis classification task, CNN-based models significantly outperformed transformer-based models. A notable decline in performance was observed when transformer-based models were trained on $40\times$ magnification and then tested on other magnifications. A similar drop in accuracy was also noted for the MLP-Mixer when tested at $40\times$ magnification.

To address the potential impact of input resolution, we conducted additional experiments with higher resolutions for MLP-Mixer, ViT, and Swin-transformer. However, these adjustments did not yield any improvement over the initially reported results.

3.2 Pre-trained Backbone Performance

Among the pre-trained computer vision backbones we evaluated, a total of eleven models were tested. Among these, WaveMix, ResNet, MobileNetV3, and RegNet emerged as top performers at specific magnification levels as shown in Table 5. Notably, while MobileNetV3 showed strong performance at two magnifications and other models excelled at different magnifications, none achieved top performance consistently across all magnification levels. However, when considering the average accuracy across the four magnifications, WaveMix and EfficientNetV2 demonstrated the best overall performance among all models. This indicates that these two models maintain robust performance across varying magnifications.

Table 5. Class-weighted accuracy on the BreakHis dataset using popular computer vision backbones. The highest accuracy for each magnification is shown in bold, and the second highest accuracy is underlined.

Backbone	Breakhis Class Weighted Accuracy				
	40×	100×	200×	400×	total
WaveMix-192/16 (level 3)	99.38	99.38	98.35	**99.31**	**99.11**
ResNet-50	97.90	**99.51**	99.22	98.39	98.76
ConvNeXt-Tiny	94.94	90.43	88.28	88.70	90.59
Swin-Tiny	86.76	92.13	88.64	78.41	86.49
SwinV2-Tiny	88.24	90.18	87.46	83.67	87.39
EfficientNetV2-S	99.11	99.26	99.07	98.98	**99.11**
DenseNet-161	98.18	99.06	99.22	97.98	98.61
MobileNetV3-Large	99.53	98.02	**99.47**	98.91	98.98
RegNetY-3.2GF	**99.82**	99.18	**99.47**	97.93	99.10
ResNeXt-50 32×4d	99.43	99.14	99.32	98.02	98.98
ShuffleNetV2 ×2.0	99.36	98.59	99.20	97.92	98.77

Our analysis further reveals that the top-performing ImageNet pre-trained backbones do not exhibit the same level of performance in the medical domain, particularly with histopathology dataset. Specifically, models like ConvNeXt and Swin Transformer, which demonstrate high performance on natural images, do not show good fine-tuning performance on the BreakHis dataset. This discrepancy highlights the challenges and limitations of applying pre-trained models to specialized medical imaging tasks, indicating a need for models that can be more effectively adapted to the nuances of medical datasets.

The superior performance of WaveMix can be attributed to the inclusion of the 2D discrete wavelet transform, which enables the capture of low-frequency components from the images, unlike regular convolutional operations that focus more on high-frequency components. Additionally, the rapid expansion of the receptive field in WaveMix facilitates global information mixing, a feature absent in the other convolutional models. The lack of superior performance by the ConvNeXt architecture, which is a convolutional model with a large kernel depth-wise convolution, underscores that merely increasing the receptive field through large kernels is insufficient to enhance global token mixing and capture the detailed image features essential for medical image applications. This finding suggests that other factors, such as the ability to process low-frequency components also play a crucial role in achieving high performance in histopathological image analysis. Conversely, transformer-based models (Swin and SwinV2) performed poorly compared to other models, highlighting that even pre-trained transformer models struggle with fine-tuning tasks involving small medical images.

4   Conclusions

In our research, we examined the resilience of various deep learning models used for histopathological image analysis when subjected to different testing magnifications. We conducted a comparison across multiple architectures, including ResNet, MobileNet, Vision Transformers, Swin Transformers, FourierNet (FNet), ConvMixer, MLP-Mixer, and WaveMix, utilizing the BreakHis dataset [24]. The findings indicated that the WaveMix architecture, which naturally integrates multi-resolution features, consistently demonstrated superior robustness to variations in inference magnification, maintaining an accuracy of 87% or higher in all test conditions. The ability of WaveMix to focus on the low resolution features compared to other CNN models also contribute their superior performance. Furthermore, we assessed the effectiveness of fine-tuning ImageNet pre-trained computer vision backbones specifically for histopathology images. These insights emphasize the importance of adopting robust models like WaveMix in both histopathological and broader medical image analysis. By employing such architectures, the accuracy of deep learning systems is preserved despite the presence of anatomical features at varying scales, thereby enhancing the reliability of diagnostic outcomes in clinical environments.

References

1. Alkassar, S., Jebur, B.A., Abdullah, M.A., Al-Khalidy, J.H., Chambers, J.A.: Going deeper: magnification-invariant approach for breast cancer classification using histopathological images. IET Comput. Vision **15**(2), 151–164 (2021)
2. Chakraborty, S., Mali, K.: An overview of biomedical image analysis from the deep learning perspective. In: Research Anthology on Improving Medical Imaging Techniques for Analysis and Intervention, pp. 43–59 (2023)
3. Chan, H.P., Samala, R.K., Hadjiiski, L.M., Zhou, C.: Deep learning in medical image analysis. In: Deep Learning in Medical Image Analysis: Challenges and Applications, pp. 3–21 (2020)

4. Cherian Kurian, N., Sethi, A., Reddy Konduru, A., Mahajan, A., Rane, S.U.: A 2021 update on cancer image analytics with deep learning. Wiley Interdisc. Rev. Data Min. Knowl. Disc. **11**(4), e1410 (2021)

5. Dosovitskiy, A., et al.: An image is worth 16x16 words: transformers for image recognition at scale. In: International Conference on Learning Representations (2021). https://openreview.net/forum?id=YicbFdNTTy

6. Duncan, J.S., Ayache, N.: Medical image analysis: progress over two decades and the challenges ahead. IEEE Trans. Pattern Anal. Mach. Intell. **22**(1), 85–106 (2000)

7. Gupta, R.K., Nandgaonkar, S., Kurian, N.C., Rane, S., Sethi, A.: Egfr mutation prediction of lung biopsy images using deep learning. arXiv preprint arXiv:2208.12506 (2022)

8. Gupta, V., Bhavsar, A.: Breast cancer histopathological image classification: is magnification important? In: Proceedings of the IEEE Conference on Computer Vision and Pattern Recognition Workshops, pp. 17–24 (2017)

9. Hassani, A., Walton, S., Shah, N., Abuduweili, A., Li, J., Shi, H.: Escaping the big data paradigm with compact transformers (2021)

10. He, K., Zhang, X., Ren, S., Sun, J.: Deep residual learning for image recognition. In: Proceedings of the IEEE Conference on Computer Vision and Pattern Recognition, pp. 770–778 (2016)

11. Howard, A., et al.: Searching for mobilenetv3 (2019). https://arxiv.org/abs/1905.02244

12. Howard, A.G., et al.: MobileNets: efficient convolutional neural networks for mobile vision applications (2017)

13. Huang, G., Liu, Z., van der Maaten, L., Weinberger, K.Q.: Densely connected convolutional networks (2018). https://arxiv.org/abs/1608.06993

14. Jeevan., P., Kurian., N., Sethi., A.: Magnification invariant medical image analysis: A comparison of convolutional networks, vision transformers, and token mixers. In: Proceedings of the 17th International Joint Conference on Biomedical Engineering Systems and Technologies - BIOIMAGING, pp. 216–222. INSTICC, SciTePress (2024). https://doi.org/10.5220/0012362900003657

15. Jeevan, P., Viswanathan, K., S, A.A., Sethi, A.: Wavemix: a resource-efficient neural network for image analysis (2023)

16. Lee-Thorp, J., Ainslie, J., Eckstein, I., Ontanon, S.: Fnet: mixing tokens with Fourier transforms. arXiv preprint arXiv:2105.03824 (2021)

17. Li, Q., Cai, W., Wang, X., Zhou, Y., Feng, D.D., Chen, M.: Medical image classification with convolutional neural network. In: 2014 13th International Conference on Control Automation Robotics & Vision (ICARCV), pp. 844–848. IEEE (2014)

18. Liu, Z., et al.: Swin transformer v2: scaling up capacity and resolution (2022). https://arxiv.org/abs/2111.09883

19. Liu, Z., et al.: Swin transformer: hierarchical vision transformer using shifted windows. In: Proceedings of the IEEE/CVF International Conference on Computer Vision, pp. 10012–10022 (2021)

20. Liu, Z., Mao, H., Wu, C.Y., Feichtenhofer, C., Darrell, T., Xie, S.: A convnet for the 2020s (2022). https://arxiv.org/abs/2201.03545

21. Ma, N., Zhang, X., Zheng, H.T., Sun, J.: Shufflenet v2: practical guidelines for efficient cnn architecture design (2018). https://arxiv.org/abs/1807.11164

22. Maintainers, T., et al.: Torchvision: pytorch's computer vision library (2016). https://github.com/pytorch/vision

23. Radosavovic, I., Kosaraju, R.P., Girshick, R., He, K., Dollár, P.: Designing network design spaces (2020). https://arxiv.org/abs/2003.13678

24. Spanhol, F.A., Oliveira, L.S., Petitjean, C., Heutte, L.: A dataset for breast cancer histopathological image classification. IEEE Trans. Biomed. Eng. **63**(7), 1455–1462 (2015)

25. Tan, M., Le, Q.V.: Efficientnetv2: smaller models and faster training (2021). https://arxiv.org/abs/2104.00298

26. Tolstikhin, I.O., et al.: Mlp-mixer: an all-mlp architecture for vision. Adv. Neural. Inf. Process. Syst. **34**, 24261–24272 (2021)

27. Trockman, A., Kolter, J.Z.: Patches are all you need? arXiv preprint arXiv:2201.09792 (2022)

28. Wightman, R.: Pytorch image models (2019). https://github.com/rwightman/pytorch-image-models. https://doi.org/10.5281/zenodo.4414861

29. Yu, W., et al.: Metaformer is actually what you need for vision. In: Proceedings of the IEEE/CVF Conference on Computer Vision and Pattern Recognition, pp. 10819–10829 (2022)

Cross-Domain Evaluation of Few-Shot Classification Models: Natural Images vs. Histopathological Images

Ardhendu Sekhar[(✉)], Aditya Bhattacharya, Vinayak Goyal, Vrinda Goel, Aditya Bhangale, Ravi Kant Gupta, and Amit Sethi

Department of Electrical Engineering, Indian Institute of Technology Bombay, Mumbai, India
ardhendusekhar.playstore@gmail.com

Abstract. In this study, we investigate the performance of few-shot classification models across different domains, specifically natural images and histopathological images. We first train several few-shot classification models on natural images and evaluate their performance on histopathological images. Subsequently, we train the same models on histopathological images and compare their performance. We incorporated four histopathology datasets and one natural images dataset and assessed performance across 5-way 1-shot, 5-way 5-shot, and 5-way 10-shot scenarios using a selection of state-of-the-art classification techniques. Our experimental results reveal insights into the transferability and generalization capabilities of few-shot classification models between diverse image domains. We analyze the strengths and limitations of these models in adapting to new domains and provide recommendations for optimizing their performance in cross-domain scenarios. This research contributes to advancing our understanding of few-shot learning in the context of image classification across diverse domains.

Keywords: Few-shot classification · Deep learning · Medical imaging

1 Introduction

Few-shot learning has emerged as a powerful paradigm for addressing the challenges of classification tasks in scenarios where labeled data is scarce. By leveraging a small number of annotated examples, few-shot classification models can generalize effectively to new classes or domains. This capability holds significant promise for various real-world applications, particularly in medical imaging where labeled data is often limited and costly to obtain. However, the effectiveness of few-shot learning across diverse domains remains a topic of ongoing investigation. In this study, we explore the transferability and generalization capabilities of few-shot classification models across different domains, focusing specifically on natural images and histopathological images. Natural images, representative of everyday scenes and objects, present diverse visual characteristics, while histopathological images depict tissue samples at a microscopic level, typically used for medical diagnoses. Understanding how few-shot classification models perform when transitioning between these distinct domains is crucial for assessing

© The Author(s), under exclusive license to Springer Nature Switzerland AG 2026
M. P. Guarino et al. (Eds.): BIOSTEC 2024, CCIS 2546, pp. 134–148, 2026.
https://doi.org/10.1007/978-3-031-96899-0_9

their practical utility in real-world applications. Our investigation involves training several state-of-the-art few-shot classification models on natural image datasets and evaluating their performance on histopathological images. We then repeat the process in the reverse direction, training the same models on histopathological images and testing them on both natural and histopathological image datasets. By comparing the performance of these models across different domains, we aim to uncover insights into their adaptability and robustness in cross-domain classification tasks.

In this study, we conducted evaluations of several state-of-the-art few-shot classification techniques using histopathology medical datasets and a natural image dataset. Specifically, we utilized a dataset prepared by Komura et al. [6], FHIST [11] and Mini-Imagenet [22] for our experiments. Mini-Imagenet dataset is a standard natural image dataset meant for few-shot classification techniques. The FHIST dataset encompasses multiple histology datasets, including CRC-TP [3], NCT-CRC-HE-100K [4], LC25000 [1], and BreakHis [13]. For our experiments, we focused on CRC-TP, NCT-CRC-HE-100K, and LC25000 datasets. CRC-TP is a colon cancer dataset with six classes, while NCT-CRC-HE-100K is another colon cancer dataset with nine classes. LC25000 contains both lung and colon cancer images, featuring five classes. Additionally, we utilized a histology dataset introduced by Komura et al. [6], which comprises approximately 1.6 million cancerous image patches from 32 different organs in the body. The classes in this dataset are categorized based on distinct organ sites. We employed the datasets by Komura et al. [6] adn miniimagenet to train our few-shot classification models, which were subsequently evaluated on various FHIST datasets.

In our thorough investigation of few-shot classification methodologies, we have systematically integrated a range of state-of-the-art techniques to ensure a comprehensive evaluation. The methodologies employed in our experiments encompass Prototypical Networks [12], SimpleShot [16], LaplacianShot [20], DeepEMD [19] and DeepBDC [21]. Prototypical Networks [12], a cornerstone technique in few-shot learning, utilize prototypes as representative embeddings for each class. By minimizing the distance between query examples and class prototypes, this model excels in quickly adapting to new classes with limited labeled data. SimpleShot [16] emphasizes simplicity in few-shot learning, relying on straightforward yet effective techniques. This highlights the efficacy of simplicity in addressing complex classification tasks with limited data. LaplacianShot [20] introduces Laplacian regularization to enhance few-shot learning performance. By integrating this regularization technique, the model aims to enhance generalization and robustness across diverse classes. DeepEMD [19] learns image representations by quantifying the discrepancy between joint characteristics of embedded features and the product of the marginals, facilitating comprehensive understanding of image similarities. DeepBDC [21], an advanced version of prototypical networks which uses a Brownian Distance Covriance matrix, realised in the form of a CNN module, calculates the prototypes of the classes in episodes of few-shot setting. Then the distance between the query examples and the support prototypes is minimised.

This research contributes to advancing the understanding of few-shot learning algorithms and their applicability in diverse image classification scenarios. The findings from our study hold implications for various fields, including medical imaging, where the ability to transfer knowledge across domains can significantly enhance diagnostic accuracy and efficiency.

2   Related Work

Over recent years, there has been a significant upsurge in research efforts dedicated to overcoming the challenges of few-shot learning within specialized areas of medical imaging. This section provides insights into various contributions in this field, highlighting how researchers have employed diverse few-shot learning techniques to address a range of medical diagnostic problems. For instance, Mahajan et al. [7] focused on skin disease identification in their study. They explored the effectiveness of two well-known few-shot learning methods, Reptile [9] and Prototypical Networks [12], in distinguishing between different skin diseases. Another notable study by Medela et al. [8] tackled the challenge of transferring knowledge across different tissue types. Their approach involved training a deep Siamese neural network to transfer knowledge from a dataset containing colon tissue to another dataset encompassing colon, lung, and breast tissue. Teng et al. [15] proposed a specialized few-shot learning algorithm based on Prototypical Networks, specifically designed for classifying lymphatic metastasis of lung carcinoma from Whole Slide Images (WSIs). In a different approach, Chen et al. [2] adopted a two-stage framework for the critical task of COVID-19 diagnosis from chest CT images. They first captured expressive feature representations using an encoder trained on publicly available lung datasets through contrastive learning. Subsequently, in the second stage, the pre-trained encoder was utilized within a few-shot learning paradigm, leveraging the Prototypical Networks method. Yang et al. [17] introduced an innovative approach by incorporating contrastive learning (CL) with latent augmentation (LA) to build a few-shot classification model. Here, contrastive learning learns significant features without requiring labels, while Latent Augmentation transfers semantic variations from one dataset to another without supervision. The model was trained on publicly available colon cancer datasets and evaluated on PAIP [5] liver cancer Whole Slide Images. Additionally, Shakeri et al. [11] introduced the FHIST dataset along with evaluations of various few-shot classification methodologies, which serve as a catalyst for further exploration in this domain. The scope of few-shot learning extends beyond image classification, as evidenced by [10]'s introduction of a few-shot semantic segmentation framework to reduce reliance on labeled data during training. Likewise, [18] explores medical image segmentation using the location-sensitive local prototype network, integrating spatial priors to improve segmentation accuracy.

3   Methodology

Few-shot classification tackles the challenge of working with limited data instances, such as in medical datasets where rare classes may only have a handful of examples, typically around five images per class. Training deep learning (DL) models with such a small dataset can be exceedingly difficult and may lead to overfitting. Furthermore, since these classes are rare, it's probable that pre-trained models have not encountered similar images during their training phase. Consequently, traditional transfer learning approaches may not be effective in this scenario, prompting the adoption of few-shot models that follow an episodic-training paradigm (Fig. 1).

In few-shot training, the training and test sets are disjoint. The training set, denoted as D_{Train}, comprises pairs $(X_{Train}, Y_{Train})_{i=1}^{M}$, where X_{Train} represents the images

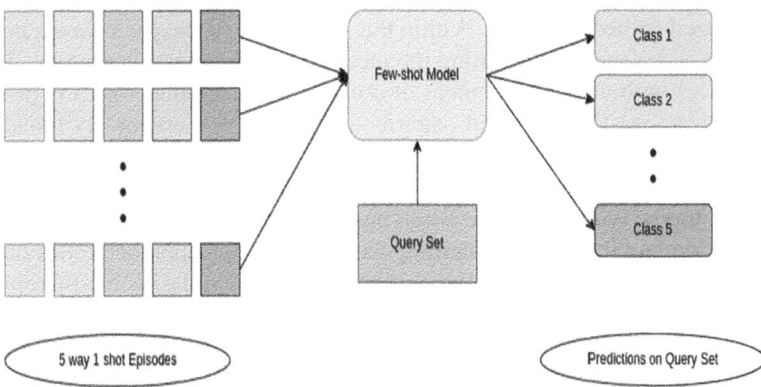

Fig. 1. The diagram depicts a few-shot learning model, demonstrating its capability to generalize effectively and recognize classes within an unlabeled query set using only a limited number of support examples. In the illustration, five different colors in the support set represent five distinct classes (ways), each having one sample (shot). [23].

and Y_{Train} denotes the corresponding labels. Here, M denotes the number of classes. In episodic training, the extensive labeled training dataset is divided into multiple episodes. Each episode consists of a support set(S) and a query set(Q). These episodes are characterized by the K-way N-shot Q-query setup. Essentially, for each episode, K classes are randomly chosen from the total M classes. Within each of these K classes, N images are designated for the support set, while Q images are reserved for the query set. Consequently, the support set comprises N×K images, while the query set comprises Q×K images. The few-shot model is then trained to learn from the support set in order to accurately predict the labels of the query set. Following training, the model's performance is evaluated on the test set.

$$D_{Train} = (X_{Train}, Y_{Train}) \tag{1}$$

$$S := (X_i, Y_i)_{i=1}^{K \times N} \tag{2}$$

$$Q := (X_i, Y_i)_{i=1}^{K \times Q} \tag{3}$$

$$D_{Test} = (X_{Test}, Y_{Test}) \tag{4}$$

$$S := (X_i, Y_i)_{i=1}^{K \times N} \tag{5}$$

$$Q := (X_i) \tag{6}$$

$$Y_{Train} \cap Y_{Test} = \Phi \tag{7}$$

3.1 Prototypical Networks

The fundamental principle behind Prototypical Networks [12] lies in the recognition that data points, which exhibit closeness to a singular prototype representation for each class, contribute significantly to a meaningful embedding. To translate this concept into practice, an essential step involves a non-linear mapping that transforms the input data into a specialized embedded space. Within this embedded space, each class's prototype representation is derived by computing the mean of its respective support set. The process commences with the establishment of a non-linear mapping, which is pivotal for capturing intricate relationships and patterns within the data, effectively transforming the original input data into a specialized embedded space. Within this space, a prototype representation is defined for each category, serving as a central point representing the class. This prototype is computed by averaging the feature vectors of all instances in the support set belonging to that class. During classification, the approach relies on identifying the nearest distance between the embedded query and the prototype representation of each class. The class associated with the closest prototype is then assigned to the query, thereby determining its classification. The support set S comprises K labeled examples, represented as $S=[(X_1,Y_1),...,(X_K,Y_K)]$ where X_i denotes a D-dimensional feature vector for each image and Y_i represents the corresponding label of X_i. Within the support set, there are N classes, with the number of examples within each class denoted as S_N.

Prototypical Networks employ an embedding function, typically a Convolutional Neural Network (CNN), denoted as f_Φ, to estimate an M-dimensional representation C_N for each class. Here, C_N represents the mean vector of the support points belonging to each class. The parameters Φ are learned during the training process, allowing the network to adapt and optimize its embedding function to effectively capture the underlying structure and characteristics of the data.

$$f_\Phi : R^D - > R^M \tag{8}$$

$$C_N \in R^M \, Rellungcarc \tag{9}$$

$$C_N = \frac{1}{|S_N|} \sum_{(X_i,Y_i)\in S} f_\Phi(X_i) \tag{10}$$

Prototypical Networks generate a probability distribution across classes for a given query example X. This distribution is computed by applying a softmax function to the distances between the query example and other prototypes in the embedding space. Specifically, the softmax function normalizes these distances, transforming them into a probability distribution that indicates the likelihood of the query belonging to each class represented by the prototypes.

$$P_\Phi(Y = N|X) = \frac{\exp(-d(f_\Phi(X), C_N))}{\sum_{N'} \exp(-d(f_\Phi(X), C_{N'}))} \tag{11}$$

The model learns by minimizing the negative log probability $J(\Phi)$ of the true class N using the Adam solver.

$$J(\Phi) = -\log(P_\Phi(Y = N|X)) \tag{12}$$

3.2 SimpleShot

SimpleShot [16] is a straightforward non-episodic few-shot learning approach that leverages transfer learning and the nearest-neighbor rule. Initially, a large-scale deep neural network is trained on a set of training classes, effectively learning rich representations of the data. During testing, the trained deep neural network serves as a feature encoder. The nearest-neighbor rule is then applied to the images of the test episodes using these learned features. This process enables SimpleShot to make predictions for new classes based on their similarity to the learned representations of the training classes, without requiring the episodic training paradigm typically employed in other few-shot learning methods.

The training set, denoted as D_{Train}, consists of image-label pairs, where X represents the images and Y denotes the corresponding labels. This training set is used to train a Convolutional Neural Network (CNN) using the cross-entropy loss function. In the context where f_θ represents the Convolutional Neural Network (CNN), W represents the weights of the classification layer, and L represents the cross-entropy loss function, the training process involves optimizing the parameters θ of the CNN to minimize the loss function L.

$$D_{Train} = [(X_1, Y_1), (X_2, Y_2), ..., (X_N, X_N)] \tag{13}$$

$$argmin_\theta \sum_{(X,Y) \in D_{Train}} l(W^T f_\theta(X), Y) \tag{14}$$

Testing involves utilizing the nearest neighbor rule for classification. Initially, an image's features are extracted by feeding it through the CNN, resulting in feature representation denoted as Z. Subsequently, classification via nearest neighbor rule is executed, employing Euclidean distance calculations between Z and the feature representations of test set episodes.

$$Z = f_\theta(X) \tag{15}$$

In a one-shot setting, the support set S of the test set comprises one labeled example from each of the N classes.

$$S = ((\hat{X}_1, 1), ..., (\hat{X}_N, N)) \tag{16}$$

Utilizing the Euclidean distance measure, the nearest neighbor rule assigns the query image $\hat{X}$ to the class of the most similar support image.

$$Y(\hat{X}) = argmin_{N \in (1,2,..,N)} d(\hat{Z}, \hat{Z}_N) \tag{17}$$

In a multi-shot setting, $\hat{Z}$ and $\hat{Z}_N$ represent the CNN features of the query and support images, respectively. Specifically, $\hat{Z}_N$ is computed as the average feature vector of each class in the support set.

3.3 Laplacianshot

LaplacianShot [20] presents a novel methodology for addressing few-shot tasks: transductive Laplacian regularized interference. This approach is centered around minimizing a quadratic binary assignment function that consists of two crucial components. The first component, a unary term, is responsible for assigning query samples to their nearest class prototypes. Meanwhile, the second component, the pairwise-Laplacian term, serves to encourage consistent label assignments among neighboring query samples.

Similar to the methodology employed in SimpleShot, the training dataset, denoted as D_{Train}, is utilized. In this approach, the training dataset is fed into a convolutional neural network (CNN) and trained using a basic cross-entropy loss function. Notably, this methodology does not incorporate any episodic or meta-learning strategies.

$$argmin_\theta \sum_{(X,Y) \in D_{Train}} l(W^T f_\theta(X), Y) \tag{18}$$

Below are the regularization equations utilized during few-shot test inference:

$$E(Y) = N(Y) + \lambda \frac{1}{2} L(Y) \tag{19}$$

$$N(Y) = \sum_{q=1}^{N} \sum_{c=1}^{C} y_{q,c} d(z_q - m_c) \tag{20}$$

$$L(Y) = \frac{1}{2} \sum_{q,p} w(z_q, z_p) ||y_q - y_p||_2^2 \tag{21}$$

In this task, we aim to minimize two components. The first component, denoted as N(Y), is minimized by assigning each query point to the class of its nearest prototype m_c from the support set. This assignment is made using a distance metric like Euclidean distance. The second component, L(Y), serves as the Laplacian regulariser and is given by tr($Y^T LY$). Here, L represents the Laplacian matrix, which corresponds to the affinity matrix W = $w(z_q, z_p)$. This matrix quantifies the similarity between feature vectors z_q and z_p using a kernel function. Specifically, z_q and z_p denote the feature vectors of query images x_p and x_q, respectively.

3.4 DeepEMD

In DeepEMD [19], the Earth Mover's Distance (EMD) is employed as a metric to compute the structural distance between dense image representations, thereby assessing image similarity. By facilitating optimal matching flows between structural elements, EMD minimizes the matching cost, which in turn serves as an indicator of image distance for classification purposes. To establish crucial weights for elements within the EMD framework, a cross-reference mechanism is introduced. This mechanism helps alleviate the impact of clustered backgrounds and intra-class variations. For K-shot classification tasks, a structured fully connected layer is utilized, enabling direct classification of dense image representations using EMD.

The Earth Mover's Distance functions as a distance metric between two sets of weighted objects or distributions, drawing upon the core concept of distance between individual objects. It mirrors the structure of the Transportation Problem within Linear Programming. In this problem, a set of suppliers S = ($S_i | i = 1, 2....m$) is tasked with transporting goods to a set of demanders ($d_j | j = 1, 2.... k$). Here, S_i denotes the supply unit of supplier i, while d_j indicates the demand of demander j. The cost of transporting one unit from supplier i to demander j is denoted by c_{ij}, and the quantity of units transported is represented by x_{ij}. The primary objective of the transportation problem is to determine the least-expensive flow of goods $\tilde{x} = (\tilde{x}_{ij}|i = -1, 2,..., m, j = 1, 2...., k)$ from each supplier to each demander.

$$\underset{x_{ij}}{\text{minimize}} \quad \sum_{i=1}^{m} \sum_{j=1}^{k} c_{ij} x_{ij} \tag{22}$$

In few-shot classification, determining the similarity between support and query images involves passing the images through a fully convolutional network (FCN) to generate image features for both the support set (denoted as S) and the query set (denoted as Q).

$$\mathbf{S} \in \mathbb{R}^{H \times W \times C} \tag{23}$$

$$\mathbf{Q} \in \mathbb{R}^{H \times W \times C} \tag{24}$$

The matching cost between the two sets of vectors is indicative of the similarity between the images. The cost between the two embeddings s_i and q_j is determined by:

$$c_{ij} = 1 - \frac{\mathbf{s}_i^T \mathbf{q}_j}{\|\mathbf{s}_i\| \|\mathbf{q}_j\|}, \tag{25}$$

In a support set, when the shot is greater than 1, the learnable embedding consists of a group of image features for each class rather than a single vector. Subsequently, the mean of these features is computed to obtain a single image feature. This process is akin to calculating the prototype of a class within the support set. The fully connected network serves as a feature extractor, and the Stochastic Gradient Descent (SGD) optimizer is employed to update the weights by sampling few-shot episodes from the dataset.

3.5 DeepBDC

In Standard few-shot learning, the process is conducted episodically across various tasks. Each task is typically structured as an N-way K-shot classification challenge, where N represents the number of classes, K denotes the number of support images per class, and Q represents the number of query images per class. These tasks are performed on a support set and a query set. During training, a learner is trained on the support set, learning to classify images into their respective classes. Following training, the learner is evaluated by making predictions on the query set, determining its ability to generalize and classify unseen images accurately.

In DeepBDC [21], the model learns a metric space where classification is achieved by computing distances to the prototype of each class. For a given task (with support set D_{sup} and query set D_{que}), we feed each image z_j to the network to generate the Bilateral Distance Covariance (BDC) matrix $A_\theta (z_j)$.

$$\mathbf{P}_k = \frac{1}{K} \sum_{(\mathbf{z}_j, y_j) \in \mathcal{S}_k} \mathbf{A}_\theta (\mathbf{z}_j) \tag{26}$$

S_k represent the set of examples in the support set D_{sup} labeled with class k. To generate a distribution over classes, a softmax function is computed over the distances from the query examples to the prototypes of the support classes. This softmax operation assigns probabilities to each class based on their similarity to the query examples. The loss function is formulated as the following:

$$\arg\min_{\theta} - \sum_{(\mathbf{z}_j, y_j) \in \mathcal{D}_{\text{que}}} \log \frac{\exp\left(\tau \operatorname{tr}\left(\mathbf{A}_{\ominus}\left(\mathbf{z}_j\right)^T \mathbf{P}_{y_j}\right)\right)}{\sum_k \exp\left(\tau \operatorname{tr}\left(\mathbf{A}_{\theta}\left(\mathbf{z}_j\right)^T \mathbf{P}_k\right)\right)} \tag{27}$$

4 Experiments and Results

(See Fig. 2).

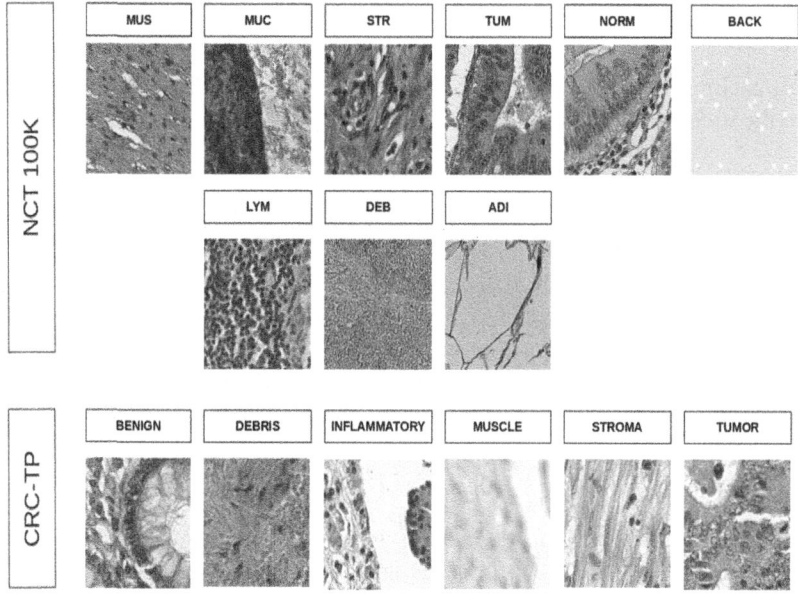

Fig. 2. The NCT dataset is illustrated by the sample images in the top two rows, whereas the CRC-TP dataset is represented by the sample images in the bottom row. [23].

4.1 Dataset

The dataset created by Komura et al. [6] comprises histology images extracted from uniform tumor regions in The Cancer Genome Atlas Program whole slide images [14]. The TCGA dataset encompasses tissue slides from 32 cancer types across various human body sites. From this extensive dataset, Komura et al. generated a collection of 1,608,060 image patches, encompassing six different magnification levels ranging from 0.5μ/pixel to 1.0μ/pixel. Given that these images originate from 32 distinct cancer types, they are categorized into corresponding 32 classes. The Mini-Imagenet dataset, proposed by Vinyals et al. [22], comprises

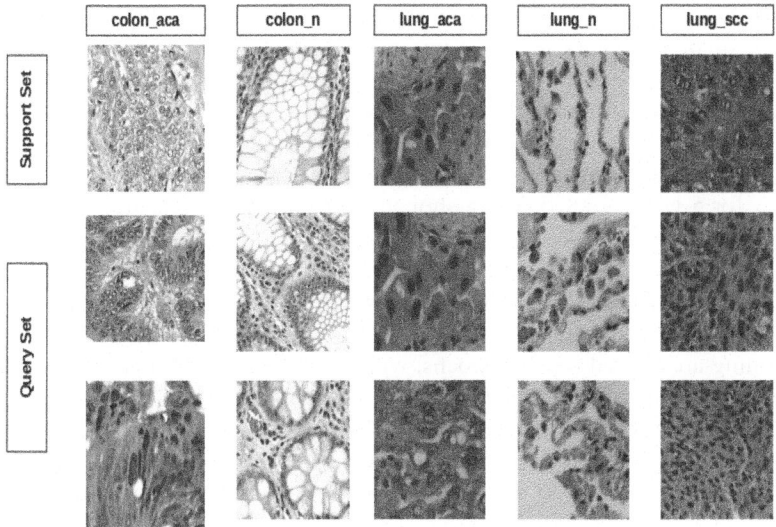

Fig. 3. 5-way 1-shot 2-query episode with support set images from five LC25000 dataset classes in the first row and query set images in the last two rows. [23].

of 64,000 images, evenly distributed among 100 classes. Each image in mini-Imagenet has a resolution of 84×84. The NCT dataset [4] consists of 100,000 image patches of human colorectal cancer, extracted from Hematoxylin and Eosin stained histological images, alongside normal tissue samples. These images, with a resolution of 224×224, are classified into seven classes: Adipose (ADI), background (BACK), debris (DEB), lymphocytes (LYM), mucus (MUC), smooth muscle (MUS), normal colon mucosa (NORM), cancer-associated stroma (STR), and colorectal adenocarcinoma epithelium (TUM). LC25000 [1], or the Lung and Colon Histopathological dataset, consists of 25,000 image patches. As the name implies, it includes images from both lung and colon cancer. With a resolution of 768×768, these images are categorized into five classes, three of which belong to lung cancer and the remaining two to colon cancer. The classes include benign colon tissues, colon adenocarcinoma, lung squamous cell carcinoma, and benign lung tissues. CRC-TP [3] is yet another colon cancer dataset, comprising 280,000 image patches categorized into six classes: tumor, stroma, complex stroma muscle, debris, inflammatory, and benign. These images have dimensions of 150×150. Mini-Imagenet dataset and the dataset prepared by Komura et al. serves as the training dataset due to their substantial size, suggesting the potential for robust few-shot backbone network training. Conversely, the remaining datasets are utilized as the testing set, adhering to the standard practice in few-shot learning where the test and training sets are disjoint.

4.2 Results and Discussion

The experiments were conducted on an NVIDIA A100 using PyTorch, employing two distinct training approaches: episodic training and standard training. Standard training involves training across the entire dataset with ample examples per class, while episodic training, tailored for few-shot learning, enables the model to quickly generalize from small episodes containing minimal examples of new classes. Methods like Protonet, DeepEMD, and DeepBDC adopt episodic training, whereas SimpleShot and LaplacianShot adhere to standard training procedures.

During episodic training, the methods undergo training for 120 epochs. Each epoch involves selecting 600 random episodes from the training set. The models are trained separately for 5-way 1-shot, 5-way 5-shot, and 5-way 10-shot scenarios, with the number of query images set to 15 in all cases. The initial learning rate is set to 1e-3, with a γ value of 0.1. The batch size is configured to accommodate one episode, with the number of images in a batch calculated as 80, 100, and 125 for 5-way 1-shot, 5-way 5-shot, and 5-way 10-shot training, respectively. Conversely, few-shot methods employing standard CNN training are trained for 150 epochs, with a batch size of 512. The initial learning rate and weight decay are initialized to 0.05 and 5e-4, respectively. ResNet18 serves as the backbone network in both episodic and standard training procedures. All trained models undergo meta-testing, wherein 5000 episodes are randomly sampled from the CRC-TP, NCT, and LC25000 datasets. Regardless of the K-shot testing scenario, the number of query images remains fixed at 15 in each episode. The results on 1-shot, 5-shot, 10-shot models on different datasets trained on dataset proposed by Komura et al. [6] and Mini-Imagenet dataset [22] are reported in the Table 1 and Table 2 respectively (Figs. 3, 4 and 5).

Table 1. Accuracy(%) on three different datasets; CRC-TP [3], NCT [4] and LC25000 [1]. Komura et al. [6] proposed the dataset used to train the few-shot models. [23].

Method	Training Method	CRC-TP		
		5-way 1-shot	5-way 5-shot	5-way 10-shot
ProtoNet [12]	Episodic	43.8	63.6	68.3
DeepEMD [19]	Episodic	47.3	64.6	68.6
DeepBDC [21]	Episodic	47.7	65.3	70.2
SimpleShot [16]	Standard	47.9	66.9	71.4
LaplacianShot [20]	**Standard**	**48.5**	**68.0**	**72.8**
Method	Training Method	NCT		
		5-way 1-shot	5-way 5-shot	5-way 10-shot
ProtoNet [12]	Episodic	62.6	80.9	84.9
DeepEMD [19]	Episodic	68.5	84.0	86.0
DeepBDC [21]	Episodic	69.3	84.7	87.5
SimpleShot [16]	Standard	71.2	85.5	88.2
LaplacianShot [20]	**Standard**	**71.8**	**86.9**	**89.5**
Method	Training Method	LC25000		
		5-way 1-shot	5way 5-shot	5-way 10-shot
ProtoNet [12]	Episodic	67.2	84.8	86.2
DeepEMD [19]	Episodic	73.8	85.3	86.4
DeepBDC [21]	Episodic	74.7	85.8	86.9
SimpleShot [16]	Standard	66.4	83.6	87.2
LaplacianShot [20]	**Standard**	**67.5**	**84.2**	**87.9**

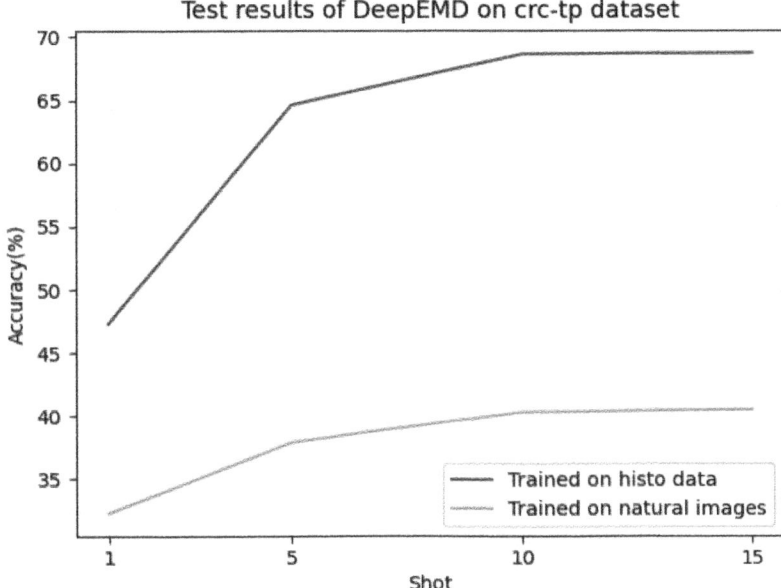

Fig. 4. Performance of DeepEMD on crc-tp dataset with different training conditions.

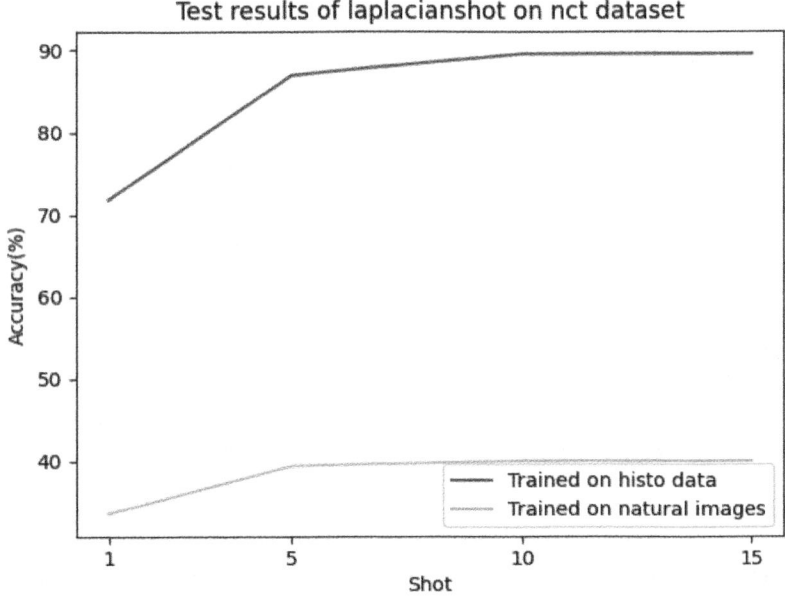

Fig. 5. Performance of laplacianshot on nct dataset with different training conditions.

Table 2. Accuracy(%) on three different datasets; CRC-TP [3], NCT [4] and LC25000 [1]. The few-shot models are trained on Mini-Imagenet [22].

Method	Training Method	CRC-TP		
		5-way 1-shot	5-way 5-shot	5-way 10-shot
ProtoNet [12]	Episodic	28.9	36.3	39.3
DeepEMD [19]	Episodic	32.3	37.9	40.3
DeepBDC [21]	Episodic	31.9	36.5	41.2
SimpleShot [16]	Standard	32.4	**44.7**	**49.3**
LaplacianShot [20]	Standard	**34.0**	39.3	40.4
Method	Training Method	NCT		
		5-way 1-shot	5-way 5-shot	5-way 10-shot
ProtoNet [12]	Episodic	26.3	33.9	37.4
DeepEMD [19]	Episodic	28.9	34.6	38.5
DeepBDC [21]	Episodic	30.1	34.5	39.8
SimpleShot [16]	Standard	32.3	**44.9**	**49.1**
LaplacianShot [20]	Standard	**33.6**	39.4	40.0
Method	Training Method	LC25000		
		5-way 1-shot	5way 5-shot	5-way 10-shot
ProtoNet [12]	Episodic	30.2	35.5	41.1
DeepEMD [19]	Episodic	29.5	35.9	39.7
DeepBDC [21]	Episodic	31.3	35.7	40.7
SimpleShot [16]	Standard	32.5	**44.8**	**49.2**
LaplacianShot [20]	Standard	**33.9**	39.2	40.1

When trained on Mini-Imagenet i.e. natural images' dataset, the few-shot models did not exhibit promising performance. On testing these models on histopathology data, their accuracies and general capabilities are significantly low. This suggests that the feature encoders learned from natural images dataset might not adequately capture the unique characteristics and complexities present in histopathology images. Conversely, when trained directly on histopathology data, the same few-shot classification models demonstrated significantly improved performance across all tested scenarios (5-way 1-shot, 5-way 5-shot, and 5-way 10-shot). The enhanced results indicate that training the models on domain-specific data enables them to learn feature representations that are better suited for histopathology image classification tasks. By directly optimizing the feature encoder on histopathology data, the models can effectively capture the intricate patterns and subtle nuances characteristic of histopathological images, leading to improved classification accuracy and robustness. As expected, few-shot methodologies employing standard fine-tuning methods like SimpleShot and LaplacianShot demonstrated superior performance when compared to episodic training approaches such as ProtoNet, DeepEMD, and DeepBDC. This could be attributed to the fact that the standard training techniques allowed these models to leverage the extensive dataset provided by Komura et al., encompassing cancer image patches from 32 distinct organ classes. In 10-shot test scenarios, the accuracies of all methods across all datasets, except for CRC-TP, ranged from 85% to 90%.

5   Conclusion

Upon conducting rigorous experiments with a range of few-shot classification techniques, including SimpleShot, LaplacianShot, Prototypical Networks, DeepEMD, and DeepBDC, across different training and testing datasets, it became apparent that training these models on histopathology data resulted in significantly improved performance compared to training on natural images. This notable improvement underscores the critical role of obtaining a specialized feature encoder tailored specifically for histopathology data. Histopathology images possess unique characteristics and complexities that differ from natural images, such as varied tissue structures, cellular compositions, and staining patterns. By training the models on histopathology data, the feature encoder becomes adept at capturing and extracting relevant discriminative features inherent to histopathological images, leading to enhanced classification accuracy and robustness. Overall, these findings underscore the importance of training few-shot classification models on domain-specific data to obtain a good feature encoder tailored to the target application domain. Therefore, investing efforts in developing and optimizing feature encoders specifically designed for histopathology data is essential for achieving superior performance in few-shot classification tasks within the domain of medical imaging.

References

1. Borkowski, A.A., Bui, M.M., Thomas, L.B., Wilson, C.P.L., Del, L.A., Mastorides, S.M.: Lung and colon cancer histopathological image dataset (lc25000) (2019)
2. Chen, X., Yao, L., Zhou, T., Dong, J., Zhang, Y.: Momentum contrastive learning for few-shot covid-19 diagnosis from chest ct images. Pattern Recogn. **113**, 107826 (2021)
3. Javed, S., Mahmood, A., Werghi, N., Benes, K., Rajpoot, N.: Multiplex cellular communities in multi-gigapixel colorectal cancer histology images for tissue phenotyping. IEEE Trans. Image Process. **29**, 9204–9219 (2020)
4. Kather, J.N., et al.: Predicting survival from colorectal cancer histology slides using deep learning: a retrospective multicenter study. PLoS Med. **16**(1), e1002730 (2019)
5. Kim, Y.J., et al.: Paip 2019: liver cancer segmentation challenge. Med. Image Anal. **67**, 101854 (2021)
6. Komura, D., Ishikawa, S.: Histology images from uniform tumor regions in TCGA whole slide images. Cell Rep. **38**(9), 110424 (2021)
7. Mahajan, K., Sharma, M., Vig, L.: Metadermdiagnosis: few-shot skin disease identification using meta-learning. In: Proceedings of the IEEE/CVF Conference on Computer Vision and Pattern Recognition Workshops, pp. 730–773 (2020)
8. Medela, A., et al.: Few-shot learning in histopathological images: reducing the need of labeled data on biological datasets. In: 2019 IEEE 16th International Symposium on Biomedical Imaging (ISBI 2019), pp. 1860–1864. IEEE (2019)
9. Nichol, A., Schulman, J.: Reptile: A scalable metalearning algorithm. arXiv preprint arXiv:1803.02999 (2018)

10. Ouyang, C., Biffi, C., Chen, C., Kart, T., Qiu, H., Rueckert, D.: Self-supervision with super-pixels: training few-shot medical image segmentation without annotation. In: Vedaldi, A., Bischof, H., Brox, T., Frahm, J.-M. (eds.) ECCV 2020. LNCS, vol. 12374, pp. 762–780. Springer, Cham (2020). https://doi.org/10.1007/978-3-030-58526-6_45
11. Shakeri, F., et al.: Fhist: A benchmark for few-shot classification of histological images. arXiv (2022)
12. Snell, J., Swersky, K., Zemel, R.: Prototypical networks for few-shot learning. In: Advances in Neural Information Processing Systems (NeurIPS) (2017)
13. Spanhol, F.A., Oliveira, L.S., Petitjean, C., Heutte, L.: A dataset for breast cancer histopatho-logical image classification. IEEE Trans. Biomed. Eng. **63**(7), 1455–1462 (2016)
14. https://www.cancer.gov/ccg/research/genomesequencing/tcga . Accessed 30 Nov 2023
15. Teng, H., et al.: Few-shot learning on the diagnosis of lymphatic metastasis of lung carci-noma. Research Square (2021)
16. Wang, Y., Chao, W.-L., Weinberger, K.Q., van der Maaten, L.: Simpleshot: revisiting nearest neighbor classification for few-shot learning. arXiv preprint arXiv:1911.04623 (2019)
17. Yang, J., Chen, H., Yan, J., Chen, X., Yao, J.: Towards better understanding and better gen-eralization of few-shot classification in histology images with contrastive learning. arXiv preprint arXiv:2202.09059 (2022)
18. Yu, Q., Dang, K., Tajbakhsh, N., Terzopoulos, D., Ding, X.: A location-sensitive local pro-totype network for few-shot medical image segmentation. In: 2021 IEEE 18th International Symposium on Biomedical Imaging (ISBI), pp. 262–266. IEEE (2021)
19. Zhang, C., Cai, Y., Lin, G., Shen, C.: Deepemd: few-shot image classification with differen-tiable earth mover's distance and structured classifiers. In: Conference on Computer Vision and Pattern Recognition (CVPR) (2020)
20. Ziko, I.M., Dolz, J., Granger, E., Ben Ayed, I.: Laplacian regularized few-shot learning. In: International Conference on Machine Learning (ICML) (2020)
21. Xie, J., Long, F., Lv, J., Wang, Q., Li, P.: Joint distribution matters: deep brownian distance covariance for few-shot classification (CVPR) (2022)
22. Vinyals, O., Blundell, C., Lillicrap, T., et al.: Matching networks for one shot learning. In: Advances in Neural Information Processing Systems, pp. 3637–3645 (2016)
23. Sekhar, A., Gupta, R., Sethi, A.: Few-shot histopathology image classification: evaluating state-of-the-art methods and unveiling performance insights. In: Proceedings of the 17th International Joint Conference on Biomedical Engineering Systems and Technologies, vol. 1, pp. 244–253 (2024), ISBN 978-989-758-688-0. ISSN 2184-4305. https://doi.org/10.5220/0012568000003657

Bioinformatics Models, Methods and Algorithms

Modeling the Mechanism of Sprouting Angiogenesis in Tumor Using Petri Nets

Adéla Šterberová[1], Andreea Dincu[1], Stijn Oudshoorn[1], Vincent van Duinen[2], and Lu Cao[1(✉)] (iD)

[1] Leiden Insisute of Advanced Computer Science, Leiden University, 2333 CC Leiden, The Netherlands
l.cao@liacs.leidenuniv.nl
[2] Leiden University Medical Center, 2333 ZA Leiden, The Netherlands

Abstract. Sprouting angiogenesis is the most representative process of tumor angiogenesis. It is featured as the formation of new vascular branches from blood vessels towards tumor. These new vascular branches are made to supply the necessary nutrients for the further growth of existing tumor tissue. The entire process of angiogenesis is highly complex. It involves production and utilization of biomolecules, transition between subtypes of endothelial cells. In addition, it incorporates cell interaction, division and migration. In order to understand the mechanism of sprouting angiogenesis, microfluidic cell culture platform has been used in combination with human induced pluripotent stem cell derived endothelial cells (iPSC-ECs) to form a physiological relevant micro-environment. In this paper, we explore the possibility of using bio-modeling technique to model sprouting angiogenesis in microfluidic cell culture platform and to conduct *in silico* experiment. We utilize Petri nets for modeling the cell transition and associated constraints. The environmental and spacial factors are realized using custom 2-dimensional grids. The model is able to capture the essence of endothelial cell transition and migration in sprouting angiogenesis using this abstract computational solution.

Keywords: Sprouting angiogenesis · Petri Nets · Endothelial cell transition · VEGF gradient

1 Introduction

Angiogenesis is the process of developing new blood vessels. It plays an important role in cancer development since these new blood vessels deliver oxygen, nutrients and growth factors to tumor [1]. Sprouting angiogenesis is the most observed type of angiogenesis and is a process involving formation and outgrowth of sprouts (tip cells) from preexisting blood vessels [2, 18]. The formation of blood vessels into tumors has also been shown to influence metastasis and growth rates [7, 12, 27].

In recent years, stem cell technology became influential for disease modeling, drug discovery and toxicity/safety screening [5, 6, 16, 24, 25]. Microfluidic system has been introduced to culture various types of cells differentiated from stem cells. For example,

M. P. Guarino et al. (Eds.): BIOSTEC 2024, CCIS 2546, pp. 151–166, 2026.
https://doi.org/10.1007/978-3-031-96899-0_10

angiogenesis study using iPSC-ECs has been realized using microfluidic platform to create a physiological relevant cellular micro-environment with controlled perfusion and gradients [11]. In this paper, we concentrated on modeling sprouting angiogenesis in a microfluidic environment induced by vascular endothelial growth factor (VEGF) which is originally released by tumor cells under hypoxic conditions.

2   Related Work

Several mathematical and computational models have been developed to study various aspects of angiogenesis [20]. A discrete mathematical model, incorporating cell-mixing behavior and temporal length generating behavior of the blood vessel, was designed to examine the dynamics of vascular endothelial cells in angiogenic morphogenesis [19]. Another mathematical model was created to replicate the tumour-induced vascular networks going through stages of growth, regression and regrowth [29]. The model manages to capture capillaries at full scale and the dynamics of vessel networks at long time range. A mathematical formalism was developed to simulate the early stages of angiogenesis based on a 3D in vitro model, accounting for dynamic interactions and interchange of different endothelial cell phenotypes [3]. In addition, the model takes into account several biomolecules that play roles in the interaction. A hybrid model was designed to facilitate *in silico* experiment for tumor growth and angiogenesis [21]. This model treats each cell as an agent, incorporating phenotypic transitions of both tumor cell and endothelial cell. It also allows VEGF and nutrient fields to impact the dynamics. A numerical model was proposed to mimic the chemoatrractant effect of VEGF in stimulating sprouting angiogenesis. The work mainly focuses on modeling endothelial cell migration and branching process so as to obtain a realistic capillary network [13].

These mathematical models are highly powerful but they lack standardization for comparison which further hampers reproducibility. We seek for a unified and versatile framework for modeling biological systems. Petri nets is a graphical and mathematical formalism used for modeling and analyzing concurrent, asynchronous and distributed systems [9]. It is proven to be a promising mathematical tool for describing and studying the relationships and interactions within various parts of biological systems such as metabolic pathways, organelles, cells, and organisms [8,17,28]. In addition, multiple variants of the initial formalism (e.g. stochastic, timed, hybrid, coloured) have been developed to analyze dynamic properties of complex processes, from either a qualitative or a quantitative perspective [10].

In this paper, we utilized Petri nets to simulate the transitions of iPSC-ECs during tumor angiogenesis within a microfluidic cell culture platform. We designed a complex pipeline to model the diffusion and consumption of VEGF, as well as the migration of the cells in response to the VEGF gradient.

3   Biological Details

When the tumor cells encounter a depletion of nutrients like oxygen, they induce the growth in quiescent arteries. This growth induction is thus triggered in hypoxic cells, leading them to release VEGF. Subsequently, VEGF diffuses to the surrounding environment and causes the formation of phalanx. Endothelial cells, that make up the artery, start turning into tip cells under the influence of VEGF. Additionally, VEGF acts as a chemoattractant for tip cells, which in turn inhibit neighboring cells from becoming tip cells through Notch signalling [23]. These neighboring cells instead turn into stalk cells. Stalk cells proliferate and follow the nearby tip cell. The tip cells inhibit the stalk cells from reverting to phalanx cells within a certain distance. When the distance between a tip cell and a stalk cell is long enough, the stalk cell can turn into phalanx cell to stabilise the growing artery structure. In Fig. 1, an example of this stage in angiogenesis is shown.

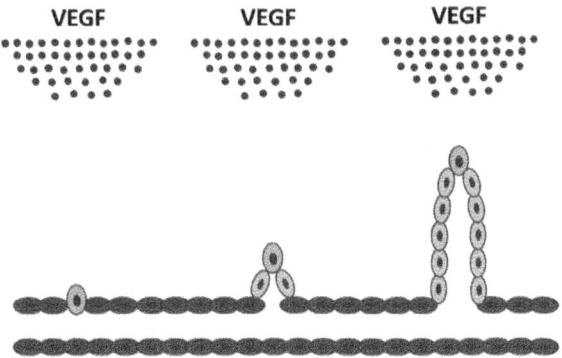

Fig. 1: A visualization of the sprouting process. Red cells are phalanx cells. Brown cells are tip cells and light brown cells are stalk cells [30] (Color figure online).

New physiologically relevant *in vitro* screening was recently developed [11] utilizing iPSC-ECs within a microfluidic cell culture platform, to model sprouting angiogenesis in response to a VEGF gradient. This method serves as a simplified representation of vessel growth near tumors, replacing hypoxic tumor cells with a VEGF gradient. In this paper, we simulate vessel formation *in silico*, aiming to develop a model which encompasses cell transition, migration, differentiation and VEGF consumption. Moreover, the model realizes formation of new blood vessels, incorporating several cell types with different roles. The methods designed to realize these processes are detailed in the following sections.

4   Method

We developed a hybrid model consisting a central Petri net and two grid matrices. The central Petri net controls the transition of subtypes of endothelial cells. One grid matrix deals with spatially connected features, such as the cell positioning and movement. The other grid matrix manages the distribution of the growth vector (i.e. VEGF) concentrations.

4.1   Endothelial Cell Transition Model

The transition of endothelial cell subtypes is modeled using a timed hybrid Petri net so as to incorporate division/growing time, distance to the closest tip cell and VEGF concentration for each cell. The scheme, originally from [21] and illustrated in Fig. 2, is designed to mimic the movement of the tip cell according to the gradient of VEGF. This scheme fits our microfluidic environment the best. In addition, the paper provides a detailed baseline parameters to work with. It brings biologically relevant properties to our model and makes our model more realistic. In our model, the places represent all possible cell subtypes that an endothelial cell can adopt, namely: phalanx cell P, stalk cell S, and tip cell T.

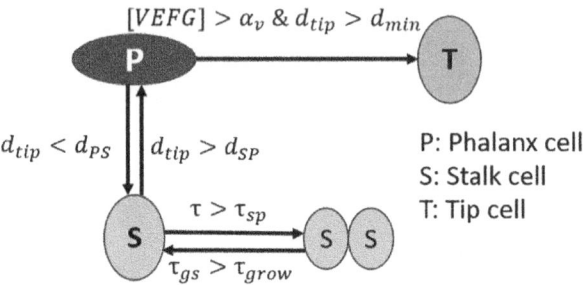

Fig. 2: Schematic illustration of endothelial cell transitions [30]. d_{tip}: the distance from the current cell to the nearest tip cell. d_{SP}: Minimum distance from the current cell to the nearest tip cell for $S \rightarrow P$ transition. d_{PS}: Maximum distance from the current cell to the nearest tip cell for $P \rightarrow S$ transition. d_{min}: Minimum distance from the current cell to the nearest tip cell for $P \rightarrow T$ transition. [VEGF]: VEGF concentration. α_v: VEGF threshold for $P \rightarrow T$ transition. τ: the amount of time that a cell spends in a given place. τ_{sp}: a predefined time interval for a stalk cell to divide. τ_{gs}: growing time of a stalk cell. τ_{grow}: mandatory growing time.

An additional place is added to represent the division of stalk cells (SS). When the connected division transition gets fired, it results in the separation of one cell into two daughter cells, generating two different tokens representing daughter cells adjacent to each other (positions (i, j) and $(i - 1, j)$). The introduction of a new token in the system has to be reflected also in the positioning grid, by filling an additional position $((i - 1, j))$ as a stalk cell. A stalk cell can divide after a predefined time interval (τ_{sp}), resulting in two daughter cells, with each being half of the size and volume of the parent cell. To be considered as integral stalk cells again, the newly divided stalk cells have to go through a growing period to increase their volume. This mandatory growing time is defined as a pre-set threshold, τ_{grow}. Although we have standardized the cell volume to a constant, the mechanisms behind the growth phase are preserved.

The transitions in our Petri net correspond to possible changes between subtypes that an endothelial cell with a given subtype can reach. Each transition has specific conditions, as shown in Fig. 2. The division of a stalk cell ($S \rightarrow SS$) and the transition of divided daughter cell back to integral stalk cell ($SS \rightarrow S$) depend on the time intervals, τ_{sp} and τ_{grow} respectively. In addition, the $S \rightarrow SS$ transition is constrained by the available space in the positioning grid. The transitions from phalanx cell P to stalk cell S ($P \rightarrow S$) and from stalk cell to phalanx cell ($S \rightarrow P$) are conditioned by the distance of a given cell to the nearest tip cell d_{tip}. For the transition from phalanx cell P to stalk cell S, the distance from a given cell to the nearest tip cell T must be less than a pre-defined threshold d_{PS}. Conversely, for the transition from stalk cell S to phalanx cell P, the distance to the nearest cell T must exceed another pre-defined threshold d_{SP}. Finally, the transition from phalanx cell P to tip cell T ($P \rightarrow T$) occurs only when no other tip cell is within a certain immediate vicinity (d_{min}) and the VEGF concentration at the location of the cell exceeds a certain threshold α_v. The distance to the nearest tip cell d_{tip} is calculated based on the positioning grid, while the VEGF concentration is retrieved from the VEGF grid. The thresholds used in the implementation can be found in Table 1. These parameters are derived from baseline set of model parameter values in [21] after unifying both tumor and endothelial cell radii to 1, ensuring the biological relevance of our model.

Table 1: Table with the fixed parameters in our simulation [30].

Parameter	Meaning	Value
α_v	VEGF threshold for $P \rightarrow T$ transition	0.1
γ	Consumption rate	$10h^{-1}$
d_{SP}	Minimum distance from tip cell for $S \rightarrow P$ transition	1.55
d_{PS}	Maximum distance from tip cell for $P \rightarrow S$ transition	1.55
d_{min}	Minimum distance from tip cell for $P \rightarrow T$ transition	20
R	Endothelial cell radius	1
S_delay	Stalk cell may divide after this delay	4
SS_delay	Stalk cell growth time	3

To prevent transition conflicts in our Petri net during simulation, choices need to be made between several enabled transitions in conflict with each other. We designed the firing order of transitions, which is based on biological reasoning. The $S \rightarrow SS$ transition fires first, as biologically, there is no inhibition for cell division when division conditions are met. The $SS \rightarrow S$ transition fires second, as cells, reached to the full volume of a stalk cell, should be immediately assigned to that subtype. Once the divisions of stalk cells are handled, the transition from remaining stalk cells S to phalanx cells P can proceed. Two transitions $P \rightarrow T$ and $P \rightarrow S$ are executed at last. Although these transitions are generally not concurrent, in case such a situation occurs due to the set values of d_{min} and d_{PS}, the transition to a tip cell T is prioritized when VEGF conditions are met. By defining a clear ordering, transition conflicts are effectively mitigated.

The final component of Petri nets that needs to be explained is the token. In our model, a token represents a specific subtype of endothelial cell. The token encapsulates various features of the defined cell. The token's internal representation is {x, y, d_{tip}, $VEGF$, τ}. x and y define the position of the cell in the positioning matrix. d_{tip} specifies the distance from the current cell to the nearest tip cell computed using the positioning matrix. $VEGF$ indicates the VEGF concentration at the cell's position (x,y) retrieved from the VEGF grid and τ stores the amount of time that the cell spends in a given place.

The Petri net is implemented using the Python library SNAKES [22], which provides flexibility in modeling options and feature extensions. The source code is available at https://github.com/LuLIACS/angiogenesis-modeling. The net scheme is illustrated in Fig. 3, where the places for each endothelial cell subtype are marked by circles. The net includes two types of transitions: one for transitions between different subtypes and the other representing time. The time is applied only to the places S and SS. In all transitions, $t[i]$ refers to specific information stored in the token at position i.

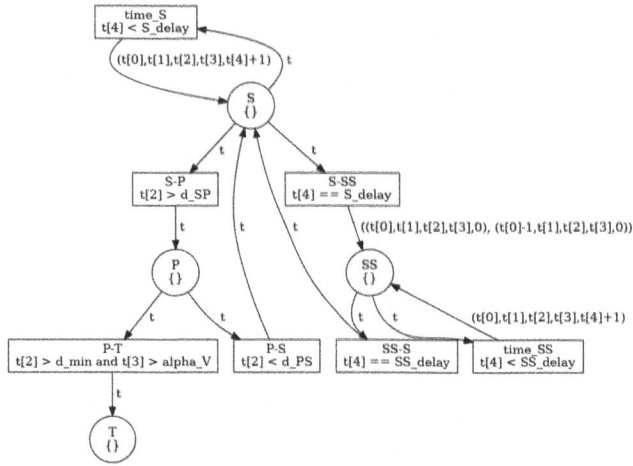

Fig. 3: Schematic illustration of the Petri net [30].

4.2   Positioning and VEGF Grid

As previously mentioned, our model needs to determine the distance between two cells. To define a proper distance metric, we firstly have to define the space in which the cells are placed. We chose to model this environment as a 2-dimensional space, using Euclidean distance as the distance metric. This approach preserves the integrity of the biological concepts and allows for a straightforward extension to 3-dimensional space. This spatial representation can be seen as a projection of the original 3-dimensional environment.

The grid was implemented as a 2-dimensional NumPy [14] matrix with a configurable size (H, W). Each position in the matrix can hold a cell or a zero value when it is empty. This implementation implies that all cells have the same volume and, consequently, the same growth factor consumption rate γ. Cells are designed as objects initialized with the endothelial cell subtype (phalanx, stalk, or tip). Various cell-related functions are implemented on this matrix, such as cell movement (changing positions of cells), cell transition (changing cell subtypes), calculating the distance to the nearest tip cell, and stalk cell division. These functions are integrated with the Petri net and enabled by firing related transitions. In order to simulate the formation of new blood vessels, the matrix is initially empty, except for the bottom row, which is filled with phalanx cells P. This row represents a section of the micro-vessel culture in a microfluidic chip.

The VEGF grid is similar to the positioning grid and must match its configured size. It was implemented as a 2-dimensional NumPy matrix that contains the VEGF concentration at each position. Initially, the VEGF grid has non-zero concentrations only in the first row on the top to simulate the existence of tumor cells emitting the VEGF signal. At each time step, a diffusion model is applied to simulate VEGF diffusion in our system. We implemented two types of diffusion models. The first one is normal diffusion. The portion of VEGF diffused from the central position to neighboring position with a lower VEGF concentration is determined by a diffusion factor f_d, which is set to 0.1 in our implementation. Therefore, the VEGF concentration in the center position and the VEGF concentration in the neighboring position can be updated by

$$VEGF_{center} = VEGF_{center} - f_d \cdot VEGF_{center}, \qquad (1)$$

$$VEGF_{neighbor} = VEGF_{neighbor} + f_d \cdot VEGF_{center}. \qquad (2)$$

However, normal diffusion is too orderly and predictable for a natural phenomenon. Therefore, we implemented a second type of diffusion that introduces some level of randomness. In this model, for each position in the grid, we randomly determine the amount of VEGF that diffuses in each direction [15]. For each element in the VEGF matrix, a random portion of VEGF is diffused into each neighboring position.

In addition, cells continuously consume VEGF according to their consumption rate γ. Consequently, the VEGF grid has to be continuously updated to reflect this consumption.

4.3 Cell Movement

Regarding the cell movement, we adopt a simplified model where cells only move upwards. When a cell transitions to a tip cell, and if the tip cell is surrounded by stalk cells, the tip cell is allowed to update its position. Another type of movement occurs during stalk cell S division. The parent cell has to be replaced by two new tokens representing the two smaller daughter cells. In order to create space for these two tokens, all cells in the previous rows shift one row up, provided that there is space. If there is no space, cell division and movement do not take place. This approach particularly helps naturally end the simulation, preventing continuous cell division and pushing cells outside the grid. This design choice can be adjusted as needed.

4.4 Time Integration

As illustrated in Fig. 2, certain transitions of the endothelial cell subtypes are time constrained. Furthermore, cell movement and VEGF diffusion need to be discretized in order to be integrated into the model. An intuitive way is to use time as the sampling factor, updating both cell positions and VEGF concentrations once per time step. Thus, time is an essential component of our model.

To better match the biological scenario, we introduced a custom time modeling approach. Each cell (token) has an internal timer τ which resets to 0 when the token enters into a new place. This timer increases independently for each cell until it reaches the time constraint necessary for the connected transitions (e.g. for the $S \rightarrow SS$, the condition is $\tau > \tau_{sp}$). When the condition is met, the transition is fired, and the timer of the token resets. The timer increment can be integrated into the Petri net using a loop transition, which increments the τ variable inside the token representation until a set threshold (e.g. τ_{sp}). This loop transition should be fired at the start of each time step. This approach ensures that the biological model remains functional when implementing the time aspect, allowing cells to transition simultaneously if needed.

5   Experiments and Results

The experiments and results presented in this paper are extended from our previous work [30], where we did the experiments using a 11 × 15 grid. The main drawback that we observed was scalability. The running time of our model increased exponentially, when the grid size is logarithmically increased. Furthermore, the small grid size hampers the sensitivity analysis, making it difficult to learn the sensitivity of the model to the choice of parameters. To address these issues, we employed multiprocessing package in Python to enable parallel computing and alleviate computational demands. Our following experiments used a larger grid size of 20 × 60 to better mimic the shape of Microfluidic Chip. The enlarged grid contain 1200 blocks to contain cells, compared to 165 blocks in the 11 × 15 grid. We perform 300 iterations for the larger grid.

5.1   Diffusion Simulations

We firstly compared two types of diffusion using the same matrix initialization. The simulation results, when the first tip cells form and when the final movement is made, are shown in Figs. 5 and 6 for normal and random diffusion, respectively.

In the simulation with the normal diffusion, 11 tip cells form and are evenly distributed in the center of the grid at the same time as shown in (a) of Fig. 5. When these tip cells move upwards and enough distance is accumulated, two additional tip cells form at time step 101 and 105 on both sides of the grid. Following the same pattern, one last tip cell forms at time step 175 on the right side of the grid. The number of cells throughout the simulation is depicted for each cell subtype in Fig. 4(a). The graph shows that each time the number of tip cells increases, there is a consistent rise in the number of phalanx cells and stalk cells.

The simulation with random diffusion, as shown in Fig. 6, has only one phalanx cell transitioned to tip cell at time step 75. This first tip cell positions on one side of the grid, which happens 32 time steps later than in the normal diffusion simulation. The count of different cell subtypes for this experiment is shown in Fig. 4(b). There are roughly three stages of cell number increases, each followed by the formation of new tip cells. The first stage happens when two new tip cells form at time steps 75 and 80. The second stage occurs at time steps 135, 140 and 146 when three more tip cells form. The final stage is at time steps 215 and 216, with the formation of two last new tip cells. In total, there are 7 tip cells formed over 300 iterations. The number of cells is significantly lower comparing to the simulation of normal diffusion. However, the distribution of tip cells and stalk cells is more balanced and less overcrowded than in the normal diffusion scenario.

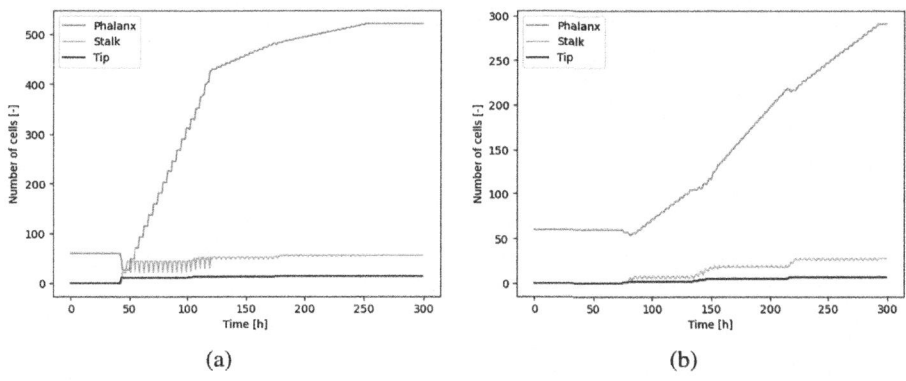

Fig. 4: The number of cells shown per type for the normal and random diffusion experiments.

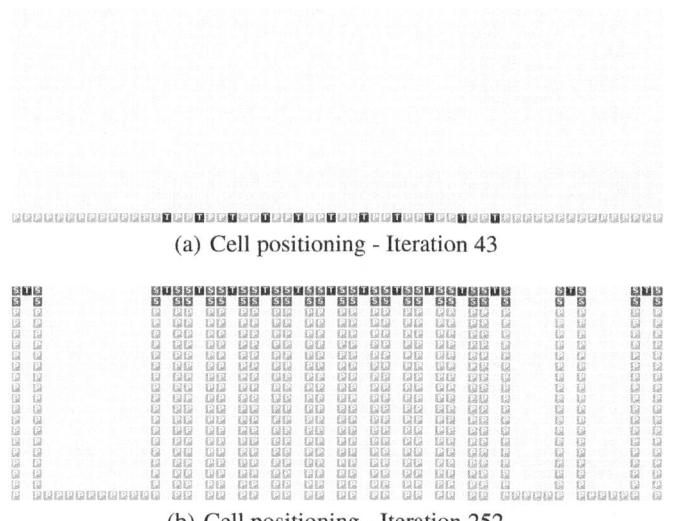

(a) Cell positioning - Iteration 43

(b) Cell positioning - Iteration 252

Fig. 5: The cell matrix during the normal diffusion experiment when the first tip cells form and when the final movement is made in the grid. The time step is shown below the figures.

The corresponding VEGF matrices for the normal and random diffusion are shown in Figs. 7 and 8. The first state shows the concentrations at the time of the first transition to tip cells, while the second state is from the moment the last tip cell reaches the top of the grid. A structured gradient is observed in the simulation of normal distribution. As random diffusion is not deterministic, the same initial state could reach to different end states. We notice that the spreading patterns of the concentrations look similar at the same phase (iteration 43) despite using different diffusion models. We observe different patterns at time step 252 because more cells are formed during normal diffusion and, consequently, more VEGF is consumed by cells.

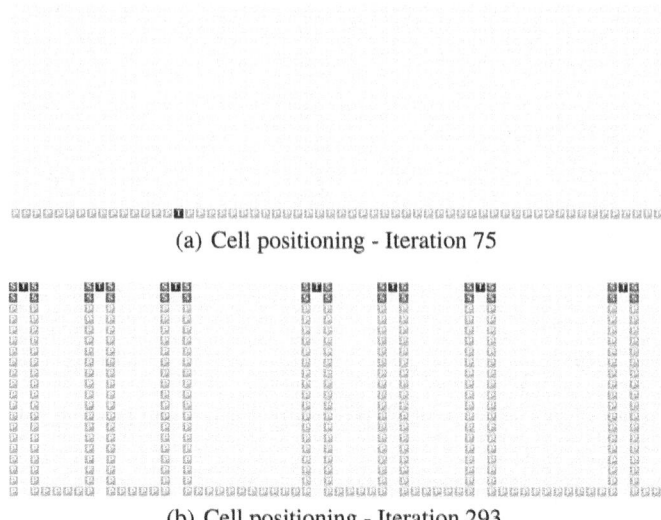

(a) Cell positioning - Iteration 75

(b) Cell positioning - Iteration 293

Fig. 6: The cell matrix during the random diffusion experiment when the first tip cell forms and when the final movement is made in the grid. The time step is shown below the figures.

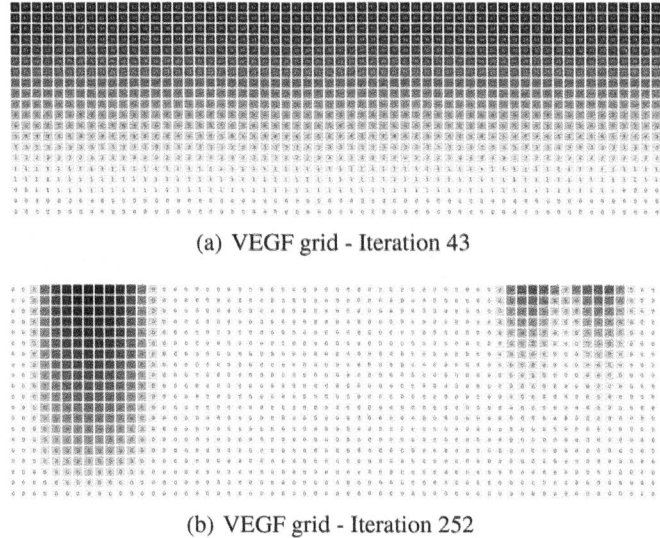

(a) VEGF grid - Iteration 43

(b) VEGF grid - Iteration 252

Fig. 7: The VEGF concentrations for the normal diffusion experiment, where the first frame shows the matrix when the first tip cell has formed and the second shows the matrix when the last tip cell reaches the top of the matrix.

We calculated the average time step at which the described events take place, and the average number of branches with their standard deviations for both normal and random diffusion as shown in Table 2. The experiment repeated 10 times for each diffusion

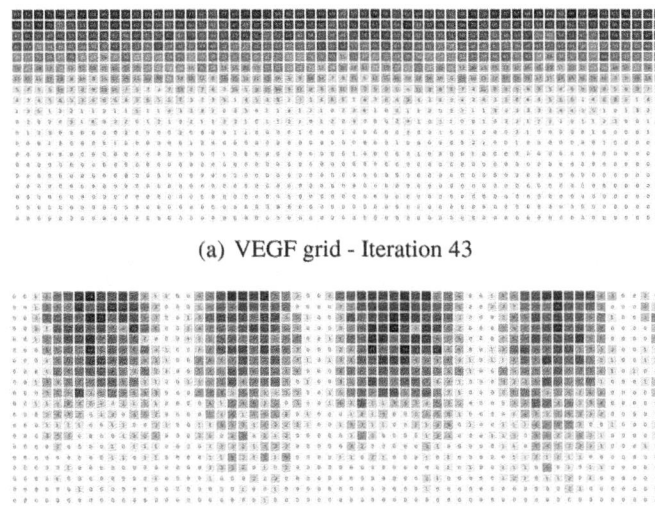

(a) VEGF grid - Iteration 43

(b) VEGF grid - Iteration 252

Fig. 8: The VEGF concentrations in the random diffusion experiments at the same time steps as in the normal diffusion in Fig. 7.

Table 2: The average time step at which the described events take place, and the average number of branches are shown with their standard deviations.

Measurement ($\mu \pm \sigma$)	Normal Diffusion	Random Diffusion
First tip cell	43.0 ± 0	67.9 ± 9.49
Number of branches	14.0 ± 0	7.0 ± 0.63
Last grown branch	252.0 ± 0	289.8 ± 16.10

model. The average number of branches in random diffusion is observed to be half of the number in the normal diffusion simulation. In addition, with normal diffusion, the simulation result is quite stable without any deviations. Therefore, random diffusion model is able to incorporate stochastic nature in biology better.

5.2 VEGF Amount Experiments

VEGF amount experiments were designed to investigate the influence of the initial VEGF concentration introduced into our model. From biological perspective, it can be assumed that the environment closer to the tumor contains higher VEGF levels than the environment more distant from the tumor. Therefore, a small amount of VEGF in the model may be seen as representing angiogenesis influenced by a distant tumor.

We performed these experiments with the same initial settings, varying only the initial VEGF concentration. We used the grid size 20×60 to ensure sufficient space for cell growth. Parameter d_{min} was set to 20. Moreover, we performed 300 iterations with each value of VEGF inserted into the grid. All experiments were conducted for both types of diffusion.

Table 3: Table of results from experiments with different initial VEGF values, with random diffusion and normal diffusion.

VEGF	First transition		number of branches		Last branch	
	random	normal	random	normal	random	normal
50	62	–	7	–	299	–
100	77	72	6	14	264	219
150	87	58	8	17	298	209
200	76	51	8	17	298	202
300	75	43	7	14	293	252
400	76	39	7	14	289	182
500	73	37	8	16	297	114
600	69	35	6	16	228	112
700	68	33	7	16	299	184
800	64	32	8	17	299	183
900	60	31	8	17	284	182
1000	69	30	8	17	298	181

The results from the experiments are shown in Table 3, with random diffusion and normal diffusion. The first column ("VEGF") shows the amount of initial VEGF. The second column ("First transition") indicates at which iteration the first transition of the cell subtype occurred. In our model, the first transition is mostly made by transition from phalanx cell to tip cell. The third column ("Number of branches") shows the number of branches that is grown in total. The last column ("Last branch") tells at which iteration the last branch is fully grown. If the value is noted by '–', the situation does not occur at all.

Regarding to normal diffusion, we observe that the minimum amount of VEGF needed for cell transition is 100. Otherwise, the amount of VEGF, that diffuses to the positions of initial phalanx cells, is trivial. We can also observe a relation between the amount of VEGF and iterations needed to have the first transition. After exceeding the limit amount necessary for the first transition, the time step at which the first transition takes place decreases. The time step at which the last branch is fully grown decreases as well. The number of branches is more stably increased while the amount of VEGF increases. But it does not hold in all cases. On the other hand, with random diffusion, we can not observe similar relation. The time steps for the first transition and the last branch growth are all in certain ranges. There are no obvious increasing trends as observed in normal diffusion. However, it takes much more iterations to have the first transition and the last branch growth. The number of branches is halved comparing to normal diffusion. No pattern can be observed in a number of branches related to the amount of VEGF.

5.3 Sensitivity Analysis

Some of the parameters 1 used in our model such as α_v, γ, d_{SP} and d_{PS} are carefully estimated in [21]. Others, such as d_{min}, R, S_delay and ss_delay, are fine-tuned to fit

Table 4: Parameter range for sensitivity analysis.

Parameter	range
α_v	[0, 3]
d_{SP}	[0.5, 2.5]
d_{min}	[19, 30]

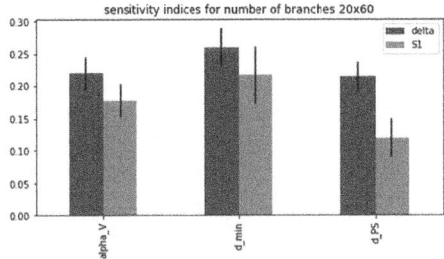

(a) sensitivity indices for number of branches

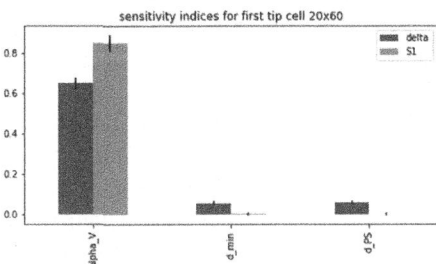

(b) sensitivity indices for first tip cell

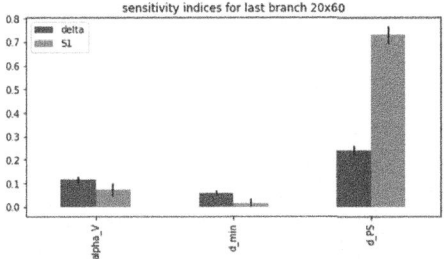

(c) sensitivity indices for last branch

Fig. 9: Results of sensitivity analysis.

the scale of our model. Nevertheless, it is unclear whether iPSC-ECs behave the same way during angiogenesis as endothelial cells derived from adult mice or humans. Therefore, the parameters need to be adjustable and we are interested in understanding the model's sensitivity to these choices. We selected three parameters, which have space to adjust in our model, for a sensitivity analysis. We set a range for each parameter to ensure cell transition occurs within 300 iterations and that branch growth remains reasonable. A reasonable manner means having only one tip cell on top of a branch while growing and no single column branch that can grow without a tip cell. Considering all factors, we define the ranges for the three parameters in Table 4.

We selected three features as the output of the model: the time step for the first tip cell, the time step for the last grown branch, and the total number of branches. The model simulation is conducted using random diffusion. For sensitivity analysis, we use Delta Moment-Independent Measure [4], a global sensitive indicator that evaluates the influence of input uncertainty on the entire output distribution. Furthermore, this method returns first-order Sobol index, which is a variance-based sensitivity [26]. We set number of samples equal to 1024 in total.

The sensitive indices are shown in Fig. 9. We observed that all three parameters contribute to the number of branches, with d_{min} contributing the most with a delta value of 0.26 and an S1 value of 0.22. But they are all not very influential to the output as the number of branches. For the first tip cell transition, α_v contributes the most with a delta score of 0.65 and an S1 score of 0.85. By definition, α_v is the VEGF concentration threshold for the transition of phalanx cells to tip cells. Undoubtedly, it contributes the most for number of iterations needed for the transition of the first tip cell. Interestingly, d_{min} does not contribute much for the transition of the first tip cell. Because, in default, the distance to the nearest tip cell for each phalanx cell is set to infinite before the first tip cell forms. Thus, there is no influence in the formation of the first tip cell. For the time step of the last growth branch, d_{SP} contributes the most with a delta value of 0.24 and an S1 value of 0.73. d_{SP} is the minimum distance to the nearest tip cell for transition from stalk cells to phalanx cells. In our model, d_{SP} and d_{PS} share the same threshold. Thus, if the threshold is too small, it prevents the phalanx cells to transform to stalk cells. Consequently, it prevents the tip cells to move upwards in the grid and prolongs the branch growth.

6   Conclusion

In this paper, we modeled the subtype transitions that iPSC-ECs undergo during sprouting angiogenesis in a microfluidics environment. We used a larger grid size of 20×60 compared to our previous work presented in [30]. The angiogenesis was guided by a VEGF grid. We tested the model's behaviour under various scenarios including normal and random diffusion models and varying initial VEGF concentrations. Moreover, we conducted a sensitivity analysis to evaluate the model's performance.

Two diffusion models were compared to find the most realistic one for model simulation. The normal diffusion simulation produced 14 overcrowded branches in a 20×60 grid. Furthermore, the number of branches is consistent following 10 repetitions. On the other hand, random diffusion resulted in roughly half of the number of branches, averaging 7. However, the number of branches, as well as the time steps for the first tip cell and the last grown branch, varied across 10 repeated simulations. This suggests that random diffusion better captures the stochastic nature of biological process. In addition, we found that the initial amount of VEGF does not affect the speed of angiogenesis with random diffusion. However, it is a crucial parameter for normal diffusion, where increasing VEGF concentration speeds up angiogenesis, and insufficient initial VEGF can prevent the angiogenesis from starting.

New insights were gained during sensitivity analysis with a larger grid size. The number of branches was influenced by all three parameters: α_v, d_{SP} and d_{min}. α_v and d_{min} had slightly greater impact compared to d_{SP}. The time step for first tip cell transition was mostly affected by α_v, with no observed influence from d_{min}. For the time step of the last growth branch, d_{SP} has the most significant contribution. Tip cells need stalk cells to move upwards. Low values of d_{SP} and d_{PS} inhibit the transformation of phalanx cells into stalk cells, thereby extending the time needed for branch growth or even stopping the process when the value is too low.

In this work, we addressed the scalability problem of our model by implementing parallel computing, allowing for simulations on a larger grid size. However, several limitations remain. Our model simplifies cell movement by only permitting upward movement. Lateral movement of tip cells should be included in the future to make the model more realistic. Furthermore, the direction of movement should be influenced by the concentration of VEGF while maintaining contact with stalk cells.

Acknowledgments. This research has received no external funding.

Conflicts of interest. The authors declare that they have no conflict of interest.

References

1. Al-Ostoot, F.H., Salah, S., Khamees, H.A., Khanum, S.A.: Tumor angiogenesis: current challenges and therapeutic opportunities. Cancer Treat. Res. Commun. **28**, 100422 (2021). https://doi.org/10.1016/j.ctarc.2021.100422
2. Beter, M., et al.: Sproutangio: an open-source bioimage informatics tool for quantitative analysis of sprouting angiogenesis and lumen space. Sci. Rep. **13**(1) (2023). https://doi.org/10.1038/s41598-023-33090-6
3. Bookholt, F.D., Monsuur, H.N., Gibbs, S., Vermolen, F.J.: Mathematical modelling of angiogenesis using continuous cell-based models. Biomech. Model. Mechanobiol. **15**(6), 1577–1600 (2016). https://doi.org/10.1007/s10237-016-0784-3
4. Borgonovo, E.: A new uncertainty importance measure. Reliabil. Eng. Syst. Saf. **92**(6), 771–784 (2007). https://doi.org/10.1016/j.ress.2006.04.015
5. Cao, L., der Meer, A.D.v., Verbeek, F.J., Passier, R.: Automated image analysis system for studying cardiotoxicity in human pluripotent stem cell-derived cardiomyocytes. BMC Bioinf. **21**(1) (2020). https://doi.org/10.1186/s12859-020-3466-1
6. Cao, L., Schoenmaker, L., Ten Den, S.A., Passier, R., Schwach, V., Verbeek, F.J.: Automated sarcomere structure analysis for studying cardiotoxicity in human pluripotent stem cell-derived cardiomyocytes. Microsc. Microanal. **29**(1), 254–264 (2022). https://doi.org/10.1093/micmic/ozac016
7. Carmeliet, P., Jain, R., Carmeliet, P., Jain, R.K.: Angiogenesis in cancer and other disease. Nature **407**, 249–57 (2000). https://doi.org/10.1038/35025220
8. Carvalho, R.V., Verbeek, F.J., Coelho, C.J.: Bio-modeling using petri nets: a computational approach. In: Alves Barbosa da Silva, F., Carels, N., Paes Silva Junior, F. (eds.) Theoretical and Applied Aspects of Systems Biology. CB, vol. 27, pp. 3–26. Springer, Cham (2018). https://doi.org/10.1007/978-3-319-74974-7_1
9. Chaouiya, C.: Petri net modelling of biological networks. Brief. Bioinf. **8**(4), 210–219 (2007). https://doi.org/10.1093/bib/bbm029
10. Chaouiya, C., Remy, E., Thieffry, D.: Petri net modelling of biological regulatory networks. J. Disc. Algor. **6**(2), 165–177 (2008). https://doi.org/10.1016/j.jda.2007.06.003
11. van Duinen, V., et al.: Standardized and scalable assay to study perfused 3d angiogenic sprouting of ipsc-derived endothelial cells in vitro. J. Visual. Exp. **153** (2019). https://doi.org/10.3791/59678
12. Folkman, J.: Role of angiogenesis in tumor growth and metastasis. Seminars Oncol. **29**(6, Supplement 16), 15–18 (2002).https://doi.org/10.1016/S0093-7754(02)70065-1. https://www.sciencedirect.com/science/article/pii/S0093775402700651

13. Guerra, A., Belinha, J., Mangir, N., MacNeil, S., Natal Jorge, R.: Sprouting angiogenesis: a numerical approach with experimental validation. Ann. Biomed. Eng. **49**(2), 871–884 (2020). https://doi.org/10.1007/s10439-020-02622-w

14. Harris, C.R., et al.: Array programming with NumPy. Nature **585**(7825), 357–362 (2020). https://doi.org/10.1038/s41586-020-2649-2

15. Hill, C.: A very simple 2-d diffusion model (2017). https://scipython.com/blog/a-very-simple-2-d-diffusion-model/

16. Hoang, D.M., et al: Stem cell-based therapy for human diseases. Signal Transd. Targeted Therapy **7**(1) (2022). https://doi.org/10.1038/s41392-022-01134-4

17. Liu, F., Heiner, M., Gilbert, D.: Coloured Petri nets for multilevel, multiscale and multidimensional modelling of biological systems. Brief. Bioinf. **20**(3), 877–886 (2017). https://doi.org/10.1093/bib/bbx150

18. Lugano, R., Ramachandran, M., Dimberg, A.: Tumor angiogenesis: causes, consequences, challenges and opportunities. Cell. Mol. Life Sci. **77**(9), 1745–1770 (2019). https://doi.org/10.1007/s00018-019-03351-7

19. Matsuya, K., Yura, F., Mada, J., Kurihara, H., Tokihiro, T.: A discrete mathematical model for angiogenesis. SIAM J. Appl. Math. **76**(6), 2243–2259 (2016). https://doi.org/10.1137/15M1038773

20. Peirce, S.: Computational and mathematical modeling of angiogenesis. Microcirculation (New York, N.Y. : 1994) **15**, 739–51 (2008). https://doi.org/10.1080/10739680802220331

21. Phillips, C.M., Lima, E.A.B.F., Woodall, R.T., Brock, A., Yankeelov, T.E.: A hybrid model of tumor growth and angiogenesis: In silico experiments. Plos One **15**(4) (2020). https://doi.org/10.1371/journal.pone.0231137

22. Pommereau, F.: SNAKES: a flexible high-level petri nets library (tool paper). In: Devillers, R., Valmari, A. (eds.) PETRI NETS 2015. LNCS, vol. 9115, pp. 254–265. Springer, Cham (2015). https://doi.org/10.1007/978-3-319-19488-2_13

23. Sainson, R., Harris, A.: Regulation of angiogenesis by homotypic and heterotypic notch signalling in endothelial cells and pericytes: from basic research to potential therapies. Angiogenesis **11**, 41–51 (2008). https://doi.org/10.1007/s10456-008-9098-0

24. Schwach, V., et al.: A safety screening platform for individualized cardiotoxicity assessment. iScience **27**(3), 109139 (2024). https://doi.org/10.1016/j.isci.2024.109139

25. Sharma, A., Sances, S., Workman, M.J., Svendsen, C.N.: Multi-lineage human IPSC-derived platforms for disease modeling and drug discovery. Cell Stem Cell **26**(3), 309–329 (2020). https://doi.org/10.1016/j.stem.2020.02.011

26. Sobol', I., Kucherenko, S.: Derivative based global sensitivity measures and their link with global sensitivity indices. Math. Comput. Simul. **79**(10), 3009–3017 (2009). https://doi.org/10.1016/j.matcom.2009.01.023

27. Toi, M., Bando, H., Ogawa, T., Muta, M., Hornig, C., Weich, H.: Significance of vascular endothelial growth factor (vegf)/soluble vegf receptor-1 relationship in breast cancer. Int. J. Cancer **98**, 14–18 (2002). https://doi.org/10.1002/ijc.10121.abs

28. Valentim, R.A.M., et al.: Stochastic petri net model describing the relationship between reported maternal and congenital syphilis cases in brazil. BMC Med. Inf. Decis. Making **22**(1) (2022). https://doi.org/10.1186/s12911-022-01773-1

29. Vilanova, G., Colominas, I., Gomez, H.: A mathematical model of tumour angiogenesis: growth, regression and regrowth. J. R. Soc. Interface **14**(126), 20160918 (2017). https://doi.org/10.1098/rsif.2016.0918

30. Šterberová, A., Dincu, A., Oudshoorn, S., van Duinen, V., Cao, L.: Modeling ipsc-derived endothelial cell transition in tumor angiogenesis using petri nets. In: Proceedings of the 17th International Joint Conference on Biomedical Engineering Systems and Technologies. SCITEPRESS - Science and Technology Publications (2024). https://doi.org/10.5220/0012268800003657

A Linear Algorithm For Efficient Representation of k-mer Sets Using De Bruijn Graphs

Enrico Rossignolo and Matteo Comin$^{(\boxtimes)}$

Department of Information Engineering, University of Padova, 35131 Padua, Italy
{enrico.rossignolo,matteo.comin}@unipd.it

Abstract. A fundamental operation in computational genomics is the reduction of input sequences into their constituent k-mers. Developing space-efficient methods to represent a collection of k-mers is crucial for enhancing the scalability of bioinformatics analyses. A common strategy is to transform the set of k-mers into a de Bruijn graph and then create a streamlined representation by identifying the smallest path cover.

In this article, we introduce USTAR2, a novel algorithm for compressing k-mers. USTAR2 leverages node connectivity principles in the de Bruijn graph for more efficient path selection in constructing the path cover. We tested USTAR2 on real read datasets and compared it with several other tools. USTAR2 demonstrated superior performance in terms of compression, requiring less memory and being significantly faster (up to 96x).

The code of USTAR2 is available at the repository https://github.com/CominLab/USTAR2.

Keywords: k-mer set · Compression · Bruijn graphs

1 Introduction

The field of computational genomics significantly benefits from the utilization of k-mer-based tools, which present numerous advantages over methodologies that directly process reads or read alignments. These tools primarily work by converting input sequence data, which can vary in length according to the sequencing technology employed, into a collection of k-mers—fixed-length sequences—accompanied by their respective counts. This conversion facilitates a more streamlined and effective analysis of genomic data.

k-mer-based methods have always exhibited superior performance across a range of applications. For instance, in genome assembly, tools such as Spades [2] utilize k-mer-based techniques to reconstruct entire genomes from reads with high accuracy.

In metagenomics, Kraken [35] excels at classifying microorganisms in complex environmental samples using k-mers, offering a speedup of $900\times$ compared to MegaBLAST. As a result, many tools for metagenomic classification are now

M. P. Guarino et al. (Eds.): BIOSTEC 2024, CCIS 2546, pp. 167–191, 2026.
https://doi.org/10.1007/978-3-031-96899-0_11

k-mer-based [1,5,23,32]. In genotyping, several tools [9,17,18,34] utilize k-mers instead of alignments to identify genetic variations in individuals and populations. In phylogenomics, Mash [19] employs k-mers to estimate distances between genomes and metagenomes, facilitating the reconstruction of evolutionary relationships among organisms. In database searching, a wide array of k-mer-based methods [3,11,16,20,33] have been developed to efficiently search sequences. k-mer-based methods have revolutionized multiple aspects of bioinformatics and have become indispensable for analyzing large-scale genomic data. To handle the vast modern sequencing datasets, these tools often rely on specialized and efficient data structures for representing sets of k-mers.

Storing sets of k-mers can be space-intensive, particularly for large databases. Conway and Bromage [8] found that, in the worst case, at least $\binom{\log 4^k}{n}$ bits are required to losslessly store a set of n k-mers. However, k-mer sets derived from sequencing experiments often exhibit a spectrum-like property [6] and contain many redundant information. Consequently, efficient data structures can significantly optimize this storage requirement [7].

Given the substantial space requirements for storing k-mer sets, reducing their size is essential. For instance, the dataset used to evaluate the BIGSI [24] index occupies roughly 12 TB of storage even in compressed form.

Given the vast volume of data accessible to bioinformaticians, the need for efficient data representation becomes imperative. With the ongoing advancements in sequencing technologies, the amount of genomic data is expected to grow substantially in the coming years. Therefore, analyzing this data will increasingly require serious computational resources.

Nevertheless, this challenge can be mitigated by using a solid k-mers representation that reduces RAM usage and accelerates analysis tools, allowing for the execution of more extensive pipelines with less computational effort. To achieve this objective, a compact, plain text representation has emerged as the most reasonable solution.

Formally, a plain text representation embodies a set of strings that includes every k-mer derived from the input sequences, whether in their forward or reverse-complemented forms, while excluding any other k-mers. This set, which may contain k-mer repetitions, is referred to as a Spectrum-Preserving String Set (SPSS), according to Schmidt et al. [30]. It is noteworthy that this definition diverges from the one proposed by Rahman and Medvedev [24], who additionally require that each k-mer appears at most once within the set.

A plain text representation offers significant advantages in certain tools, such as Bifrost's query [12], which can utilized a plain text representation as a index without requiring any modifications. Furthermore, a plain text form does not require decompression that causes overhead in the entire pipeline.

In this paper, we introduce USTAR2[1], an algorithm for k-mer set compression that leverages the correspondence between a path cover in a De Bruijn graph and its k-mer set representation. The tool exploits the graph's node connectivity and intelligently reuses nodes to minimize the impact of the representation.

---

[1] A preliminary version of USTAR2 has been presented at BIOINFORMATICS 2024 [28].

1.1   Related Works

Rahman and Medvedev [24], along with Břinda, Baym, and Kucherov [4], independently explored the concept of storing a set of k-mers in plain text without repetitions to achieve a more compact representation. They named this concept respectively "Spectrum-Preserving String Set" (SPSS) [24] and "simplitigs" [4]. To avoid confusion with the new definition of SPSS, we refer to this concept as simplitigs.

Both Rahman and Medvedev with UST and Břinda, Baym, and Kucherov with ProphAsm propose algorithms that involve greedily joining consecutive unitigs to create such a representation. UST operates on the node-centric de Bruijn graph constructed from the input strings. It identifies arbitrary paths within this graph, starting from arbitrary nodes. Each node is visited by one path, and if a path cannot be extended forward, either due to a dead-end or all successor nodes having been visited, a new path begins from a new node. If, before starting a new path, any successor node of the finished path denotes the start of a different path, these two paths are merged. During traversal, the unitigs of the visited nodes are concatenated, ensuring that k-1 overlapping characters are not repeated. These concatenated strings constitute the final output.

ProphAsm does not construct a de Bruijn graph. Instead, the approach involves collecting all k-mers into a hash table and then extending each k-mer in both forward and backward directions as far as possible without repetition.

These heuristic approaches significantly minimize the number of strings (string count, SC) and the total length of these strings (cumulative length, CL) required to store a k-mer set. The reduction in CL directly leads to lower memory usage for string storage. Additionally, a decrease in SC is beneficial as it reduces the size of the index structure needed to store the strings, making the overall storage more efficient.

Břinda, Baym, and Kucherov showed that using simplitigs significantly reduces both the SC and CL in tangled de Bruijn graphs, such as those derived from single large genomes with short k-mer lengths and pangenome graphs with many genomes. They highlighted the benefits of simplitigs in downstream applications, like faster k-mer query run times with BWA [15]. Moreover, they found that storing simplitigs with a general-purpose compressors requires less space compared to compressed unitigs.

Similarly, the authors of UST reported substantial reductions in SC and CL across various datasets and noted that simplitigs occupy less space than unitigs when compressed.

Additionally, Khan et al. [13] provided a comprehensive overview of simplitigs applications to various genomic datasets, including a human gut metagenome.

Both the authors of UST and ProphAsm established a lower bound on the cumulative length of simplitigs and demonstrated that their heuristics produce representations with a cumulative length close to this bound for typical k values, such as 31. However, for smaller k values (e.g., <20), which result in denser de Bruijn graphs, their heuristics do not approach the lower bound as closely.

Recently, a new heuristic called USTAR (Unitig STitch Advanced constRuction) was proposed in [26,27]. USTAR employs a strategy based on graph connectivity to explore de Bruijn graphs more effectively. By leveraging the density of the de Bruijn graph and node connectivity, USTAR enhances path selection for constructing the path cover, resulting in better compression, especially for denser de Bruijn graphs.

Several existing tools utilize simplitigs. For example, Cuttlefish2, a compacted de Bruijn graph builder [13], includes functionality to output simplitigs rather than maximal unitigs. Additionally, there has been a recent proposal for a standardized file format for k-mer sets that specifically supports simplitigs [10] and other plain text representations.

All these authors have investigated whether computing minimum simplitigs without repeating k-mers might be NP-hard. However, Schmidt and Alanko [31] recently proved that simplitigs with minimum cumulative length, named "eulertigs", can be computed in polynomial time. Their algorithm constructs a bidirected arc-centric de Bruijn graph in linear time using a suffix tree, followed by eulerization and the computation of a bidirected Eulerian circuit in the eulerized graph. Eulertigs optimally represent simplitigs by concatenating consecutive unitigs without repeating k-mers.

Interestingly, Eulertigs are only slightly smaller than the strings produced by previous heuristics, indicating that significant further improvements may be limited when k-mer repetitions are not allowed in a plain text representation.

In a recent study [30], the authors introduced the first algorithm for finding an SPSS of minimum size (CL) that allows for repeated k-mers. The compression advantage of SPSS compared to simplitigs and Eulertigs is significant. They demonstrated that finding a minimum SPSS with repeated k-mers is polynomially solvable, utilizing a many-to-many min-cost path query and a min-cost perfect matching approach. However, this optimal algorithm, called Matchtigs, requires $O(n^3m)$ time, where n is the number of nodes and m is the number of arcs in the de Bruijn graph, making it impractical for large datasets.

To address this, the same authors proposed a greedy heuristic for generating a compact SPSS, called Greedy Matchtigs, which gives up the optimal matching to improve efficiency.

In the next sections, we introduce USTAR2, a faster and more memory-efficient greedy heuristic designed to generate a compact SPSS for large datasets. USTAR2 is based on the USTAR paradigm [26,27], but it allows for repeated k-mers and can explore the de Bruijn graph more deeply, resulting in improved compression.

2   USTAR2: Unitig STitch Advanced ConstRuction 2

2.1   Definitions

In the context of this paper, we consider a string composed of characters from the set $\Sigma = \{A, C, T, G\}$. A string with a length of k is referred to as a "k-mer". Its "reverse complement", denoted as $rc(\cdot)$, is derived by reversing the k-mer and substituting each character with its complementary base, such as $A \mapsto T$, $C \mapsto G$, $T \mapsto A$, and $G \mapsto C$. Since the origin DNA strand is unknown, we treat a k-mer and its reverse complement as identical.

Given a string $s = \langle s_1, \ldots, s_{|s|} \rangle$, we use $pref_i(s)$ to denote the first i characters of s, and $suf_i(s)$ for the last i characters. We introduce the "glue" operation between two strings, u and v, where $suf_{k-1}(u)$ matches $pref_{k-1}(v)$. This operation concatenates u with the suffix of v:

$$u \odot^{k-1} v = u \cdot suf_{|v|-(k-1)}(v)$$

For example, given two 3-mers, $u = CTG$ and $v = TGA$, their gluing results in $u \odot^2 v = CTGA$.

A collection of k-mers can be graphically represented by a de Bruijn graph, where we introduce a node-centric definition, indicating that the connections (arcs) are implicitly defined by the nodes. Therefore, we use the terms k-mers set and $dBG(K)$ interchangeably.

For a given set of k-mers $K = \{m_1, \ldots m_{|K|}\}$, a de Bruijn graph of K is a directed graph, $dBG(K) = (V, A)$, with the following attributes:

1. $V = \{v_1, \ldots, v_{|K|}\}$
2. Each node v in V has a label $lab(v_i) = m_i$
3. Each node v in V has two distinct sides $s_v \in \{0, 1\}$, where $(v, 1)$ is visually represented with a tip
4. A node side (v, s_v) is spelled as:

$$spell(v, s_v) = \begin{cases} lab(v) & \text{if } s_v = 0 \\ rc(lab(v)) & \text{if } s_v = 1 \end{cases} \qquad (1)$$

5. An arc exists between two node sides (v, s_v) and (u, s_u) if and only if there are spellings that share a $(k-1)$-mer. In particular, this condition holds:

$$((v, s_v), (u, s_u)) \in A \iff$$

$$suf_{k-1}(spell(v, 1 - s_v)) = pref_{k-1}(spell(u, s_u))$$

This right-hand condition is also known as the (v, u)-oriented-overlap [24].

It's important to note that the notion of node sides allows for treating a k-mer and its reverse complement as the same node entity.

A path $p = \langle (v_1, s_1), \ldots, (v_l, s_l) \rangle$ is spelled by concatenating the spellings of its node sides:

$$spell(p) = spell(v_1, s_1) \odot^{k-1} \cdots \odot^{k-1} spell(v_l, s_l)$$

A path p is considered a "unitig" if its internal nodes have both in-degree and out-degree equal to 1. Additionally, a unitig is said "maximal" if it cannot be extended on either end. To reduce memory usage, a $dBG(K)$ can be "compacted" by replacing maximal unitigs with single nodes labeled with the spellings of the unitigs.

An example of a compacted dBG(K), with $k = 4$, is presented in Fig. 1. In this example, the maximal unitig $(CGAA, GAAA)$ has been replaced with the node $CGAA$.

2.2   Fast and Succint k-mer Set Compression

A k-mer set K can be compressed by creating a representation S consisting of strings of arbitrary length, such that the set of all k-mers extracted from S precisely matches the original set K.

The "spectrum" of a set of strings S is defined as the set of all k-mers and their reverse complements that occur in at least one string $s \in S$, formally

$$spec_k(S) = \{t \in \Sigma^k | \exists s \in S : t \text{ or } rc(t) \text{ is substring of } s\}$$

Consider a set of input strings K, each composed of k characters. Our goal is to find a minimal collection of strings that maintains a particular spectrum. Formally, this can be defined as follows:

Definition 1. *A Spectrum Preserving String Set (SPSS) for the input set of k-mers K is a collection of strings, denoted as S, where each string in S has a length of at least k, and such that $spec_k(K) = spec_k(S)$.*

The key property of the SPSS is its ability to contain the same collection of k-mers as the original input set K, including both the k-mers themselves and their reverse complements. Notably, our definition permits the repetition of k-mers and their reverse complements, whether within a single string or spread across multiple strings.

A straightforward method to assess the size of a string set S is by computing its *cumulative length* defined as the sum of all the string lengths:

$$CL(S) = \sum_{s \in S} |s|$$

where $|s|$ is the length of the string s.

Problem 1. Given as input a k-mer set K, find the Spectrum Preserving String Set S with minimum $CL(S)$.

Essentially, our objective is to identify the smallest possible set of strings, each at least k characters long, that preserves the k-mer spectrum of the original input strings. This means that k-mers and their reverse complements may be repeated within or across these strings. This approach differs from simplitigs, which impose an additional constraint on the repetition of k-mers.

It has been shown in [30] that Problem 1 can be solved exactly in polynomial time. The authors introduced an algorithm that utilizes a many-to-many minimum-cost path query combined with a minimum-cost perfect matching strategy. However, this optimal algorithm, named Matchtigs, demands $O(n^3 m)$ time complexity, where n represents the number of nodes in the de Bruijn graph and m the number of arcs, making it impractical for processing large datasets.

The objective of our study is to develop an effective heuristic capable of handling large datasets efficiently while achieving high-quality compression of k-mers.

Consider again the example in Fig. 1. From the path $p = (GGAA, GAAT, AATC)$ we can compute its spell $spell(p) = GGAATC$ that contains all the

4-mers *GGAA*, *GAAT* and *AATC* in p, with a saving of 6 bases. Thus from a set of paths P that contains all the nodes in dBG(K) we can derive a set S of strings that represent all the k-mers in K, that is, an SPSS of K. Therefore a path cover can be used in order to compute S and thus compress the k-mer set. Note that the paths can pass through the same node more than once.

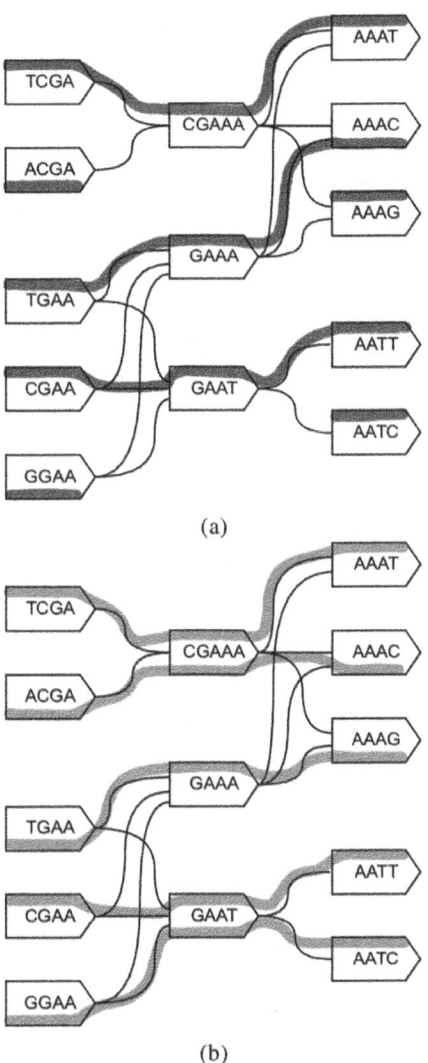

Fig. 1. An example of a compacted de Bruijn graph with $k = 4$ is shown. Nodes are labeled with k-mers. In Figure (a), simplitigs are represented by the red disjoint path cover, where each node is traversed only once, resulting in a total cumulative length (CL) of 35. In Figure (b), an SPSS is represented by the green path cover computed by USTAR2, where nodes can be reused, leading to a total CL of 32. Figure reported also in [29] (Color figure online).

In the context of simplitigs, where k-mers are not allowed to be reused, various greedy and non-optimal algorithms have been proposed. ProphAsm [4] employs a straightforward heuristic: it selects an arbitrary k-mer from the de Bruijn graph (dBG(K)), attempts to extend it both forwards and backwards as much as possible, and repeats this process until all k-mers have been covered. Similarly, UST [24] uses the compacted dBG(K) generated by BCALM2. It starts with an arbitrary node, extends it forward as far as possible, and then restarts with available nodes, ultimately merging linked paths. Both methods follow a comparable approach of selecting an initial k-mer and extending it without taking the entire graph structure into account.

For instance, as illustrated in Fig. 1, ProphAsm and UST, by choosing nodes arbitrarily, may generate simplitigs similar to those shown in Fig. 1(a). When computing the spelling of each path, we obtain the set of 7 strings $S = \{TCGAAAT, ACGA, TGAAAC, AAAG, CGAATT, GGAA, AATC\}$ with a cumulative length $CL(S) = 35$.

To solve Problem 1 and construct a minimum SPSS using the Matchtigs algorithm, the time complexity will be $O(n^3 m)$. As discussed by the authors, this exact algorithm is impractical for large datasets. In the case of simplitigs, it is evident that both ProphAsm and UST are not optimal algorithms. However, their underlying structure is quite efficient, as each node is processed only once, resulting in linear complexity.

In this work, we present USTAR2 (Unitig STitch Advanced constRuction) a linear compression algorithm that exploits the connectivity of the dBG graph, to ensure a good compression ratio, while efficiently traversing the graph.

USTAR2 employs a heuristic to approximate a minimum SPSS, similarly to UST, leveraging the compacted de Bruijn graph generated by BCALM2. Like UST and ProphAsm, USTAR2 begins by choosing a seed node from the graph and attempts to construct a path starting from this node. The path is built by linking adjacent nodes until extension is no longer possible. The process is repeated with new seed nodes until every node is covered by a path. The effectiveness of USTAR2 hinges on two crucial operations: selecting an optimal seed node and extending the path using available connections.

The pseudocode of USTAR2 is shown in Algorithm 1.

In order to select a good seed node, we need to ensure that this node will be part of an optimal path for the SPSS problem. We define the imbalance of a node, $Imb(v) = |OutDegree(v) - InDegree(v)|$, as the absolute difference between the out-degree and in-degree of the node v. In general, if a node is balanced, that is $Imb(v) = 0$, it is very likely to be traversed by one or more paths. However, as proved in [30], if a node is imbalanced $Imb(v) \neq 0$, it must be the starting or ending point of some optimal path. Therefore, balanced nodes should be avoided as starting points; instead, only nodes with imbalances should be chosen as seed nodes. To capitalize on this insight, USTAR2 selects the most imbalanced node, i.e. the one with the highest $Imb(v)$ value, as the seed node at each iteration.

The topological properties of the de Bruijn graph are important, not only for the identification of good seed nodes but also for the construction of a path from this node.

Algorithm 1. USTAR2.

Data: de Bruijn graph *dBG*; parameter D
Result: SPSS *S*
begin

    $S = \emptyset$
    seed-nodes = sort nodes by $Imb(node)$
    for *seed* $\in$ *seed-nodes* **do**
        if *seed is not visited* **then**
            visit (*seed*)
            contig = Extend (*seed*) to the right
            contig = Extend (*contig*) to the left
            $S = S \cup \{contig\}$

    return S

Function Extend (*contig*) :

    L = {non-visited neighbors of contig head}
    while *L not empty* **do**
        v = less connected node in L
        visit (*v*)
        contig = merge(v, contig)
        L = {non-visited neighbors of v}

    L = {neighbors of contig head}
    level = 1
    found new node = false;
    while *level<=D and not found new node* **do**
        L = {neighbors of all nodes in L}
        level=level+1
        L = Filter (L)
        L' = {non-visited nodes in L}
        if L' *not empty* **then**
            k = less connected node in L'
            visit (*k*)
            found new node = true;
            p = path from k to contig head
            contig = merge(p, contig)

    if *found new node* **then**
        return Extend (*contig*)
    else
        return contig

Function Filter (*L*) :

    for $v \in L$ **do**
        p = path from v to contig head
        if *length(p) > 2k - 2* **then**
            remove v from L

    return L

In constructing the path cover for simplitigs, we have noted that both UST and ProphAsm may select highly connected nodes [26]. Since these nodes become unavailable in subsequent iterations, such choices can result in isolated nodes, thereby increasing the cumulative length. As illustrated in Fig. 1(a), the path cover for simplitigs creates four isolated nodes, which contribute significantly to the high CL value. This issue persists in the context of SPSS, even though nodes can be visited multiple times.

In USTAR2, we aim to prevent this issue by adopting a different strategy. During each iteration, we extend the current path by selecting the node with fewer connections, ensuring that highly connected nodes remain available for later use. This approach helps reduce the CL by producing fewer, longer strings, which minimizes the likelihood of generating isolated nodes. Just like in UST, USTAR2 extends the current seed node first to the right and then to the left to construct a contig.

When the current contig can no longer be extended due to all neighboring nodes having been visited, we attempt to reuse one of these nodes to connect to an unvisited node. This search is conducted using a breadth-first search (BFS) with a depth limit D to restrict the exploration range. During each iteration, we prune the search space by eliminating branches that would increase the cumulative length (CL). Specifically, we discard nodes that would produce a path longer than $2k - 2$, as extending beyond this length would not improve the CL and would be better served by creating two separate contigs. If multiple unvisited nodes are available, we select the one with fewer connections to maintain consistency with our previous strategy.

In terms of running time, this algorithm will traverse efficiently the de Bruijn graph. In order to efficiently implement the above algorithm, we can take advantage of efficient data structures to store the most important information. For example, the list of seed nodes can be ordered in $O(n)$ time, where n is the number of nodes, using radix sort, since we know the maximum imbalance of a node. Also, the nodes can be ordered by the number of connections so that we can select the less connected node in constant time. Since we are dealing with DNA sequences, the alphabet is composed of only 4 bases and consequently, each node in the de Bruijn graph can have at most 4 neighbors. Thus, in the breadth-first search at level D we can visit at most 4^D nodes. However, in real cases, the distribution of k-mers will produced a sparse de Bruijn graph. Moreover, the filtering step will reduced the number of visited nodes and thus this value is only an upper bound. Overall, in the traversal of the graph with the function *Extend* each iteration takes constant time, where the constant is at most 4^D. In summary, the above algorithm runs in linear time on n, the number of nodes in the graph.

In the example in Fig. 1(b), we can see that allowing multiple traversals of a node enables USTAR2 to construct a minimum-sized SPSS. USTAR2 ensures that the most connected node, $GAAA$, is initially avoided while building the first paths. This results in a path cover (shown in green) of the de Bruijn graph, forming a set of five strings: $S' = \{TCGAAAT, ACGAAAC, TGAAAG,$

$CGAATT, GGAATC\}$. The cumulative length of S' is $CL(S') = 32$. Overall we obtain

$$CL(S') = 32 < CL(S) = 35 < CL(K) = 53$$

In this scenario, the uncompressed k-mer set would require a cumulative length of $CL(K) = 53$. With simplitigs, the k-mer set can be compressed to $CL(S) = 35$, whereas the SPSS computed by USTAR2 achieves a more efficient compression with $CL(S') = 32$.

3   Results

In this section, we present the results of a series of experiments designed to determine the most effective tool for compressing k-mers. To evaluate the performance of our tool, USTAR2, we conducted comparative assessments against several existing tools: UST [24], USTAR [26], Matchtigs, and Greedy Matchtigs [30].

To conduct our assessments, we utilized a collection of real read datasets obtained from the NCBI's Sequence Read Archive that was selected by previous studies [4, 7, 14, 21, 25]. A summary of the properties of these datasets is provided in Table 1.

Table 1. A summary of the read datasets used in the experiments. Datasets are downloaded from NCBI's Sequence Read Archive.

Dataset	Description	Read Length	#Reads	Size [GB]
SRR001665	Escherichia coli	36	20,816,448	9.304
SRR061958	Human Microbiome 1	101	53,588,068	3.007
SRR062379	Human Microbiome 2	100	64,491,564	2.348
SRR10260779	Musa balbisiana RNA-Seq	101	44,227,112	2.363
SRR11458718	Soybean RNA-seq	125	83,594,116	3.565
SRR13605073	Broiler chicken DNA	92	14,763,228	0.230
SRR14005143	Foodborne pathogens	211	1,713,786	0.261
SRR332538	Drosophila ananassae	75	18,365,926	0.683
SRR341725	Gut microbiota	90	25,479,128	1.254
SRR5853087	Danio rerio RNA-Seq	101	119,482,078	3.194
SRR957915	Human RNA-seq	101	49,459,840	3.671

For each dataset, we computed all k-mers for different values of k (see Table 7 in the Appendix); the k-mer lengths considered are 15, 21, 31, and 41. All the tools in examination require the preliminary construction of a compacted de Bruijn graph (dBG) and an input file in the format proposed by the authors of

BCALM2 [7]; for this reason all datasets are preprocessed by BCALM2 once for all. For USTAR2 we use the default parameter $D = 7$.

The following experiments are executed on a server equipped with Intel(R) Xeon(R) Platinum 8260 CPU @ 2.40 GHz and 100 GB of RAM, bounding the maximum amount of memory available.

Table 2. Considering $k = 21$, the datasets are processed with the following tools: UST, USTAR, USTAR2, Greedy Matchtigs, and Matchtigs. For each tool, the cumulative length (CL) is provided. Note that Matchtigs was only able to process four datasets due to out-of-memory errors with the others. The average CL across all experiments is shown in the final row in which USTAR obtained the best value and it is highlighted in bold.

K = 21	CL				
	UST	USTAR	USTAR2	Greedy Matchtigs	Matchtigs
SRR001665_1	36,357,928	36,324,848	33,638,588	33,858,376	33,380,903
SRR001665_2	45,751,142	45,694,102	41,864,643	42,201,273	41,478,989
SRR061958_1	623,862,618	191,039,506	178,434,526	179,301,460	
SRR061958_2	767,654,838	211,459,109	198,026,097	198,820,674	
SRR062379_1	252,418,995	248,519,235	226,998,129	228,491,551	
SRR062379_2	246,073,774	241,478,754	220,352,087	221,708,614	
SRR10260779_1	188,012,488	184,854,088	170,629,253	171,477,677	
SRR10260779_2	214,245,523	210,202,663	192,382,255	193,409,534	
SRR11458718_1	189,827,141	185,070,581	170,218,475	171,003,884	
SRR11458718_2	202,891,014	196,865,834	179,815,285	180,632,752	
SRR13605073_1	86,006,020	84,974,720	81,822,046	81,970,005	
SRR14005143_1	19,355,339	19,020,479	17,477,215	17,546,167	17,376,011
SRR14005143_2	42,328,593	41,492,693	37,213,243	37,481,708	36,908,792
SRR332538_1	18,649,027	18,382,747	17,615,333	17,688,889	
SRR332538_2	49,648,910	46,689,430	41,053,913	41,226,736	
SRR341725_1	245,548,134	243,816,714	236,221,721	236,557,911	
SRR341725_2	258,344,641	256,477,401	247,741,588	248,138,629	
SRR5853087_1	587,246,289	551,618,109	484,650,727	486,008,368	
SRR957915_1	377,292,074	366,210,794	325,707,476	327,968,686	
SRR957915_2	579,294,390	562,058,930	501,809,029	505,129,713	
average	251,540,444	197,112,537	**180,183,581**	181,031,130	

In the first experiment, we ran UST, USTAR, USTAR2, Greedy Matchtigs and Matchtigs using the k-mer sets of all datasets with $k = 21$. The results are presented in Table 2 in which are reported the cumulative length (CL) of the sequences computed with each tool. We were able to run Matchtigs only for the datasets with the smaller number of $k - mers$, since for the other datasets it gave out-of-memory errors, meaning that 100GB of RAM were not sufficient to run the program. This behavior was expected, since also the authors of Matchtigs [30] reported the problem. To bypass this problem, we included in the analysis also the greedy version of Matchtigs that produces very similar results to the optimal counterpart.

As anticipated, Matchtigs' algorithm, being exact, generates the optimal k-mers representation. USTAR2 ranks second, consistently outperforming all other tools and achieving the most compact representations for all datasets, coming close to the optimal.

Table 3. File size of k-mers (with $k = 21$) after compression using MFCompress. Dataset SRR5853087_1 encountered a compression error. Several Matchtigs computations failed previously due to out-of-memory errors.

k = 21	Compression				
	UST	USTAR	USTAR2	Greedy Matchtigs	Matchtigs
SRR001665_1	12,641,658	12,332,551	8,700,726	8,813,736	8,845,254
SRR001665_2	15,492,263	15,109,673	10,860,629	11,003,600	10,876,474
SRR061958_1	194,173,905	185,905,825	45,319,763	45,454,536	
SRR061958_2	235,657,588	225,975,765	50,305,926	50,486,848	
SRR062379_1	82,713,766	79,283,723	58,666,732	58,566,163	
SRR062379_2	80,164,746	76,708,406	56,647,674	56,882,630	
SRR10260779_1	64,644,700	61,724,139	43,092,171	43,311,649	
SRR10260779_2	72,772,294	69,375,320	48,707,100	48,574,622	
SRR11458718_1	64,694,925	61,236,404	42,574,564	42,645,409	
SRR11458718_2	68,982,466	65,438,050	44,755,366	44,708,191	
SRR13605073_1	25,833,347	24,546,244	20,112,062	20,144,454	
SRR14005143_1	6,419,520	6,220,215	4,208,321	4,179,654	4,194,213
SRR14005143_2	13,117,896	12,655,430	8,983,371	8,932,076	8,980,170
SRR332538_1	5,737,778	5,599,034	4,378,514	4,393,504	
SRR332538_2	14,410,775	13,528,977	9,813,628	9,712,821	
SRR341725_1	80,436,678	78,193,253	60,734,955	61,160,751	
SRR341725_2	84,250,689	81,877,574	63,841,063	64,009,811	
SRR5853087_1					
SRR957915_1	122,748,678	116,872,195	83,085,402	82,631,218	
SRR957915_2	182,073,051	172,757,385	129,433,290	130,303,345	
average	75,103,512	71,860,009	**41,801,119**	41,890,264	

We can observe that tools based on simplitigs, such as UST and USTAR, are unable to compress k-mers effectively due to the k-mer uniqueness constraint. In contrast, USTAR2 and Greedy Matchtigs, which use the more general SPSS approach allowing k-mer reuse, achieve significantly better results in terms of CL. Among USTAR2's competitors, Greedy Matchtigs stands out as the top performer, particularly in scenarios where Matchtigs cannot be run due to memory limitations.

In evaluating the quality of compression, we utilized two separate metrics: CL (Cumulative Length), as described in Sect. 2.2, which evaluates quality prior to compressing k-mers; and *compression*, which refers to the size of the file containing the string representation of k-mers after compression using the dedicated compressor MFCompress [22].

In our subsequent experiment, we evaluated the compressibility of different representations by comparing their file sizes after compression. The results are detailed in Table 3. As previously stated, Matchtigs failed to run on several datasets due to out-of-memory errors; furthermore, MFCompress crashed when processing dataset SRR5853087_1. Overall, Greedy Matchtigs emerged as the most effective compressor, with USTAR2 performing nearly as well, while USTAR and UST showed significantly poorer results.

The length of k-mers is a crucial parameter in many bioinformatics applications. In several studies [1,17,34,35], a k-mer length of 31 is used, balancing the need to capture sequence context with computational efficiency. Therefore, we investigated the behavior of CL and *compression* across different k-mer lengths ($k \in \{15, 21, 31, 41\}$). The average results for CL and *compression* are presented in Tables 4 and 5, respectively. Matchtigs was excluded from these experiments as it could only be run on a limited subset of the datasets.

USTAR2 consistently showed superior CL across various k-mer sizes, outperforming other tools except for $k = 15$. Notably, it achieved the best compression results for all k-mer lengths except $k = 15$. In contrast, UST and USTAR consistently demonstrated significantly lower compression performance, with UST producing an average 44% larger files compared to USTAR2. This comparative analysis underscores the dominance of USTAR2 and Greedy Matchtigs over UST and USTAR in terms of both CL and compression metrics. Specifically, at $k = 31$, the most commonly used k-mer size, USTAR2 exhibited the highest CL and *compression* performances among all evaluated tools.

Table 4. Average Cumulative Length (CL) across datasets for different values of $k \in \{15, 21, 31, 41\}$ among UST, USTAR, USTAR2, and Greedy Matchtigs. Except for $k = 15$, USTAR2 achieved the highest CL (highlighted in bold), followed by Greedy Matchtigs, USTAR, and UST.

Cumulative Length			
k	UST	USTAR	USTAR2	Greedy Matchtigs
15	389,526,197	225,048,269	122,088,205	**118,257,100**
21	251,540,444	197,112,537	**180,183,581**	181,031,130
31	296,999,909	293,947,184	**217,688,497**	218,851,662
41	366,686,084	364,249,733	**269,841,393**	271,412,813

Table 5. Average *compression*, measured as the size reduction of the fasta file using MFCompress, across all datasets for different values of $k \in \{15, 21, 31, 41\}$ among UST, USTAR, USTAR2, and Greedy Matchtigs.

	Compression			
k	UST	USTAR	USTAR2	Greedy Matchtigs
15	114,627,914	69,954,835	30,659,296	**29,313,703**
21	75,103,512	71,860,009	**41,801,119**	41,890,264
31	68,297,756	68,585,282	**49,427,296**	49,672,063
41	70,445,678	71,874,051	**50,595,570**	51,137,503

3.1 Time and Memory Usage

In the previous experiments, we identified USTAR2 and Greedy Matchtigs as the best performing compression algorithms. However, it's important to note that Greedy Matchtigs is based on the exact algorithm of Matchtigs, which may pose efficiency challenges from a computational point of view.

To study the computational performances of these tools, we conducted a comprehensive analysis of their time and memory usage. Currently, USTAR2 runs in a single-threaded mode, whereas Greedy Matchtigs leverages multi-threading capabilities. Initially, we compared these tools under their respective single-threaded configurations.

In the previous tests, we also collected the time and memory consumption across all datasets while varying the k-mer size. The average computational times are depicted in Fig. 2, and the corresponding memory requirements are illustrated in Fig. 3.

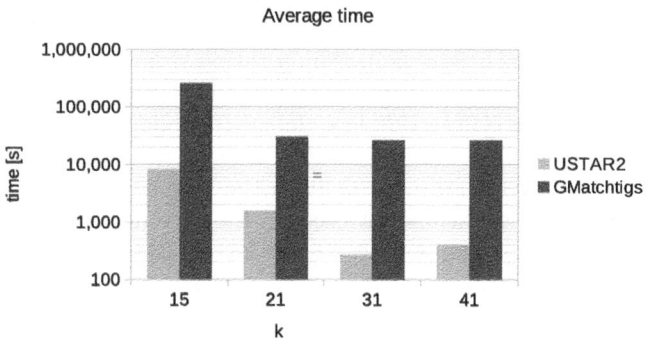

Fig. 2. Average time in seconds (single-thread) used by USTAR2 and Greedy Matchtigs for different k-mer lengths, in a logarithmic scale. USTAR2 execution time is consistently much lower compared to Greedy Matchtigs, resulting in a 96× maximum speedup. Figure reported also in [29].

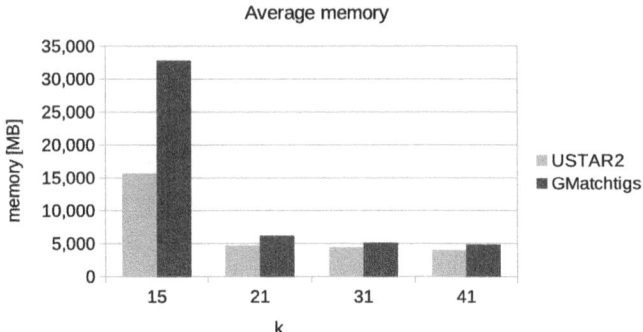

Fig. 3. Average memory in megabyte used by USTAR2 and Greedy Matchtigs for different k-mer lengths. USTAR2 memory usage is generally lower compared to Greedy Matchtigs; in particular, it reaches a peak for $k = 15$, where it consumes half the memory of the competitor. Figure reported also in [29].

From Figs. 2 and 3 we can note that there is a notable peak in both time and memory usage when $k = 15$ due to dense de Bruijn graphs at smaller k values. However, USTAR2 shows a decreasing trend in computing time as k increases, whereas Greedy Matchtigs exhibits a plateau after $k = 21$. Conversely, memory requirements decrease with larger values of k for both tools. When comparing the efficiency of the two tools, USTAR2 emerges as more resource-efficient than Greedy Matchtigs. Specifically, at $k = 15$, USTAR2 runs 30 times faster than Greedy Matchtigs while using less than half the memory. At the commonly used $k = 31$, USTAR2 achieves a remarkable speedup of 96 times compared to Greedy Matchtigs.

Given that Greedy Matchtigs supports multi-threading while USTAR2 does not, we investigated whether parallelization could improve the time performance of Greedy Matchtigs. This comparison is detailed in Fig. 4. Running Greedy Matchtigs with 16 threads reduces its computation time compared to its single-threaded version. However, even with 16 threads, Greedy Matchtigs remains significantly slower than USTAR2. For the widely adopted $k = 31$, USTAR2 (single-threaded) is still 15 times faster than Greedy Matchtigs (16-threaded).

In conclusion, USTAR2 not only delivers the best compression performance but also excels in resource efficiency. Moreover, the current single-threaded implementation of USTAR2 has the potential to be further optimized with parallelization techniques.

3.2 Varying Paramenter D: Changing BFS Depth

In this section we evaluate the behavior of USTAR2 varying the parameter D. Recall that, given a de Bruijn graph, the USTAR2 algorithm begins by selecting a seed and then generates a path by choosing adjacent, unvisited nodes with fewer connections. When no such nodes are available, the algorithm switches to a Breadth First Search (BFS) until it finds an unvisited node or reaches a

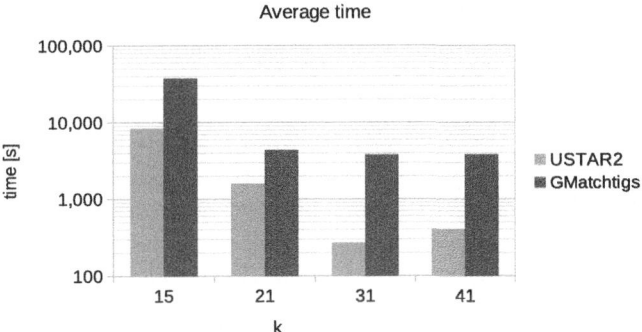

Fig. 4. Average time in seconds used by USTAR2 (single-thread) and Greedy Matchtigs (multi-thread) with different k in logarithmic scale. Even with the advantage of 16 threads, Greedy Matchtigs remains slower than its competitor. In particular, for $k = 31$, USTAR2 gains a 15× speedup. Figure reported also in [29].

depth threshold D. The search also stops if the contig formed from the visited nodes exceeds a length of $2k - 2$, at which point the same CL is achieved as if a new seed were selected. Here, we study the effect of the parameter D by testing various values and analyzing the corresponding performance. USTAR2 has been executed for different values of D and the same k-mer length $k = 21$ (Tables 8, 9, 10 in the Appendix contains the complete results). A summary of the results is reported in Table 6.

Table 6. Average results obtained by USTAR2 changing the depth parameter D and considering $k = 21$. The best *compression* and *string count* is achieved with $D = 10$ at the cost of processing time. The minimum CL is obtained with $D = 7$.

$k = 21$	USTAR2 -D3	USTAR2 -D5	USTAR2 -D7	USTAR2 -D10	GMatchtigs
CL	182,168,049	180,481,558	180,183,581	180,218,872	181,031,130
SC	2,638,074	2,427,589	2,339,810	2,278,069	2,217,643
compression [bytes]	42,817,578	42,115,904	41,801,119	41,654,047	41,890,264
time [s]	80	843	1,583	3,580	30,265
memory [MB]	4,535	4,601	4,699	4,534	6,062

A side effect of the BFS is a reduction in the number of sequences (also known as *sequence count*, SC) in the SPSS. When the BFS successfully finds a suitable node, it extends the current path rather than starting a new one, thus preventing an increase in SC. This relationship is illustrated in Appendix Table 9, and in Table 6 highlighting the decreasing trend of SC as the parameter D (BFS depth) increases. USTAR2 has been executed with different values of D and the results confirmed the previously mentioned effect; indeed the highest value of D achieved the lower SC on average.

The same experiment has been done monitoring the *compression* of the file. Even in this case, the best value found is $D = 10$, showing a possible relation between SC and *compression*.

It is important to note that a high value of D is not necessarily optimal. The purpose of the BFS in USTAR2 is to locate an isolated node or a node with neighbors on only one side, which helps extend the contig effectively. However, if the BFS identifies a node with neighbors on both sides, it can prevent the optimization of the CL, as this situation doesn't allow for the best possible extension of the path. Furthermore, increasing D will necessarily increase the execution time (see the summary Table 6). Thus, selecting an appropriate D is crucial to balancing the search depth and minimizing the CL. Accepting a tradeoff between compression ratio and execution time, we selected $D = 7$ as the best depth parameter for USTAR2.

3.3   The Relationship of CL, SC and Compression

The primary goal of the BFS in USTAR2 is to solve Problem (1) and to minimize the CL by leveraging existing links between sequences, even if this results in repeating k-mers. We aim to demonstrate that a smaller CL significantly benefits final compression, despite the associated SPSS being redundant and containing repeated strings.

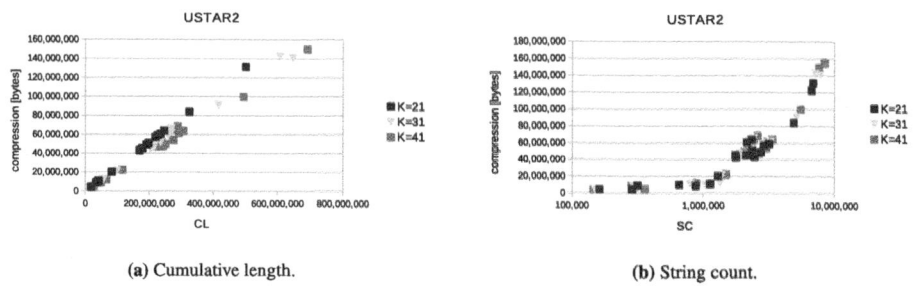

(a) Cumulative length.   (b) String count.

Fig. 5. Correlation between *compression* and CL and between *compression* and SC. In Figure (a) the *compression* has a clear linear relation with the CL for all values of k. Figure (b) shows an increasing trend with SC, in particular, the slope of the curve emphasizes the difficulty of compressing a high number of sequences.

As observed in Tables 4 and 5, tools that achieve a smaller CL also attain superior compression results. This correlation is further highlighted in Fig. 5a, which reveals a clear linear relationship between CL and compression for various k-mer lengths. This linear relationship underscores the critical importance of minimizing CL to enhance compression efficiency.

Moreover, we explore the relationship between the string count (SC) and final compression. Figure 5b illustrates that reducing SC has a more significant impact when SC is high, as indicated by the steeper slope of the curve. This suggests that optimizing SC can substantially improve compression, particularly in scenarios with a high string count.

The correlations presented in Figs. 5 indicate that both CL and SC play crucial roles in optimizing sequence file compression. Since optimal compression is achieved with both low CL and low SC, it is essential to minimize both metrics. Currently, all tools are based on Problem (1) and they only focus on minimizing CL. However, to further enhance compression performance, additional research is needed to develop strategies for effectively minimizing SC as well.

4 Conclusions

In this paper, we present USTAR2, an advanced software tool developed for the compression of k-mer sets. Our method tackles the path cover problem on a de Bruijn graph to find an optimal representation of the k-mer set, focusing on minimizing the cumulative length of the compressed data. By strategically making decisions based on node connectivity and reusing previously traversed nodes, USTAR2 achieves compression ratios that significantly outperform established tools like UST and USTAR that do not allow repeated k-mer. Additionally, USTAR2 demonstrates greater efficiency in k-mer set representation compared to Greedy Matchtigs, excelling in both cumulative length and compression across most k values.

We conducted a comprehensive performance evaluation of USTAR2 using various datasets and performed a comparative analysis with alternative tools, including Matchtigs and Greedy Matchtigs. The results consistently demonstrate the superiority of our approach, with USTAR2 outpacing Greedy Matchtigs in terms of both time and memory utilization. While USTAR2 and Greedy Matchtigs achieve similar compression ratios, USTAR2 exhibits a remarkable speed advantage, being 52 times faster on average and requiring less memory, particularly for lower k-mer lengths. For the commonly used value of $k = 31$, this speed advantage rises to 96 times. Even when Greedy Matchtigs utilizes multithreading, USTAR2 maintains a significant performance advantage, remaining 15 times faster when executed with a single thread.

The BFS phase is a crucial step in the algorithm that permits an effective reuse of k-mers and a reduction in the string count. By selecting the right depth D, USTAR2 achieves a good compromise between compression and execution time that can be adapted to enhance compression. The current single-threaded operation suggests potential for improved performance through parallelization, which needs further investigation. Thus USTAR2 offers an effective and resource-efficient solution for compressing k-mer sets.

Lastly, the clear correlations of cumulative length and sequence count with final compression highlight the importance of minimizing the number of sequences in addition to cumulative length. Currently, the problem definition and the proposed solution do not focus on the reduction of SC but only of CL. We proved that, not only a string data structure with an index can greatly benefit from a low string count as stated by [30], but even the final compression. Therefore developing strategies that minimize both factors at the same time could further enhance compression ratios for many bioinformatics pipelines based on k-mers.

Acknowledgements. Authors are supported by the Project funded under the National Recovery and Resilience Plan (NRRP), Mission 4 Component 2 Investment 1.4 - Call for tender No. 3138 of 16 December 2021, rectified by Decree n.3175 of 18 December 2021 of Italian Ministry of University and Research funded by the European Union âĂŞ NextGenerationEU.

A   Appendix

Table 7. Number of k-mers for each dataset varying $k \in \{15, 17, 21, 31, 41\}$.

dataset	#15-mers	#21-mers	#31-mers	#41-mers
SRR001665_1	13,889,837	14,286,068	10,343,472	–
SRR001665_2	16,371,558	16,895,362	12,058,109	–
SRR061958_1	225,788,025	388,490,798	404,149,685	392,492,657
SRR061958_2	265,935,616	482,235,278	495,804,915	475,405,235
SRR062379_1	109,810,585	152,875,155	160,692,477	160,746,342
SRR062379_2	108,958,432	151,987,994	159,905,793	158,802,318
SRR10260779_1	84,250,397	113,667,728	123,624,245	127,090,699
SRR10260779_2	93,032,179	128,074,943	139,633,894	143,150,103
SRR11458718_1	89,998,269	126,431,861	137,995,280	143,397,012
SRR11458718_2	94,018,791	134,997,414	150,549,990	159,144,668
SRR13605073_1	43,488,336	54,085,000	55,764,573	54,682,553
SRR14005143_1	11,307,338	13,223,059	15,005,192	16,272,583
SRR14005143_2	23,691,810	28,456,533	31,850,681	33,872,511
SRR332538_1	10,624,064	11,404,027	11,382,816	10,666,430
SRR332538_2	18,741,106	25,674,930	28,880,136	27,477,871
SRR341725_1	132,442,790	188,913,254	185,618,107	176,391,089
SRR341725_2	136,484,353	196,035,961	192,133,588	181,970,438
SRR5853087_1	159,744,051	316,438,109	382,773,071	399,026,650
SRR957915_1	126,236,121	208,110,514	239,200,400	250,988,377
SRR957915_2	188,867,779	335,926,750	364,597,018	361,352,380

Table 8. Variations on the Cumulative Length (CL) considering different depths D for the BFS. On average, the best depth found is 7 for $k = 21$.

$k = 21$	CL				
	USTAR2 -D3	USTAR2 -D5	USTAR2 -D7	USTAR2 -D10	GMatchtigs
SRR001665_1	33,724,442	33,614,577	33,638,588	33,652,878	33,858,376
SRR001665_2	42,032,844	41,820,857	41,864,643	41,899,248	42,201,273
SRR061958_1	179,344,739	178,475,353	178,434,526	178,487,472	179,301,460
SRR061958_2	199,043,149	198,089,216	198,026,097	198,076,635	198,820,674
SRR062379_1	229,141,863	227,227,918	226,998,129	227,098,559	228,491,551
SRR062379_2	222,577,626	220,639,776	220,352,087	220,410,452	221,708,614
SRR10260779_1	172,152,568	170,834,391	170,629,253	170,647,128	171,477,677
SRR10260779_2	194,447,448	192,687,883	192,382,255	192,380,954	193,409,534
SRR11458718_1	171,631,152	170,388,945	170,218,475	170,274,600	171,003,884
SRR11458718_2	181,438,971	179,994,380	179,815,285	179,918,803	180,632,752
SRR13605073_1	82,100,544	81,868,639	81,822,046	81,829,909	81,970,005
SRR14005143_1	17,533,686	17,474,598	17,477,215	17,481,274	17,546,167
SRR14005143_2	37,495,157	37,210,386	37,213,243	37,231,963	37,481,708
SRR332538_1	17,727,239	17,614,331	17,615,333	17,649,124	17,688,889
SRR332538_2	42,042,031	41,234,073	41,053,913	41,098,324	41,226,736
SRR341725_1	236,443,128	236,226,834	236,221,721	236,225,336	236,557,911
SRR341725_2	248,023,531	247,749,586	247,741,588	247,744,041	248,138,629
SRR5853087_1	494,958,774	486,601,863	484,650,727	484,842,177	486,008,368
SRR957915_1	331,279,876	326,641,472	325,707,476	325,639,350	327,968,686
SRR957915_2	510,222,204	503,236,086	501,809,029	501,789,219	505,129,713
average	182,168,049	180,481,558	180,183,581	180,218,872	181,031,130

Table 9. USTAR2 execution with different values of search depth D. The number of sequences (SC) is reported. As expected, the SC decreases with D, showing $D = 10$ as the best value when we optimize the SC.

k = 21	SC				
	USTAR2 -D3	USTAR2 -D5	USTAR2 -D7	USTAR2 -D10	GMatchtigs
SRR001665_1	916,105	885,924	879,448	877,672	872,755
SRR001665_2	1,193,991	1,146,533	1,133,937	1,130,235	1,123,195
SRR061958_1	2,306,853	2,161,535	2,117,504	2,099,684	2,072,990
SRR061958_2	2,545,347	2,394,518	2,347,407	2,327,499	2,299,075
SRR062379_1	3,504,235	3,247,734	3,150,431	3,092,370	3,035,170
SRR062379_2	3,229,276	2,976,275	2,876,695	2,812,434	2,747,027
SRR10260779_1	2,678,185	2,503,565	2,439,910	2,400,804	2,358,361
SRR10260779_2	3,032,485	2,809,268	2,724,523	2,671,897	2,617,288
SRR11458718_1	2,000,191	1,828,965	1,765,388	1,725,923	1,688,024
SRR11458718_2	2,030,450	1,828,201	1,750,189	1,700,710	1,660,098
SRR13605073_1	1,335,525	1,307,461	1,295,437	1,286,375	1,278,422
SRR14005143_1	178,560	165,370	162,631	161,845	159,507
SRR14005143_2	382,346	331,453	317,210	312,625	304,930
SRR332538_1	305,365	292,844	288,003	285,088	283,401
SRR332538_2	773,969	696,268	654,081	616,584	579,922
SRR341725_1	2,196,104	2,150,288	2,141,741	2,138,635	2,131,142
SRR341725_2	2,392,955	2,337,448	2,326,873	2,322,642	2,313,111
SRR5853087_1	8,118,590	7,174,067	6,690,760	6,259,528	5,829,696
SRR957915_1	5,630,951	5,094,097	4,865,589	4,711,944	4,575,254
SRR957915_2	8,009,999	7,219,964	6,868,448	6,626,887	6,423,501
average	2,638,074	2,427,589	2,339,810	2,278,069	2,217,643

Table 10. Size of the compressed sequences in bytes. The file is compressed with the dedicated compressor MFCompress. On average, the smallest size is obtained with the higher search depth $D = 10$, highlighted in bold. Dataset SRR5853087_1 crashed the compressor.

k = 21	compression				
	USTAR2 -D3	USTAR2 -D5	USTAR2 -D7	USTAR2 -D10	GMatchtigs
SRR001665_1	8,870,191	8,728,852	8,700,726	8,694,128	8,813,736
SRR001665_2	11,137,855	10,915,321	10,860,629	10,845,768	11,003,600
SRR061958_1	46,185,168	45,510,962	45,319,763	45,249,118	45,454,536
SRR061958_2	51,493,232	50,801,622	50,305,926	50,229,209	50,486,848
SRR062379_1	60,234,098	59,070,721	58,666,732	58,440,424	58,566,163
SRR062379_2	58,171,336	57,036,189	56,647,674	56,409,550	56,882,630
SRR10260779_1	44,200,753	43,373,952	43,092,171	42,930,594	43,311,649
SRR10260779_2	50,121,123	49,077,343	48,707,100	48,489,648	48,574,622
SRR11458718_1	43,609,615	42,840,309	42,574,564	42,422,045	42,645,409
SRR11458718_2	45,993,597	45,077,154	44,755,366	44,565,472	44,708,191
SRR13605073_1	20,254,872	20,149,898	20,112,062	20,092,184	20,144,454
SRR14005143_1	4,294,726	4,222,948	4,208,321	4,204,745	4,179,654
SRR14005143_2	9,327,582	9,056,375	8,983,371	8,960,433	8,932,076
SRR332538_1	4,438,589	4,393,161	4,378,514	4,371,049	4,393,504
SRR332538_2	10,210,659	9,930,431	9,813,628	9,737,762	9,712,821
SRR341725_1	60,952,863	60,766,288	60,734,955	60,723,741	61,160,751
SRR341725_2	64,106,507	63,879,557	63,841,063	63,826,940	64,009,811
SRR5853087_1	Error				
SRR957915_1	86,252,130	83,947,935	83,085,402	82,520,075	82,631,218
SRR957915_2	133,679,087	131,423,152	129,433,290	128,714,001	130,303,345
average	42,817,578	42,115,904	41,801,119	**41,654,047**	41,890,264

References

1. Andreace, F., Pizzi, C., Comin, M.: Metaprob 2: metagenomic reads binning based on assembly using minimizers and k-mers statistics. J. Comput. Biol. **28**(11), 1052–1062 (2021). https://doi.org/10.1089/cmb.2021.0270
2. Bankevich, A., et al.: Spades: a new genome assembly algorithm and its applications to single-cell sequencing. J. Comput. Biol. **19**(5), 455–477 (2012)
3. Bradley, P., Den Bakker, H.C., Rocha, E.P., McVean, G., Iqbal, Z.: Ultrafast search of all deposited bacterial and viral genomic data. Nat. Biotechnol. **37**(2), 152–159 (2019)
4. Břinda, K., Baym, M., Kucherov, G.: Simplitigs as an efficient and scalable representation of de Bruijn graphs. Genome Biol. **22**(1), 1–24 (2021)

5. Cavattoni, M., Comin, M.: Classgraph: improving metagenomic read classification with overlap graphs. J. Comput. Biol. **30**(6), 633–647 (2023). https://doi.org/10.1089/cmb.2022.0208. pMID: 37023405
6. Chikhi, R., Holub, J., Medvedev, P.: Data structures to represent a set of k-long DNA sequences. ACM Comput. Surv. (CSUR) **54**(1), 1–22 (2021)
7. Chikhi, R., Limasset, A., Medvedev, P.: Compacting de Bruijn graphs from sequencing data quickly and in low memory. Bioinformatics **32**(12), i201–i208 (2016)
8. Conway, T.C., Bromage, A.J.: Succinct data structures for assembling large genomes. Bioinformatics **27**(4), 479–486 (2011)
9. Denti, L., Previtali, M., Bernardini, G., Schönhuth, A., Bonizzoni, P.: Malva: genotyping by mapping-free allele detection of known variants. Iscience **18**, 20–27 (2019)
10. Dufresne, Y., et al.: The K-mer file format: a standardized and compact disk representation of sets of k-mers. Bioinformatics **38**(18), 4423–4425 (2022)
11. Harris, R.S., Medvedev, P.: Improved representation of sequence bloom trees. Bioinformatics **36**(3), 721–727 (2020)
12. Holley, G., Melsted, P.: Bifrost: highly parallel construction and indexing of colored and compacted de Bruijn graphs. Genome Biol. **21**, 249 (2020). https://doi.org/10.1186/s13059-020-02135-8
13. Khan, J., Kokot, M., Deorowicz, S., Patro, R.: Scalable, ultra-fast, and low-memory construction of compacted de Bruijn graphs with cuttlefish 2. Genome Biol. **23**, 190 (2022)
14. Kokot, M., Długosz, M., Deorowicz, S.: KMC 3: counting and manipulating k-mer statistics. Bioinformatics **33**(17), 2759–2761 (2017)
15. Li, H., Durbin, R.: Fast and accurate short read alignment with Burrows-Wheeler transform. Bioinformatics **25**(14), 1754–1760 (2009)
16. Marchet, C., Iqbal, Z., Gautheret, D., Salson, M., Chikhi, R.: REINDEER: efficient indexing of k-mer presence and abundance in sequencing datasets. Bioinformatics **36**(Supplement_1), i177–i185 (2020)
17. Marcolin, M., Andreace, F., Comin, M.: Efficient k-mer indexing with application to mapping-free SNP genotyping. In: Lorenz, R., Fred, A.L.N., Gamboa, H. (eds.) Proceedings of the 15th International Joint Conference on Biomedical Engineering Systems and Technologies, BIOSTEC 2022, Volume 3: BIOINFORMATICS, 9–11 February 2022, pp. 62–70 (2022)
18. Monsu, M., Comin, M.: Fast alignment of reads to a variation graph with application to SNP detection. J. Integr. Bioinform. **18**(4), 20210032 (2021)
19. Ondov, B.D., et al.: Mash: fast genome and metagenome distance estimation using minhash. Genome Biol. **17**(1), 1–14 (2016)
20. Pandey, P., Almodaresi, F., Bender, M.A., Ferdman, M., Johnson, R., Patro, R.: Mantis: a fast, small, and exact large-scale sequence-search index. Cell Syst. **7**(2), 201–207 (2018)
21. Pandey, P., Bender, M.A., Johnson, R., Patro, R.: Squeakr: an exact and approximate k-mer counting system. Bioinformatics **34**(4), 568–575 (2018)
22. Pinho, A.J., Pratas, D.: MFCompress: a compression tool for FASTA and multi-FASTA data. Bioinformatics **30**(1), 117–118 (2014)
23. Qian, J., Comin, M.: MetaCon: unsupervised clustering of metagenomic contigs with probabilistic k-mers statistics and coverage. BMC Bioinform. **20**(367) (2019). https://doi.org/10.1186/s12859-019-2904-4
24. Rahman, A., Medvedev, P.: Representation of k-mer sets using spectrum-preserving string sets. In: International Conference on Research in Computational Molecular Biology, pp. 152–168. Springer (2020)

25. Rizk, G., Lavenier, D., Chikhi, R.: DSK: k-mer counting with very low memory usage. Bioinformatics **29**(5), 652–653 (2013)
26. Rossignolo, E., Comin, M.: USTAR: Improved compression of k-mer sets with counters using de Bruijn graphs. In: Guo, X., Mangul, S., Patterson, M., Zelikovsky, A. (eds.) Bioinformatics Research and Applications, pp. 202–213. Springer, Singapore (2023)
27. Rossignolo, E., Comin, M.: Enhanced compression of k-mer sets with counters via de Bruijn graphs. J. Comput. Biol. **31**(6), 524–538 (2024). https://doi.org/10.1089/cmb.2024.0530
28. Rossignolo, E., Comin, M.: Ustar2: Fast and succinct representation of k-mer sets using de Bruijn graphs. In: Proceedings of the 17th International Joint Conference on Biomedical Engineering Systems and Technologies - Volume 1: BIOINFORMATICS, pp. 368–378. INSTICC, SciTePress (2024). https://doi.org/10.5220/0012423100003657
29. Rossignolo, E., Comin, M.: USTAR2: fast and succinct representation of k-mer sets using de Bruijn graphs. In: BIOSTEC (1), pp. 368–378 (2024)
30. Schmidt, S., Khan, S., Alanko, J.N., Pibiri, G.E., Tomescu, A.I.: Matchtigs: minimum plain text representation of k-mer sets. Genome Biol. (Online) **24** (2023). https://doi.org/10.1186/s13059-023-02968-z
31. Schmidt, S., Alanko, J.N.: Eulertigs: minimum plain text representation of k-mer sets without repetitions in linear time. Research square, p. rs.3.rs—2581995 (2023). https://doi.org/10.21203/rs.3.rs-2581995/v1
32. Storato, D., Comin, M.: K2Mem: discovering discriminative k-mers from sequencing data for metagenomic reads classification. IEEE/ACM Trans. Comput. Biol. Bioinf. **19**(1), 220–229 (2022). https://doi.org/10.1109/TCBB.2021.3117406
33. Sun, C., Harris, R.S., Chikhi, R., Medvedev, P.: Allsome sequence bloom trees. J. Comput. Biol. **25**(5), 467–479 (2018)
34. Sun, C., Medvedev, P.: Toward fast and accurate SNP genotyping from whole genome sequencing data for bedside diagnostics. Bioinformatics **35**(3), 415–420 (2019)
35. Wood, D.E., Salzberg, S.L.: Kraken: ultrafast metagenomic sequence classification using exact alignments. Genome Biol. **15**(3), 1–12 (2014)

Hematoxylin and Eosin Stained Images Artificially Generated by StyleGAN Model Conditioned on Immunohistochemical Ki67 Index

Lucia Piatriková[✉][iD], Ivan Cimrák[iD], and Dominika Petríková[iD]

Faculty of Management Science and Informatics, University of Žilina, Žilina, Slovakia
{Lucia.Piatrikova,Ivan.Cimrak,Dominika.Petrikova}@fri.uniza.sk

Abstract. Analysing tissue sections is crucial in cancer diagnosis, influencing tumour classification and treatment decisions. Hematoxylin and Eosin (HE) staining is widely used; however, it captures only basic morphological structures, prompting pathologists to use Immunohistochemistry (IHC) for more detailed information, such as the Ki67 index, which indicates cell proliferation. However, IHC is more time- and resource-consuming. Deep learning models offer potential enhancements in medical diagnosis by providing consistent and cost-effective decisions. For clinical application, these models must be explainable. A generative model can provide additional information that can help to explain predictions. This paper presents a conditional StyleGAN model to generate synthetic HE-stained images conditioned on the Ki67 index. We evaluate three StyleGAN models: one trained on an unfiltered dataset, another on a filtered dataset that includes only higher-quality HE-stained images with a sufficient number of cells, and a third model trained on the filtered dataset with extended training duration. We analyse the results in terms of training progress and the quality of generated images. Results indicate that models trained on the filtered dataset generate more realistic images, and the model with the extended training duration produces indistinguishable images from real samples validated by the expert pathologist.

Keywords: Hematoxylin and Eosin · Ki67 · Conditional GAN · StyleGAN · Digital pathology

1 Introduction

Analysing tissue sections is an essential step in cancer diagnosis, significantly influencing tumour classification and subsequent treatment decisions. Tissue sections are stained with specific dyes to differentiate various tissue components. For cancer diagnosis, pathologists examine stained tissue sections under a microscope or through images obtained from digital scanners.

Hematoxylin and Eosin (HE) staining is commonly used in cancer diagnosis [4]. However, HE staining captures only essential morphological structures [19]. For this reason, pathologists often use Immunohistochemistry (IHC) to obtain more information from a tissue. In particular, IHC staining allows pathologists to evaluate a specific

M. P. Guarino et al. (Eds.): BIOSTEC 2024, CCIS 2546, pp. 192–212, 2026.
https://doi.org/10.1007/978-3-031-96899-0_12

protein's expression in a tissue. One such protein, Ki67, serves as an indicator of cell proliferation. The Ki67 index measures its expression by calculating the percentage of Ki67-positive cells. Although Ki67 staining provides deeper insights into tissue characteristics compared to HE staining, it demands more time and resources.

Deep learning models have the potential to enhance medical diagnoses by providing prompt, consistent, and cost-effective decisions. Nonetheless, these models must be explainable before they are applied in clinical practice for multiple reasons. Especially, errors in medical contexts can have life-threatening consequences. Additionally, the General Data Protection Regulation (GDPR) [17] by the European Union requires the transparency of an algorithm as a prerequisite for its utilisation in patient care.

A generative model added to a deep learning model can yield extra information that serves as explanations for deep learning model predictions. For instance, it allows for the generation of counterfactual examples. A counterfactual example is a result of minimal modifications of the original data that led to a reversal in the model's prediction, e.g., a change in the label from healthy to unhealthy in medical image analysis.

Generative Adversarial Network (GAN) is a deep learning model introduced by Goodfellow et al. [3]. It can learn to generate novel, realistic samples from the high-dimensional distribution of training data. GAN consists of two main components: a generator that produces new samples and a discriminator that evaluates whether the generated samples resemble those in the training set. Conditional GAN [10] incorporates extra information about training samples, allowing both the generator and the discriminator to utilise these additional details.

StyleGAN is an enhanced GAN model developed by Karras et al. [8], which features an improved architecture for both the generator and the discriminator. It employs the principle of progressive growing, enabling the generation of high-resolution images. StyleGAN automatically disentangles high-level image features, thereby constructing a latent space with higher interpretability.

The goal of our research is an explainable model for predicting the Ki67 index from HE-stained histopathological images. We employ generative models to add explainability to our solution and scrutinise the underlying relationship between HE and Ki67 staining. We are currently exploring the use of a conditional StyleGAN model to generate synthetic HE-stained images conditioned on the Ki67 index. For this purpose, we utilise a histopathological image dataset [14] comprising pairs of adjacent HE and Ki67-stained tissue sections with Ki67 indexes.

The paper presents the results of three StyleGAN models in order to analyse the influence of two factors: the quality of the training dataset and the length of the training. To scrutinise the first factor, we filtered the dataset to include only higher-quality HE-stained images with a sufficient number of cells, and secondly, we extended the training length. The first of three models, previously introduced in [15], was trained on the unfiltered dataset containing a variety of HE-stained images. The second model was trained on the filtered dataset. The third model was also trained on the filtered dataset but for approximately twice the duration as the first two models. In the paper, we analyse the results in terms of training progress and the quality of the generated images. Furthermore, all three models were evaluated by an expert pathologist.

The structure of the paper is as follows: Sect. 2 discusses related studies that apply a generative model to histopathology image generation. Section 3 describes datasets and model implementation. Section 4 presents results, discusses training progress, and analyses generated images. Finally, Sect. 5 offers the conclusion and discusses directions for future research.

2 Related Work

Several studies have leveraged generative models for applications in histopathology. One such study [16] introduces PathologyGAN, a model designed to generate 224×224 patches of HE-stained histopathological images from an interpretable latent space. PathologyGAN combines BigGAN architecture [1] with selected features from Style-GAN model. Utilising linear interpolation between two latent vectors, the researchers demonstrated a realistic transition from benign to malignant tissue with the increasing number of cancer cells.

In another study, Schutte et al. [18] employ StyleGAN model alongside a Convolutional Neural Network (CNN) as an encoder. Using a trained logistic regression classifier, their model can generate a series of synthetic images that depict the evolution of pathology. Specifically, it generates images by traversing the shortest path in latent space between two vectors with opposite model predictions. One application presented in the study involves shifting the tumour probability in HE-stained image patches. However, the model struggles to reconstruct reliable histopathological images.

Although Moghadam et al. [11] does not employ GAN but a diffusion probabilistic model, it generates realistic brain histopathology images validated by expert pathologists. Their work demonstrates the successful use of diffusion models in generating histopathological images. Authors state that their model outperforms Progressive GAN [6], which is the predecessor of StyleGAN.

The research conducted by Daroach et al. [2] uses the model of StyleGAN2 [9], which is an improved version of the original StyleGAN [8], to generate HE-stained prostatic histology images. Their model produces high-quality 1024×1024 image patches validated by expert pathologists. Additionally, the paper presents various experiments, e.g., grouping generated samples into classes, which reveals that the class mean in latent space represents specific morphological information. In the next experiment, researchers explore the impact of latent space representations at different levels of Style-GAN generator on histologic morphologies. Another experiment with interpolation between latent vectors of images with different histologic labels concludes that while the generated images appear reliable, they do not imitate legitimate physical transitions. Nevertheless, Daroach et al. proved that StyleGAN model can generate high-resolution histopathological images.

In this paper, we adopt a similar approach as Daroach et al. [2], but we use conditional StyleGAN3 model, which is conditioned on the Ki67 index of HE-stained image patches.

3 Methods

This study demonstrates the application of conditional StyleGAN model to generate HE-stained tissue images corresponding to specific Ki67 indexes. We present three models that differ either in the training dataset or in the length of training.

3.1 Dataset

The original unprocessed dataset was provided by the Department of Pathology, Jessenius Medical Faculty of Comenius University and University Hospital. It comprises HE and Ki67-stained whole slide images (WSI) of seminoma, testicular tumuor. This dataset includes 77 pairs of HE-stained and Ki67-stained tissue scans. Each pair of HE and Ki67-stained images was created from adjacent tissue sections. Although not matching at the cellular level, we assume that the tissue sections made in the same region share similar characteristics.

Since the original dataset contains no labels, we first needed to annotate it. For this purpose, we employed the improved semi-automated approach based on [13], involving three main steps: tissue registration, clustering into dominant colours, and Ki67 index quantification. In the preprocessing step, because of the large size of tissue scans and limited computational resources, we created patches from the first level of whole slide images, i.e., with the second-highest resolution, keeping the corresponding pairs of HE and Ki67-stained patches at the same position together. Each HE patch was then labelled with the Ki67 index derived from the corresponding Ki67 patch. Figure 1 illustrates an example of patches cut from the same position: on the left, the HE patch, followed by the original Ki67 patch and the clustered Ki67 patch, which is the result of the clustering into dominant colours. These clustered Ki67 patches were used to calculate Ki67 indexes as a proportion of brown pixels in patches.

For the training of StyleGAN models, we used two versions of this processed dataset. Both datasets consist of 256×256 square patches of HE-stained images, each labelled with the Ki67 index. Firstly, the unfiltered dataset, where we filtered only empty white patches or nearly white patches. The unfiltered dataset includes 49 tissue scans cut into 189 602 patches. Secondly, the filtered dataset has been processed using more advanced filtering techniques. Specifically, we have combined edge detection, blur detection, blob detection and clustering techniques in our filter to keep only higher-quality patches with a sufficient number of cells. Therefore, the filtered dataset is less variable than the unfiltered dataset, which contains a greater variety of tissue components. We created the filtered dataset from 271 407 patches cut from 77 scans. It contains 177 907 patches, while our filter excluded 93 500 patches. Hence, the filtered dataset includes a similar number of patches cut from the higher number of tissue scans. Figure 2 provides an example of HE patches with Ki67 labels included in the filtered dataset. In contrast, Fig. 3 shows an example of patches excluded by the filter.

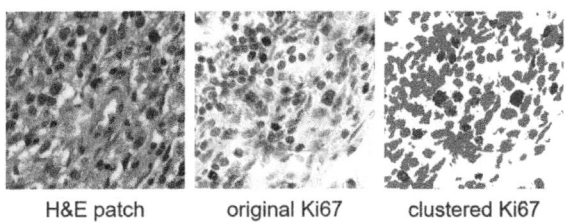

H&E patch   original Ki67   clustered Ki67

Fig. 1. Example of corresponding HE and Ki67 patches from the dataset [15].

Ki67=0.1   Ki67=0.3   Ki67=0.5   Ki67=0.7   Ki67=0.9

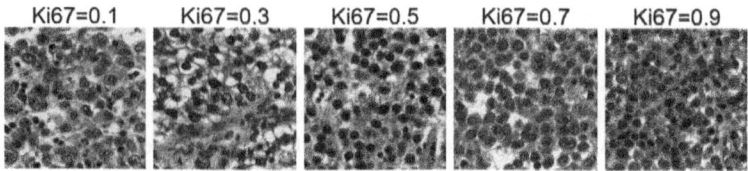

Fig. 2. Example of HE patches with Ki67 index labels from the filtered dataset.

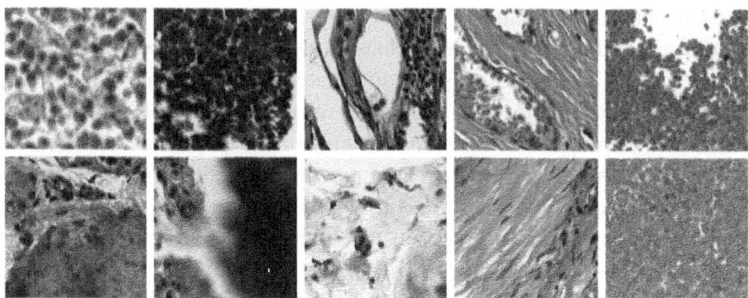

Fig. 3. Example of HE patches excluded by our filter.

3.2 Model

StyleGAN enables the generation of high-resolution images, which is crucial for microscopic histopathology images. We employ conditional StyleGAN model for generating HE image patches conditioned on the Ki67 index. It means that StyleGAN generates an HE-stained image patch starting from an input latent vector and the specified Ki67 index. The model is illustrated in Fig. 4. We utilise pairs of HE patches with their corresponding Ki67 indexes for the training. Our goal is that pathologists are unable to distinguish between real and synthetically generated HE images.

Specifically, we adopt StyleGAN3 [7], which maintains equivariance to translation and rotation. We trained the translation and rotation equivariant StyleGAN3-R variant from the official NVlabs GitHub repository [12]. For all models, we set the regularisation parameter gamma to 2 and enabled adaptive discriminator augmentation (ADA). All models were trained on two GPUs: NVIDIA GeForce RTX 3090 and NVIDIA GeForce RTX 3080 Ti.

4 Results

This Section provides the results of three StyleGAN models. The first model, presented in the paper [15], was trained on the unfiltered dataset for 5343 kimgs, meaning it processed 5 34 3000 image patches during training. Hence, the model iterated through the entire dataset approximately 28 times. The training process took 3 days and 8 h. The second model was also trained for 5343 kimgs, but the filtered dataset was used; thus, the model viewed the dataset about 30 times. Finally, the third model was trained on

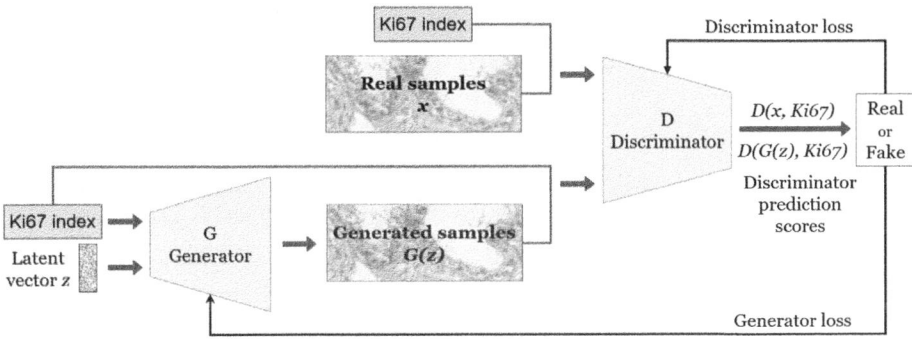

Fig. 4. StyleGAN model.

the filtered dataset, and the training started from the second model. It further ran for 4657 kimgs; thus, for 10 000 kimgs in total, that is about two times more kimgs than the other two models. Considering together with the second model, the training of the third model ran for 6 days and 4 h and iterated the dataset about 56 times.

Figures 17, 18, and 19 show samples of images generated by the first, the second and the third model with corresponding Ki67 indexes indicated above images. The images in samples are arranged according to the increasing value of the Ki67 index.

4.1 Training Progress

During the training process, we calculated generator and discriminator losses following the original formula by Goodfellow et al. [3]. We also recorded discriminator prediction scores for real and synthetic images where positive values indicate real images and, vice versa, negative values identify synthetic images. Additionally, we selected two metrics to assess the quality of generated images and latent space. Firstly, Fréchet Inception Distance (FID) [5] compares generated images to the real data distribution, thereby evaluating both the quality and diversity. Specifically, we computed the FID score for the entire training dataset and 50 000 generated images. The second metric was Perceptual Path Length (PPL) introduced with StyleGAN model [8]. It measures the disentanglement of the latent space by calculating the interpolation between latent vectors. We computed the PPL score as an average over 50 000 samples. Lower values of FID and PPL indicate more realistic generated images and a higher quality of latent space.

Figures 5 and 6 illustrate the training progress of the first model (unfiltered dataset, 5343 kimgs) in the left columns and the second model concatenated with the third model (filtered dataset, 10 000 kimgs) in the right columns. Since the third model started from the second model, their progress is concatenated in the figures; thus, the first 5343 kimgs belong to the training of the second model, and the rest belongs to the third model. The vertical line in the figures indicates the model's switching at 5343 kimg.

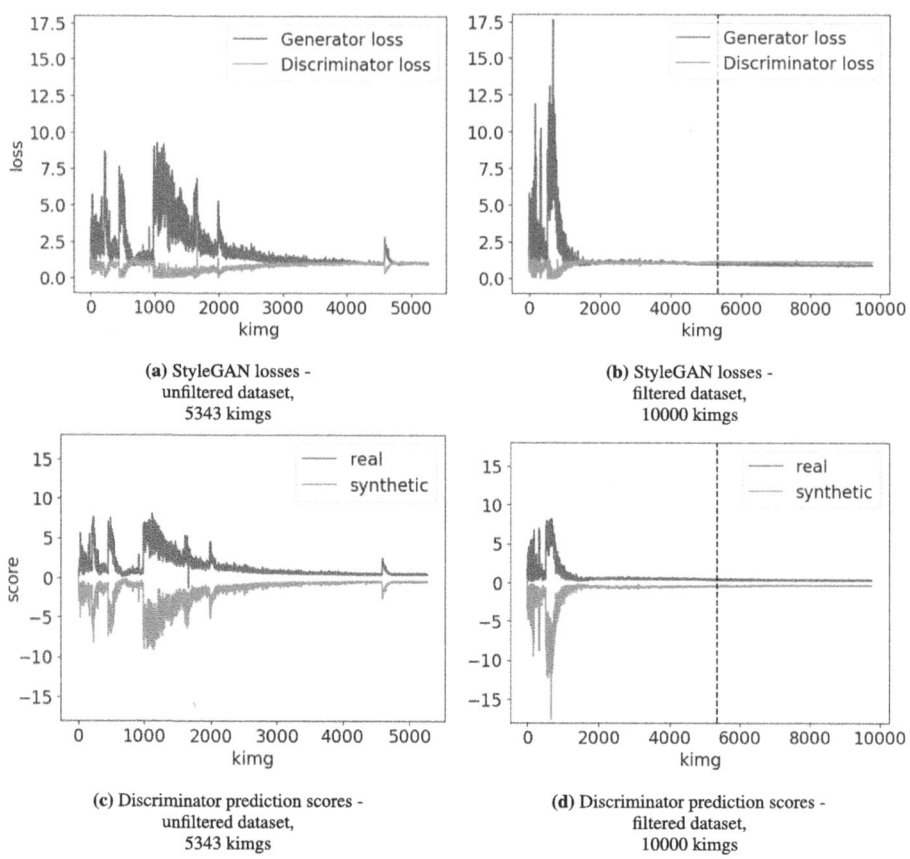

(a) StyleGAN losses -
unfiltered dataset,
5343 kimgs

(b) StyleGAN losses -
filtered dataset,
10000 kimgs

(c) Discriminator prediction scores -
unfiltered dataset,
5343 kimgs

(d) Discriminator prediction scores -
filtered dataset,
10000 kimgs

Fig. 5. Training progress of StyleGAN generator and discriminator.

Figure 5 shows StyleGAN generator and discriminator training progress. We observe that the right model stabilises in approximately 1800 kimgs, significantly sooner than the left model, and remains stable. Furthermore, in the right model, the generator loss slightly outperforms the discriminator, and discriminator prediction scores are closer to zero than in the left model. Hence, the results indicate that the less variable filtered dataset results in more stable training and higher-quality generated images.

Figure 6 depicts the training progress by FID and PPL metric calculated after every 200 kimgs. Similarly, as in Fig. 5, the FID score of the right model stabilises sooner than the left model's FID. The final FID score of the first model is 16.62, the second model is 5.5, and the third model is 3.34. Although the right model achieves lower FID scores, these scores are not fully comparable due to the different data used for the FID calculation. On the contrary, the right model's PPL scores are several times higher than those of the left model and increase during training. The first model's final PPL is 118.74, the second model's is 1541.35, and the third model's is 1957.03. Higher PPL scores indicate a lower-quality latent space constructed by the model. Therefore, we

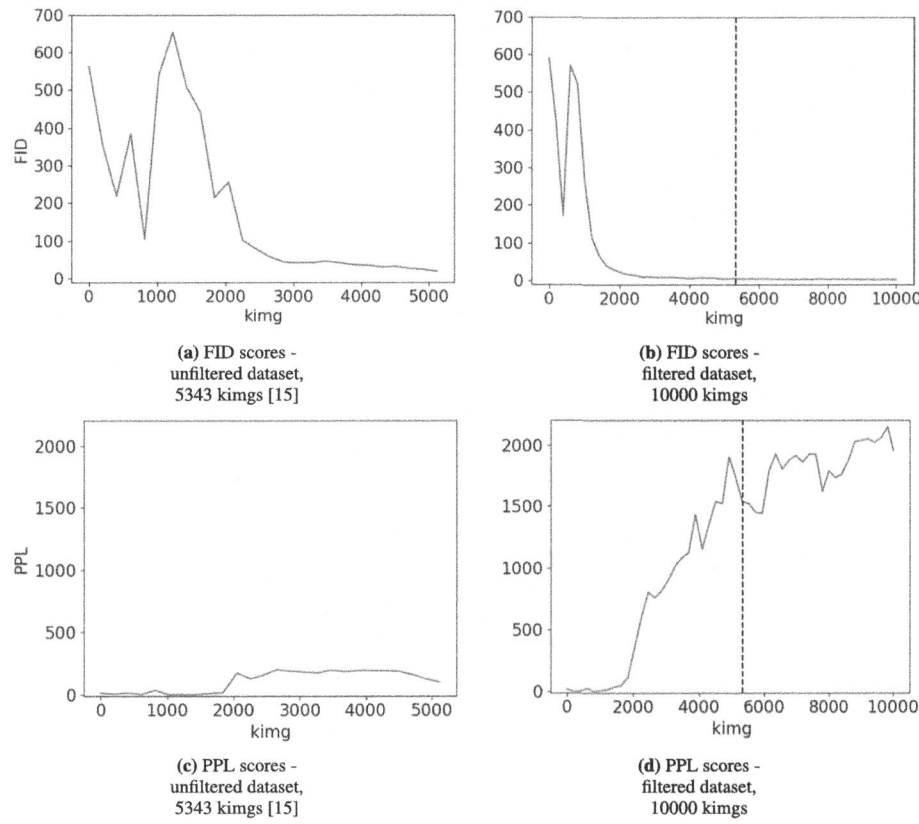

Fig. 6. Training progress of FID and PPL metrics.

conclude that although the filtered dataset enhances the image quality and stabilises the training, it results in more entangled latent space. Additionally, we compared the FID and PPL scores with models from the work of Daroach et al. [2]. First, their best FID model achieved a FID value of 2.86 and a PPL of 139.34. Secondly, their best PPL model has a FID of 3.69 and a PPL of 33.25. The researchers mostly obtained better results, especially for PPL. However, these values are not fully comparable because the models were trained on different datasets; thus, the metrics were calculated on different data.

4.2 Evaluation by the Pathologist

The quality of the generated images was validated by an expert pathologist from the Department of Pathology, Jessenius Medical Faculty of Comenius University and University Hospital. We generated a random sample of 30 synthetic and 30 real images for this purpose. The evaluation was conducted in two phases: fast estimation and slow estimation. In the fast estimation, the pathologist evaluated images at first glance, just briefly looking at each image. In the slow estimation, the pathologist had unlimited time to analyse images. In both fast and slow estimation, the pathologist classified each image into one of five categories: certainly real, rather real, certainly synthetic, rather synthetic, or could not decide.

Tables 1, 3 and 5 summarise fast and slow estimation results for all three models. We processed results from these tables into confusion matrices presented in Tables 2, 4 and 6, with Undecided category omitted and Certain and Rather categories merged. Finally, Table 7 shows pathologist accuracies and recalls computed based on confusion matrices.

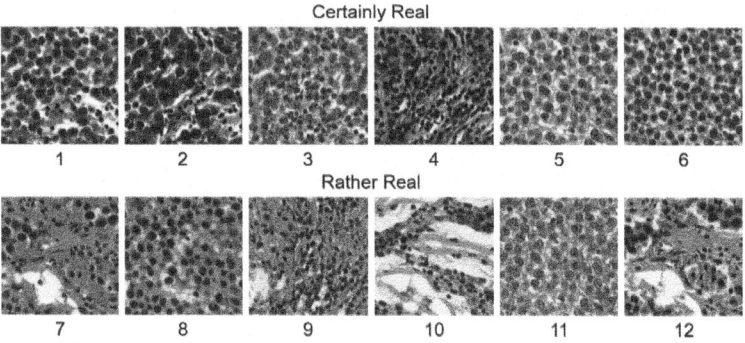

Fig. 7. Best-ranking synthetic images of the first model (unfiltered dataset, 5343 kimgs) from the fast estimation [15].

Considering Table 1 of the first model and fast estimation, the pathologist classified six synthetic images as certainly real, another six synthetic images as rather real and could not decide about three synthetic images. In summary, 15 synthetic images convinced the pathologist that they were real or left undecided and 15 synthetic images were correctly identified as synthetic. The 12 best-ranking images from fast estimation are shown in Fig. 7. However, the pathologist correctly identified nearly all synthetic images in the slow estimation, while only two were labelled as rather real. Regarding real images, the pathologist correctly identified almost all samples in both fast and slow estimations. In summary, in the fast estimation of the first model, the pathologist achieved an accuracy of 69.23% and recall of 55.56%, indicating uncertainty in synthetic images. However, in slow estimation, the pathologist demonstrated a high confidence level with an accuracy of 96.36% and recall of 93.33%. Therefore, we conclude that images generated by the first model trained on the unfiltered dataset can deceive the pathologist at first glance, but a more detailed analysis allows for their detection.

Table 1. Pathologist results - unfiltered dataset, 5343 kimgs [15].

	Certainly Real	Rather Real	Undecided	Rather Synthetic	Certainly Synthetic
Fast Pathologist Estimation					
Real	11	10	5	4	0
Synthetic	6	6	3	7	8
Slow Pathologist Estimation					
Real	16	9	5	0	0
Synthetic	0	2	0	2	26

Table 2. Pathologist Confusion Matrix - unfiltered dataset, 5343 kimgs [15].

	Fast Pathologist Estimation	
	EstimatedReal	EstimatedSynthetic
ActualReal	21	4
ActualSynthetic	12	15

	Slow Pathologist Estimation	
	EstimatedReal	EstimatedSynthetic
ActualReal	25	0
ActualSynthetic	2	28

Table 3. Pathologist results - filtered dataset, 5343 kimgs.

	Certainly Real	Rather Real	Undecided	Rather Synthetic	Certainly Synthetic
Fast Pathologist Estimation					
Real	11	13	2	3	1
Synthetic	0	5	1	12	12
Slow Pathologist Estimation					
Real	16	7	2	5	0
Synthetic	0	2	0	7	21

Table 3 illustrates the results of the second model trained on the filtered dataset. Considering the fast estimation of the second model, only five synthetic images were evaluated as rather real, one as undecided, and none as certainly real. Altogether, only six synthetic images were labelled as either real or undecided, while the pathologist correctly identified 24 synthetic images. We conclude that the results of the fast estimation are worse than the first model trained with the same number of kimgs. Consequently, the pathologist's accuracy and recall are higher, 84.21% and 82.76% respectively. However, the results of the slow estimation for synthetic images are quite similar, maintaining the same recall value of 93.33%. The decrease in accuracy can be attributed to the pathologist's errors in evaluating the real images. To conclude, some images generated by the second model can deceive the pathologist at first glance.

Pathologist results on the third model trained on the filtered dataset for 10 000 kimgs are shown in Table 5. In fast estimation, the pathologist evaluated three synthetic images as certainly real, seven as rather real and could not decide about five synthetic images. Similarly to the first model fast estimation, 15 synthetic images were categorised as either real or undecided, and 15 synthetic images were identified as synthetic. However,

Table 4. Pathologist Confusion Matrix - filtered dataset, 5343 kimgs.

	Fast Pathologist Estimation			Slow Pathologist Estimation	
	EstimatedReal	EstimatedSynthetic		EstimatedReal	EstimatedSynthetic
ActualReal	24	4	ActualReal	23	5
ActualSynthetic	5	24	ActualSynthetic	2	28

Table 5. Pathologist results - filtered dataset, 10000 kimgs.

	Certainly Real	Rather Real	Undecided	Rather Synthetic	Certainly Synthetic
	Fast Pathologist Estimation				
Real	8	10	2	7	3
Synthetic	3	7	5	5	10
	Slow Pathologist Estimation				
Real	10	11	1	7	1
Synthetic	9	5	1	4	11

Table 6. Pathologist Confusion Matrix - filtered dataset, 10000 kimgs.

	Fast Pathologist Estimation			Slow Pathologist Estimation	
	EstimatedReal	EstimatedSynthetic		EstimatedReal	EstimatedSynthetic
ActualReal	18	10	ActualReal	21	8
ActualSynthetic	10	15	ActualSynthetic	14	15

Table 7. Pathologist Accuracy and Recall.

	Accuracy		Recall	
	Fast	Slow	Fast	Slow
unfiltered dataset 5343 kimgs [15]	**69.23%**	96.36%	**55.56%**	93.33%
filtered dataset 5343 kimgs	84.21%	87.93%	82.76%	93.33%
filtered dataset 10000 kimgs	**62.26%**	**62.07%**	**60.00%**	**51.72%**

the third model has comparable results even for slow estimation, with nearly identical accuracies of 62.26% for fast estimation and 62.07% for slow estimation. Nevertheless, six additional synthetic images were considered certainly real compared to fast estimation. Consequently, the recall for slow estimation is 51.72%, which surpasses the 60% achieved in fast estimation. Furthermore, the pathologist committed more errors in assessing real images than in the other two models. These results indicate that the pathologist was unable to recognise synthetic images generated by the third model even after a more detailed analysis. Therefore, the third model, trained on the filtered dataset for 10 000 kimgs, generates images of the highest quality, almost unrecognisable from real images.

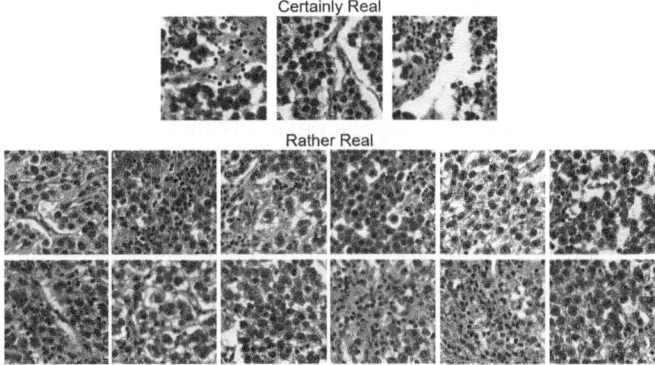

Fig. 8. Best-ranking synthetic images of the second and the third model (filtered dataset) in the fast estimation.

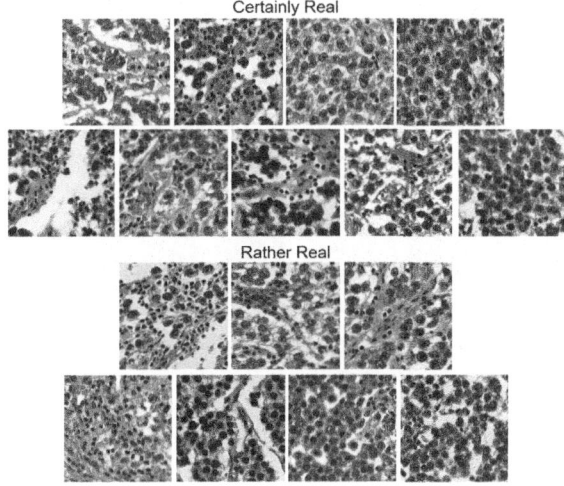

Fig. 9. Best-ranking synthetic images of the second and the third model (filtered dataset) in the slow estimation.

Additionally, we observe that accuracy and recall are more consistent between the fast and slow estimations when the model is trained on the filtered dataset, in contrast to the first model, which exhibits a significant discrepancy between the fast and slow estimations. Based on all the presented results, we conclude that the filtered dataset significantly improved the image quality. Although the second model's results were worse than the first model in fast estimation, we attribute it to the pathologist's improved ability to detect synthetic images. The best-ranking images of the second and the third model in fast estimation are shown in Fig. 8 and in slow estimation in Fig. 9.

4.3 Analysis of Generated Images

When we study synthetic images in more detail, we can observe undesirable structures and patterns. First, we analyse images generated by the first model. It was trained
on the unfiltered dataset, which has higher variability than the filtered dataset. Hence,
the model had to learn more diverse tissue components. For this reason, the quality of
synthetic image structure and tissue components is lower. Figure 10 depicts undesirable patterns, where synthetic images are positioned in the left column and similar real
images in the right column. Both have one or two zoomed-in parts next to the image for
comparative analysis. In the first row, it can be observed that synthetic tumour cells have
similar structures and are significantly more regular compared to real cells. The second
row illustrates cells arranged in regular formations, such as circles or arcs, which are
rare in real HE images.

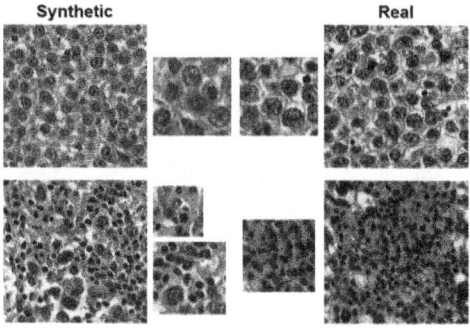

Fig. 10. Undesirable patterns - the first model (unfiltered dataset, 5343 kimgs) [15].

   In the following images, we highlight problematic parts using black circles or
squares. Another undesirable structures generated by the first model are illustrated in
Fig. 11. Generated images often contain symmetric parts. In Fig. 11, image 2 has a symmetric layout, and image 3 contains symmetric cells. Since the unfiltered dataset contains images of lower quality, the first model learned to generate them. For example, the
model generates blurred images where, in some parts, we can not identify any cells, as
illustrated in Fig. 11 - images 1, 2 and 4. Furthermore, the model also generates images
without any live cells, as shown in Fig. 11 - image 4. Additionally, there is another
undesirable phenomenon where the layout of several synthetic images resembles each
other. An example of generated images with similar layouts demonstrating this issue is
presented in Fig. 12.
   Secondly, we analyse images generated by the second and the third model, trained
on the higher-quality filtered dataset. The pathologist observed that the images generated by the second and the third model, trained on the filtered dataset, exhibit a higher
level of realism, enhanced quality, and improved cell structure and overall image structure compared to the first model trained on the unfiltered dataset. All tissue components

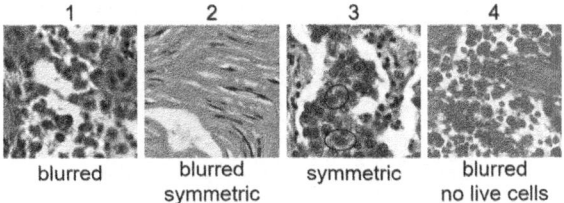

Fig. 11. Undesirable image structure - the first model (unfiltered dataset, 5343 kimgs).

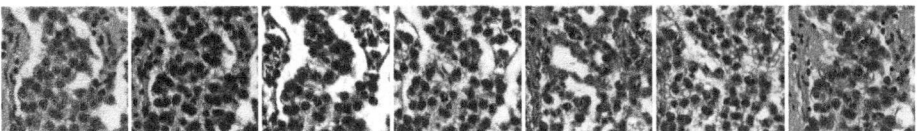

Fig. 12. Undesirable repeating layout - the first model (unfiltered dataset, 5343 kimgs) [15].

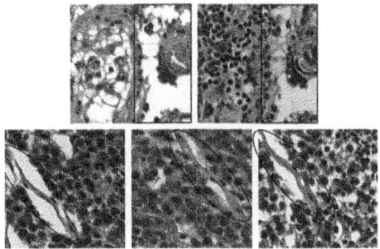

Fig. 13. Similar image parts - the second and the third model (filtered dataset).

appear convincing, with tumour cells showing realistic variability and irregularity. Particularly concerning the third model, there were minimal differences between the real and synthetic images, which were not immediately apparent.

There is no similar layout among the generated images. Only smaller, comparable image regions are present, as shown in Fig. 13. Next, only a minimal number of regular patterns found in the first model's results appear in the generated images. Furthermore, fully blurred images have disappeared; instead, only smaller blurred areas of images occasionally appear. These blurred areas, typically located at the edges of images, seem to be incompletely generated, as in Fig. 14.

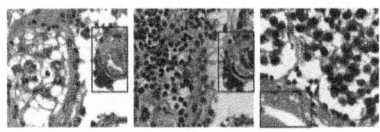

Fig. 14. Blurred parts of images - the second and the third model (filtered dataset).

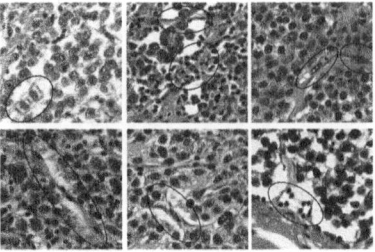

Fig. 15. Symmetric image parts - the second and the third model (filtered dataset).

Another undesirable phenomenon frequently observed in the generated images from the second or the third model is radial or point symmetry, depicted in Fig. 15. However, this symmetry is local, in contrast to the first model, where the symmetry often extends globally across the entire image. Another unrealistic pattern involves repeating cell groups. In reality, cells are randomly spread within tissue. Examples of repeating cell groups are shown in Fig. 16, where, for instance, erythrocytes are repeatedly positioned around cells.

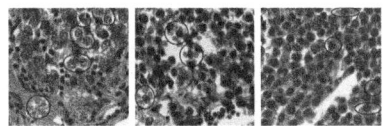

Fig. 16. Repeating cells - the second and the third model (filtered dataset).

5   Conclusion

Building on our previous model, which was trained on the unfiltered dataset [15], we presented two new models trained on the higher-quality, filtered dataset. The updated results provide a deeper analysis of the training progress and the quality of generated images. The first new model achieved comparable results to the old model with the same length of training; however, the pathologist described its images as more realistic than the old model's images. The second new model, which has been trained for approximately two times longer, outperformed the old model and learned to generate realistic HE-stained histopathology images to the extent that the pathologist could not recognise them.

This new model, trained on the filtered dataset for twice the duration, demonstrates significant improvements over the old model trained on the unfiltered dataset considering various aspects. The new model's training stabilises faster and maintains stability, as evidenced by the progress of generator and discriminator losses and discriminator prediction scores. The filtered dataset's contribution to a more stable training process and superior image quality is also reflected in the faster stabilisation and lower values of the FID score. However, higher PPL scores indicate a less optimal latent space with higher entanglement.

The pathologist's evaluation highlights that while the old model can deceive at first glance, the new model's images remain indistinguishable from real images even under detailed analysis. This is further supported by consistent accuracy and recall rates between fast and slow estimations for the new model, contrasting with the old model's discrepancies. Especially, the pathologist's recall on the new model for slow estimation is 51.72%, proving that the generated images were indistinguishable from real images to the pathologist.

The pathologist's observations confirm the new model's ability to produce more realistic and varied cell structures with fewer undesirable patterns like symmetry, repeating layout, and blur, prevalent in the old model's outputs. These patterns still appear, but more on a local rather than global scale. Therefore, the filtered dataset significantly enhances the quality of the synthetic images, making them more realistic and less distinguishable from real tissue images.

In the following research, we will analyse the Ki67 index within StyleGAN latent space and its influence on the quality of results. We assume that incorporating Ki67 information improves the structure of latent space and image quality. Additionally, we will utilise our model to scrutinise the relationship between HE and Ki67 staining.

Acknowledgements. This research was supported by the Ministry of Education, Science, Research and Sport of the Slovak Republic under the contract No. VEGA 1/0369/22. Gratitude is extended to K. Tobiášová for her assessment of generated images and to L. Plank and K. Tobiášová for their collaboration in the preparation of the dataset.

A   Appendix

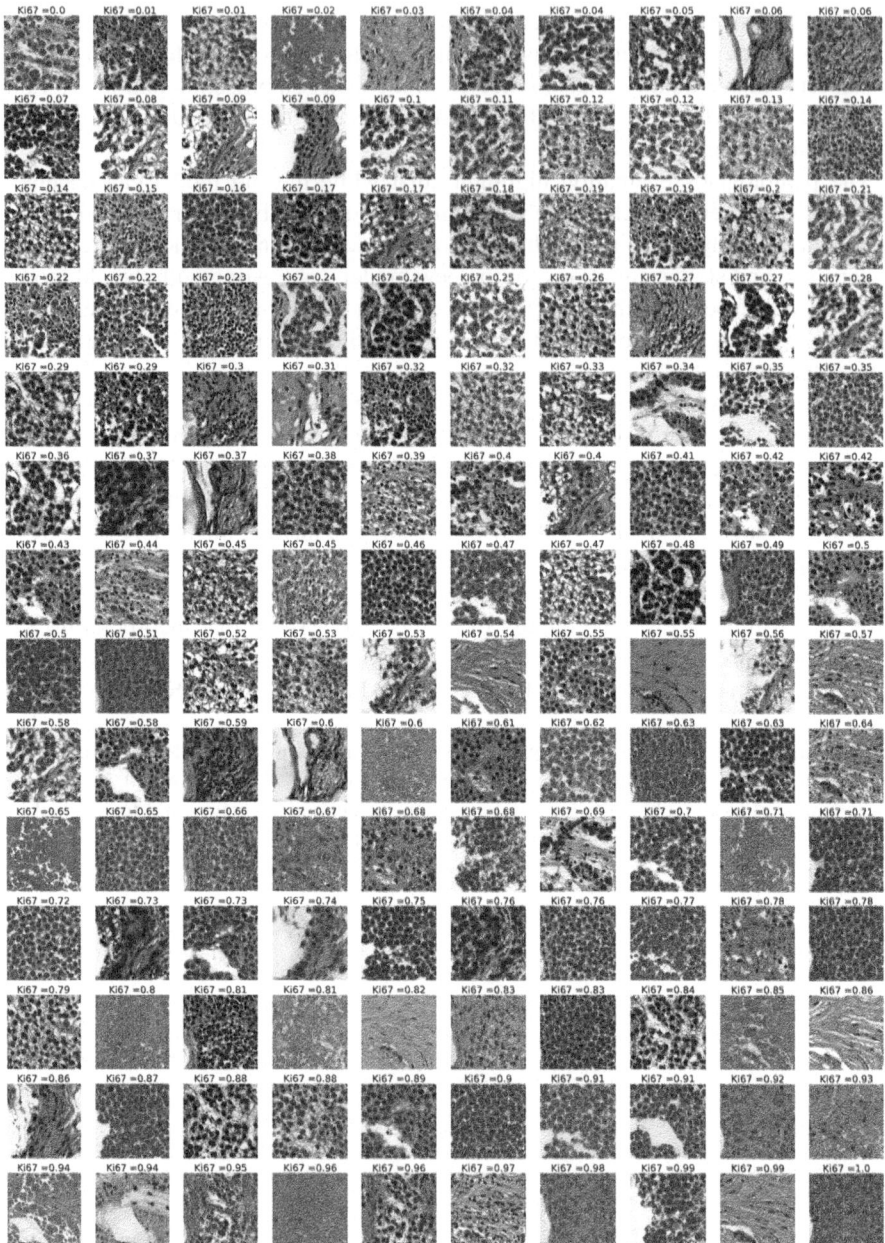

Fig. 17. Sample of generated images - not filtered dataset and 5343 kimgs [15].

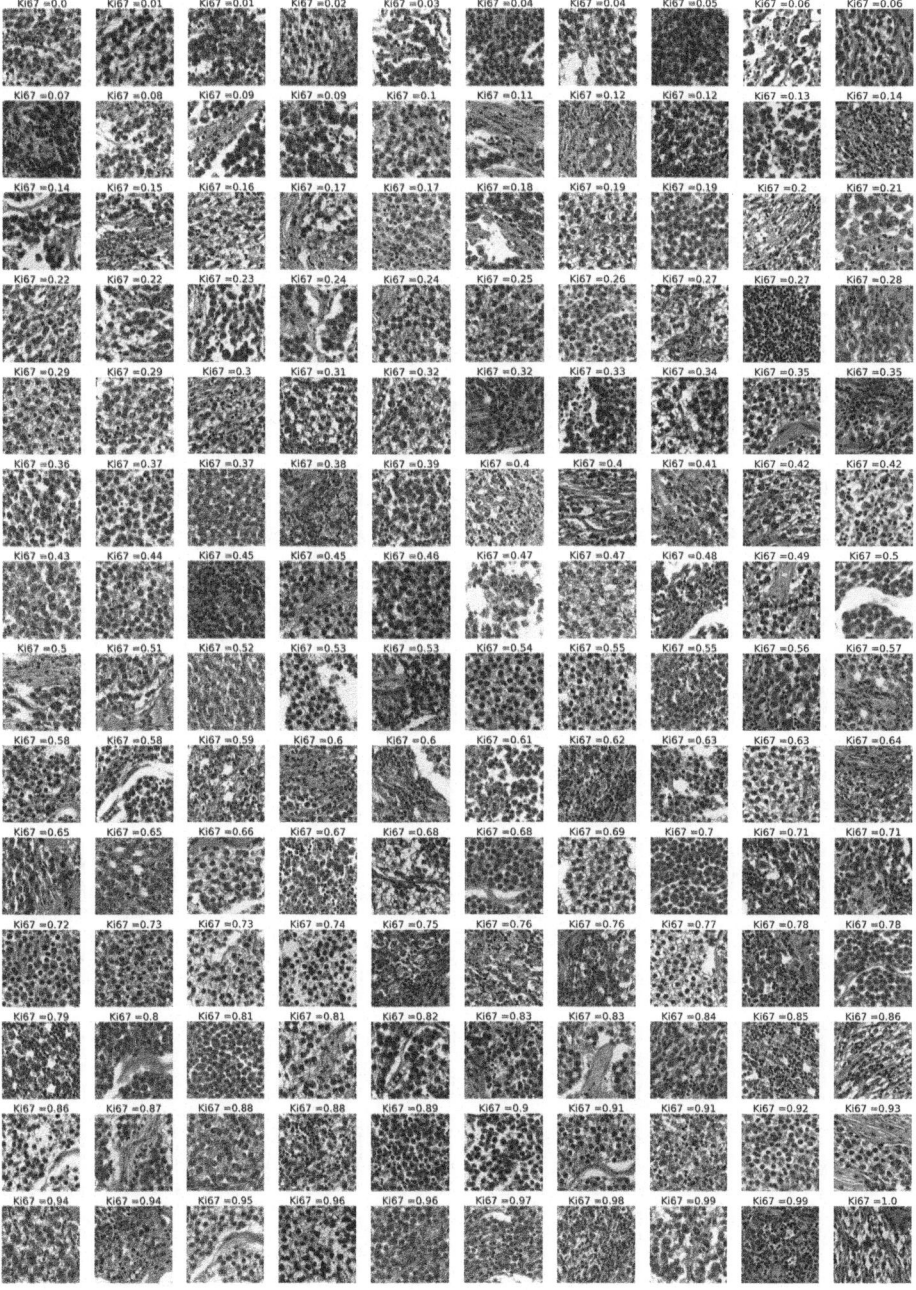

Fig. 18. Sample of generated images - filtered dataset and 5343 kimgs.

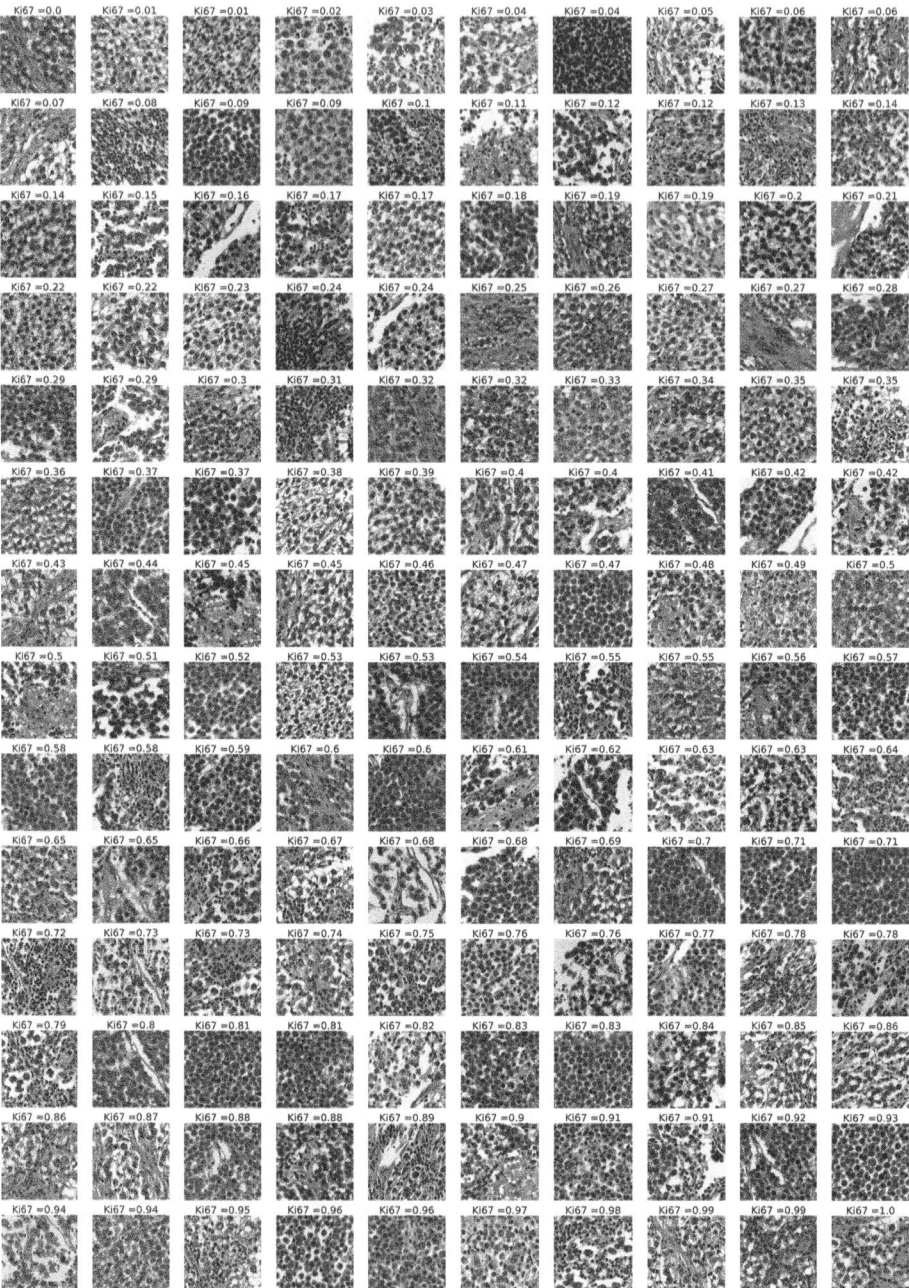

Fig. 19. Sample of generated images - filtered dataset and 10 000 kimgs.

References

1. Brock, A., Donahue, J., Simonyan, K.: Large scale GAN training for high fidelity natural image synthesis. arXiv preprint arXiv:1809.11096 (2018)
2. Daroach, G.B., Yoder, J.A., Iczkowski, K.A., LaViolette, P.S.: High-resolution controllable prostatic histology synthesis using StyleGAN. BIOIMAGING **11** (2021)
3. Goodfellow, I., et al.: Generative adversarial nets. In: Ghahramani, Z., Welling, M., Cortes, C., Lawrence, N., Weinberger, K. (eds.) Advances in Neural Information Processing Systems, vol. 27. Curran Associates, Inc. (2014). https://proceedings.neurips.cc/paper_files/paper/2014/file/5ca3e9b122f61f8f06494c97b1afccf3-Paper.pdf
4. Gurcan, M.N., Boucheron, L.E., Can, A., Madabhushi, A., Rajpoot, N.M., Yener, B.: Histopathological image analysis: a review. IEEE Rev. Biomed. Eng. **2**, 147–171 (2009)
5. Heusel, M., Ramsauer, H., Unterthiner, T., Nessler, B., Hochreiter, S.: GANs trained by a two time-scale update rule converge to a local nash equilibrium. In: Advances in Neural Information Processing Systems, vol. 30 (2017)
6. Karras, T., Aila, T., Laine, S., Lehtinen, J.: Progressive growing of GANs for improved quality, stability, and variation. arXiv preprint arXiv:1710.10196 (2017)
7. Karras, T., et al.: Alias-free generative adversarial networks. In: Proceedings of the NeurIPS (2021)
8. Karras, T., Laine, S., Aila, T.: A style-based generator architecture for generative adversarial networks. In: Proceedings of the IEEE/CVF Conference on Computer Vision and Pattern Recognition, pp. 4401–4410 (2019)
9. Karras, T., Laine, S., Aittala, M., Hellsten, J., Lehtinen, J., Aila, T.: Analyzing and improving the image quality of StyleGAN. In: Proceedings of the IEEE/CVF Conference on Computer Vision and Pattern Recognition, pp. 8110–8119 (2020)
10. Mirza, M., Osindero, S.: Conditional generative adversarial nets. arXiv preprint arXiv:1411.1784 (2014)
11. Moghadam, P.A., et al.: A morphology focused diffusion probabilistic model for synthesis of histopathology images. In: Proceedings of the IEEE/CVF Winter Conference on Applications of Computer Vision, pp. 2000–2009 (2023)
12. NVlabs: Alias-Free Generative Adversarial Networks (StyleGAN3) - Official PyTorch implementation of the NeurIPS 2021 paper (2023). https://github.com/NVlabs/stylegan3
13. Petríková, D., Cimrák, I., Tobiášová, K., Plank, L.: Semi-automated workflow for computer-generated scoring of Ki67 positive cells from HE stained slides. In: BIOINFORMATICS. pp. 292–300 (2023)
14. Petríková, D., Cimrák, I., Tobiášová, K., Plank, L.: Histopathology pairs of hematoxylin-eosin and Ki67 stainings of testicular seminoma (2024). https://doi.org/10.5281/zenodo.11218961
15. Piatriková, L., Cimrák, I., Petríková, D.: Generation of H&E-stained histopathological images conditioned on Ki67 index using StyleGAN model. In: Proceedings of the 17th International Joint Conference on Biomedical Engineering Systems and Technologies - BIOINFORMATICS, pp. 512–518. INSTICC, SciTePress (2024). https://doi.org/10.5220/0012464200003657
16. Quiros, A.C., Murray-Smith, R., Yuan, K.: PathologyGAN: learning deep representations of cancer tissue. arXiv preprint arXiv:1907.02644 (2019)
17. Regulation, G.D.P.: Art. 22 GDPR. Automated individual decision-making, including profiling. Intersoft Consulting (2020). https://gdpr-info.eu/art-22-gdpr

18. Schutte, K., Moindrot, O., Hérent, P., Schiratti, J.B., Jégou, S.: Using StyleGAN for visual interpretability of deep learning models on medical images. arXiv preprint arXiv:2101.07563 (2021)
19. Wittekind, D.: Traditional staining for routine diagnostic pathology including the role of tannic acid. 1. Value and limitations of the hematoxylin-eosin stain. Biotechnic Histochem. **78**(5), 261–270 (2003)

Patch Based Analysis with Machine Learning to Aid Breast Cancer Recurrence Prediction

Madison Rose[1]([envelope]) [iD], Joseph Geradts[2,3] [iD], and Nic Herndon[1] [iD]

[1] Department of Computer Science, East Carolina University, Greenville, NC 27858, USA
rosem19@students.ecu.edu, herndonn19@ecu.edu
[2] Department of Pathology, Brody School of Medicine, East Carolina University, Greenville, NC 27858, USA
[3] Department of Pathology, University of California San Francisco, San Francisco, CA 94143, USA

Abstract. Since the introduction of whole slide scanners, machine learning research has become a popular area of interest in digital pathology. Many studies have attempted to use machine learning to aid pathology tasks such as breast cancer diagnosis and metastasis detection. However, one area that has less available research is in applying machine learning to predict patient recurrence risk categories as a surrogate of patient outcome. Since H&E-stained images are routinely collected for diagnostic purposes, creating an image-based recurrence prediction method could help increase accessibility and lower cost for recurrence risk category assessment for breast cancer patients. In this study, patches were extracted from a dataset of 102 whole slide images to train a machine learning model to predict slide level breast cancer Oncotype DX risk category using only H&E-stained images with no additional clinical data or region of interest annotations. Differences in accuracy were also analyzed based on multiple patch size and quantity combinations. Patches were extracted from each whole slide image and feature extraction was performed before the features were aggregated together to create a bag of features for each case. These bags were then used to train a logistic regression model. The best scoring model used 2,000 patches of size 256×256 pixels. This model scored 0.628 ± 0.044 accuracy on 5-fold cross validation across the entire dataset.

Keywords: Machine learning · Breast cancer · Image classification

1 Introduction

Breast cancer is one of the most common cancers among women worldwide. Although incidence rates have increased in recent years, survival rates are also up [21]. One factor that could be contributing to better survival rates is the use of more personalized treatment plans. One way treatment plans can be personalized is with chemotherapy. Oncologists can decide if a patient would benefit from chemotherapy based on their recurrence score, which is an indicator of how aggressive the cancer is and how likely it is to recur. Most often, the Oncotype DX (ODX) Recurrence Test is used to evaluate recurrence risk. The Oncotype DX Recurrence Test is a 21 gene assay which outputs an integer between 0 and 100, also known as a recurrence score [22]. Generally,

M. P. Guarino et al. (Eds.): BIOSTEC 2024, CCIS 2546, pp. 213–226, 2026.
https://doi.org/10.1007/978-3-031-96899-0_13

scores of 26 or higher are considered to be high-risk and scores below 26 are considered to be non-high risk, which includes low- and intermediate risk cases. In general, only breast cancers with a high recurrence score were found to benefit from adjuvant chemotherapy [26]. The ODX test is performed on breast cancer biopsies or excisions. The ODX recurrence score has been shown to be strongly correlated with risk of breast cancer recurrence within 10 years. However, these tests are costly and not available in resource-poor countries.

Since whole slide scanners capable of digitizing stained tissue slides from breast biopsies have become more common, there is a strong research interest to use machine learning to aid in digital pathology tasks. Image-based machine learning has been applied to tasks such as breast cancer diagnosis, tissue segmentation, and metastasis detection with very accurate results [12, 16]. However, there is not as much available research focused on using image-based machine learning methods to predict patient recurrence risk.

Some studies have focused on predicting recurrence with non image data including clinical data and electronic health records and have produced good results [2]. There are fewer studies attempting to predict recurrence with images. However, if recurrence could be predicted from images, such as hematoxylin and eosin-stained whole slide images, which are routinely collected for diagnosis, then less laboratory work would be needed [20]. This could also help keep costs lower since no additional information would need to be collected from the patient. Many works that focus on image-based prediction of breast cancer recurrence from H&E-stained images use pathologist tumor region of interest annotations which are extremely helpful in determining the area within the whole slide image that is most relevant. Additionally, some studies combine H&E-stained images with clinical data or also investigate recurrence prediction using whole slide images stained with other materials [23].

This study investigates machine learning model performance on predicting breast cancer recurrence based on the associated Oncotype DX recurrence score, given only H&E stained slides, with no additional clinical data or region of interest annotations. Patch size and quantity selection are also investigated as to their impact on overall model accuracy. The patch sizes 512×512 pixels and 256×256 pixels were selected for analysis as these are commonly used image sizes [12, 15]. Understanding the impact of patch size and patch quantity on overall model accuracy could assist more researchers when selecting patches for their work. If it were possible to predict the recurrence score with only the H&E-stained image, tumor region of interest annotations would not be needed and this would reduce the time needed for image annotation by pathologists. Ultimately, machine learning could provide a tool to assist with recurrence risk assessment which could hopefully increase access to more personalized treatment options for breast cancer patients.

2 Background

2.1 Digital Pathology Tasks

Within digital pathology, there has been a focus centered around three main image analysis tasks: classification, segmentation, and object detection [19]. With classification, images are given a label or sorted into a class. This can be done with binary classification, where there are only two possible classes, or multi-class classification, where there are three or more possible labels [10]. A study by Araujo et al. [3] demonstrated both types of classification. This study used CNNs to classify whole slide images into binary classes of carcinoma and non-carcinoma and then multi-class classes of normal, benign, in situ carcinoma, and invasive carcinoma. While having more specific labels, such as in multi-class classification, can be helpful for medical diagnosis, it also can impact accuracy due to having more classes and a higher chance of predicting the wrong label. An example can be seen in the previously mentioned study. The binary classification model achieved 77% accuracy compared to 65% accuracy by the multi-class model [3].

2.2 Whole Slide Image Annotations

Whole slide images are typically annotated in one of three ways – pixel (also called patch) level, slide level, and patient level. Each annotation level has tasks they are better suited for as well as unique drawbacks. Pixel level annotations are the most specific type of annotation and provide the most information about the image. In pixel level, each individual pixel has a label associated with it. Pixel level annotations are most helpful in tasks such as segmentation or object detection. Examples of pixel level annotations include segmentation masks or bounding boxes [4]. The drawback to pixel level annotations is that they are extremely time consuming as a pathologist must take the time to label each part of the whole slide image. The next type of annotation, slide level, is less time consuming but also less specific. In this case, each slide is given a single label, for example a slide may be labeled as carcinoma or non-carcinoma [3]. Slide level labels are commonly used in classification tasks. However, since these are less specific than pixel level labels, there is room for error. When using slide level labels, if a patching approach is used to analyze the whole slide images, then it is possible for a patch to not match its slide level label [7]. The final type of annotation is patient level. This is the least time consuming and least specific annotation level. In this case, each patient would have several associated whole slide images. The collection of slides would be labeled based on the patient [16]. In this case, the concern is that an entire slide may be mislabeled [7].

2.3 Challenges and Techniques

One challenge in digital pathology is the lack of available, well annotated data. Deep learning techniques require large amounts of data. Annotating datasets is time consuming and requires domain knowledge. To overcome this limitation, techniques such as transfer learning are used. Transfer learning is inspired by the psychology idea that knowledge from one task can aid in another task [13]. A common example of transfer learning is the use of the ImageNet dataset to pretrain convolutional neural networks [6]. CNNs are very time consuming to train and require abundant amounts of training data. Pretrained CNNs can later be finetuned using domain specific data. Later, the model can be fine tuned with domain specific data to update the weights for only a few layers [1]. This greatly reduces the total amount of training time needed.

Image size is another common issue when attempting to apply machine learning techniques for whole slide image analysis. These scans are extremely large at around 100,000 by 100,000 pixels per whole slide image [7]. Machine learning tools such as CNNs take input around 224×224 pixels in size [5]. This large disparity in image sizes causes difficulties when using machine learning on whole slide images. While image compression would be a helpful tool, there are drawbacks when using image compression for medical images. Compression can distort markers that are important for diagnosis. Studies have shown a significant decrease in classification of benign and malignant breast tissue once compression reaches levels greater than 32:1 [14]. Often, the large whole slide image is broken into many smaller images that are more suitable in size for machine learning [11].

One common approach when using whole slide images for machine learning is to perform some type of patching of the whole slide image. This can be used to address the image size issue. With patching, a collection of smaller patches is typically retrieved from each image, and these are used instead since they are smaller and easier to work with. Often studies vary on patching techniques. A wide variety of patches may be used by various studies, including overlapping vs non overlapping, varying image sizes, varying number of images, and their selection methods.

However, using patches instead of the whole slide image presents new challenges. First, there is the possibility that an individual patch's label will not match the slide level label. Secondly, even once patch level labels are obtained, aggregation is needed to generate a level for the entire slide [7]. This is most notable in classification problems as these generally look for a slide or patient level label as opposed to segmentation tasks that predict at the patch/pixel level. One common approach to address this is by using convolutional neural networks to extract features from image patches first [13]. This can be followed by a number of techniques, but recently multiple instance learning has started to emerge as a popular choice. In multiple instance learning, patch features would be grouped together according to the slide they came from. These features would become instances and their slide group would be considered a bag. In multiple instance learning, instances (and their combination) inside a bag are used to predict the entire bag's label [9].

2.4 Masking Techniques

When using a patching method to work with whole slide images, there are thousands or even hundreds of thousands of possible patches to choose from, depending on the image size and selected patch size. Not all patches are created equal and some do not contain useful information. In fact, some patches may contain only background data or whitespace and create noise if used for machine learning [24]. The method of patch selection varies between studies with selection methods ranging from algorithmic to random selection [11]. However, most of these patch selection methods aim to remove patches containing only background data from consideration. Removing irrelevant patches is often done as a preprocessing step. One preprocessing technique that can be used to separate background from foreground is thresholding or masking, which separates foreground from background [17]. This allows for only patches with significant amounts of relevant foreground data to be considered for selection.

3   Related Works

One study focused on identifying patients who were considered high-risk for early breast cancer recurrence. Early recurrence was defined to be the return of a primary tumor within three years of diagnosis. Instead of using recurrence scores, patients were followed for confirmed recurrence. The dataset used in this case contained 704 images from 202 patients. The dataset was balanced among the classes with 101 of the patients having recurrence within 3 years while the other 101 were non-recurrent. In this paper, VGG16 was used as a feature extractor and was combined with support vector machines to make final predictions. The cross-validation accuracy for predicting recurrence was 62.4%. The model performed better at predicting early-recurrence for low to intermediate grade tumors [20].

Another study looked to predict ODX risk from whole slide histopathology images annotated with tumor region of interests by pathologists. In this work, a novel sampling method for patches was introduced to select the most discriminative patches from the image tumor regions for use. The framework was analyzed for both H&E-stained slides and Ki67 stained slides. Overall, the Ki67 slides had better results, with a 0.800 accuracy when evaluated with leave two out cross validation. The H&E-stained slides set achieved 0.700 ± 0.030 accuracy across 5-fold cross validation [23].

Another study looked to predict recurrence risk categories using H&E-stained slides with pathologist annotated regions of interest (ROIs). Once patches were extracted from the ROIs, nuclei detection was performed and then was combined with a model to perform epithelial/stromal separation. Next, feature extraction was performed and a classification model was used to predict patch level recurrence risk. Finally, a patch-based voting method was implemented to predict the patient level risk category. This proposed model scored between 76% and 85% for all tests performed. The authors of this work proposed that these results indicated that it could be possible for recurrence risk to be predicted from H&E-stained images [25].

A related work looked to predict recurrence risk based on a 70 gene signature risk score. Multiple convolutional neural networks were evaluated on the training data and Xception scored the highest, so it was selected for testing. Using Xception, an accuracy of 87% was achieved without region of interest labeling. A patch size of 512×512 pixels was originally sampled from the whole slide images but was later resampled to fit the model architecture [18].

4   Methods

The approach in this work uses only H&E-stained images to train a machine learning model to predict breast cancer recurrence. No tumor ROI annotations or clinical data were included in the dataset. A total of 424 breast cancer cases were collected from ECU Health. For each case, tissue sections from biopsies or excisions were sectioned, and then stained with hematoxylin and eosin. All slides were prepared in the Department of Pathology at ECU Health. Each tissue section was scanned using Philips IntelliSite Pathology 760001 Ultra-Fast Scanner 1.8. All images were uploaded to Philips Digital Pathology Solution. All images were saved using a scan factor of 40x (magnification) and were saved using the TIFF format. Each case was assigned a recurrence

Table 1. Dataset statistics. Tumor details for the samples used (left table), and patient demographics (right table).

Tumor Statistic	Low	High		Demographic	Low	High
Tumor Grade				Age Range		
1	7	4		≤ 30	0	1
2	22	22		31–40	2	2
3	22	25		41–50	6	6
No. of Lymph Nodes				51–60	17	17
0	28	35		61–70	15	16
1	10	9		71–80	10	8
2	4	4		81–90	1	1
Other	9	3		Race		
				Black	25	25
				Hispanic	2	2
				White	24	24

score between 0 and 100. The cases were sorted into recurrence risk categories based on this score. Recurrence scores of 25 or less were deemed non-highrisk while cases with recurrence scores of 26 or greater were sorted into the high-risk category. Due to the lower natural occurrence of high-risk scores, only 51 of these cases were high-risk. All available high-risk cases were used. A handpicked group of 51 non-high risk cases was selected for a total of 102 cases. These cases were handpicked rather than randomly selected to ensure the data was consistent among a variety of factors for the low and high-risk groups. The data in both categories was balanced on patient age group, tumor grade, race, and number of lymph nodes impacted. The exact breakdowns for these categories across the low and high-risk groups can be seen in Table 1. These were kept consistent across both the low and high-risk groups to reduce the chance the model would be influenced by factors other than recurrence.

Due to the large size of whole slide images, image patches were used in place of the whole slide image for each case. Multiple patch sizes and patch quantities were extracted so their impact on the model accuracy could be analyzed. After cases were selected to be included in the dataset, they were analyzed for patch quality based on the total amount of tissue available in each patch. The code to analyze patch quality was modified from code that is publicly available at https://github.com/deroneriksson/python-wsi-preprocessing [8]. Code from this repository was updated to fix some bugs and errors, as well as to customize file paths and analysis variables before being used. New code was written to extract the top tiles from each image using the CSV data.

Each slide was filtered to remove background, errant pen markings, and other irrelevant information on the slide. Any image data determined to not be tissue was mapped to a black value using masking to get a clear picture of the tissue within the image. An example of a whole slide image from the dataset before and after filtering can be seen

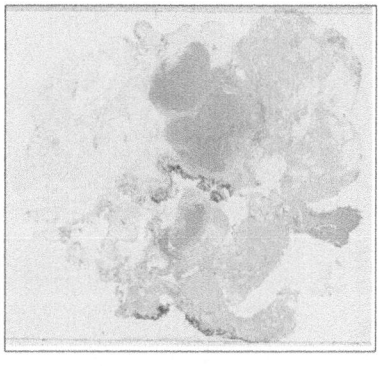
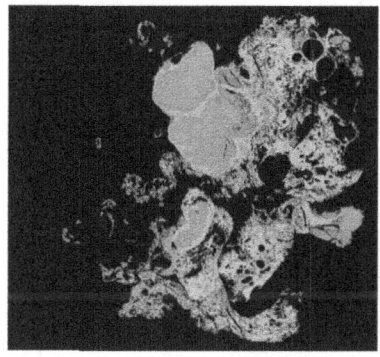

a) Original RGB WSI   b) WSI after filters

Fig. 1. Original RGB and filtered images. Image (a) is a compressed and downsized version of a whole slide image used in the dataset. Image (b) shows the image after all filters have been applied. Any pixels not mapped to 0 (black) are now considered tissue and impact each tile's score. (Color figure online)

in Fig. 1. Each possible patch was scored based on a number of factors including tissue percentage, tissue quantity factor, color factor, and saturation and value factor [8].

The tissue quantity per patch was determined by what percentage of pixels were not 0 after the filter masks were applied. High and low tissue thresholds were set to 75% and 10% respectively. Patches with a tissue percentage at least equal to the high threshold were marked as "High" tissue quantity. Patches with tissue percentages between the high and low thresholds were considered to have "Medium" tissue quantity. Patches with less tissue percentage than the low threshold but more than 0% were considered "Low", and patches with 0% were considered "None". Each patch received a quantity factor based on the amount of available tissue. The values for high, medium, low, and none tissue quantities are as follows, respectively: 1.0, 0.2, 0.1, 0.0. A color factor was also determined for each patch. The color factor favors patches that contain more purple (hematoxylin) values. Lastly, the saturation and value factor is used to reduce the scores of patches with small standard deviations of HSV saturation and HSV values. This can help eliminate blurred patches as significant patches often have broad standard deviations [16]. Once the tissue quantity factor, color factor, and saturation and value factor were all computed, they were multiplied together to get a combined factor to be used in the final score calculation.

Patches were considered high quality if they had a score of 75% or better. An example of an image patch scoring can be seen in Fig. 2. For both patch sizes, the top 1,000 and top 2,000 scoring patches were extracted for analysis. Later, a set of 3,000 tiles of size 256 × 256 pixels were extracted from each image. If an image had less than 3,000 patches that were considered high quality, then first all high quality patches were extracted. Then, these patches were oversampled until a total of 3,000 patches were extracted for each whole slide image. Data on the total number of patches and high quality patch statistics can be found in Table 2.

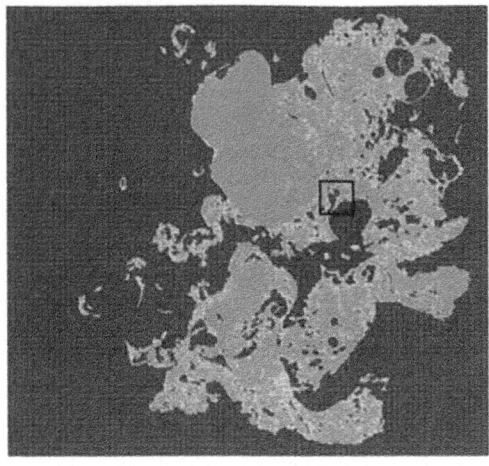 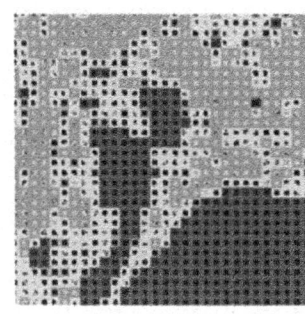

a) Whole Slide Patch Summary   b) Section Patch Summary

Fig. 2. Patch overlay. This shows the same whole slide image as shown in Fig. 1. Here, the patch summary overlay is placed on top of the image. The smaller squares each represent a patch and their outline color represents the tissue quantity per patch. Green indicates high amounts of tissue, yellow indicates medium, orange indicates low and red indicates no tissue. (Color figure online)

Table 2. Patch Statistics. Patch statistics are shown for high quality tiles for patch sizes 256 × 256 pixels and 512 × 512 pixels. Patches are considered "high quality" if their overall score is at least 75%.

Measurement/Patch Size	256 × 256	512 × 512
Smallest # High Quality Patches	538	51
Largest # High Quality Patches	60,371	15,113
Average # High Quality Patches	17,651	4,306
Standard Deviation of High Quality Patches	11,724	3,025

Once patches had been extracted from each whole slide image, the patches were sorted into subfolders "high" and "non-high" based on their recurrence risk category. A convolutional neural network was used to extract features from each image. The CNN used for feature extraction was ResNet-18. Feature extraction via ResNet-18 was done using the Python library Img2Vec. Each image yielded 512 features regardless of image size. For each patch processed, the patch features, slide level label, and case number were saved. Feature extraction was performed on a Tesla T4 GPU and averaged approximately 8.5 iterations (images processed) per second. The total time to process feature extractions for each dataset varied based on the patch size and number of patches per whole slide. After feature extraction, patches were sorted into bags based on their original cases. The data bags were split into 80% training and 20% testing for holdout testing.

The data underwent preprocessing to convert the three-dimensional arrays into two dimensional arrays for analysis. Data was standardized using the Python library Standard Scalar. Once the data was preprocessed, it was fed into a logistic regression model. Grid search was used to determine the best parameters for each dataset for logistic regression. The parameters used for the best scoring dataset were C=10.0, penalty= 'l1', and scorer= 'liblinear'. After the models were created, they were tested on a variety of measurements including accuracy, F1 score, and AUC. Cross validation of the training dataset as well as cross validation of the entire dataset was also used to evaluate their ability to generalize the training data in addition to the testing data. The code used in this work is publicly available and can be accessed at https://github.com/mad-rose/breastcancerrecurrence-prediction.

5   Results

Table 3. Holdout testing results. Results from holdout testing for each patch type are reported across multiple metrics including accuracy, F1 score, AUC, and cross-validation of the training data.

Patch Type	Accuracy	F1	AUC	Training Cross Validation
256 × 3,000	0.524	0.540	0.676	0.481 ± 0.104
256 × 2,000	**0.714**	**0.750**	**0.736**	**0.640 ± 0.067**
256 × 1,000	0.619	0.636	0.704	0.530 ± 0.078
512 × 2,000	0.571	0.640	0.593	0.517 ± 0.080
512 × 1,000	0.571	0.609	0.630	0.518 ± 0.066

Model performance was evaluated in two main ways. First, holdout testing was performed with 20% of the data that was originally selected for testing using the train test split function from Sci-kit learn. The logistic regression model was evaluated on this data. The model's accuracy, F1 score, and AUC were evaluated. These results are displayed in Table 3. 5-fold cross validation was performed on the training set to assess the model's ability to generalize across the training data. Due to the size of the dataset being relatively small (n = 102), 5-fold cross validation on the entire dataset was performed. These results can be seen in Table 4. Due to the size of the dataset, this cross validation is likely more indicative of the model's overall performance on the entire dataset. When performing cross validation on the dataset, 5-fold cross validation was used and was measured on accuracy and F1 score. The results for each model are indicated for the model's best parameters as determined by grid search. The best performing patch type across all evaluations was the patch size 256 × 256 pixels with 2,000 patches per whole slide image. Generally, a patch size of 256 × 256 pixels performed better than a patch size of 512 × 512 pixels, with the exception of the 256 × 256 × 3,000 model that used patch oversampling. A larger patch quantity of 2,000 patches appeared to perform better in comparison to only using 1,000 patches for the patch size 256 × 256. However, the

3,000 patch model performed more poorly than both the 1,000 and 2,000 patch models. The performance of both the 1,000 and 2,000 patch models was similar for the patch size 512 × 512.

Table 4. 5-fold cross-validation testing results. Accuracy and F1 scores are reported for each patch type when the entire dataset (102 cases) was used for 5-fold cross-validation.

Patch Type	Accuracy	F1
256 × 3,000	0.462 ± 0.075	0.471 ± 0.095
256 × 2,000	**0.628 ± 0.044**	**0.639 ± 0.060**
256 × 1,000	0.588 ± 0.044	0.596 ± 0.037
512 × 2,000	0.521 ± 0.117	0.521 ± 0.126
512 × 1,000	0.529 ± 0.053	0.515 ± 0.072

6 Discussion

Overall, the patching method of using 2,000 patches of size 256 × 256 performed the best across all measurements. This includes both the holdout testing and the 5-fold cross validation of the entire dataset. The lower scores for cross validation when compared to the accuracy for the holdout data could suggest that the selected holdout data was easier to predict or may be more similar to the training data used. The cross-validation scores for the entire datasets are likely a better indicator of overall model performance since multiple folds of testing were completed. Interestingly, the 256 × 256 × 3,000 images using oversampling had the lowest accuracy and cross validation scores. There are a few reasons this method might have performed so poorly. First, if the relevant patches needed for recurrence prediction were already captured within the first 2,000 patches extracted, extracting 3,000 patches may have only introduced extra noise into the dataset. The oversampling method might have also caused some irrelevant patches to be oversampled which would also introduce noise into the dataset.

In the 5-fold cross validation for the entire dataset, the standard deviation values for the 256 × 256-pixel sized patch datasets, excluding the 256 × 3,000 oversampling model, are smaller than the standard deviation for the datasets of the 512 × 512-pixel sized patches. This could suggest that the models using the 256 × 256 patch size are able to generalize better across more data, since the scores for each fold are closer to the cross validation mean. One reason for this could be that the smaller patches may be able to capture important information near the tissue edge. When a larger patch size is used, this could become a lower quality patch due to increased background presence since the tissue is right at the edge between the sample and the background.

One factor that could be hindering the model performance is the varying size of tissue samples in each case. These statistics can be seen in Table 2. The number of available patches of high quality (patches with a score of at least 75%) varied greatly among cases. With the patch size of 256 × 256 pixels, the whole slide image with the fewest number of high quality patches contained 538 high quality patches. The image that contained the most high quality patches had 60,371 high quality patches. This is a range of 59,833 patches. Given the average number of high quality patches at 17,651 and the standard deviation of 11,724, it can be concluded that there is high variability of high quality patches amongst the images in the dataset. For the patch size of 512 × 512 pixels, the smallest and largest number of high quality patches from images in the dataset were 51 and 15,113 respectively. This represents a range of 15,062 patches. The average number of high quality patches for this dataset was 4,306 and the standard deviation was 3,025. These high standard deviations contribute to a large difference in the total high quality patches available for analysis, which can make it difficult to determine the total number of patches that should be extracted from each image.

Both ends of this spectrum present their own challenges. On the smaller side, for cases with fewer available high quality patches, the number of these available patches is sometimes less than the total number of patches used in each dataset for training. This would result in some patches being included in the dataset that are of lower quality and include more irrelevant data. This could introduce noise into the dataset which could impact model accuracy. On the other side, having such a large number of high quality tiles makes it less likely that a sample of 1,000 or 2,000 patches would include the tumor region of the image. This could mean that the selected patches are not as relevant to recurrence and important patches for predicting recurrence were not captured in the dataset which could also impact the model's accuracy.

Some limitations of this study include the data availability. The dataset used was relatively small (n = 102). While more cases were available, all available high-risk cases were used, and a select number of non-high risk cases were used to keep the dataset balanced. Since high-risk cases are less common, this was the limiting factor on the dataset. Another limitation is the data used in this study came from one hospital and one whole slide image scanner. More analysis is needed using data from multiple hospitals and multiple whole slide image scanners to increase variability.

7 Conclusion

Since whole slide image scanners were introduced, there has been a strong push towards using machine learning methods within digital pathology. Great strides have been made on tasks such as breast cancer diagnosis and metastasis detection, however there is not as much research into outcome predictions, including recurrence risk. Many studies that attempt to predict recurrence scores or categories use clinical data or image data containing region of interest annotations. If an image-based model could be developed, this could greatly decrease the cost associated with recurrence score testing since H&E-stained images are routinely collected for breast cancer diagnosis [20]. Additionally, if these predictions could be done without the need for pathologist annotations of tumor regions of interest, additional pathology work could be reduced.

Within this research area there are many potential future work opportunities. One thing that would be interesting would be to use a CNN finetuned on the patches themselves to perform feature extraction. This might increase model accuracy by allowing the CNN to extract more relevant features from each of the image patches. It would also be interesting to investigate more patch sizes. Since in this study, the smaller patch size generally performed better, more investigation should be done into even smaller patch sizes, possibly even as small as one cell per patch, to see if an improvement in accuracy continues. Additionally to add onto this work, one future possibility is obtaining more varied data from different hospitals and scanners to test. If this were done it is possible techniques for color normalization would be needed to be added to account for this variability. Also, including available patient data such as age and tumor grade may also help the model perform better with its predictions.

Despite not having any region of interest annotations from a pathologist in this dataset, another possible avenue for future work could include using this dataset with preexisting models available for tumor segmentation. This way, a region of interest map/mask could be used without requiring extra work from a pathologist. This could allow for better patch selection.

In summary, in this study a dataset containing only H&E-stained images was used to train a machine learning model with the goal of predicting breast cancer recurrence risk category. Image patches were collected from each whole slide image and features were extracted from each image patch using a ResNet-18 architecture. Image features were then aggregated together into bags, where each slide represented a bag and the patch features represented instances inside the bag. These bags were used to train a logistic regression model which was evaluated across multiple metrics including accuracy, and F1. The best scoring model across all metrics used 2,000 patches of size 256 $\times$ 256 pixels from each whole slide image. This model observed a mean accuracy of 0.628 ± 0.044 in 5-fold cross validation across the entire available dataset. Analysis of various patch sizes and patch quantities is also performed to determine their impact on the overall accuracy of the model. A few possible factors that could contribute to poorer model performance are discussed in this study, including high variance amongst available tissue in each whole slide image. Also, the dataset used in this study was limited in size and variance due to coming from only one hospital and one whole slide image scanner. More research is needed across larger and more varied datasets to further assess the possibilities of using only H&E-stained images for ODX recurrence risk category prediction.

References

1. Classification of breast cancer histopathological images using densenet and transfer learning. Comput. Intell. Neurosci. **2022** (2022). https://doi.org/10.1155/2022/8904768
2. Alzu'bi, A., Najadat, H., Doulat, W., Al-Shari, O., Zhou, L.: Predicting the recurrence of breast cancer using machine learning algorithms. Multimed. Tools Appl. **80**, 13787–13800 (2021). https://doi.org/10.1007/s11042-020-10448-w
3. Araújo, T., et al.: Classification of breast cancer histology images using convolutional neural networks. PLoS ONE **12**(6), 1–14 (2017). https://doi.org/10.1371/journal.pone.0177544
4. Ciga, O., Martel, A.L.: Learning to segment images with classification labels. Med. Image Anal. **68** (2021). https://doi.org/10.1016/j.media.2020.101912
5. Ciga, O., Xu, T., Nofech-Mozes, S., Noy, S., Lu, F.I., Martel, A.L.: Overcoming the limitations of patch-based learning to detect cancer in whole slide images. Sci. Rep. **11** (2021). https://doi.org/10.1038/s41598-021-88494-z

6. Deng, J., Dong, W., Socher, R., Li, L.J., Li, K., Fei-Fei, L.: ImageNet: a large-scale hierarchical image database (2010). https://doi.org/10.1109/cvpr.2009.5206848
7. Dimitriou, N., Arandjelović, O., Caie, P.D.: Deep learning for whole slide image analysis: an overview. Front. Med. **6** (2019). https://doi.org/10.3389/fmed.2019.00264
8. Eriksson, D.: python-wsi-preprocessing. GitHub repository (2017). https://github.com/deroneriksson/python-wsi-preprocessing.git
9. Gadermayr, M., Tschuchnig, M.: Multiple instance learning for digital pathology: a review of the state-of-the-art, limitations & future potential. Comput. Med. Imaging Graph. **112**, 102337 (2024). https://doi.org/10.1016/j.compmedimag.2024.102337
10. Gupta, V., Mishra, V.K., Singhal, P., Kumar, A.: An overview of supervised machine learning algorithm. In: 2022 11th International Conference on System Modeling & Advancement in Research Trends (SMART) (2022). https://doi.org/10.1109/SMART55829.2022.10047618
11. Hou, L., Samaras, D., Kurc, T.M., Gao, Y., Davis, J.E., Saltz, J.H.: Patch-based convolutional neural network for whole slide tissue image classification. In: IEEE Conference on Computer Vision and Pattern Recognition (2016). https://doi.org/10.1109/CVPR.2016.266
12. Khened, M., Kori, A., Rajkumar, H., Krishnamurthi, G., Srinivasan, B.: A generalized deep learning framework for whole-slide image segmentation and analysis. Sci. Rep. **11** (2021). https://doi.org/10.1038/s41598-021-90444-8
13. Kim, H.E., Cosa-Linan, A., Santhanam, N., Jannesari, M., Maros, M.E., Ganslandt, T.: Transfer learning for medical image classification: a literature review. BMC Med. Imaging **22**(1) (2022). https://doi.org/10.1186/s12880-022-00793-7
14. Krupinski, E.A., Johnson, J.P., Jaw, S., Graham, A.R., Weinstein, R.S.: Compressing pathology whole-slide images using a human and model observer evaluation. J. Pathol. Inform. **3**, 17 (2012). https://doi.org/10.4103/2153-3539.95129
15. Li, J., et al.: Signet ring cell detection with a semi-supervised learning framework. In: Chung, A.C.S., Gee, J.C., Yushkevich, P.A., Bao, S. (eds.) IPMI 2019. LNCS, vol. 11492, pp. 842–854. Springer, Cham (2019). https://doi.org/10.1007/978-3-030-20351-1_66
16. Litjens, G., et al.: 1399 H&E-stained sentinel lymph node sections of breast cancer patients: the CAMELYON dataset. GigaScience **7** (2018). https://doi.org/10.1093/gigascience/giy065
17. Otsu, N.: Threshold selection method from gray-level histograms. IEEE Trans. Syst. Man Cybern. **9**(1), 62–66 (1979). https://doi.org/10.1109/tsmc.1979.4310076
18. Phan, N.N., Hsu, C.Y., Huang, C.C., Tseng, L.M., Chuang, E.Y.: Prediction of breast cancer recurrence using a deep convolutional neural network without region-of-interest labeling. Front. Oncol. **11** (2021). https://doi.org/10.3389/fonc.2021.734015
19. Rose, M., Geradts, J., Herndon, N.: Deep learning in digital breast pathology. In: Proceedings of the 17th International Joint Conference on Biomedical Engineering Systems and Technologies, vol. 1, pp. 404–414 (2024). https://doi.org/10.5220/0012576100003657
20. Shi, Y., et al.: Predicting early breast cancer recurrence from histopathological images in the Carolina breast cancer study. NPJ Breast Cancer **9**, 92 (2023). https://doi.org/10.1038/s41523-023-00597-0
21. Siegel, R.L., Miller, K.D., Wagle, N.S., Jemal, A.: Cancer statistics, 2023. CA: Cancer J. Clin. **73**(1), 17–48 (2023). https://doi.org/10.3322/caac.21763
22. Sparano, J.A., Paik, S.: Development of the 21-gene assay and its application in clinical practice and clinical trials. J. Clin. Oncol. **26**, 721–728 (2008). https://doi.org/10.1200/JCO.2007.15.1068
23. Su, Z., et al.: BCR-net: a deep learning framework to predict breast cancer recurrence from histopathology images. PLoS ONE **18**(4) (2023). https://doi.org/10.1371/journal.pone.0283562
24. Veta, M., Pluim, J.P., Diest, P.J.V., Viergever, M.A.: Breast cancer histopathology image analysis: a review. IEEE Trans. Biomed. Eng. **61**(5), 1400–1411 (2014). https://doi.org/10.1109/TBME.2014.2303852

25. Whitney, J., et al.: Quantitative nuclear histomorphometry predicts oncotype dx risk categories for early stage ER+ breast cancer. BMC Cancer **18**, 610 (2018). https://doi.org/10.1186/s12885-018-4448-9
26. Zujewski, J.A., Kamin, L.: Trial assessing individualized options for treatment for breast cancer: the TAILORx trial. Future Oncol. **4**, 603–610 (2008). https://doi.org/10.2217/14796694.4.5.603

Bio-inspired Systems and Signal Processing

Advancements in Camera-Based Oxygen Desaturation Monitoring in Sleep Apnea Patients

Belmin Alić[1]([⊠])(iD), Wang Liao[2], Samuel Tauber[3], Chen Zhang[2],
Sarah Dietz-Terjung[4,5], Alina Wildenauer[4], Jose Guillermo Ortiz Sucre[5],
Gerhard Weinreich[5], Sivagurunathan Sutharsan[5], Christoph Schöbel[4], Gunther Notni[2],
Reinhard Viga[1], Christian Wiede[3], and Karsten Seidl[1,3]

[1] Chair of Electronic Components and Circuits, University of Duisburg-Essen,
Duisburg, Germany
belmin.alic@uni-due.de
[2] Department of Mechanical Engineering, Ilmenau University of Technology, Ilmenau,
Germany
[3] Fraunhofer Institute for Microelectronic Circuits and Systems, Duisburg, Germany
[4] Chair of Sleep and Telemedicine, University Medicine Essen-Ruhrlandklinik,
University of Duisburg-Essen, Essen, Germany
[5] Department of Pulmonary Medicine, Division of Cystic Fibrosis, University Medicine
Essen-Ruhrlandklinik, University of Duisburg-Essen, Essen, Germany

Abstract. Recurrent apneic episodes lead to a decrease in blood oxygen levels and eventually hypoxemia. Persistent hypoxemic SpO_2 values during sleep are linked to severe health risks, including organ damage, heart failure, tachycardia, and shortness of breath. Oxygen desaturation events are usually detected during polysomnography (PSG) in sleep laboratories. A PSG involves a high number of contact-based sensors, which may lead to patient discomfort and biased measurement results. In this work, a contactless camera-based oxygen desaturation monitoring method based on the analysis of multispectral videos is proposed. The method is built on the extraction and analysis of remote photoplethysmography (rPPG) signals at wavelengths of 780 and 940 nm from the forehead and a breath temperature signal via far-infrared (FIR) thermography from the subnasal region. A manual feature extraction is implemented to gather pertinent medical and physiological parameters from the obtained signals. These parameters are used to design a fully connected feed-forward neural network-based classifier, which distinguishes between periods with and without desaturation. A patient dataset consisting of 23 sleep apnea patients is collected for evaluation. The classification accuracy between desaturation events and periods without a desaturation based on the leave-one-patient-out cross-validation metric is 95.4%. The oxygen desaturation index (ODI) is estimated with a mean average error (MAE) of 2.9 $\frac{events}{hour}$, while a correct ODI stage prediction is given for 21 of the 23 patients. The regression of the exact SpO_2 value during desaturation results in an MAE of 1.79%.

Keywords: Contactless · Camera-based · Oxygen saturation · Desaturation monitoring · Sleep apnea · Feature extraction · Remote photoplethysmography

© The Author(s), under exclusive license to Springer Nature Switzerland AG 2026
M. P. Guarino et al. (Eds.): BIOSTEC 2024, CCIS 2546, pp. 229–252, 2026.
https://doi.org/10.1007/978-3-031-96899-0_14

1   Introduction

Sleep apnea syndrome (SAS) is a sleep disorder marked by repeated interruptions in airflow during sleep, resulting in various symptoms such as daytime drowsiness, concentration issues, and heightened cardiovascular disease risk [28]. These recurrent interruptions cause blood oxygen levels to drop, leading to hypoxemia [25]. Hypoxemia episodes during sleep are known as oxygen desaturation events [31], defined by a decrease in oxygen saturation of at least 3% [6]. The oxygen desaturation index (ODI), which measures the average number of desaturation events per hour of sleep, summarizes the prevalence of these events. Along with the apnea-hypopnea index (AHI), the ODI is a crucial indicator of SAS severity [25].

The gold standard for diagnosing SAS is cardiorespiratory polysomnography (PSG), a multi-parametric measurement performed in sleep laboratories. PSG uses a large number of contact-based sensors, causing patient discomfort and unnatural sleeping behavior, which may result in biased measurements [32]. To measure peripheral oxygen saturation (SpO$_2$), a PSG usually includes a pulse oximeter placed on the index finger. A contactless alternative to PSG could mitigate the aforementioned drawbacks and enable sleep diagnostics outside sleep laboratories. One promising approach for contactless sleep diagnostics is camera-based solutions.

In this article, we reintroduce the method for oxygen desaturation detection and ODI estimation based on the analysis of multispectral videos, which was previously presented in our conference publication [3]. Furthermore, we introduce a novel method for the regression of the exact SpO$_2$ value and provide a clinical perspective to the proposed methods and results. The article is structured in the following way. In Sect. 2, we elaborate on related work on contactless SpO$_2$ measurement and oxygen desaturation detection, highlighting the current state-of-the-art and identifying existing research gaps. In Sect. 3, we introduce the proposed methods for oxygen desaturation detection and the regression of the SpO$_2$ value. In Sect. 4, we present the results of our patient study conducted at the Center for Sleep Medicine, University Medicine Essen. In Sect. 5, we discuss the results and provide a clinical perspective. Finally, in Sect. 6, we conclude and propose further research steps.

2   Related Work

The first method for measuring a photoplethysmography (PPG) signal without direct contact with human skin was proposed in Ref. [18]. Light from two infrared LEDs (760 nm and 880 nm) was emitted through the index finger, and a CMOS camera 40 cm away measured the transmitted light. Later that year, in Wieringa et al. [39], the concept for a contactless PPG-based measurement of SpO$_2$ via remote PPG (rPPG) was introduced. Between 2005 and 2023, twelve studies on the contactless measurement of SpO$_2$ have been identified in a literature screening conducted as part of this study. An overview of these studies, including the related topic, the region of interest (ROI) denoting the body region from which the measurement data originates, and information on the test subject sample is provided in Table 1.

Ten studies involved camera-based methods built on analyzing rPPG signals from multiple wavelengths, while two were based on respiratory movement analysis via

Table 1. Overview of related studies on contactless SpO_2 measurement [3].

Publication	Study topic	ROI	Test subjects
Wieringa et al., 2015 [39]	Proof of concept study	Hand	Healthy, awake
Lingqin et al., 2013 [21]	SpO_2 regression via rPPG	Face	Healthy, awake
Tsai et al., 2014 [35]	SpO_2 regression via rPPG	Hand	Healthy, awake
Guazzi et al., 2015 [16]	SpO_2 regression via rPPG	Face	Healthy, awake
Shao et al., 2016 [29]	SpO_2 regression via rPPG	Face	Sick, awake
Addison et al., 2017 [1]	Hypoxia detection via rPPG	Face	Healthy, awake
Vogels et al., 2018 [37]	SpO_2 regression via rPPG	Face	Healthy, asleep
Tran et al., 2019 [34]	SpO_2 regression via Radar	Torso	Sick, asleep
Rosa et al., 2020 [27]	SpO_2 regression via rPPG	Face	Healthy, awake
Toften et al., 2021 [33]	SpO_2 regression via Radar	Torso	Sick, asleep
Wieler et al., 2021 [38]	SpO_2 regression via rPPG	Face	Healthy, awake
Liao et al., 2023 [20]	SpO_2 regression via rPPG	Hand	Healthy, awake

radar. The ROI for the signal source varied between the hand [20, 35, 39] and the face [1, 16, 21, 27, 29, 37, 38] for rPPG methods, and the torso [33, 34] for Doppler effect-based methods. All studies introduced a regression analysis method to determine the SpO_2 value, except [1], where hypoxia detection was performed. Three studies involved sleeping subjects [33, 34, 37], with the latter two involving symptomatic SAS patients.

Based on the overview of related work, the following observations and conclusions are made: (1) regression of the SpO_2 value via contactless methods is a non-trivial task; (2) there are insufficient patient studies for conclusive evidence on the medical applicability of the proposed methods; (3) the majority (9 out of 12) of studies are conducted with healthy test subjects, with only three including measurements in the hypoxemic range; (4) all studies have a small number of test subjects (in the one-digit or low double-digit range), which is insufficient for conclusive proof of principle concerning demographic variability; (5) none of the listed studies dealt with detecting oxygen desaturation events or estimating the ODI score; and (6) there is an evident necessity for further work in this area.

3 Methods

3.1 Selection of Biosignals

SpO_2 is the percentage of oxyhemoglobin (HbO_2) in the total hemoglobin. Oxyhemoglobin and deoxyhemoglobin (Hb) have different light absorption behaviors, as shown in Fig. 1 [24]. To determine the amount of HbO_2 in the blood, at least two rPPG signals at distinct wavelengths are required. The first wavelength should have a higher absorption ratio for HbO_2 than Hb, and vice versa for the second wavelength. Further details on this principle are provided in Ref. [22].

An external light source is essential for continuous SpO_2 measurement during the night with a camera. To avoid disturbing the sleeping person, the light source and the wavelengths of the rPPG signals should be in the near-infrared (NIR) spectrum. By

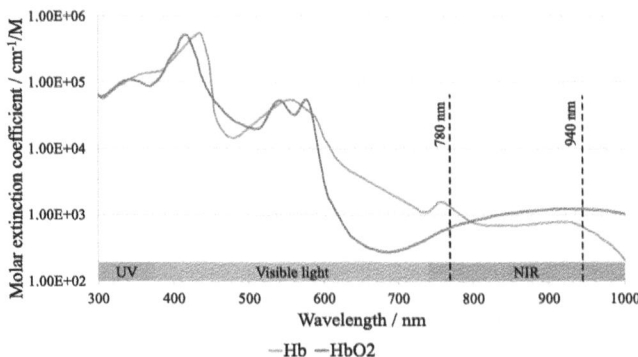

Fig. 1. Absorption behavior of Hb (orange) and HbO$_2$ (blue) with respect to the wavelength of the incident light [3]. (Color figure online)

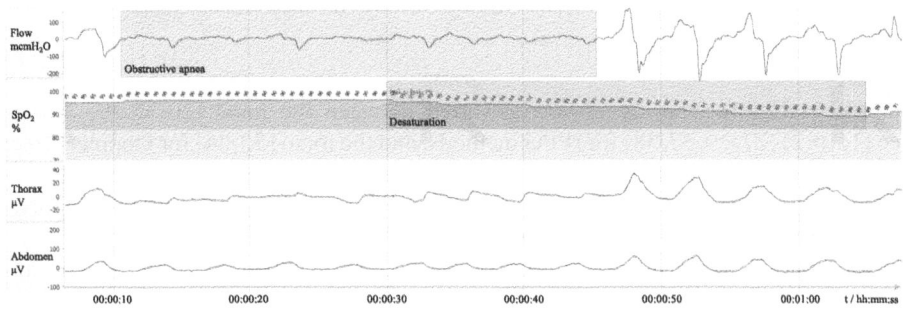

Fig. 2. A section of a PSG recording in Noxturnal consisting of (from top to bottom): 1) Respiratory flow signal with a labeled obstructive apnea; 2) SpO$_2$ signal with a labeled desaturation event; 3) thorax; and 4) abdomen movement signal [3].

analyzing the Hb and HbO$_2$ absorption behavior from Fig. 1, considering the selection criteria, and the specifications of available optical components, a combination of 780 and 940 nm wavelengths is selected.

Oxygen desaturation events often occur directly after an apneic event due to the cessation of breathing. Figure 2 shows a section of a PSG measurement from a patient in this study, displaying four biosignals: 1) airflow measured with a nasal cannula; 2) SpO$_2$ measured with a pulse oximeter at the fingertip; 3) thorax movement measured with an inductive respiration sensor; and 4) abdomen movement measured with an inductive respiration sensor. An obstructive apnea is detected and labeled (orange marked section) on the airflow signal, while a desaturation event is labeled (green marked section) on the SpO$_2$ signal. The desaturation event starts approximately 20 s after the apnea begins and ends approximately 20 s after the apnea ends, restoring the baseline SpO$_2$ level. This correlation between nocturnal respiratory events and oxygen saturation is significant for detecting desaturation events. Therefore, in addition to the two rPPG signals, a new biosignal is introduced: the respiratory airflow signal, measured in the subnasal region (equivalent to the nasal cannula location during PSG) via far-infrared (FIR) thermography.

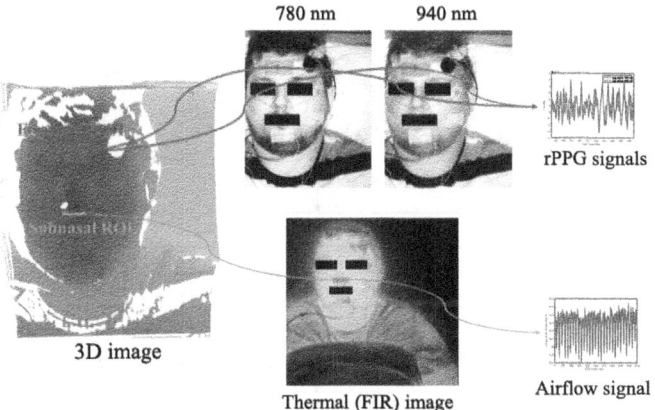

Fig. 3. Extraction of time series signals by detecting and tracking the ROIs in the 3D image and projecting the ROI on the forehead onto the 2D NIR 780 and 940 nm images to extract two rPPG signals and the ROI in the subnasal region onto the 2D thermal FIR image to extract the respiratory airflow signal [3].

3.2 Image Acquisition and Image Processing

To acquire the three selected biosignals, a multi-modal camera system is utilized, comprising: 1) a real-time NIR 3D sensor for assessing head motion; 2) a NIR camera with a central wavelength of $\lambda_c = 780$ nm and a full width at half maximum bandwidth of FWHM $= 10$ nm; 3) a NIR camera with $\lambda_c = 940$ nm and FWHM $= 10$ nm; 4) an FIR thermography camera with a noise equivalent temperature difference of NETD < 0.05 °C at 30 °C/50 mK; and 5) one LED with $\lambda_c = 780$ nm and FWHM $= 28$ nm, and three LEDs with $\lambda_c = 940$ nm and FWHM $= 37$ nm. The additional NIR LEDs enable an irritation-free illumination of the patient. All cameras are clock-synchronized and operate at a frame rate of 15 frames per second (FPS). Further technical specifications can be found in previous publications [4,5,41].

The image sequences are anonymized by blacking out irrelevant facial regions and reduced by extracting only valid image sequences (where the patient is in bed and facing the camera). Two ROIs are identified and monitored in the 3D image sequences: one on the forehead for extracting rPPG signals and another in the subnasal region for respiratory airflow extraction. These 3D ROIs are then projected onto the 2D images from the NIR and FIR cameras. The rPPG signals are extracted using the method outlined in Ref. [41], employing Eulerian video magnification [40]. The respiratory airflow signal is derived by averaging temperature values pixel-wise within the ROI in each frame captured by the FIR camera. Figure 3 illustrates this signal acquisition process. The three raw time series are then used for two separate applications: (1) the detection of oxygen desaturation events; and (2) the regression of the oxygen saturation value. The methodology for both applications is introduced in separate subsections below.

3.3 Detection of Oxygen Desaturation Events

In order to distinguish episodes with an oxygen desaturation event (OD) and with no oxygen desaturation event (NOD), the three raw time series extracted from the image

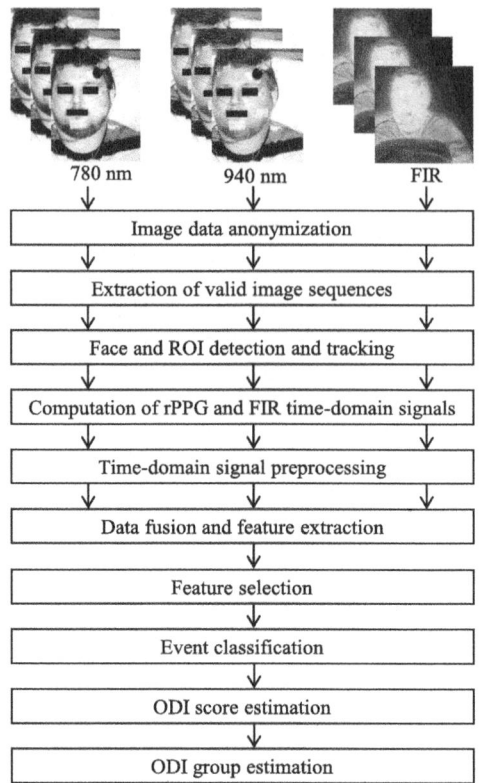

Fig. 4. List of all steps in the proposed data processing chain for oxygen desaturation event detection and ODI score estimation beginning with the image acquisition and processing, followed by time domain signal processing and concluding with event classification and ODI estimation.

sequences are subjected to a series of data processing steps. An overview of these steps is provided in Fig. 4. The first stages in the data processing chain, including the image acquisition and the image processing are already described in Subsect. 3.2. The remaining steps of the data processing chain are elaborated in the following subsections.

Time Domain Preprocessing. Time domain preprocessing starts by extracting valid time domain sequences via system clock alignment with the labeled PSG reference data. We then generate an event dataset consisting of data snippets with a variable time duration t_v, equal to the duration of the desaturation event as labeled in the PSG data. Furthermore, an approximately equal number of periods with stable saturation are labeled as NOD events to create a balanced dataset. Resaturation periods are currently excluded from the classification.

Besides the current time window of the event, one preceding and one succeeding non-overlapping time window with a fixed window length of $t_w = 30$ s, are added to the event database. With the preceding and succeeding windows, the physiological pro-

Table 2. Characterization of the applied finite impulse response band-pass filters.

Frequency spectrum	$f_{c,low}$ (Hz)	$f_{c,high}$ (Hz)	Abbreviation
RR components	0.1	0.5	RR
HR components	0.8	1.5	HR
Extended HR and RR spectrum	0.0667	3	Ext_HR_RR

cesses before and after the desaturation event are to be analyzed. A desaturation event is likely to occur 10 to 30 s after the beginning of an apneic event [8]. Consequently, the analysis of the respiratory activity before an event may contribute to the distinction between desaturation events and stable SpO_2 periods. An example of a desaturation event following an apneic event with a delay of approximately 20 s is shown in Fig. 2. On the other hand, due to the restoration of respiratory activity after the end of the apneic event, higher respiratory activity is to be expected during and directly after desaturation events. Furthermore, we account for the resaturation periods in the window after the event. In the next step, the snippets are detrended via mean subtraction to remove superimposed DC signal components. The DC components may differ during one or between measurements due to changes in environmental and lighting factors, movement, and head rotation.

After detrending, the snippets are subjected to selective band-pass filtering with finite impulse response filters, where different frequency spectra are extracted to separately analyze selected physiological responses, including heart rate (HR) and respiratory rate (RR) components. A list of the applied filters with their respective lower and upper cut-off frequencies, $f_{c,low}$ and $f_{c,high}$, is given in Table 2. We analyze the 780 and 940-nm rPPG and FIR signals in the RR spectrum and the 780 and 940-nm rPPG signals in the HR spectrum. Besides heart rate, it is possible to observe respiratory rate in an rPPG signal. The rPPG signal is influenced by respiratory-induced variations in the cardiovascular system, which may manifest through respiratory sinus arrhythmia, thoracic pressure changes, and variations in blood oxygen saturation [10, 30].

Data Fusion and Feature Extraction. The preprocessed and filtered snippets from the three time series are fused together to perform a feature extraction. The goal of the feature extraction stage is to manually generate medically significant features, with which it will be possible to distinguish OD and NOD events. A total of 142 features is designed in this stage and a small subset of selected features is described below. The feature set consists of features from all three signals. To demonstrate the impact of all signals, we introduce a few selected features from all three signals.

Oxygen desaturation events often take place after a patient experiences an apneic event with a delay of 10 to 30 s, due to the continued cessation in breathing [8]. Figure 2 shows a section of a PSG measurement with a labeled obstructive apnea and oxygen desaturation. By examining the timing of these two events, it can be noticed that the desaturation event starts approximately 20 s after the end of the apnea. Furthermore, the desaturation event ends approximately 20 s after the end of the apnea, leading to a resaturation period. This correlation between nocturnal respiratory events and oxygen

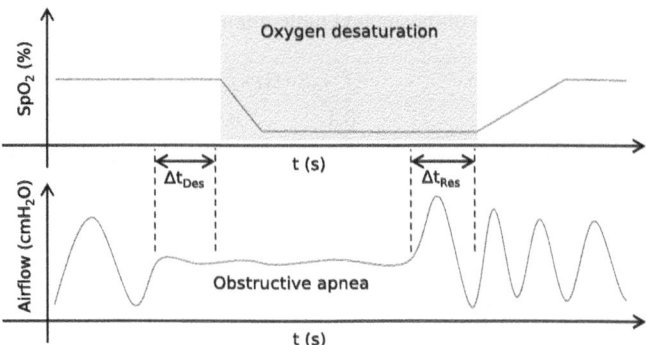

Fig. 5. Graphical representation of the expected time delay between an apneic event and a desaturation event. The upper graph depicts an SpO₂ signal with a labeled desaturation event, while the lower graph depicts a respiratory airflow signal with a labeled obstructive apnea.

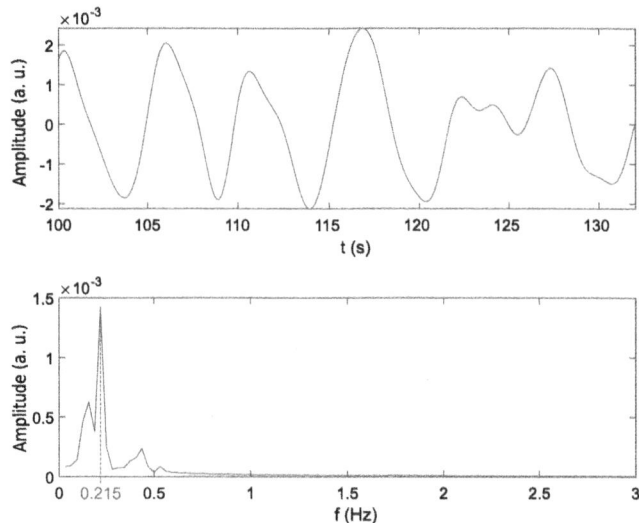

Fig. 6. A time domain (above) and frequency domain (below) representation of a 30-s-long snippet of a 780-nm rPPG signal during normal breathing, filtered in the RR spectrum ($f_{c,low}$ = 0.1 Hz, $f_{c,high}$ = 0.5 Hz). The peak in the frequency spectrum indicates the estimated respiratory rate [3].

desaturation events may therefore be a significant tool to detect oxygen desaturation events. This correlation is depicted in Fig. 5, where Δt_{Des} is the time delay between the end of the apneic event and the beginning of the desaturation event and Δt_{Res} is the time delay between the end of the apneic event and the start of the resaturation period (increase in SpO₂ value).

To qualitatively examine the correlation between respiratory rate and oxygen desaturation, a 30-second-long snippet of a 780-nm rPPG signal in the RR spectrum is

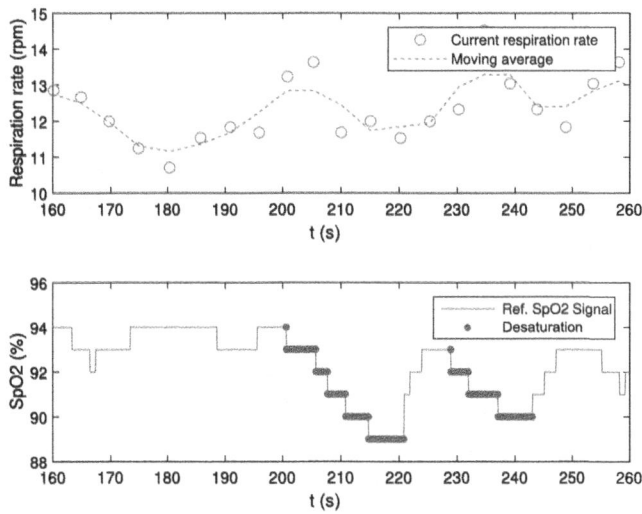

Fig. 7. Instantaneous and averaged respiratory rate estimated by computing the peak in the frequency spectrum of a 780-nm rPPG signal (above) and reference SpO₂ signal with two desaturation and resaturation periods (below) during a 100-s-long sample [3].

selected and an FFT is applied to it to detect the respiratory rate. The respiratory rate is assumed to be the highest peak in the frequency spectrum. This rPPG signal section and its frequency spectrum are presented in Fig. 6. The highest peak in the frequency spectrum is located at $f = 0.215$ Hz, which is equal to 12.9 respirations per minute (rpm) and in correspondence with the reference breathing rate. We then increase the signal length to a 100-second-long sample during which two desaturation and resaturation events occur. We estimate the instantaneous respiratory rate by computing the highest peak in the frequency spectrum and applying a moving average filter (with a window size of four samples) to estimate the change in respiratory rate over time. Figure 7 shows the change in instantaneous respiratory rate and the SpO₂ level of the 100-second-long sample. We observe a decreased respiratory activity before and an increased respiratory activity during the desaturation events, confirming the aforementioned correlation between respiratory rate and oxygen saturation.

Figure 8 shows six selected features for the classification between OD and NOD. The probability density functions of the features are shown as Kernel Density Estimation (KDE) plots with the area under the curve for the probability density function of each event type equal to one. The features are normalized in the value range between zero and one. The names of the features are shown above the KDE plots in the following form: *Feature name [signal type; frequency spectrum; time window]*. In signal types, we differentiate between 780-nm rPPG (*780*), 940-nm rPPG (*940*), and FIR respiratory airflow (*FIR*) signals. The frequency spectra are abbreviated according to Table 2. In time windows, we differentiate between the current window (*during*), the preceding window (*before*), and the succeeding window (*after*). Subplots A) to C) show the distribution of the peak-to-peak (P-P) distance of the FIR signal in the RR spectrum before

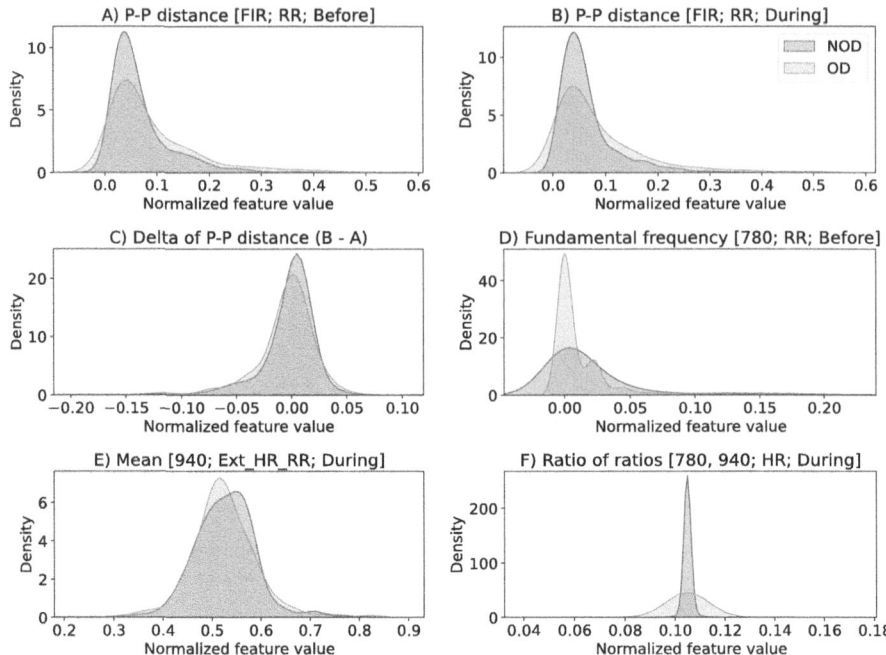

Fig. 8. Six selected features from the oxygen desaturation event classification: A) P-P distance of the FIR signal in the RR spectrum before the event; B) P-P distance of the FIR signal in the RR spectrum during the event; C) difference in P-P distance during and before the event (B - A); D) fundamental frequency of the 780-nm signal in the RR spectrum before the event; E) mean value of the 940-nm signal in the extended HR and RR spectrum during the event; and F) ratio of ratios of the 780 and 940-nm signals in the HR spectrum during the event.

and during the event, and the difference between the two time windows (the value of the preceding is subtracted from the value in the current time window). The P-P distance is a measure of the average time difference between two signal peaks (in this scenario analogous to exhalations) in a given time period. If we follow the analogy observed in Fig. 7 on the correlation between the change in respiration rate and the SpO$_2$ level, we would expect a lower respiration rate before the event and a higher respiration rate during the event. The P-P distance is inversely proportional to the respiration rate so we would expect a higher distance before the event than during the event for oxygen desaturation events. This would mean that in Subplot C) we expect a lower value for the class OD and a more dominant probability density distribution on the left-hand side of the KDE plot. Indeed, if we observe Subplot C), we confirm both of these hypotheses.

Subplot D) shows the distribution of the fundamental frequency of the 780-nm rPPG signal in the RR spectrum before the event. The fundamental frequency is defined as the lowest non-zero frequency component after noise cancellation. In the RR spectrum, this frequency should correspond with the respiration rate. Hence, we expect to confirm the observations from Subplots A) to C) regarding the relation between respiration rate

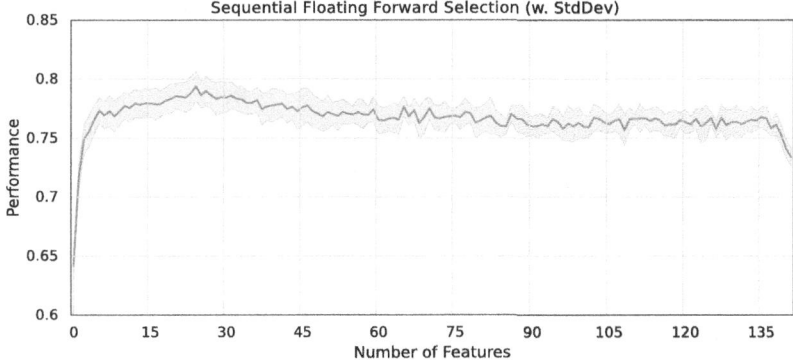

Fig. 9. Results of the SFFS for the oxygen desaturation detection. The dark blue curve indicates the mean performance (classification accuracy) for each iteration (increase in the number of features), while the light blue shows the standard deviation within the 4-fold cross-validation. (Color figure online)

and desaturation events before the event. Indeed, we see that the distribution for class OD is in a lower value range as compared to class NOD, indicating a tendency for a lower respiration rate before oxygen desaturation events.

Subplot E) shows the distribution of the mean value of the 940-nm rPPG signal in the extended HR and RR spectrum during the event. Gil et al. [15] reported that Decrease in Amplitude fluctuation of PPG (DAP) events can be accurately detected in the PPG signal and that DAP events are most prevalent in the post-apnea period with a 15% higher incidence compared to the pre-apnea period. Under the hypothesis that desaturation events often occur after an apneic event and the higher incidence of DAP events in the post-apnea period, we expect a lower mean value in the rPPG signals during desaturation events. By analyzing the KDE plots of the mean value for both NOD and OD classes, we see a very high overlap with a slight tendency for lower values for the class OD, which aligns with the previously introduced expectations.

Subplot F) shows the distribution of the ratio of ratios (RoR) of the 780 and 940-nm rPPG signals in the HR spectrum during the event. The RoR method is generally used to directly compute the SpO_2 level from two PPG signals. We expect fluctuations in the RoR value during OD events due to the change in SpO_2 value, whereas we do not expect significant fluctuations during NOD events. This hypothesis is confirmed in Subplot F) where we observe a narrow distribution for class NOD and a wide distribution for class OD.

Feature Selection. To reduce the number of features, a feature selection stage is introduced before the classification stage. The feature selection is performed with the sequential floating forward selection (SFFS) algorithm. A random forest (RF) classification model with a 4-fold cross-validation is used for evaluation. Figure 9 shows the SFFS results for the classification between OD and NOD events. The best feature subset found by SFFS has $k = 25$ features, reducing the number of features by a factor of

Table 3. Best feature subset for the classification between OD and NOD events.

Feature	Signal	Spectrum	Time window
P-P distance	FIR	RR	Before
P-P distance	FIR	RR	During
Fundamental frequency	780	RR	Before
Fundamental frequency	780	RR	After
Fundamental frequency	FIR	RR	After
RoR	780, 940	HR	During
Mean	940	Ext_RR_HR	During
Mean	FIR	Ext_RR_HR	During
Mean	940	Ext_RR_HR	Before
Mean	FIR	Ext_RR_HR	Before
Fundamental frequency	780	HR	After
Fundamental frequency	940	HR	After
Median	940	Ext_RR_HR	During
Median	FIR	Ext_RR_HR	During
Spectral slope	940	Ext_RR_HR	During
Spectral centroid	940	Ext_RR_HR	During
Spectral kurtosis	FIR	Ext_RR_HR	During
Spectral entropy	780	Ext_RR_HR	During
Spectral entropy	FIR	Ext_RR_HR	During
Total energy	780	Ext_RR_HR	During
Autocorrelation	780	Ext_RR_HR	During
Total energy	940	Ext_RR_HR	During
Spectral distance	780	RR	Before
Spectral distance	940	RR	Before
Spectral distance	FIR	RR	Before

5.7. It is observed that with an increased number of features with $25 < k < 135$ the model performance steadily decreases, while with a very large number of features with $k > 135$, the performance rapidly drops, likely due to overfitting [26]. A list of features from the selected subset is given in Table 3.

Event Detection and ODI Estimation. For the classification between OD and NOD, a fully connected feed-forward neural network (FCNN) classifier is designed. The number of input neurons is equal to the number of features in the optimal subset (25), while there is a single neuron in the output layer. The network topology and hyper-parameter optimization are performed iteratively with the $keras$ and $scikit - learn$ machine-learning libraries in Python. The best-performing network topology is shown to be a two-hidden-layer structure with 64 and 32 neurons in the first and second hidden layer respectively. The activation function in both hidden layers is the rectified linear unit ($ReLU$), while a $Sigmoid$ activation function is used for the output neuron. The optimal hyper-parameter set and the trial range for each hyper-parameter is listed in Ref. [3]. Model accuracy is assessed using leave-one-patient-out cross-validation (LOPOCV).

The detected events are used in the next step to estimate the ODI value. The ODI estimation is performed with a linear regression analysis based on forming the quotient of the number of detected desaturation events n_{desat} and the recorded sleep duration t_{rec}. The mathematical description of the regression model is given in Eq. 1. The coefficients a and b are computed in the training phase. The evaluation of the model is based on LOPOCV.

$$ODI_{Est} = a \cdot \frac{n_{desat}}{t_{rec}} + b \tag{1}$$

In a recent study [36], the ODI score is found to have a good correlation with the SAS severity stage. Therefore, the ODI score is grouped into four groups analogous to the grouping of the AHI score [4]: (1) normal ($ODI_{Est} < 5$); (2) mild ($5 \leq ODI_{Est} < 15$); (3) moderate ($15 \leq ODI_{Est} < 30$); and (4) severe ($ODI_{Est} \geq 30 \; \frac{events}{hour}$).

3.4 Oxygen Saturation Regression

To estimate the exact SpO$_2$ values from the captured facial video, especially during desaturation events, we propose a deep learning-based approach. As introduced in Sect. 3.2, all 2D modal images are registered based on the 3D information provided by the point cloud, and the ROIs are thus also tracked. For each registered and tracked NIR image sequence, as shown in Fig. 10, we extract the forehead ROI to estimate oxygen saturation values. This forehead NIR ROI sequence is firstly spatially preprocessed. Since we are more interested in the global information rather than texture information in the ROI across both channels, we apply Gaussian filtering. Specifically, a 5×5 Gaussian kernel is used to reduce noise and epidermis texture details effectively. Then, the two channels' forehead ROI are spatially averaged to obtain rPPG signals of NIR 780 nm and NIR 940 nm. For each rPPG signal $I(t)$ with n time points, we decompose this signal into a low-frequency trend component (DC) and a high-frequency pulsatile component (AC). The trend component is obtained by fitting a third-order polynomial function $T(t) = a_3t^3 + a_2t^2 + a_1t + a_0$ by minimizing the mean squared error (MSE) as shown in Eq. 2. The detrended component can be derived as $D(t) = I(t) - T(t)$.

$$(a_0, a_1, a_2, a_3) = \underset{a_0, a_1, a_2, a_3}{\mathrm{argmin}} \sum_{i=1}^{n} \left(I(t_i) - \left(a_0 + a_1 t_i + a_2 t_i^2 + a_3 t_i^3 \right) \right)^2 \tag{2}$$

Thus, we separate the two NIR rPPGs into trend parts and detrended parts and concatenate them into a new preprocessed four-row array. The array is temporally sliced into non-overlapping time windows, with each time window consisting of 15 sample points, equivalent to one second. We use these time windows as samples for the neural network input. Each point within the time window is flattened and fed into the long short-term memory (LSTM) network [17] as one time step. After the LSTM processes all the time steps within a time window, it produces a feature representation that will pass into the regressor, which consists of two fully connected layers, to obtain the SpO_2 value for this time window.

The LSTM model used in this work was pre-trained. To train this LSTM model, we recruited 23 healthy individuals. Their ages ranged from 23 to 40 years and Fitzpatrick skin types ranged from II to V [14]. All participants signed informed consent. We captured two 4-min multimodal videos of each healthy participant using our camera system. During each data collection session, participants held their breath to voluntarily produce a desaturation event. A commercial pulse oximeter PO-200 (Pulox, Cologne, Germany) was used to record the reference SpO_2 values in synchronization with the camera system. By holding the breath, the SpO_2 value dropped below 90% or even 85%. A total of 10,112 s of data were captured and the ground truth SpO_2 values ranged from 80% to 99%. More than 40% of the total time, the ground truth SpO_2 was below 95%, indicating that our data distribution includes many instances of desaturation. This 10,112 s of data mean that we can obtain 10,112 time windows for neural network input after preprocessing. We used these time windows and their corresponding SpO_2 labels for supervised learning to obtain the pre-trained model used in this work. MSE is used as loss function and *Adam* is chosen as the optimizer. To prevent overfitting, a dropout layer with a rate of 0.3 is applied to the regressor. The training hyper-parameters are determined empirically.

3.5 Patient Study

To collect data and evaluate the proposed methods, a patient study was conducted at the Center for Sleep Medicine, University Medicine Essen. The multi-modal camera system is installed in a dedicated room within the sleep laboratory. Patients undergoing a PSG are simultaneously filmed with this camera system. The measurement setup is illustrated in Ref. [3]. The sensor head is positioned perpendicularly to the pillow at a distance of 150 cm from the mattress. This placement allows for successful signal extraction while patients sleep on their backs. However, signal extraction is not possible if the patient's head is completely rotated to the side or if the patient sleeps on their stomach, resulting in "blind" measurement periods.

A total of 40 patients are recruited for the study between April 2022 and April 2023. All patients were referred to the Center for Sleep Medicine due to suspected SAS. The patients slept without any therapeutic devices, such as continuous positive airway pressure (CPAP) machines or oral appliances. The study yielded 23 successful measurements with sleeping periods recorded by the camera system. Four measurements were unsuccessful due to camera failure, and no useful image sequences could be extracted from 13 measurements. During the recorded time, the mean ODI was 35.9 (SD = 28.5) $\frac{events}{hour}$. The average age was 53.6 years (SD = 11.8 years) and 30% of patients were female. The total amount of recorded OD events is 796. The average number of events per patient was 34.6 (SD = 48.9). An additional 799 NOD events are included to form a balanced dataset. The shortest event length is 7 s, the longest is 90 s, and the mean event duration is 30 s. This study was approved by the Ethics Committee of the Faculty of Medicine, University of Duisburg-Essen (approval no. 21-10312-BO).

4 Results

The event classification yielded a mean LOPOCV accuracy of 95.4% with a perfect classification in 13 patients, eight patients with accuracies above 90.0%, and two outliers at 75.0% and 62.0%. The distribution of classification accuracy for all 23 patients is presented in the form of a boxplot in Fig. 11. An increased false positive rate of 0.54 and 0.81 is noticed in the two outliers, leading to an overestimation in OD events for these two patients.

The ODI score estimation resulted in a mean absolute error (MAE) of 2.9 $\frac{events}{hour}$ and a root mean square error (RMSE) of 4.0 $\frac{events}{hour}$, while the mean estimated ODI is 36.1 $\frac{events}{hour}$ and the mean reference ODI is 35.9 $\frac{events}{hour}$. The Pearson correlation is equal to $\rho = 0.99$. Figure 12 shows the Bland-Altman plot of the ODI estimation. The plot shows a minor negative bias of 0.22 and limits of agreement (LoA) between 7.87 and -8.30. Only two measurements lie beyond, while 21 measurements lie within the LoA. The estimation of the ODI group resulted in a correct prediction with 21 out of the 23 patients (91%). Figure 13 shows the true and predicted ODI groups for all 23 patients. Patients with IDs 11 and 20 are the only two patients whose ODI group is not predicted correctly. However, in both of these cases, the difference between the true and predicted group is off by one. For patient 20 a moderate ODI is predicted, while the reference system indicates a mild ODI. On the other hand, for patient 11 a severe ODI is predicted, while the reference system indicated a moderate ODI. In both cases, the estimation algorithm overestimated the ODI group of the patients.

For all 796 recorded oxygen desaturation events, using the method introduced in Sect. 3.4, we can estimate the exact SpO_2 values during each desaturation event. Typically, during an oxygen desaturation event, the SpO_2 level remains below the normal threshold of 95%, and fluctuations may occur during the event. Among all 796 desaturation events, the distribution of SpO_2 values recorded by PSG is shown in Fig. 14(a). Of these values, 68.14% are below the normal SpO_2 threshold (95%). With the pre-trained model, we successfully detect these low values, as demonstrated by the histogram of estimated values in Fig. 14(b), which shows a distribution similar to the PSG recordings, with 67.66% of the estimated SpO_2 values below the normal threshold.

The MAE between the estimated SpO_2 values and the ground truth values during all oxygen desaturation events is 1.79%. A patient-wise MAE distribution is shown in Fig. 11. The Bland-Altman plot in Fig. 15 illustrates the agreement between the estimated values and ground truth. There is a slight positive bias of 0.12%, and the 95% LoA range from -5.30% to 5.55%. The vast majority of scatter points lie within the 95% LoA. The points that exceed the 95% LoA typically correspond to very low ground truth SpO_2 values, likely because our training data distribution includes very few instances of such low SpO_2 values. Acquiring data with extremely low SpO_2 levels is challenging, especially with healthy participants, even when they hold their breath. Based on Fig. 16, we do a correlation analysis between our estimation and ground truth. The diagonal dashed line represents perfect agreement (where estimated SpO_2 equals ground truth SpO_2). The majority of the scatter points lie close to this line, indicating a good correlation. The overall analysis shows that the model generally estimates SpO_2 values accurately, especially for normal and mildly desaturated values.

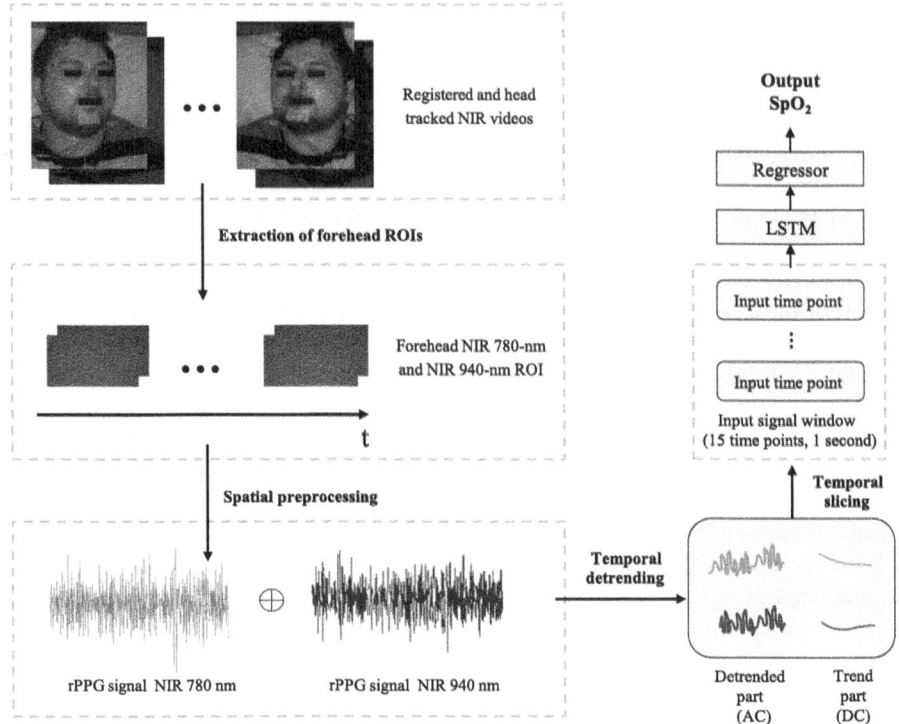

Fig. 10. Overview of the approach to estimate oxygen saturation values from captured facial video.

To more intuitively present the results of the estimated SpO_2, we selected the first 8 out of 23 patients (Par#1 to Par#8) as examples. In Fig. 17, we show the time series of the estimated SpO_2 values and the ground truth SpO_2 values for one desaturation event per patient. Additionally, the MAE and Pearson correlation coefficient (ρ) are provided. The MAE results range from 0.86% to 1.99%, while the Pearson correlation coefficient ranges from 0.50 to 0.94. Despite some fluctuations and slight deviations, the estimated SpO_2 values generally track the actual SpO_2 values well. The plots highlight the performance of our method to capture the trend of SpO_2 changes over time and demonstrate the robustness in estimating SpO_2 across different individuals and varying desaturation events, as evidenced by the consistently low MAE and good correlation.

5   Discussion

This work focuses on detecting oxygen desaturation events and distinguishing them from non-desaturation periods. Additionally, we present a method for SpO_2 regression during desaturation periods. Previous studies do not include contactless oxygen desaturation detection so there is no baseline for comparison. In a study comparing the desaturation detection accuracy of three sleep scoring tools for PSG on a sample of 100

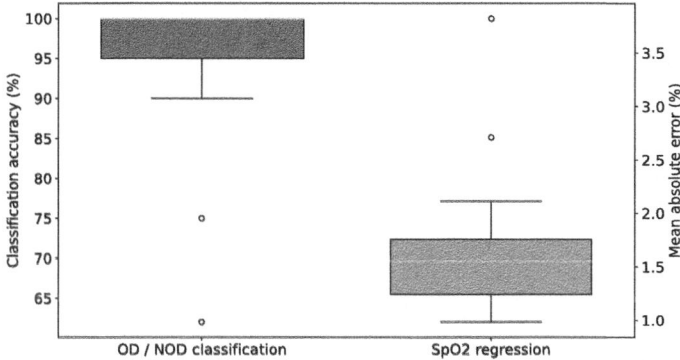

Fig. 11. Boxplot of the LOPOCV classification accuracy for oxygen desaturation event detection (blue) and MAE of patient-wise SpO$_2$ regression (orange). (Color figure online)

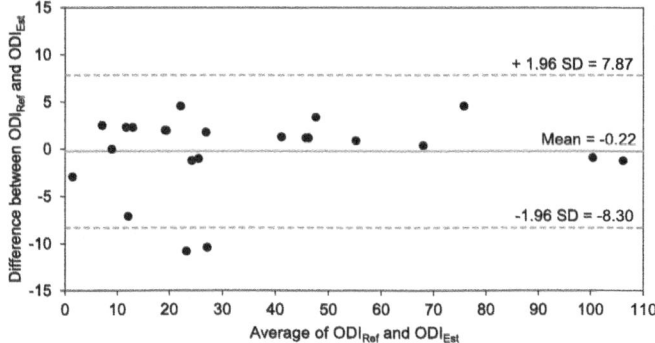

Fig. 12. Bland-Altman plot comparing the estimated and reference value of ODI$_{Est}$ and ODI$_{Ref}$ [3].

patients, the following accuracies were reported: Noxturnal (97.3%), ABOSA (97.1%), and Profusion (96.1%) [19]. The contactless approach in this paper achieved a 95.4% accuracy on a sample of 23 patients, just 1.9% below the best performer Noxturnal. This indicates that the proposed method is comparable to validated and commercially distributed systems used in sleep laboratories worldwide.

The core of the presented desaturation detection method is expert knowledge-based feature extraction. We include 30-second-long periods before and after an event in the feature analysis due to the expected physiological responses presented in the section Methods. The best feature subset from Table 3 confirms that the periods before and after the event have a valuable contribution to the classification. Therefore, it can be

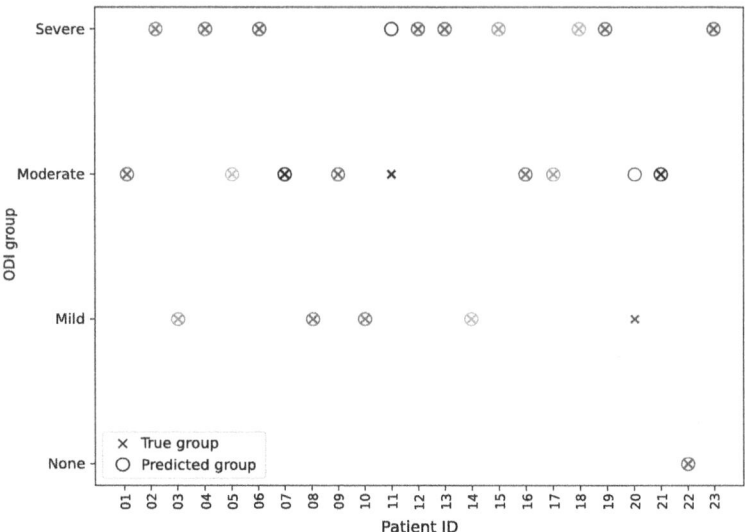

Fig. 13. Comparison of the predicted and true ODI groups [3].

concluded that the presented method can detect physiological changes occurring before, during, and after an event, and these changes significantly contribute to the detection of desaturation events. Another novelty is the selective band-pass filtering to analyze respiratory and heart rate components. We have demonstrated that both are valuable additions to the feature extraction stage.

Persistent hypoxemic SpO_2 values during sleep are linked to severe health risks, including organ damage, heart failure, tachycardia, persistent headaches, shortness of breath and neurological illnesses [7, 13]. They are also associated with cognitive deficits, memory issues, and impaired visuospatial and decision-making abilities [9, 11]. These risks highlight the need for monitoring SpO_2 and diagnosing sleep-related breathing disorders (SRBD) early. However, many SRBD remain undiagnosed due to high costs, long waiting times for sleep lab exams, and patient unawareness [12]. Alternatives to PSG could lower the prevalence of undiagnosed SRBD by reducing cost and increasing diagnostic tool availability. While the benefits of contactless diagnostics are established [2], more research and solutions are needed, presenting both challenges and opportunities for further work in this field.

From a clinical perspective, it can be suggested that the presented method is suitable for long-term use, allowing the examination of significant sleep-related parameters in sleep apnea patients. Additionally, long-term analysis of sleep quality could be a valuable tool not only for sleep disorders but also for chronic diseases, as disrupted sleep

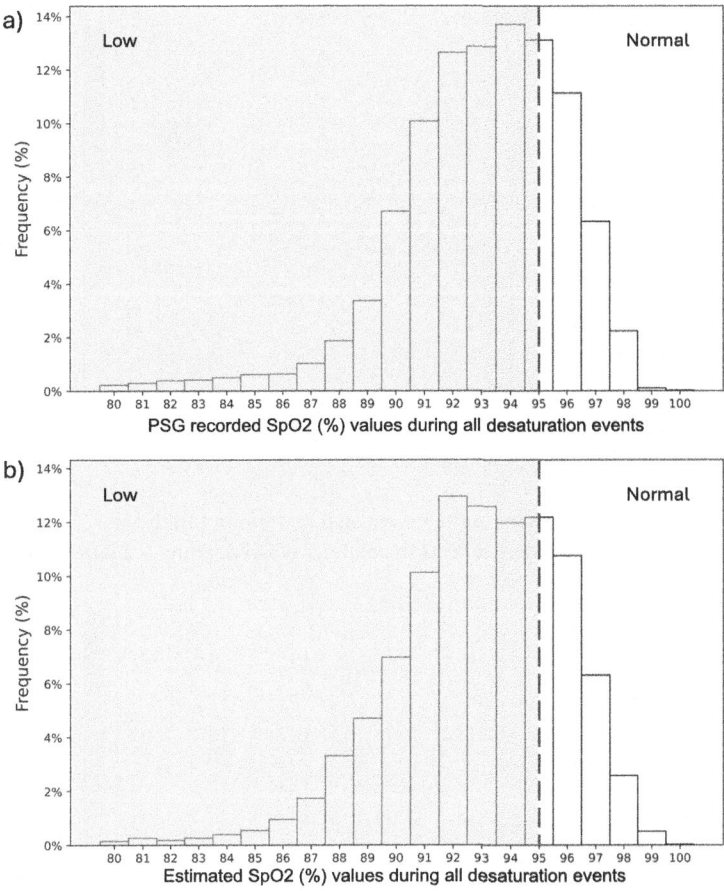

Fig. 14. Histograms of SpO$_2$ value distribution during all recorded desaturation events: a) Ground truth from PSG and b) our estimated values.

appears to be an important predictor of disease progression [23]. Moreover, this method appears to be well integrated into the clinical setting and can be considered a convenient screening method for the patient in the context of step-wise diagnostics if advancements regarding body movement tracking and secure ROI detection are pursued. Furthermore, based on the results presented here, it can be suggested that the technology presented here can be very effectively used for contactless monitoring of infectious patients or for controlling the success of therapy with antibiotic administration. Respiratory events can not only be detected with very high clinical quality but oxygen saturation can also be determined with a bias of 1.79%. Of course, these results need to be validated in a larger study and with patients having different lung diseases, but the results shown here are promising.

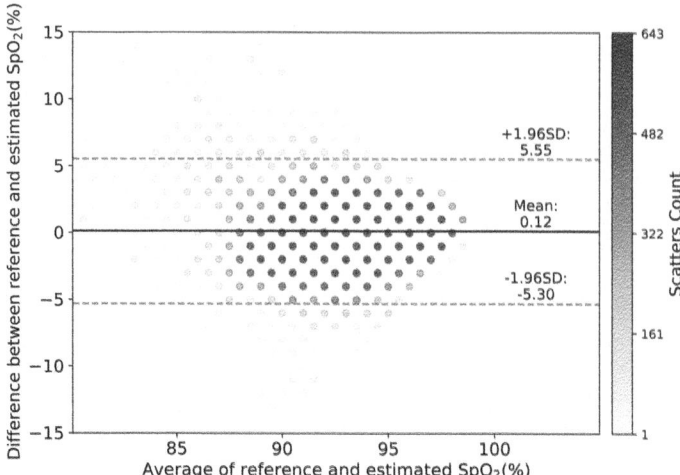

Fig. 15. Bland-Altman plot comparing the estimated and ground truth SpO_2 values. The color intensity of the solid circle markers reflects the number of overlapping scatters.

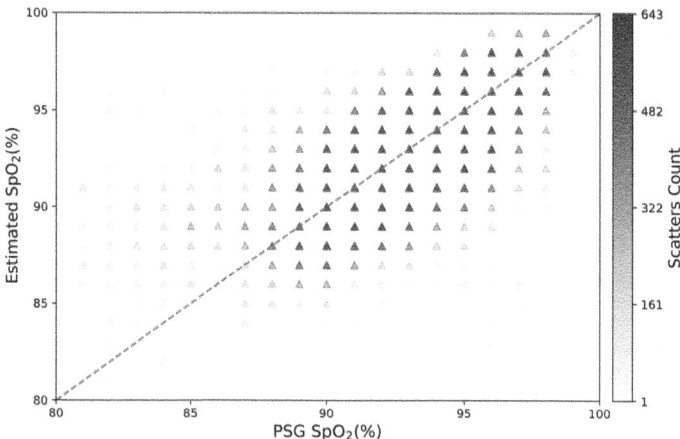

Fig. 16. Correlation plot of the estimated and ground truth SpO_2 values. The diagonal dashed line represents perfect agreement (where estimated SpO_2 equals ground truth SpO_2). The color intensity of the triangle markers reflects the number of overlapping scatters.

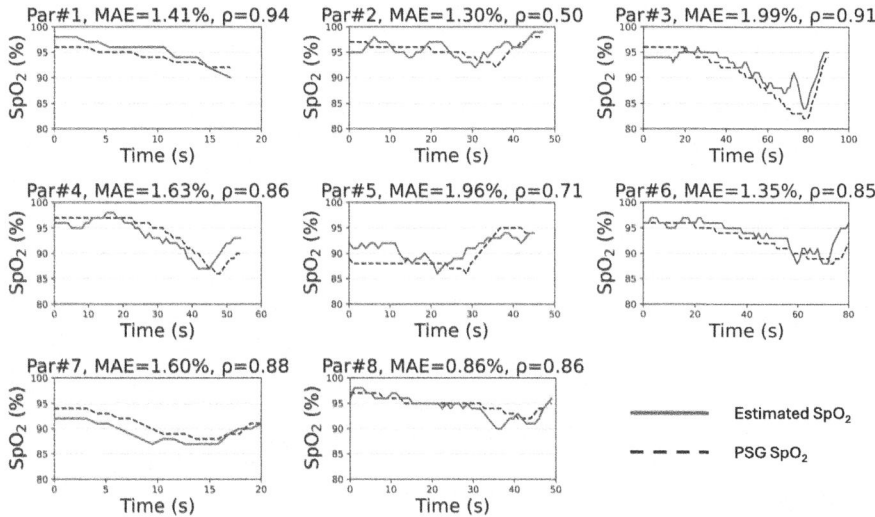

Fig. 17. Time series of estimated SpO$_2$ and ground truth of 8 patients (one desaturation event per patient).

6   Conclusion and Outlook

This work introduces an innovative approach for contactless, camera-based detection of oxygen desaturation events and the estimation of the ODI score in patients with SAS. The foundation of this approach lies in a manual feature extraction method that analyzes medically significant events in rPPG and breath temperature signals. This analysis considers not only the duration of the event but also includes 30-s periods before and after the event to capture the expected physiological responses associated with oxygen desaturation. The method is evaluated using a balanced dataset of 1595 events from a study involving 23 symptomatic SAS patients. The classification accuracy for differentiating between desaturation events and non-desaturation periods, based on the LOPOCV metric, is 95.4%, while the ODI estimation results in an MAE of 2.9 $\frac{events}{hour}$. We further introduce the regression of the exact SpO$_2$ value with a deep learning-based model pretrained on healthy test subjects and achieve an MAE of 1.79%. We have demonstrated that it is feasible to monitor oxygen desaturation in a clinical environment with a fully contactless camera-based approach.

In future work, this method will be evaluated with a larger dataset, considering the impact of various demographic parameters on classification accuracy. Additionally, the method will be enhanced to differentiate between different depths of desaturation rather than treating all levels of desaturation as a single class. Furthermore, strategies for overcoming limitations due to body position are to be addressed. Possible solutions may include a spatially distributed camera system, multiple camera systems, or adaptable ROI selection, where it would be possible to change the ROI based on the body position (e.g. visible skin on the neck or cheeks in lateral position for rPPG and side view of mouth and nostrils for the FIR signal).

Acknowledgements. This work is funded through a research grant (No.: 458611451) from the German Research Foundation (DFG).

Disclosure of Interests. The authors have no competing interests to declare that are relevant to the content of this article.

References

1. Addison, P.S., Jacquel, D., Foo, D.M.H., et al.: Video-based physiologic monitoring during an acute hypoxic challenge: heart rate, respiratory rate, and oxygen saturation. Anesth. Analg. **125**(3), 860–873 (2017). https://doi.org/10.1213/ane.0000000000001989
2. Alić, B., Zauber, T., Wiede, C., et al.: Current methods for contactless optical patient diagnosis: a systematic review. Biomed. Eng. Online **22**(1), 61 (2023). https://doi.org/10.1186/s12938-023-01125-8
3. Alić, B., Tauber, S., Viga, R., et al.: Contactless camera-based detection of oxygen desaturation events and ODI estimation during sleep in SAS patients. In: Proceedings of the 17th International Joint Conference on Biomedical Engineering Systems and Technologies - BIOSIGNALS, pp. 599–610. INSTICC, SciTePress (2024). https://doi.org/10.5220/0012349100003657
4. Alić, B., Zauber, T., Wiede, C., et al.: Contactless camera-based ahi score estimation in SAS patients. Curr. Direct. Biomed. Eng. **9**, 218–221 (2023). https://doi.org/10.1515/cdbme-2023-1055
5. Alić, B., Zauber, T., Zhang, C., et al.: Contactless optical detection of nocturnal respiratory events. In: Proceedings of the 18th International Joint Conference on Computer Vision, Imaging and Computer Graphics Theory and Applications, pp. 336–344 (2023). https://doi.org/10.5220/0011694400003417
6. Berry, R., Quan, S., Abreu, A., et al.: The AASM manual for the scoring of sleep and associated events: rules, terminology and technical specifications, version 2.6. American Academy of Sleep Medicine (2020)
7. Berry, R.B.: Chapter 22 - Sleep and obstructive lung disease. In: Fundamentals of Sleep Medicine, pp. 409–428. W.B. Saunders, Saint Louis (2012). https://doi.org/10.1016/B978-1-4377-0326-9.00022-1
8. Borer, J.: Obstructive Sleep Apnea in Adults. Karger Medical and Scientific Publishers, Basel (2011)
9. Bucks, R.S., Olaithe, M., Eastwood, P.: Neurocognitive function in obstructive sleep apnoea: a meta-review. Respirology **18**(1), 61–70 (2013). https://doi.org/10.1111/j.1440-1843.2012.02255.x
10. Charlton, P.H., et al.: Breathing rate estimation from the electrocardiogram and photoplethysmogram: a review. IEEE Rev. Biomed. Eng. **11**, 2–20 (2018). https://doi.org/10.1109/RBME.2017.2763681
11. Delazer, M., Zamarian, L., Frauscher, B., et al.: Oxygen desaturation during night sleep affects decision-making in patients with obstructive sleep apnea. J. Sleep Res. **25**(4), 395–403 (2016). https://doi.org/10.1111/jsr.12396
12. Faria, A., Allen, A.H., Fox, N., et al.: The public health burden of obstructive sleep apnea. Sleep Sci. **14**(3), 257–265 (2021)

13. Ferini-Strambi, L., Lombardi, G.E., Marelli, S., Galbiati, A.: Neurological deficits in obstructive sleep apnea. Curr. Treat. Options. Neurol. **19**(4), 1–13 (2017). https://doi.org/10.1007/s11940-017-0451-8
14. Fitzpatrick, T.B.: The validity and practicality of sun-reactive skin types I through VI. Arch. Dermatol. **124**(6), 869–871 (1988). https://doi.org/10.1001/archderm.124.6.869
15. Gil, E., María Vergara, J., Laguna, P.: Detection of decreases in the amplitude fluctuation of pulse photoplethysmography signal as indication of obstructive sleep apnea syndrome in children. Biomed. Signal Process. Control **3**(3), 267–277 (2008). https://doi.org/10.1016/j.bspc.2007.12.002
16. Guazzi, A.R., Villarroel, M., Jorge, J., et al.: Non-contact measurement of oxygen saturation with an RGB camera. Biomed. Opt. Express **6**(9), 3320 (2015). https://doi.org/10.1364/boe.6.003320
17. Hochreiter, S., Schmidhuber, J.: Long short-term memory. Neural Comput. **9**(8), 1735–1780 (1997). https://doi.org/10.1162/neco.1997.9.8.1735
18. Humphreys, K., Ward, T., Markham, C.: A CMOS camera-based pulse oximetry imaging system. In: Proceedings of IEEE Engineering in Medicine and Biology Conference. IEEE (2005). https://doi.org/10.1109/iembs.2005.1617232
19. Karhu, T., Leppänen, T., Töyräs, J., et al.: ABOSA – freely available automatic blood oxygen saturation signal analysis software: Structure and validation. Comput. Methods Programs Biomed. **226**, 107120 (2022). https://doi.org/10.1016/j.cmpb.2022.107120
20. Liao, W., Zhang, C., Sun, X., et al.: Oxygen saturation estimation from near-infrared multispectral video data using 3D convolutional residual networks. In: Proceedings of SPIE, vol. 12621 (2023). https://doi.org/10.1117/12.2673109
21. Lingqin, K., Zhao, Y., Dong, L., et al.: Non-contact detection of oxygen saturation based on visible light imaging device using ambient light. Opt. Express **21**, 17464–71 (2013). https://doi.org/10.1364/OE.21.017464
22. Mannheimer, P., Cascini, J., Fein, M., et al.: Wavelength selection for low-saturation pulse oximetry. IEEE Trans. Biomed. Eng. **44**(3), 148–158 (1997). https://doi.org/10.1109/10.554761
23. Okun, M.L.: Biological consequences of disturbed sleep: important mediators of health? Jpn. Psychol. Res. **53**(2), 163–176 (2011). https://doi.org/10.1111/j.1468-5884.2011.00463.x
24. Prahl, S.: Tabulated molar extinction coefficient for hemoglobin in water. Oregon Medical Laser Center (1998)
25. Rashid, N.H., Zaghi, S., Scapuccin, M., et al.: The value of oxygen desaturation index for diagnosing obstructive sleep apnea: a systematic review. Laryngoscope **131**(2), 440–447 (2021). https://doi.org/10.1002/lary.28663
26. Reunanen, J.: Overfitting in feature selection: pitfalls and solutions. Aalto University Publication Series Doctoral Dissertations, Helsinki (2012)
27. Rosa, A.D.F.G., Betini, R.C.: Noncontact SpO2 measurement using Eulerian video magnification. IEEE Trans. Instrum. Meas. **69**(5), 2120–2130 (2020). https://doi.org/10.1109/tim.2019.2920183
28. Rundo, J.: Obstructive sleep apnea basics. Clevel. Clin. J. Med. **86**, 2–9 (2019). https://doi.org/10.3949/ccjm.86.s1.02
29. Shao, D., Liu, C., Tsow, F., et al.: Noncontact monitoring of blood oxygen saturation using camera and dual-wavelength imaging system. IEEE Trans. Biomed. Eng. **63**(6), 1091–1098 (2016). https://doi.org/10.1109/tbme.2015.2481896
30. Shelley, K.: Photoplethysmography: beyond the calculation of arterial oxygen saturation and heart rate. Anesth. Anal. **105**, S31–6 (2008). https://doi.org/10.1213/01.ane.0000269512.82836.c9

31. Smith, M.L., Niedermaier, O.N., Hardy, S.M., et al.: Role of hypoxemia in sleep apnea-induced sympathoexcitation. J. Auton. Nerv. Syst. **56**(3), 184–190 (1996). https://doi.org/10.1016/0165-1838(95)00062-3

32. Smolley, L.: Adult Polysomnography, 2nd edn. Academic Press, Oxford (2023). https://doi.org/10.1016/B978-0-12-822963-7.00181-X

33. Toften, S., Kjellstadli, J.T., Tyvold, S.S., et al.: A pilot study of detecting individual sleep apnea events using noncontact radar technology, pulse oximetry, and machine learning. J. Sens. **2021**, 1–9 (2021). https://doi.org/10.1155/2021/2998202

34. Tran, V.P., Al-Jumaily, A.A.: A novel oxygen-hemoglobin model for non-contact sleep monitoring of oxygen saturation. IEEE Sens. J. **19**(24), 12325–12332 (2019). https://doi.org/10.1109/jsen.2019.2940228

35. Tsai, H.Y., Huang, K.C., Chang, H.C., et al.: A noncontact skin oxygen-saturation imaging system for measuring human tissue oxygen saturation. IEEE Trans. Instrum. Meas. **63**(11), 2620–2631 (2014). https://doi.org/10.1109/TIM.2014.2312512

36. Varghese, L., Rebekah, G., Priya, N., et al.: Oxygen desaturation index as alternative parameter in screening patients with severe obstructive sleep apnea. Sleep Sci. **15**, 224–228 (2022). https://doi.org/10.5935/1984-0063.20200119

37. Vogels, T., van Gastel, M., Wang, W., et al.: Fully-automatic camera-based pulse-oximetry during sleep. In: Proceedings of the IEEE Conference on Computer Vision and Pattern Recognition Workshops (2018). https://doi.org/10.1109/CVPRW.2018.00183

38. Wieler, M.E., Murphy, T.G., Blecherman, M., et al.: Infant heart-rate measurement and oxygen desaturation detection with a digital video camera using imaging photoplethysmography. J. Perinatol. **41**(7), 1725–1731 (2021). https://doi.org/10.1038/s41372-021-00967-1

39. Wieringa, F., Mastik, F., van der Steen, A.: Contactless multiple wavelength photoplethysmographic imaging: a first step toward SpO2 camera technology. Ann. Biomed. Eng. **33**, 1034–41 (2005). https://doi.org/10.1007/s10439-005-5763-2

40. Wu, H.Y., Rubinstein, M., Shih, E., et al.: Eulerian video magnification for revealing subtle changes in the world. ACM Trans. Graph. **31**(4), 8 (2012). https://doi.org/10.1145/2185520.2185561

41. Zhang, C., Gebhart, I., Kühmstedt, P., et al.: Enhanced contactless vital sign estimation from real-time multimodal 3D image data. J. Imaging **6**(11) (2020). https://doi.org/10.3390/jimaging6110123

Technical Test of a Dry Electrode Headset for EEG Measurement Under Microgravity

Judith Bütefür[1]([⊠]), Mathias Trampler[2], and Elsa Andrea Kirchner[1,2] [iD]

[1] Institute of Medical Technology Systems, University of Duisburg-Essen, Duisburg, Germany
{judith.buetefuer,elsa.kirchner}@uni-due.de
[2] Robotics Innovation Center, German Research Center for Artificial Intelligence (DFKI GmbH), Bremen, Germany
mathias.trampler@dfki.de

Abstract. In this paper we aim to test a prototype dry electrode headset during a parabolic flight in microgravity phases. We want to investigate, whether the EEG data measured with the same system during microgravity phases of a parabolic flight have the same quality as on Earth. Therefore, we conducted a study (3 operators) with an N-back task, which can be solved under both conditions. Each operator performed the experiment with the same dry electrode headset under microgravity as well as under Earth gravity to make the data comparable. The results show that it is possible to measure EEG data under microgravity with a prototype dry electrode headset. The data provide 87.5% of significant differences between workload conditions ($p < 0.02$) under microgravity and 75% of significant differences between workload conditions ($p < 0.002$) under Earth gravity, if the analysis pipeline is carried out in the same way. In conclusion, the results are promising and it is worth conducting a further study with more operators using dry electrode systems under microgravity.

Keyword: Microgravity · ZeroG · EEG frequency power · Dry Electrode headset

1 Introduction

To measure high quality EEG data without a demanding preparation time for non-experts would be very helpful in different areas. For example, to prevent permanent overload during highly demanding tasks, it would be an advantage to measure high quality EEG to detect the workload level of a person. This is important to recognize because constant stress and overwork can lead to mental disorders such as burnout [1]. Moreover, the tendency towards mental disorders increased in the past [2]. Also, safety-critical environments in particular need to be better monitored in terms of workload to protect the people who work in them. Astronauts, for example, are working in a highly safety-critical environment during their space missions. Therefore, it is important to know the workload level of each astronaut, since a higher level of workload is related to a higher risk to make mistakes [3], which can quickly end fatally under such conditions. Besides the demanding tasks and experiments an astronaut must conduct, the microgravity on

ISS and in space will likely have an impact on the overall workload, since astronauts are not used to it in general and will need time to adapt [4–6]. To determine the workload level of an astronaut, for example, the literature shows that different physiological signals could be measured and analyzed [7–10].

The following modalities are of special interest for our future research, as they can all be attached quickly:

- Electroencephalogram (EEG),
- Eye Tracking (ET),
- Electrocardiogram (ECG) and
- Respiration (RESP)

EEG and ET are very common modalities for workload estimation. ECG and RESP are very interesting for workload detection in space, as different gravity conditions have an impact to the cardiovascular system of a person as well [11]. As mentioned above ET, ECG and RESP can be attached quickly to a person.

For EEG there is still some effort needed since the preparation of EEG systems with gel electrodes can be very time consuming. Therefore, a dry electrode headset, which can be set up in a few minutes [12], could be an alternative, especially under special conditions as space missions where time and personnel is limited.

To experience microgravity on Earth and test possible systems for future applications in space, it is possible to carry out parabolic flights. For this, an airplane (A310 Zero-G) based at Mérignac International Airport in Bordeaux, France follows a given protocol (see Fig. 3). Each flight starts with a test parabola after take-off, flowed by 30 parabolas which can be used to conduct experiments. Each parabola lasts around 70s, starts with around 20-25s hyper-gravity (1.8G), followed by 21–22 s microgravity and ends up with again 20-25s hyper-gravity (1.8G). Before the next parabola starts there is a break of 90s under normal gravity (1G). After each set of 5 parabolas there is a longer break of 5 min or 8 min after 15 parabolas. [13].

The aim of this paper is to technically test a prototype dry electrode headset during a parabolic flight under microgravity phases. The goal of the technical test was to evaluate whether EEG data measured with the same system during microgravity phases have comparable quality as EEG data measured under Earth gravity and allow the analysis of human states. To test this, we conducted a study with an N-back task [14], which can be solved under both conditions. Each subject must perform the experiment with the same dry electrode headset under microgravity as well as under Earth gravity to make the data comparable. The task was not solved with the intention of being able to analyze the workload of the subject, but to be able to use comparable analysis methods and thus to be able to make a statement about the quality of the data and its potential usability for human state estimation. A pre-study, published from Bütefür et al. [15], shows the results of an EEG analysis, where EEG was measured with dry electrodes in comparison to gel electrodes – both under Earth gravity condition. This shows that EEG data recorded with dry electrodes is nearly as good as EEG data recorded with a gel electrode system to estimate workload.

2   Workload Detection Based on Electroencephalogram Under Microgravity

Since the goal of this paper was to use a paradigm that evokes a well described cognitive condition and changes in the EEG to prove the usability of dry electrodes under microgravity this section provides information from literature about the EEG recorded under Earth gravity and expected changes caused by "lower" and "higher" workload. "Lower" workload was therefore evoked by a simpler task with considerably lower demands on the working memory. In this section also literature regarding EEG measurements under microgravity will be presented.

Basically, the EEG measures brain activity with a very high time resolution by measuring the potential difference between two selected electrodes [16]. Four parameters of the EEG in the frequency domain are reported in the literature that change with different workload levels.

Klimesch et al. [17] and Andreassi et al. [18] reported a sensitivity of theta and alpha oscillations to task difficulty. Additionally, Ding et al. [19] reported a stronger alpha 1 (8–10 Hz), activity in insula but a weaker alpha 2 (10–12 Hz) activity in the anterior cingulate cortex for higher workload after source reconstruction, compared to lower workload. Ewing et al. [20] reported a change in alpha band power over parietal sites. They calculated the frequency bands for every subject individually and found a decrease in lower alpha band power (7.5–10 Hz) in the right hemisphere. For the upper alpha band power (10.5–13 Hz) they reported a decrease in power with an increase in demand.

Ewing et al. [20] as well as Bagheri et al. [21] could show an increase of theta band power (4–8 Hz) over the frontal sites during an increase of workload.

Beta band power (13–25 Hz) also increases for higher workload conditions compared to lower workload conditions. Matthews et al. [22] interprets the higher beta band power as a direct expression of attentional overload or as an indirect product of cognitive self-regulation. The higher beta frequency power was mostly found in fronto-central, temporal and occipital sites [8].

The gamma band power (25–45 Hz) was also shown to increase for higher workload conditions, compared to lower workload conditions in the same areas as beta band power [8].

There is no literature so far, which is comparing measurements of dry electrodes at parabolic flights and on Earth using the same electrodes and measuring systems during a cognitive task. But there is some literature reporting successful EEG measurements during microgravity, especially during parabolic flights. To analyse the quality of EEG studies, the resting EEG is (usually) compared.

For all studies different gel electrode systems were used [23–25]. Schneider et al. [23] investigated the influence of microgravity during closed-eye resting state to different EEG frequency bands. They could show an increase of lower beta activity (12.5–18 Hz) in-flight in frontal and medial frontal gyrus brain areas, compared to pre-flight, but no significant changes for higher beta (18–35 Hz) or both alpha activities (lower alpha: 7.5–10 Hz; higher alpha: 10–12.5 Hz). Post-flight they showed a decrease in lower beta activity in the same brain areas. Subjects from this study did not take scopolamine. [23].

Also, Cheron et al. [24] and Cebolla et al. [25] did successful EEG studies during parabolic flights and report a reduced alpha activity. Cheron et al. [24] observed this for relaxed subjects with eyes closed. Cebolla et al. [25] did a visuo-motor docking task. For both studies nothing is known about the subjects' intake of scopolamine.

Summarized we expect the following changes between different workload conditions under microgravity as well as under Earth gravity:

Table 1. Expected changes in frequency bands during different workload conditions under different gravity conditions.

Parameter	Brain area	Expected changes from lower to higher workload condition
Theta band power (4–8 Hz)	Frontal	↑
Alpha band power (8–13 Hz)	Parietal	↓
Beta band power (13–25 Hz)	Fronto-central, occipital, temporal	↑
Gamma band power (25–45 Hz)		

During parabolic flights it is common to take scopolamine, a medication to prevent motion sickness. This medication also has an influence to EEG activity. The results of the study from Reis et al. showed a significant decrease of higher alpha band activity. For theta, gamma, lower alpha and all beta frequency bands the results were not significant, which shows no influence of scopolamine to this brain activities. [26] We are aware of this influence on alpha frequency band, but it does not need to be considered in this study, as we are either comparing the data from the flight with scopolamine or the data from the lab without scopolamine within each other (Table 1).

A technical test and validation of a new prototype could also include a more general qualitative analysis of the EEG. Fiedler et al. showed that it is possible to draw conclusions about the environmental noise by means of a Power Spectral Density (PSD) analysis averaged over all channels. For this, it is necessary to measure the data with the same EEG system and experimental setup, as well as to reject strong artifacts and bad channels [27].

3 Methods

In this section the dataset in general will be presented, as well as the experimental setup and procedure. It also contains information about the data recording, pre-processing and the statistical as well as qualitative EEG analysis.

In the following, everyone who tested the headset will be mentioned as operator since the goal is to test the headset and not the person using it.

3.1 Dataset

The data were recorded in four different studies. For the pre-study (pre-study 1 & pre-study 2) the experimental setup was the same. The setup is explained in detail in Bütefür et al. [15]. For the pre-studies a dry electrode headset as well as a gel electrode cap was used.

The main study reported here consisted of two studies as well (main study 1 and main study 2). Main study 1 took place during a parabolic flight campaign organized by DLR Space Agency and Novespace. For the main studies, the setup from the pre-studies was slightly adapted to the new conditions. The experimental setup can be seen in Fig. 1A. For EEG data recording a prototype of a waveguard net with modified overall design and dry electrodes from ANT Neuro B.V. (Hengelo, Netherlands) was used. The headset and its layout can be seen in Fig. 1B and 1C.

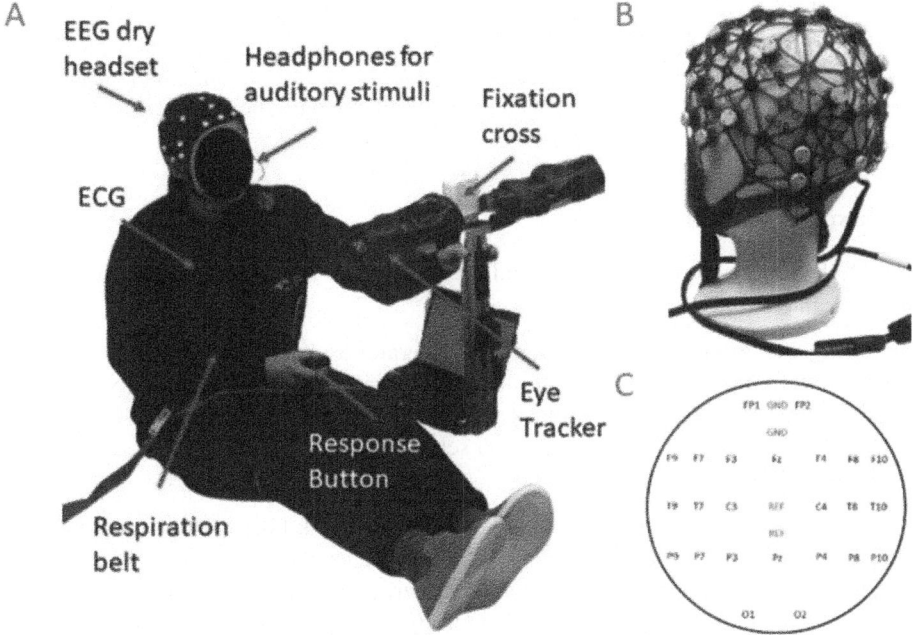

Fig. 1. A: Experimental setup; B: Dry Electrode Headset with integrated electrodes; C: Layout.

Main study 2 was performed under a control condition, i.e., recorded in our lab at the University of Duisburg-Essen. The same dry electrode headset as in main study 1 was used.

The challenges of dry electrode systems are still the signal quality and wearing comfort for the operators. Because the headset used in Bütefür et al. [15] does not fit perfectly to the operators, a further developed prototype was used for the measurements during the parabolic flight. Instead of a 3D printed corpus, a silicon net with implemented electrodes was used. The wearing comfort for all measured operators was reported to be good and none of the operators had to quit the measurement prematurely because of pain or discomfort. Due to a technical issue when saving the data stream during the parabolic flight the channels P9, P8, P10 and O1 could not be recorded.

3.2 Participants

EEG and ET data for pre-studies were measured from eight healthy operators (6 male, average age $= 29,8 \pm 6,8$). All operators gave their written consent and were told that they could stop the experiment at any time without consequences. The studies were approved by the local Ethical Committee of the University of Bremen. [15].

EEG, ECG, RESP and ET data for the main studies were measured from three healthy, native German speaking, operators (1 male, average age $= 43 \pm 12,7$, head sizes 54 – 58 cm). Main study 1 was a pure technical test of the headset; therefore, no ethic statement was needed. All operators took scopolamine (a medication to prevent motion sickness) on a voluntary basis during the parabolic flight. The control condition (main study 2) took place in Duisburg.

For the analysis, operator AE41D had to be removed, due to overlaying square wave noise in the second part of the measurement with unknown origin. The measurement also took place over two days due to technical problems with the aircraft during the first flight and was therefore not comparable.

3.3 Experimental Setting

In the following section the experimental setup of the pre-study as well as the main study will be explained.

Pre-Study. Throughout the pre-study, every operator executed four different tasks each, always in the same order. After every task the operator had to answer the NASA-TLX questionnaire [28]. Between every task and set there were short breaks between 60 s and 5 min. The difficulty increased with each set. A detailed experimental description can be found in Bütefür et al. [15].

In the following the second task, a visual N-back task [14], will be analyzed. The easiest level for the pre-study was $N = 1$, the middle level $N = 2$ and the most difficult level $N = 3$. Square figures, as shown in Fig. 2, were shown to the operators and operators were instructed to press a button if the stimulus was a target. The number of targets differ between 20 and 30 targets and the number of non-targets between 160 and 248 for every operator. This difference in total time is caused by a time limit for the task given to the operator. Within this pre-defined time operators had to process as many stimuli as possible. The presentation time for each figure was 500ms and the inter-stimulus interval 2000 ms.

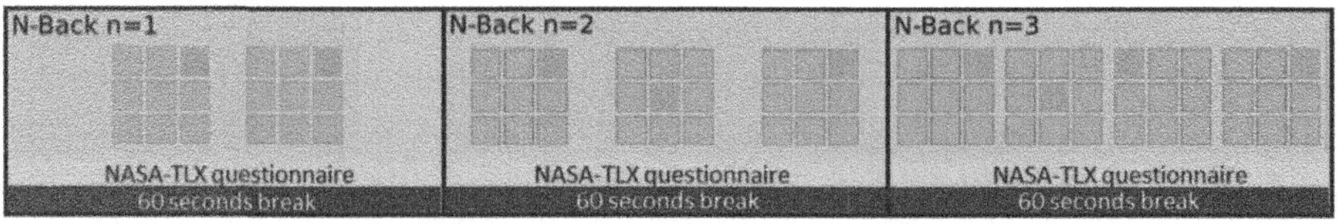

Fig. 2. Experimental design for pre-study (adapted from Bütefür et al. [15]).

Main Study. For the main study the experimental design was adapted due to the conditions inside an airplane during microgravity phases. Instead of the visual N-back task the operators had to fulfill an auditory N-back task. Therefore, the operator must listen to stimuli presented via headphones. The stimuli were the numbers 0, 3, 4, 7 and 9 spoken in German. During the first half of the study two operators performed an $N = 1$ task and the third operator performed an $N = 2$ task. During the second half the difficulty in solving the task increased. Here, every operator performed an $N = 3$ task. The relation of targets was 1:6 for 135 stimuli in total in each condition. The stimulus interval was 600ms and the inter-stimulus interval 1800ms. Each run (21–22 s microgravity during one parabola as described in Sect. 1) was followed by a break of around 90 s. Each set consisted of five runs. After each set there was a break of 5 or 8 min, where operators had to fill out the NASA-TLX questionnaire. The operators had to do 3 sets per condition which can be seen in Fig. 3.

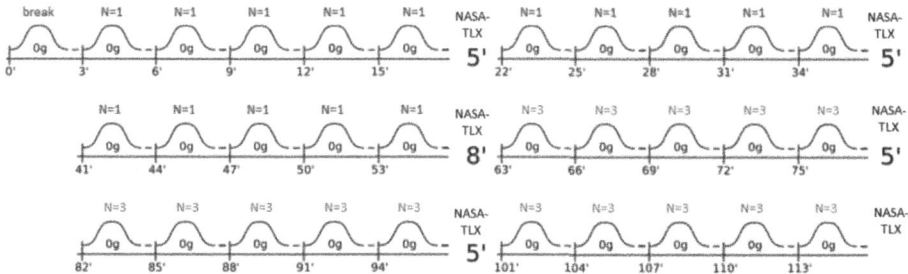

Fig. 3. Experimental design for main study (flight pattern adapted from Novespace [13]).

The procedure of the parabolic flight was copied for the control condition in the lab (main study 2). However, the breaks were shortened from 90 s to 20 s and from 5 or 8 min to 90 s.

3.4   EEG Recording and Pre-Processing

Pre-Study. For the pre-study each operator was prepared with the Pupil Core Eye Tracker from Pupil Labs (https://pupil-labs.com/products/core/) with a sampling frequency of 200 Hz @ 192x192px and an accuracy of 0.60°. Operators were also prepared with the ANT eego myLab (https://www.antneuro.com/products/eego-mylab) EEG system with a sampling rate of 500 Hz. Six operators (WK76, RR09, JR48, AA70, VA13 & BS09) were prepared with 64-channel Ag/AgCL active gel electrodes, positioned according to the 10–20 system with reference at FCz. The operator FW00 and SD50 were prepared with a 24-electrode tailor-developed headset with dry electrodes also according to the 10–20 system. For more detailed information see Bütefür et al. [15]. During the experiment, both EEG and ET were measured the entire time.

Main Study. For the main study 1 each operator was prepared with the ANT eego mini (https://www.ant-neuro.com/products/eego_24) as an EEG system. The EEG system also measured ECG and respiration with a sampling frequency of 500 Hz. ECG was measured with 3 channel lead and respiration with a respiration belt. All operators from the main study (AC07D, AE41D & BU87D) were prepared with a 24-channel dry electrode headset (see Fig. 1B), positioned according the 10–20 system with reference at Cz and CPz (see Fig. 1C). During the experiment the operator was sitting in front of the Tobii Pro Fusion Eye Tracker (https://www.tobii.com/products/eye-trackers/screen-based/tobii-pro-fusion) with a sampling frequency of 250 Hz and an accuracy of 0.3°.

For main study 2 the setup was the same as in main study 1, but ANT eego myLab (https://www.ant-neuro.com/products/eego-mylab) was used as an EEG system. Both amplifiers, ANT eego mini as well as ANT eego myLab, are technically identical except the number of channels that can be measured.

Pre-processing for all measured data was done with the MNE python-library. A bandpass filter between 0.1 and 40 Hz as well as an ICA for artifact removal was applied. For qualitative analysis the raw signal was used after removing objectively apparent artefact-ridden channels.

3.5 EEG Analysis

The detailed EEG pipeline for the pre-study analysis can be found in Bütefür et al. [15]. For the analysis of the main study the pipeline has been adapted slightly and will be presented in the following. The first step was to visually inspect the data to see whether there was suitable data over the entire microgravity phases or whether the contact of the electrodes had been lost in the meantime. Afterwards data were segmented into epochs of 5 s without any overlap and without consideration of the target- / non-target-events. Due to the different experimental conditions the segments are smaller in comparison to the pre-study [15]. This was necessary, because of higher environmental noise in the airplane and under the control condition compared to the pre-study recording (see Fig. 5). PSD in $\mu V^2/Hz$ was computed for different frequency bands using the multitaper method. The frequency bands were defined for every operator individually, as explained in detail in Bütefür et al. [15]. Basically, the peaks in fixed frequency ranges [29] were detected using the Brain Vision Analyzer 2.2 (Brain Products GmbH, Gilching, Germany).

The electrodes were chosen based on the expected changes with different levels of workload in the individual brain areas (see Sect. 2). For peak detection Fz electrode was used for theta band, Pz electrode for alpha band, as well as FCz electrode for beta and gamma band. Peak detection was done for low and high workload condition and an average of both peaks was calculated to obtain a value for defining the frequency band.

At the end the final individual frequency bands were calculated as a 2Hz band for theta and alpha with the average value as the center. For beta and gamma, a 4Hz frequency band around the average values were calculated.

After the values of all individual frequency bands were determined, the average power within these ranges was determined for each epoch individually. This was done for all electrodes listed in Table 2, considering the relevant brain areas. Due to another cap layout and other GND and REF positions the electrode selection for analyses had to be adapted. In comparison to the pre-studies [15] for calculation of theta band power Fz was used additionally, as well as Pz for alpha band calculation for the main study. This was done because of more noise during the measurements. For beta and gamma band power Fz and Cz were removed as well as O1. Cz was set to reference and could not be recalculated. Fz was removed to avoid an over representation of one brain area. O1 could not be recorded as it was one of the electrodes affected by technical problems as mentioned before (see Sect. 3.1). O2 electrode was only used for operator AC07D, as for operator BU87D the contact between the electrode and the scalp was lost.

For further analysis an outlier removal was performed, whereby the 95th percentile of data was used.

Table 2. Electrodes used for analyses in different frequency bands for the main study.

Frequency bands	Used electrodes
Theta	F3, Fz, F4
Alpha	P3, Pz, P4
Beta / Gamma	F3, F4, C3, C4, T7, T8 (O2)

Statistical Analysis. For statistical analysis the normal distribution was checked first. For this, the Kolmogorov-Smirnov test was applied. Since data were not normally distributed, the Wilcoxon signed-rank test was used to check for statistical significance. If the test shows that the data are significantly different, the absolute values for every epoch was plotted. Afterwards it was checked, if the conditions for higher or lower workload, as for example alpha power for $N = 1 > N = 3$ were fulfilled. Figure 4 shows an example.

Behavioral Analysis. A behavioral analysis was performed to find out, if the analysis brings comparable results to the behavioral data of the subject. Therefore, the precision of the subjects' responses was calculated using following equation:

$$Precision = \frac{TP}{TP + FP} \tag{1}$$

3.6 Quantitative EEG Analysis

Based on the analysis from Fiedler et al. [27] a quantitative EEG analysis was done to find differences between lab and flight conditions. To this end, the first 20 s of the first set from pre-study 1, main study 1 and main study 2 were used. The PSD analysis was done in a range of 0–60 Hz after excluding all bipolar and objectively apparent artefact-ridden channels. For visualization an average of all channels was build and the standard deviation was visualized in grey.

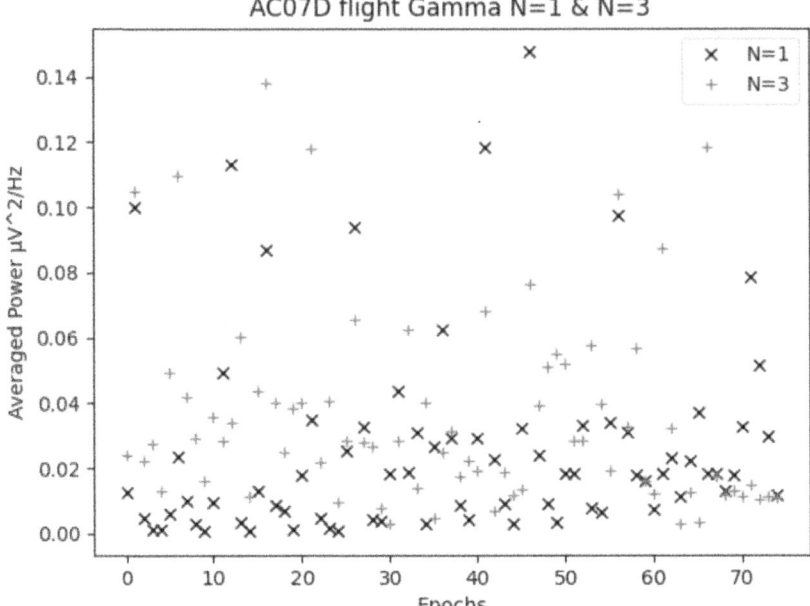

Fig. 4. Averaged PSD values for gamma band power of operator AC07D under different conditions at electrodes F3, F4, C3, C4, T7, T8, O2.

4 Results

The following section presents the results of the EEG analysis in frequency domain for the pre-study and the main study to evaluate the technical functionality of the dry electrode headset.

4.1 Results Pre-study

In the analysis, the power of the individual EEG frequency bands under different workload conditions (N = 1 and N = 3) for each operator were compared.

For theta band power the electrodes F3 and F4 were analyzed. A significant increase in theta power could be shown for four operators with gel electrodes ($p < 0.003$) and one operator with dry electrodes ($p < 0.001$). The results can be seen in Table 3.

P3, Pz and P4 were used for the analysis of alpha band power and a significant decrease in power ($p < 0.03$) could be shown for four operators. However, the four operators in which the change in the alpha band power is significant do not match the four operators that show significant changes in theta band power for different workload levels. For operators with dry electrodes, a significant decrease ($p < 0.01$) for one operator was shown. For the second operator with dry electrodes (FW00) a significant difference was shown, but alpha power was increasing from lower to higher workload condition instead of decreasing. Values where this is happening are marked with an asterisk in Table 3.

During pre-study analysis the electrodes F3, Fz, F4, C3, Cz, C4, T7, T8, O1 and O2 were used to analyze the beta and gamma band power. A significant increase in beta band power could be shown for one operator with gel electrodes ($p < 0.05$) and for one with dry electrodes ($p < 0.001$). For four of the other operators the difference in beta band power was significant under different conditions, but power decreased for higher workload condition instead of increasing. In Table 3, these values are marked with an asterisk as well.

For gamma band power a significant increase in gamma band power for three operators with gel electrodes ($p < 0.01$) and for both operators with dry electrodes ($p < 0.004$) could be shown. These results can also be seen in Table 3.

All in all, 50% of the results for gel electrodes are significant and band power is changing as expected. 37.5% of the results are not significant and 12.5% are not changing as expected. For dry electrodes 62.5% of the results are significant and band power is changing as expected. 12.5% are not significant and 12.5% are not changing as expected.

Table 3. p-values for each operator and frequency band from Wilcoxon signed-rank test 1.

Operator	θ	α	β	γ
WK76	< 0.001	< 0.001	< 0.001*	n.s
RR09	< 0.001	< 0.03	< 0.05	< 0.01
JR48	< 0.001	< 0.001	n.s	n.s
AA70	< 0.003	n.s	< 0.001*	n.s
VA13	n.s	n.s	n.s	< 0.001
BS09	n.s	< 0.001	< 0.001*	< 0.001
FW00[a]	< 0.001	< 0.001*	< 0.001*	< 0.004
SD50[a]	n.s	< 0.009	< 0.001	< 0.001

*Significantly different, but power does not change in the direction as expected.
[a]Operators measured with dry electrodes.

4.2 Results Main Study

After visual inspection of the data quality both operators (AC07D and BU87D) were analyzed.

As already mentioned in Sect. 4.1 the frequency bands under different workload and gravity conditions were compared for each operator individually. For analyses of the different conditions (flight and lab) the same electrodes were used for all frequency bands. The overall results can be seen in Table 4 and will be described in the following section.

For theta band power F3, Fz and F4 electrodes were used. During the flight a significant increase ($p < 0.02$) in theta power from lower to higher workload condition could be shown for one operator (AC07D). For the second operator the change was significant, but not as expected. For the lab condition the distribution of results was the same, but vice versa. A significant increase ($p < 0.001$) of theta band power could be shown for BU87D but for AC07D theta band decreased significantly, which was not expected.

To analyze changes in alpha band power the electrodes P3, Pz and P4 were used. Under flight condition the decrease of alpha band power was significant ($p < 0.001$) for both operators. Under lab condition the decrease of alpha band power was significant ($p < 0.001$) for AC07D. For BU87D the change was significant as well, but alpha increased from lower to higher workload condition instead of decreasing.

For beta and gamma band power F3, F4, C3, C4, T7, T8 and O2 were used. For BU87D under flight condition O2 was removed. For beta band power there was a significant increase of power for both operators under both conditions (flight: $p < 0.004$; lab: $p < 0.002$).

The increase of gamma band power under flight condition was significant ($p < 0.02$) for both operators. Under lab condition the increase of gamma band power was significant ($p < 0.001$) for both operators.

In summary, all investigated frequency bands showed significant differences between workload conditions.

All in all, for flight conditions 87.5% of the results were significant and as expected between workload conditions and 12.5% of the results were significant but the change in power was not as expected. For lab conditions 75% of the results were significant and as expected between workload conditions. 25% of the results were significant but the change in power was not as expected between workload conditions.

Table 4. p-values for each operator and frequency band in each condition from Wilcoxon signed-rank test.

Operator	Condition	θ	α	β	γ
AC07D	Flight	< 0.02	< 0.001	< 0.004	< 0.02
	Lab	< 0.001*	< 0.001	< 0.001	< 0.001
BU87D	Flight	< 0.001*	< 0.001	< 0.001	< 0.001
	Lab	< 0.001	< 0.001*	< 0.002	< 0.001

*Significantly different, but power does not change in the direction as expected.

Table 5. Behavioral analysis of both subjects.

Operator	AC07D				BU87D			
Condition	Flight		Lab		Flight		Lab	
WL level	Low	High	Low	High	Low	High	Low	High
Precision	96%	65%	100%	77%	89%	77%	100%	95%

The behavioral analysis shows a decrease of precision for higher workload level compared to lower workload level, which can be seen in Table 5. For AC07D the precision decreased from 96% for lower workload level under flight condition to 65% for higher workload level. Under lab condition the precision decreased from 100% to 77% from lower workload level to higher workload level. Subject BU87D also showed a decrease from 89% to 77% from lower to higher workload level under flight condition and from 100% to 95% under lab condition. It can also be seen that the precision under lab condition is slightly better than under flight condition. But the precision under flight condition also shows that the subjects were able to perform the task even under microgravity.

4.3   Results on EEG Signal Quality

As already described in Sect. 3.6 a PSD analysis was computed after excluding all bipolar channels. The channel O2 was excluded for operators BU87D and AC07D as it was particularly noisy. The results can be seen in Fig. 5.

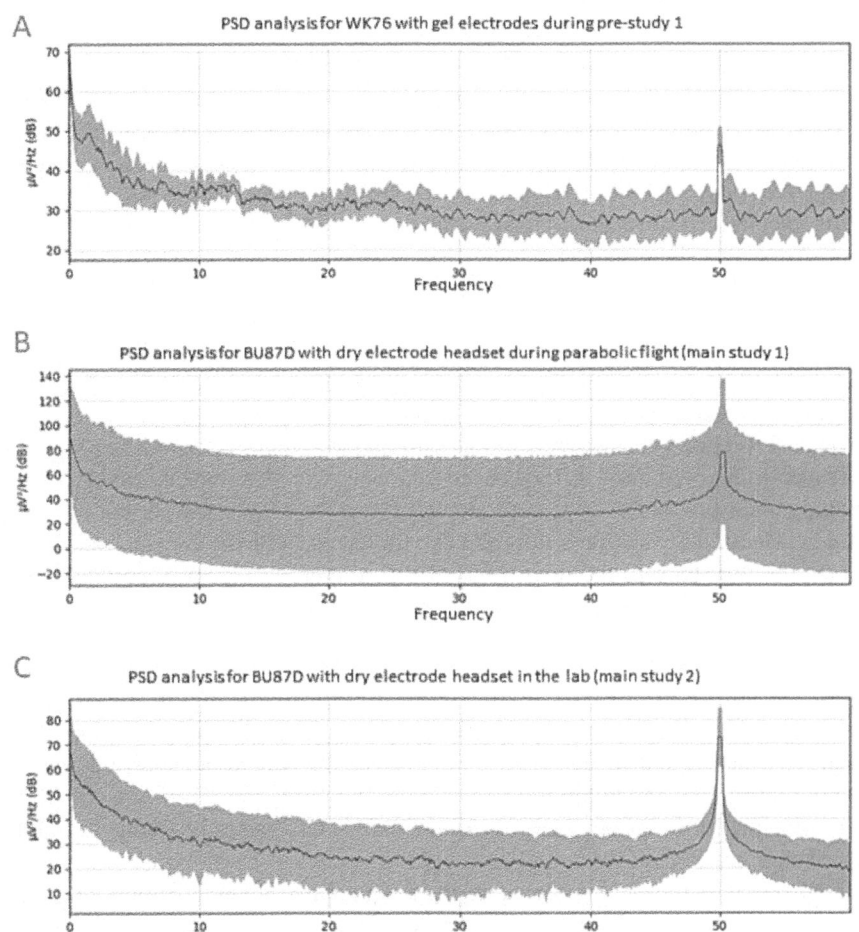

Fig. 5. A: PSD analysis for WK76 with gel electrodes during pre-study 1; B: PSD analysis for BU87D with dry electrode headset during parabolic flight (main study 1); C: PSD analysis for BU87D with dry electrode headset in the lab (main study 2).

In all subfigures of Fig. 5 the powerline interference at 50 Hz can be seen. For Fig. 5A, which shows the pre-study 1 measured with gel-electrodes, the range of standard deviation is 40 $\mu V^2/Hz$. In main study 1 measured with the prototype dry electrode headset during the parabolic flight, the range of standard deviation is 100 $\mu V^2/Hz$ (see Fig. 5B). For Fig. 5C, which shows data from main study 2 measured with the prototype of the dry electrode headset in the lab, the range of standard deviation is 60 $\mu V^2/Hz$.

5 Discussion

The main objective of this paper was, to show that it is possible to measure EEG of sufficient quality with a dry electrode headset under microgravity during a parabolic flight to even allow predictions on human states under noisy environment such as parabolic flight.

To evaluate this, we performed a pre-study as well as the main study with almost the same setup and compared the data sets. Under every setup the operators had to do an N-back task with different difficulty levels. A frequency analysis was performed to evaluate difference in the EEG signal caused by different workload levels.

In the pre-study we compared gel to dry electrodes to see, if the results of a custom-made dry electrode headset are comparable to a cap with gel electrodes. In that pre-study we found out, that the custom-made headset, which fitted one operator perfectly was not usable for more than two operators, because the data quality strongly decreased, and some operators had to quit the study because of pain. But anyway, in case that the headset did fit the operators well, the results of the dry electrodes were comparable to the results of the gel electrodes (see Table 3, as well as [15]). All in all, we could show that 50% of the results of gel electrodes were significantly changing with respect to workload in the expected direction (increase/decrease of frequency bands as reported in literature). For dry electrodes even more differences in frequency (62.5%) were significant between workload conditions and as expected. However, it must be considered that the sample size for gel electrodes was 6 operators and two for the test with the dry electrode headset.

From the pre-study to the main study the prototype was adapted so that it would fit more operators better. Instead of a 3D-printed headset, a waveguard silicon net with modified overall design and the same type of dry electrodes was used. This leads to a better fit, none of the operators had to quit the experiments due to discomfort although the head sizes differ from 54–58 cm and wearing time was up to 3 h. Based on visual inspection no loss of contact between the electrodes and the scalp was found during microgravity phases, unless for BU87D in electrode O2 where the loss of contact was before the start of the parabolic flight.

The pipeline for frequency analysis for the main study had to be changed slightly in comparison to the pre-study.

As all operators took scopolamine during the parabolic flight it is important to mention that it has no direct influence to our results, since we are just comparing data under the same condition within each other. Therefore, the influence of scopolamine to EEG Reis et al. [26] investigated, is visible in all compared data from the parabolic flight.

For the statistical analysis and the evaluation of the new prototype dry electrode headset, we tested if the frequency bands for the different difficulty conditions are significantly different within one condition (flight / lab). The results show that under flight conditions 87.5% of the results were significant and changes were as expected between the workload conditions. 12.5% of the results were significant but the change of power was not as expected. For lab conditions 75% of the results were significant and change as expected between workload conditions. 25% of the results were significant but the change in power was not as expected. The behavioral analysis that shows differences in the subjects' performance between lower and higher workload condition as expected underlines these findings. Changes in precision are supporting the differences found by EEG frequency analysis.

For the signal quality analysis of the EEG, we showed that the environmental noise in the airplane is higher than in the lab. Although this is the case, the analysis of workload effects was carried out successfully. This shows that this analysis method can also be used for noisier signal.

It can be summarized that the results provide comparable results under microgravity and Earth gravity if the analysis pipeline is carried out in the same way. It can also be summarized that it is possible to record data with this prototype dry electrode headset under microgravity and to use the recorded data to allow analysis of human states.

6 Conclusion

In this study, we investigated if it is possible to record EEG data under microgravity with a prototype of a waveguard net with modified overall design and dry electrodes from ANT Neuro B.V. (Hengelo, Netherlands). We also tested, if we can get similar results for the same measurements under Earth gravity as well as under microgravity. Our preliminary results suggest that dry electrodes can be used under microgravity and show similar sensitivity as under Earth gravity. Dry electrodes mounted in a comfortable and adjustable headset are a promising alternative to be used during space flight missions. As a next step it would be interesting to compare the data from the main study with data from the same operators, measured with gel electrodes, during the same scenario under microgravity. It would also be necessary to have a larger sample size to underline the results of our study. However, the parabolic flights do limit the number of operators. Moreover, the signal to noise ratio is still lower for data recorded with the dry electrode headset compared to data recorded with gel electrode caps. Nevertheless, it could be shown that it is possible to analyze the workload level as a human condition despite the noisier signal. These results are promising since it suggests that effects of state changes in human EEG can potentially be detected with dry electrodes even under harsh conditions such as during space flight.

Acknowledgments. We would like to express our gratitude to all the operators who participated in the studies. Also, we would like to thank the researchers from DFKI, namely Marc Tabie and Mathias Trampler, wo set up most of the experimental software and recorded the data. We would also like to thank DLR Space Agency for funding our experiments during the 42nd parabolic flight campaign in Bordeaux, France. The work was supported by the German Federal Ministry for Economic Affairs and Climate Action (BMWK) under the grant number FKZ 50RP2270A (UDE) and FKZ 50RP2270B (DFKI) in the project GraviMoKo. Experiments from pre-studies were supported by the BMWK under the grant number 16SV8023 (DFKI) in the project Kameri and 50RA1701 (DFKI) in the project TransFIT.

Disclosure of Interests. The authors declare that the research was conducted in the absence of any commercial or financial relationships that could be constructed as a potential conflict of interest.

References

1. Greif, S., Bertino, M.: Burnout: characteristics and prevention in coaching. In: Greif, S., Möller, H., Scholl, W., Passmore, J., Müller, F. (eds) International Handbook of Evidence-Based Coaching. Springer, Cham (2022). https://doi.org/10.1007/978-3-030-1938-5_9
2. World Health Organization, Mental disorders (2023). https://www.who.int/news-room/fact-sheets/detail/mental-disorders
3. Morris, C.H., Leung, Y.K.: Pilot mental workload: how well do pilots really perform? Ergonomics **49**(15), 1581–1596 (2006). https://doi.org/10.1080/00140130600857978
4. Manzey, D., Lorenz, B.: Mental performance during short-term and long-term spaceflight. Brain Res. Rev. 215–221 (1998)
5. Casler, J.G., Cook, J.R.: Cognitive performance in space and analogous environments. Int. J. Cogn. Ergon., 351–372 (1999). https://doi.org/10.1207/s15327566ijce0304_5
6. Moore, S.T., Dilda, V., Morris, T.R., Yungher, D.A., MacDougall, H.G., Wood, S.J.: Long-duration spaceflight adversely affects post-landing operator proficiency. Sci. Rep. (2019). https://doi.org/10.1038/s41598-019-39058-9
7. Fairclough, S., Mulder, L.: Psychophysiological processes of mental effort investment. In: How Motivation Affects Cardiovascular Response: Mechanisms and Applications, Washington, DC, USA, American Psychological Association, pp. 61–76 (2011)
8. Singh, G., Ponzoni Carvalho Chanel, C., Roy, R.N.: Mental workload estimation based on physiological features for pilot-UAV teaming applications. Front. Hum. Neuroscience, 22–28 (2021). https://doi.org/10.3389/fnhum.2021.692878
9. Volden, F., Alwis, E., de Viveka, Fostervold, K.-I.: Human gaze-parameters as an indicator of mental workload. In: Proceedings of the 20th Congress of the International Ergonomics Association (IEA 2018). Volume X: Auditory and Vocal Ergonomics, Visual Erfonomics, Psychophysiology in Ergonomics, Ergonomics in Advanced Imaging, pp. 209–215 (2018)
10. Ding, Y., Cao, Y., Duffy, V.G., Wang, Y., Thang, X.: Measurement and identification of mental workload during simulated computer tasks with multimodal methods and machine learning. Ergonomics **63**(7), 896–908 (2020). https://doi.org/10.1080/00140139.2020.1759699
11. Schlegel, T.T., et al.: Cardiovascular and Valsalva responses during parabolic flight. J. Appl. Physiol., 1957–1965 (1998). https://doi.org/10.1152/jappl.1998.85.5.1957
12. Trampler, M., Tabie, M., Rotonda, M., Heere, N., Kirchner, E.A.: Continuous mental state detection for mental ergonomics. In: Neuroergonomics Conference 2021 (2021)
13. Novespace, 42nd DLR parabolic flight campaign (VP179) - Practical and technical information (2011)
14. Kirchner, W.K.: Age differences in short-term retention of rapidly changing information. J. Exper. Psychol., 352–358, Band 55, Nummer 4, (1958)
15. Bütefür, J., Trampler, M., Kirchner, E.: Evaluation of gel and dry electrodes for EEG measurement to compare their suitabiloty for multimodal worklaod detection in humans. In: Proceedings of the 17th International Joint Conference on Biomedical Engineering Systems and Techologies, vol. 1, pp. 747–754 (2024). ISBN 978–989–758–688–0
16. Berger, H.: Über das elektroencephalogramm des menschen. Dtsch. Med. Wochenschr. **60**(51), 1947–1949 (1934). https://doi.org/10.1055/s-0028-1130334
17. Klimesch, W.: EEG alpha and theta oscillations reflect cognitive and memory performance: a review and analysis. Brain Res. Rev. **29**(2), 169–195 (1999)

18. Andreassi, J.L.: Psychophysiology: Human Behaviour and Physiological Responses. Lawrence Erlbaum Associates Inc. (1995)
19. Ding, H.-M., Lu, G.-Y., Lin, Y.-P., Tseng, Y.-L.: An EEG stuy of auditory working memory load and cognitive performance. In: Constantine Stephanidis (Hg.): HCI International 2016 - Posters' Extended Abstracts, pp. 181–185 (2016)
20. Ewing, K., Fairclough, S., Gilleade, K.: Evaluation of an adaptive game that uses EEG measures validated during the design process as inouts to a biocyberentic loop. Front. Hum. Neurosci., 223 (2016)
21. Bagheri, M., Power, S.D.: EEG-based detection of mental workload level and stress: the effect of variation in each state on classification of the other. J. Neural Eng. 17(5), 56015 (2020). https://doi.org/10.1088/1741-2552/abbc27
22. Matthews, G., Reinerman-Jones, L., Abich, J., Kustubayeva, A.: Metrics for individual differences in EEG response to cognitive workload: optimizing performance prediction. Pers. Individ. Differ., 22–28 (2017)
23. Schneider, S., et al.: The effect of parabolic flight on preceived physical, motivational and psychologial state in men and women: correlation with neuroendocrine stress parameters and electrocortical activity. Int. J. Biol. Stress, 336–349 (2009). https://doi.org/10.1080/102538 90802499175
24. Cheron, G., et al.: Effect of gravity on human spontaneous 10-Hz electroencephalographic oscillations during the arrest reaction. Brain Res., 104–116 (2006)
25. Cebolla, A., Petieau, M., Dan, B., Balazs, L., McIntyre, J., Cheron, G.: Cerebellar contribution to visuo-attentioanl alpha rhythm: insights from weightlessness. Sci. Rep. (2016). https://doi.org/10.1038/srep37824
26. Reis, P.M.R., Eckhardt, H., Denise, P., Bodem, F., Lochmann, M.: Localization of scopolamine induced electrocortical brain activitiy changes, in healthy humans at rest. J. Clin. Pharmacol., 619–625 (2013). https://doi.org/10.1002/jcph.83
27. Fiedler, P., et al.: Noise characteristics in spaceflight multichannel EEG. PLOS ONE (2023). https://doi.org/10.1371/journal.pone.0280822
28. Hart, S.G., Staveland, L.E.: Development of NASA-TLX (Task Load Index): results of empirical and theoretical research. In: Human Mental Workload. Advances in Psychology. 52, Amsterdam: North Holland, pp. 139–183 (1988)
29. Samima, S., Sarma, M.: EEG-based mental workload estimation. In: Annual International Conference of the IEEE Engineering in Medicine and Biology Society. IEEE Engineering in Medicine and Biology Society. Annual International Conference 2019, pp. 5605–5608 (2019). https://doi.org/10.1109/EMBC.2019.8857164
30. Nowak, K., Costa-Faidella, J., Dacewicz, A., Escera, C., Szelag, E.: Altered event-related potentials and theta oscillations index auditory working memory deficits in healthy aging. Neurobiol. Aging. Aging **108**, 1–15 (2021). https://doi.org/10.1016/j.neurobiolaging.2021.07.019

Muscle Synergy and Co-contraction Effects on Joystick Manipulation

Chuanyun Ouyang[1,2], Liming Cai[1,3(✉)], Shuhao Yan[1,2], Tianxiang Zhang[1,2], Jun Zhu[3], Li Chen[3,4], and Hui Liu[5(✉)]

[1] Suzhou Institute of Biomedical Engineering and Technology, Chinese Academy of Sciences, Suzhou 215163, Jiangsu, China
[2] School of Biomedical Engineering (Suzhou), Division of Life Sciences and Medicine, University of Science and Technology of China, Suzhou, China
[3] Academy for Engineering and Technology, Fudan University, Shanghai 200433, China
cailm@sibet.ac.cn
[4] Department of Orthopedics, Huashan Hospital, Fudan University, Shanghai, China
[5] Cognitive Systems Lab, University of Bremen, Bremen, Germany
hui.liu@uni-bremen.de

Abstract. Extracting muscle synergy from surface electromyographic (sEMG) signals has become a standard method for evaluating motor control strategies during exercise. While numerous studies have described the synergy of the upper extremity in various stretch and reach tasks, few have analyzed the relationship between task performance and muscle synergy. This study introduces an experimental device and analysis method for examining muscle coordination in joystick manipulation, specifically for pilots. In this study, eight healthy subjects performed joystick manipulation tasks involving isotonic exercises with three different load levels. EMG and acceleration data from ten muscles were recorded. The muscle synergy effect was extracted, and the correlation between muscle synergy similarity, manipulation performance, and interaction load was analyzed. The experimental data revealed that while manipulation performance varied under different loading conditions, there were no significant changes in the synergistic muscle structure. Significant correlations were found between the similarity of some synergistic muscle structures and manipulation performance. However, there was no strong correlation between individual action performance and the average similarity of their muscle synergy. The analysis indicated a fixed muscle synergy pattern during rocker manipulation, which remained independent of the rocker load level. A negative correlation was observed between muscle synergy similarity and manipulation performance, as well as between muscle co-contraction index and manipulation performance. These findings contribute to improving the ergonomics of the flight stick and suggest targeted muscle training methods to enhance the precision of flight maneuvers.

Keywords: Muscle synergy extraction · Muscle synergy similarity · Accuracy · Manipulate · Electromyography · EMG · sEMG

M. P. Guarino et al. (Eds.): BIOSTEC 2024, CCIS 2546, pp. 270–292, 2026.
https://doi.org/10.1007/978-3-031-96899-0_16

1   Introduction

Precise joystick manipulation is a critical skill for pilots, integral to both their selection and training processes [23]. This ability hinges on the coordination of the neuromusculoskeletal system, facilitated by the central nervous system (CNS), to execute fine motor movements in response to visual stimuli processed by the optic nerve [53]. The accuracy and stability required for joystick manipulation make it a fundamental aspect of flight control.

Joystick manipulation involves complex multi-joint movements, where various control strategies are employed by the human body to achieve the desired precision. These control modes can vary significantly, and consistency is often achieved through repetitive practice, as seen in professional athletes. Recent studies have focused on muscle synergy to better understand these intricate motor control patterns. Research has demonstrated that the CNS generates motor commands by combining synergistic muscle groups, which work together to perform coordinated movements [6, 7, 18]. Muscle synergy is not only essential for understanding motor control but also has practical applications in areas such as the assessment of nerve damage [48, 56], posture control [3, 46, 58], robot-assisted technology [9, 42, 49, 62], and locomotion [1, 10].

In isometric tasks, muscle synergies remain structurally stable despite variations in movement speed, although the neural commands to these synergies may change [30]. Motor control strategies can be adapted based on the accuracy requirements of specific tasks, particularly in fine motor activities where precision is crucial [21, 59]. In tasks involving isotonic contractions, the CNS can learn to adjust mechanical impedance by co-activating antagonist muscle groups, thereby refining control over muscle stiffness relative to the target size [44, 51]. This co-contraction of antagonist muscles plays a vital role in achieving precise upper limb movements [8, 22, 50].

The co-contraction index (CCI) is a key metric used to evaluate the simultaneous activation of antagonist muscle groups. CCI is crucial for maintaining joint stiffness, stability, and accuracy in fine motor tasks, thereby enhancing movement precision [50]. Beyond co-contraction, research has also explored the similarities in motor coordination across different individuals and within the same individual under varying conditions [2, 4, 20]. Studies suggest that muscle synergy patterns remain relatively consistent between elite and non-elite individuals during controlled experiments [5]. While many studies affirm the consistency of synergistic components across subjects under specific task conditions [14, 16, 28, 55, 61], the relationship between intra-subject similarity and motion accuracy under different conditions remains underexplored [10, 14]. Most studies tend to generalize findings by averaging data across trials, which can obscure detailed intra-subject variability [1, 41, 66].

This study aims to delve deeper into the relationship between muscle synergy, co-contraction, and joystick manipulation performance. By designing isotonic manipulation tasks with varying load levels, we extracted muscle synergy structures and assessed their similarities based on surface electromyography (sEMG) data. The study then analyzes how these muscle synergy structures correlate with manipulation accuracy and interaction load, providing insights into the interplay between motor control strategies and task performance. This paper is an extended version of the work initially presented at the BIOSTEC 2024 conference [10].

2   Experimental Design and Data Acquisition

2.1   Subjects and Experimental Apparatus

Eight healthy male subjects, aged 22 to 24 years, with an average height of approximately 170 cm $\pm$ 5 cm and a weight of around 68 kg $\pm$ 5 kg, participated in this study. All subjects provided informed consent and were fully briefed on the experimental procedures.

The joystick manipulation apparatus, developed by our research team, allowed for precise movements in the X and Y axes. The apparatus recorded real-time positional data using an encoder, as depicted in Fig. 1. Participants manipulated the joystick according to the upper computer interface (Fig. 2A), following a specific task completion process illustrated in Fig. 2B.

2.2   Three Tasks

Joystick manipulation requires coordinated actions involving the shoulder, elbow, wrist, and fingers. This study involved reciprocating motions under three different load conditions (Fig. 2B). Participants performed internal and external rotations while flexing and extending the elbow joint in the sagittal plane and retracting in the coronal plane. For simplicity, these movements are described as supination and pronation.

Participants underwent a brief training session before the tests began. During the experiment, they were seated upright and asked to move the joystick back and forth along the X-axis (Fig. 2A). As the joystick moved rightward along the +X axis, a blue ball on the screen would simultaneously move toward the B circle (Fig. 2B), starting from the center position.

Two black circles (diameter 2 cm) were symmetrically placed on either side of the blue ball. The joystick was set to three load levels: task 1 with a drag torque of 0.72 Nm, task 2 with 2.16 Nm, and task 3 with 6 Nm.

Participants were instructed to:

– Keep their elbows away from their thighs.
– Engage their upper limb muscles effectively.
– Make the blue ball reciprocate between the black circles.
– Focus on accuracy while gradually increasing speed.

Operating Procedures. Each participant completed 16 repetitions per set, followed by a 5-min rest before the next set. A total of 24 sets of trials were conducted, with each set comprising 16 cyclic actions.

Data Collection. Data was collected from 24 clusters of experiments across eight subjects, with each subject completing three tasks. The data includes manipulation accuracy for left and right positions and the similarity of muscle synergies.

2.3 EMG Data Acquisition

EMG signals are one of the most commonly used data for studying human activities, behaviors, and limb coordination [60,65], often used in conjunction with inertial sensors [25,26,37,38]. Manipulation performance was recorded using a self-made joystick manipulation experimental prototype with a position sampling frequency of 200 Hz.

During the subjects' performance of the movement tasks, a surface EMG system (Diese Trigno, USA DELSYS. Inc) was used to measure EMG and acceleration from 10 muscles of the upper arm (Fig. 1A). These muscles included brachioradialis (BR), the short head of biceps (BICS), long head of biceps (BICL), anterior deltoid (AD), long head of triceps (TRIL), lateral head of triceps (TRLA), pectoralis major (PM), infraspinatus (INF), teres minor (TM), and posterior deltoid (PD).

The electrode placement is depicted in Fig. 1B/C, and it adhered to the guidelines of surface EMG [27].The surface EMG was sampled at a frequency of 1249 Hz, while the acceleration was sampled at 149 Hz.

The acquired signals were recorded and imported into Matlab 2017 (The Mathworks, Natick, MA) for processing using custom routines.

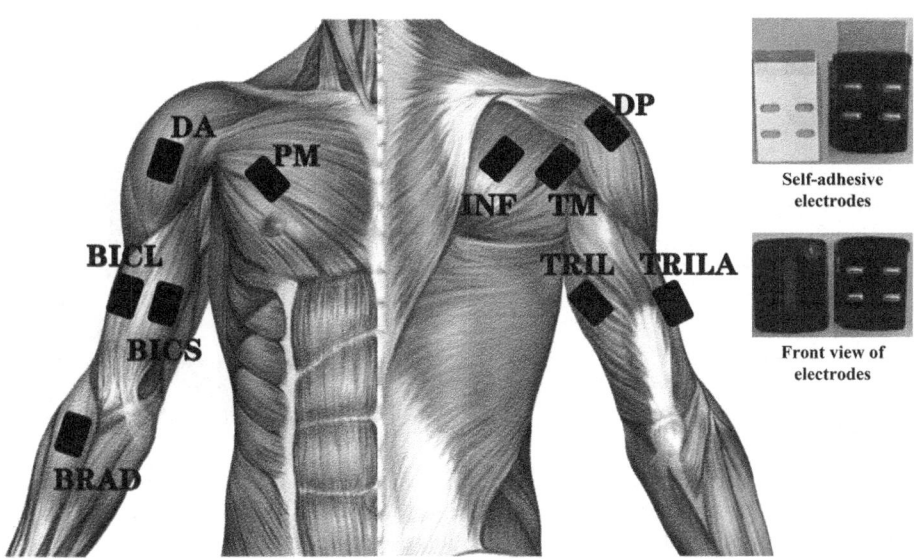

Fig. 1. Placement and sensing muscles of sEMG sensors. Top right: self-adhesive electrodes. BR: brachioradialis; BICS: the short head of biceps; BICL: the long head of biceps; PM: pectoralis major; AD: anterior deltoid; TRIP: the long head of triceps; TRLA: the lateral head of triceps; INF: infraspinatus; TM.: teres minor; PD.: posterior deltoid. (adapted from [10]).

2.4 Manipulation Performance Data

The data of manipulation was derived from the motor encoder (Fig. 2C), which was pre-processed in the following way:

a. Apply absolute value and normalization processing to the original data to determine the threshold setting.
b. Perform median filtering on the data obtained in (a) to eliminate noise (abnormal burr) interference.
c. Analyze the data, set the detection threshold, obtain the position index of data points greater than this threshold, and determine the maximum and minimum position index values to identify the start and end positions of the valid data segment.
d. Calculate and obtain the valid data from the original data based on the results of (c) and compute the mean and variance. item[e.] Quantification of Manipulation Performance:
   – **Position Deviation (P.D.):** The difference between the mean of all data and the ideal position value.
   – **Position Accuracy (P.A.):** The difference between the actual position value and the ideal position value.
   – **Position Repeatability (P.R.):** Operational repeatability, which is the variance of all actual values.
   – **Positon stability (P.E.):** Range for all manipulation data.

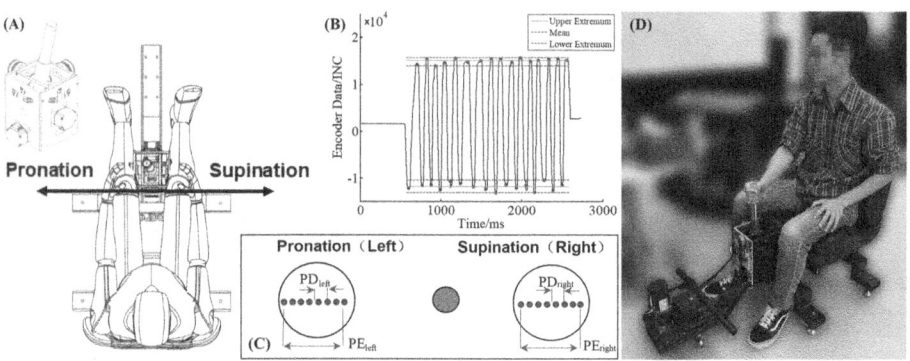

Fig. 2. Self-developed experimental device and software interface. (A) Top view of the device for experiments; (B) A screenshot of the software interface; (C) An exemplar result record. P.D.: position deviation; P.E.: extreme range of the position. (adapted from [10] and [11]).

3 Experimental Method and Result Analysis

3.1 EMG Preprocessing

The custom routines were used for the sEMG Pre-processing in Matlab. The EMG pretreatment was in the following way:

a. A mean shift was applied to eliminate baseline drifts caused by electrode shifts during the trial or by different subjects.

b. Band-pass Filtering (40–250 Hz): This step removed high-frequency noise and motion artifacts.

c. Notch Filtering: A 50 Hz and 150 Hz notch filter was used to remove fixed frequency noise.

d. Rectification: This standard method was employed to create a non-negative sEMG signal envelope

e. Low-pass Filtering (20 Hz): Applied to the rectified sEMG signals, a cutoff frequency of 0.5 Hz ensured a smooth envelope and influenced the NMF results [29,45].

f. Normalization: The signals were normalized by the maximum value recorded during the trials.

g. Segmentation: The ACC (accelerometer) signal was obtained concurrently with the EMG (electromyography) signal. However, since the sampling frequency of the ACC signal was lower than that of the EMG signal, it was necessary to interpolate the ACC signal first to match the length of the sEMG signal. After applying median filtering to the ACC signal, it was used to segment the EMG signal. For this study, data from the first 14 cycles were extracted, with each cycle including one supination and one pronation movement.

3.2 Extraction of Muscle Synergies

A Non-negative Matrix Factorization (NMF) algorithm was employed to extract muscle synergies [33]. The pre-processed signal ($V_{m \times t}$, where m represents the muscle channels and t denotes time, was decomposed into two matrices: $W_{m \times n}$ and $H_{n \times t}$. Here, n is the number of extracted muscle synergies, W is the basis matrix representing muscle activation patterns, and H is the matrix of activation coefficients for the muscle activations across m channels.

$$
\begin{aligned}
V_{m \times t} &\approx W_{m \times n} \times H_{n \times t} \\
&= W_1 \times H_1 + W_2 \times H_2 + \cdots + W_n \times H_n
\end{aligned}
\tag{1}
$$

Each vector W_i from the Muscle Synergy Matrix defines a pattern of muscle activity determined by muscle synergy. The elements of W_i range between 0 and 1 [12]. The activation coefficient matrix H_i functionally activates the muscle synergies composed by these vectors [34]. The activation coefficient represents the neural command from the CNS and determines the relative contribution to establishing the muscle synergy matrix [11,58].

The number of muscle synergies n ranged from 1 to 10. The reconstructed matrix $V'_{m \times t}$ is expressed in Eq. (2). Then, the minimum number of synergies required to adequately reconstruct the pre-processed signals $V_{m \times t}$ across all trials was selected. This was determined based on the criterion that the Variability Accounted For (VAF), shown in formula (3), exceeds 90% for each muscle data vector [56].

$$
\begin{aligned}
V'_{m \times t} &= W_{m \times n} \times H_{n \times t} \\
VAF &= 1 - \left(V_{m \times t} - V'_{m \times t} \right)^2 / V^2_{m \times t}
\end{aligned}
\tag{2}
$$

3.3   Clustering Muscle Synergies

To understand the differences in muscle-synergy vectors between subject groups, we used k-means clustering to identify representative synergy vectors for each group. This process was executed using the kmeans function in MATLAB's Statistics Toolbox, with the squared-Euclidean distance as the metric. Initial cluster centroid positions were selected uniformly at random from the vectors to be clustered. The clustering procedure was repeated 2000 times with different initial centroid positions, and the iteration with the smallest sum of point-to-centroid distances was chosen [13].

To determine the number of synergy clusters in each subject group, we computed the gap statistic. This statistic measures the compactness of the clustering compared to reference data sets that lack obvious clustering. We created reference data sets (N = 1000) by uniformly sampling within the bounds of the original muscle-synergy set. Each reference data set was clustered using k-means with 100 replicates, evaluating cluster numbers ranging from 4 to 10. The optimal number of clusters was identified as the smallest number, k, for which:

$$\text{Gap}(k) \geq \text{Gap}(k+1) - \text{sd}(k+1), \tag{3}$$

where Gap(k) is the gap statistic for k clusters, and sd(k) is the standard deviation of the clustering compactness in the reference data sets.

3.4   Calculating Co-contraction Index

To assess the level of muscle activation between different muscle pairs, we analyzed specific channels of electromyogram (EMG) data using the co-systolic index (CCI) [35,50]. The calculation of CCI involves comparing the activation levels of muscle channels within a defined time window, and the cosystolic index in this paper is calculated according to the following formula:

$$\text{CCI} = \frac{2 \times \sum \min(|M1(t)|, |M2(t)|)}{\sum |M1(t)| + \sum |M2(t)|} \tag{4}$$

In this formula, $|M1(t)|$ is the absolute activation value of the first muscle channel at time point t. $|M2(t)|$ is the absolute activation value of the second muscle channel at point in time t. $\sum \min(|M1(t)|, |M2(t)|)$ is the sum of the minimum values of the first and second muscle channel activations at all time points. $\sum |M1(t)| + \sum |M2(t)|$ is the sum of the activation values of the two channels at all points in time.

3.5   Quantitative Similarity of Muscle Synergies

To determine the similarity of synergies among tasks between clusters, we utilized the intraclass correlation coefficient (ICC) analysis [14,16,39,55,61]. Each subject performed 14 round trips for a single task. Initially, individual synergies from a single subject were grouped into one cluster. The similarity of the synergies within this cluster was then assessed using the R_{icc-wi} as indicated in formula (5), where w_i represents the synergy matrices and is defined as $[w_1, w_2, w_i, ..w_n]$. In formula (5), m denotes the number of round trips, which was 14, and i varies from 1 to n.

$$R_{icc-wi} = ICC(W_{i1}, W_{i2}, , , , , , W_{im}) \tag{5}$$

In the single cluster, r (Pearson's correlation coefficients) assessed the similarity between two muscle synergy matrices. Assume the number of trials was S for each subject. For Subject 1, the correlation coefficients were expressed as $R_{i-wi} = [r_1, r_2, ...r_{i-1}, r_{i+1}, ...r_S]$, where r_i represents the similarity of w_i from the data of the i-th trial to the other trials. The dispersion of all the averaged R_i values was then analyzed using the quartile method [56]. After filtering the data, the R_{task} muscle synergies for each subject were averaged.

$$R_{i-wi} = \frac{1}{S-1} \sum_{i=1}^{S} (r_1 \ldots + r_{i-1} + r_{i+1} + r_s)$$
$$\tag{6}$$
$$R_{task-wi} = \frac{1}{S} \sum_{i=1}^{S} (R_{1-wi} + R_{2-wi} \ldots + R_{S-wi})$$

3.6 Statistics Methods

This study's descriptive statistics included the mean and standard deviation of the experimental data. One-way ANOVA was used to evaluate the differences in R_{icc-wi}/R_i both between and within clusters, across different loadings and subjects. In this study, three different levels of significance were used, namely $p < 0.1$, $p < 0.05$ and $p < 0.01$, to determine the significance of the coefficients.

4 Results

4.1 Muscle Synergy Analysis

Muscle synergies extracted from three tasks of 8 healthy subjects are shown in Fig. 3. Four muscle synergies were recruited in these tasks. W_1 mainly reflected the activation of BR, INF, and AD; W_2 contained the activation of AD, TRIL, TRLA, and TRIL; W_3 was mainly BICL and BICS; W_4 was composed of PD, TM, INF, TRIL, TRLA, BR. When the load increased, the effect of INF decreased, and the effect of DA increased in the synergy (W_1). Notably, as a small muscle group, BR's contribution diminished in all four synergy patterns as the load increased.

Within the cluster, a pronounced structure was observed among the eight subjects. The average of R_{icc-wi} across all tasks and subjects was 0.87 ± 0.05 ($R_{icc-w2} = 0.97 \pm 0.02$, $R_{icc-w3} = 0.89 \pm 0.09$, $R_{icc-w4} = 0.96 \pm 0.03$), as shown in Fig. 4. A one-way analysis was conducted to evaluate the subjects and tasks for R_{icc-w1}. There was a significant difference in R_{icc-w2} among different subjects ($F = 3.674, p = 0.015$), and no statistical difference was found in the level of R_{icc-w1}, which is affected by different tasks. The Table 1 presents all the ICC results of muscle synergies in all trials.

In the cluster, One-way analysis was used to assess R_{icc-w1} of the subjects and tasks of. There was a significant difference in R_{icc-w1} among different subjects: R_{icc-w1} $(F = 10.754, p = 0)$; R_{icc-w2} $(F = 16.675, p = 0)$; R_{icc-w3} $(F = 43.418, p = 0)$; R_{icc-w4} $(F = 25, p = 0)$, and statistical differences in the level of R_{icc-w1} $(F = 5.903, p = 0.003)$ affected by task.

4.2   Manipulation Accuracy Analysis

During pronation, six subjects exhibited smaller manipulation errors in task 2 compared to the other two tasks. Furthermore, seven subjects had smaller manipulation errors in task 2 than in task 1, and the same seven subjects had smaller errors in task 2 than in task 3, as shown in Fig. 5A. Regarding supination, as depicted in Fig. 5B, five subjects experienced smaller manipulation errors in task 2 than in the other two tasks, and five subjects had greater errors in task 1 compared to the other tasks.

The average similarity ri of a single trial in the whole process was calculated. Meanwhile, the ri with low similarity was proposed using the four-class classification method. According to this method, the experimental results left by each subject are shown in Fig. 5 and Fig. 6; during pronation, there are seven subjects whose manipulation error of task 2 was smaller than the other two tasks. During supination, the manipulation error of task 2 with six subjects was smaller than that of the other two tasks. The number of subjects with this characteristic was higher than before the treatment.

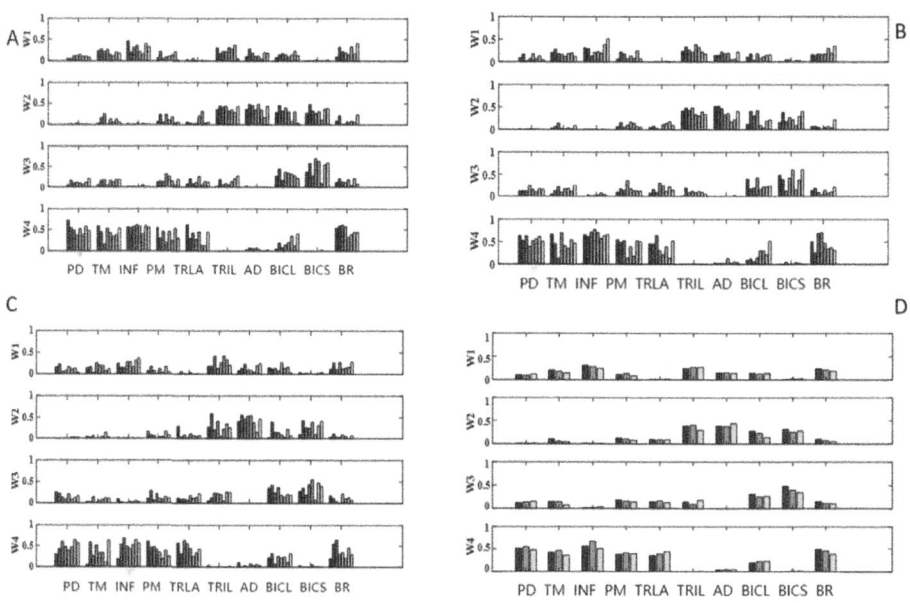

Fig. 3. Muscle synergies extracted from 8 subjects **(A)**, **(B)**, **(C)** Y-axis is the muscle synergies under the different task **(D)** the mean muscle synergies from all subjects, The horizontal axis is all corresponding to the selected ten muscles. (adapted from [10] and [11]).

One-way analysis was used in the cluster to assess manipulation accuracy P.A.-L, P.A.-R. There was a significant difference in P.A.-L among different subjects ($F = 3.374, p = 0.002$), and different loads ($F = 5.143, p = 0.006$).

4.3   Analysis of Correlation

Between the cluster, View Table 3, as shown in Fig. 8 The correlation between P.D.-L and load is -0.29 ($p = 0.168$), the r between P.D.-R and load is $-0.41*$($p = 0.05$), the r between P.R.-L and load is -0.3 ($p = 0.15$), the r between P.D.-R and load is -0.24 ($p = 0.261$), and r between P.E.-L and load is -0.32 ($p = 0.12$). The load correlation between the P.E.-R load correlation is -0.27 ($p = 0.2$).

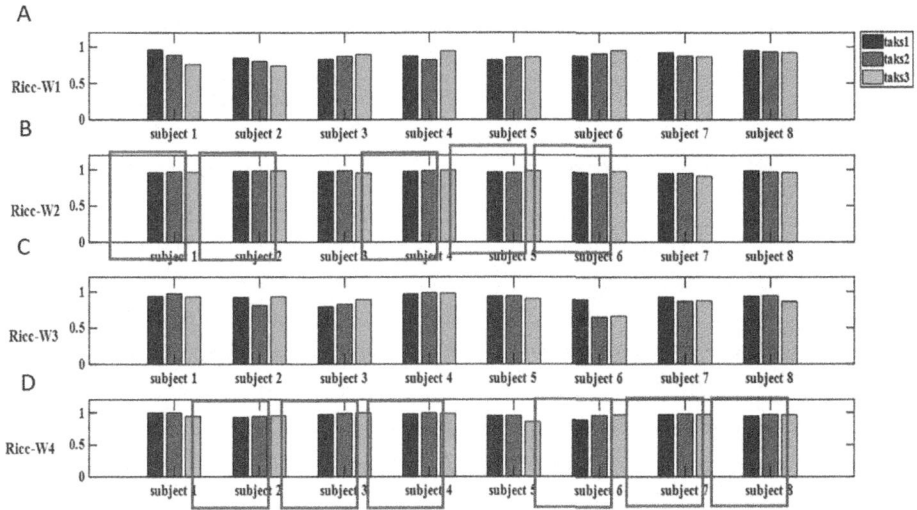

Fig. 4. Intragroup correlation coefficients of muscle synergy in three tasks, **(A)** W_1, **(B)**W_2, **(C)**W_3, **(D)**W_4. The horizontal axis represents eight subjects; The vertical axis represents the intra-group correlation coefficient of muscle synergy in the three tasks of the subjects. (adapted from [10]).

In the cluster, the relationship between the performance of a single manipulation and ri (the similarity of the muscle synergy from the single manipulation) was shown in Table 4. Among the 96 groups of correlation indicators, 18 were significant, W_4 was significant six times, W_3 and W_2 appeared four times each, and W_1 appeared three times ($p < 0.1$).

5   Discussion

In this study, when a subject manipulated a rocker with their upper limb, muscle activity from 10 channels was measured using EMG. Muscle synergy was subsequently

Table 1. ICC of muscle synergies and results of manipulation for all trials. (adapted from [10]).

	w_1	w_2	w_3	w_4	P.D.-L	P.D.-R	Task	P.R.-L	P.R.-R	P.E.-L	P.E.-R
Subject1	0.96	0.96	0.94	0.99	4.02	0.74	1	5.85	2.25	20.74	6.98
Subject1	0.89	0.97	0.98	0.99	1.02	0.32	2	3.47	3.65	15.31	11.4
Subject1	0.76	0.97	0.93	0.94	0.57	0.71	3	2.88	2.53	9.9	8.91
Subject2	0.85	0.98	0.92	0.93	4.06	1.57	1	4.02	5.35	14.12	20.76
Subject2	0.8	0.98	0.81	0.94	2.34	0.02	2	3.57	2.58	14.53	8.6
Subject2	0.74	0.99	0.93	0.95	1.76	0.29	3	3.74	3.81	14.12	14.54
Subject3	0.83	0.97	0.8	0.97	0.24	3.17	1	3.85	7.16	14.1	27.19
Subject3	0.87	0.99	0.83	0.99	0.63	0.94	2	4.44	2.77	15.19	9.74
Subject3	0.89	0.96	0.89	0.99	0.78	0.61	3	3.46	3.56	11.63	11.92
Subject4	0.87	0.97	0.97	0.98	1.49	0.77	1	4.33	4.41	17.09	15.7
Subject4	0.82	0.99	0.98	0.99	2.22	1.49	2	3.25	2.99	11.08	9.62
Subject4	0.94	0.99	0.98	0.98	2.39	1.4	3	4.15	4.07	15.43	16.31
Subject5	0.82	0.97	0.94	0.95	4.61	3.63	1	7.58	9.15	27.05	34.2
Subject5	0.85	0.96	0.94	0.96	0.78	0.67	2	3.65	6.31	13.42	27.54
Subject5	0.86	0.99	0.9	0.86	1.07	0.86	3	6.51	6.7	26.28	20.69
Subject6	0.87	0.96	0.89	0.89	1.36	0.59	1	5.63	3.71	25.03	10.41
Subject6	0.91	0.94	0.65	0.96	0.59	0.81	2	2.86	4.52	9.84	12.96
Subject6	0.95	0.97	0.67	0.96	1.56	0.64	3	3.71	5.07	14.16	18.29
Subject7	0.92	0.95	0.93	0.97	0.93	1.37	1	5.02	7.42	18.8	32.69
Subject7	0.87	0.95	0.86	0.98	1.28	0.99	2	4.02	3.51	17.04	13.3
Subject7	0.86	0.91	0.88	0.97	2.65	0.22	3	5.7	5.72	17.55	20.7
Subject8	0.95	0.98	0.94	0.94	2.86	0.48	1	4.25	3.06	14.13	12.46
Subject8	0.93	0.97	0.94	0.97	1.06	0.39	2	3.03	2.78	10.63	11.48
Subject8	0.92	0.96	0.86	0.96	2.14	1.01	3	3.39	2.62	11.97	9.05

extracted from the data. The results indicated that approximately four distinct synergistic effects were extracted from separate EMG datasets, meeting the 90% VAF criterion. Under various load conditions, the similarity between the manipulation performance and muscle synergy for each action was analyzed. This research clarified the relationship between manipulation performance and muscle synergy from the perspective of manipulation performance.

5.1   The Load and the Structure of Muscle Synergy

In this study, we found that changes in loading did not lead to differences in muscle synergy; rather, muscle synergy was remarkably consistent across subjects. This aligns with previous research indicating that changes in loading have limited effects on synergistic structures [43]. Providing the arm with a certain amount of assistance or resistance did not alter the composition of the muscle synergy utilized by the subjects during stretching. Instead, it changed the magnitude of the activation spectrum of the muscle synergy [15]. Previous studies have shown that 3 to 5 muscles collaborate in generating three-dimensional force in the upper extremity [47]. The four muscle synergies identified in our study warrant further analysis. The extracted muscle synergy is influenced by biomechanics and task constraints [57]. For instance, during pronation, the muscle weights of PD, PM, BICL, and BICS in the W_2 synergistic effect are more prominent, indicating coordinated action of these muscles in pronation. In supination, the muscle weights of PD, TM, INF, TRLA, and TRIL, forming the synergistic effects of W_4, are more substantial. We also observed that smaller muscle groups, like BR, had lower weights in all four synergistic modes under increased load.

In our study, muscle synergy similarity (R_{icc-w2}) per cluster was not significantly correlated with load ($r = 0 \sim 0.17$), which is also consistent with previous studies. For

Table 2. Co-contraction index and results of manipulation for all trials. (adapted from [10]).

	CCI1	CCI2	CCI3	P.M.-L	P.M.-R	Task	P.R.-L	P.R.-R	P.E.-L	P.E.-R
Subject1	0.83	0.82	0.87	4.02	0.74	1	5.85	2.25	20.74	6.98
Subject1	0.84	0.82	0.85	1.02	0.32	2	3.47	3.65	15.31	11.4
Subject1	0.94	0.94	0.88	0.57	0.71	3	2.88	2.53	9.9	8.91
Subject2	0.95	0.9	0.91	4.06	1.57	1	4.02	5.35	14.12	20.76
Subject2	0.91	0.94	0.92	2.34	0.02	2	3.57	2.58	14.53	8.6
Subject2	0.93	0.86	0.92	1.76	0.29	3	3.74	3.81	14.12	14.54
Subject3	0.74	0.75	0.84	0.24	3.17	1	3.85	7.16	14.1	27.19
Subject3	0.93	0.95	0.84	0.63	0.94	2	4.44	2.77	15.19	9.74
Subject3	0.95	0.91	0.96	0.78	0.61	3	3.46	3.56	11.63	11.92
Subject4	0.74	0.89	0.83	1.49	0.77	1	4.33	4.41	17.09	15.7
Subject4	0.84	0.82	0.82	2.22	1.49	2	3.25	2.99	11.08	9.62
Subject4	0.91	0.87	0.87	2.39	1.4	3	4.15	4.07	15.43	16.31
Subject5	0.76	0.84	0.79	4.61	3.63	1	7.58	9.15	27.05	34.2
Subject5	0.89	0.97	0.88	0.78	0.67	2	3.65	6.31	13.42	27.54
Subject5	0.87	0.87	0.84	1.07	0.86	3	6.51	6.7	26.28	20.69
Subject6	0.94	0.85	0.92	1.36	0.59	1	5.63	3.71	25.03	10.41
Subject6	0.91	0.96	0.92	0.59	0.81	2	2.86	4.52	9.84	12.96
Subject6	0.89	0.86	0.85	1.56	0.64	3	3.71	5.07	14.16	18.29
Subject7	0.91	0.88	0.92	0.93	1.37	1	5.02	7.42	18.8	32.69
Subject7	0.89	0.95	0.88	1.28	0.99	2	4.02	3.51	17.04	13.3
Subject7	0.90	0.85	0.86	2.65	0.22	3	5.7	5.72	17.55	20.7
Subject8	0.80	0.82	0.85	2.86	0.48	1	4.25	3.06	14.13	12.46
Subject8	0.94	0.84	0.92	1.06	0.39	2	3.03	2.78	10.63	11.48
Subject8	0.82	0.85	0.81	2.14	1.01	3	3.39	2.62	11.97	9.05

instance, a study on three-digit force generation reported that EMG coherence was not significantly affected by force levels, suggesting that the distribution of neural drive to multiple hand muscles is independent of force [52]. However, we found that manipulation performance does have a certain correlation with load ($r = -0.41$, $p < 0.05$). Numerous studies have investigated how the motor system modulates limb stiffness to achieve accurate movements in the presence of unstable force loads [8, 24].

Table 3. Pearson correlation of ICC and results of manipulation. (adapted from [10]).

	W_1	W_2	W_3	W_4	P.D.-L	P.D.-R	Task	P.R.-L	P.R.-R	P.E.-L	P.E.-R
W_1	1	-0.22	-0.14	0.23	0.08	-0.14	-0.13	0.04	-0.12	0.02	-0.09
W_2		1	0.28	-0.18	0.06	0.13	0	-0.11	-0.18	-0.02	-0.17
W_3			1	0.08	0.29	0.03	-0.17	0.21	-0.05	0.2	0.04
W_4				1	-0.04	0.05	-0.02	-0.37	-0.24	-.48*	-0.13
P.D.-L					1	0.26	-0.29	.501*	0.1	0.36	0.1
P.D.-R						1	-.41*	0.37	0.65**	0.3	0.63**
Task							1	-0.3	-0.24	-0.32	-0.27
P.R.-L								1	0.55**	0.94**	0.46*
P.R.-R									1	0.50*	0.97**
P.E.-L										1	0.39
P.E.-R											1

5.2   Manipulation Performance and the Co-contraction Index

To accomplish motor tasks, individuals use different muscle compensation strategies to achieve the same movement outcomes [10, 32]. In this study, we analyzed the co-contraction index (CCI) across three types of isometric tasks as shown in Table 2, selecting three pairs of muscles: the posterior deltoid (PD) and anterior deltoid (AD), the infraspinatus (INF) and pectoralis major (PM), and the long head of the triceps brachii (TRIL) and lateral head of the triceps brachii (TRLA) [19]. We conducted regression analyses on performance error (P.E.) and performance accuracy (P.R.) with CCI and, through Levenberg-Marquardt iterations as shown in Fig. 7, found a negative correlation between the co-contraction index and performance error across the three tasks.

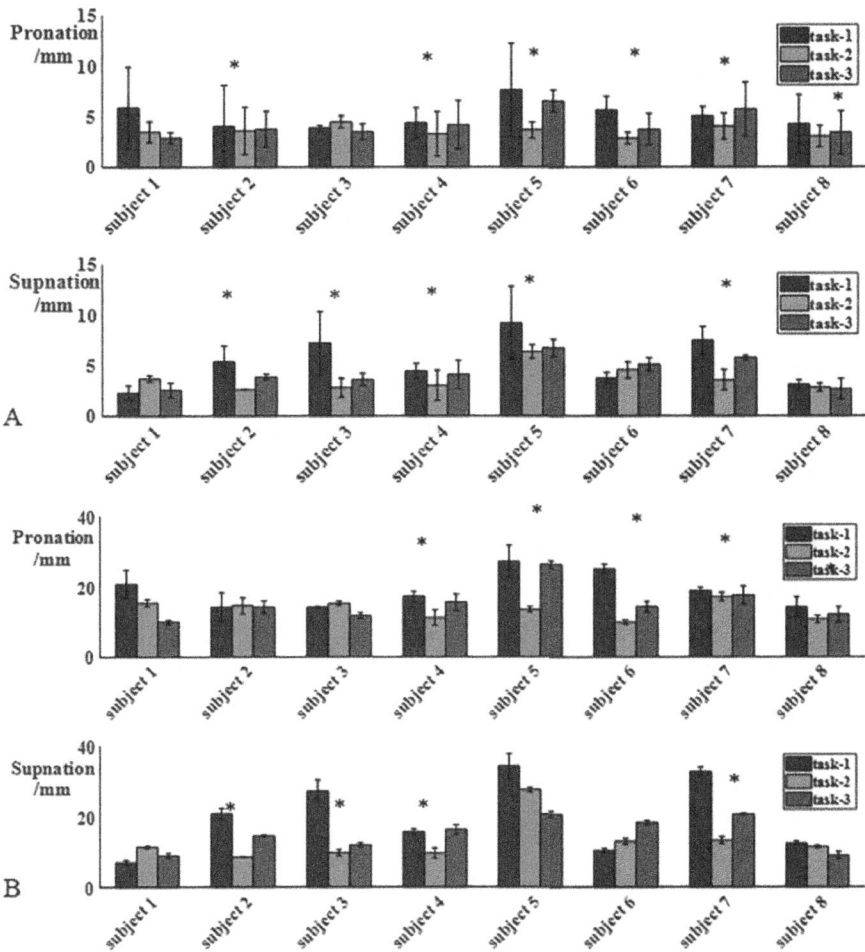

Fig. 5. Results of manipulation for three tasks, the horizontal axis represents eight subjects (**A**) P.D. during pronation, (**B**) P.E. during Supination. (adapted from [10]).

This negative correlation was particularly evident in tasks two and three. Specifically, in task two, CCI1 and PD ($r = -0.62$, $p < 0.1$) and CCI3 and P.R. ($r = -0.66$, $p < 0.1$) showed significant differences. In task three, CCI1 and P.R. ($r = -0.68$, $p < 0.1$), CCI2 and PD ($r = -0.69$, $p < 0.1$), CCI2 and P.R. ($r = -0.81$, $p < 0.01$), and CCI3 and P.R. ($r = -0.58$, $p < 0.1$) also showed significant differences.

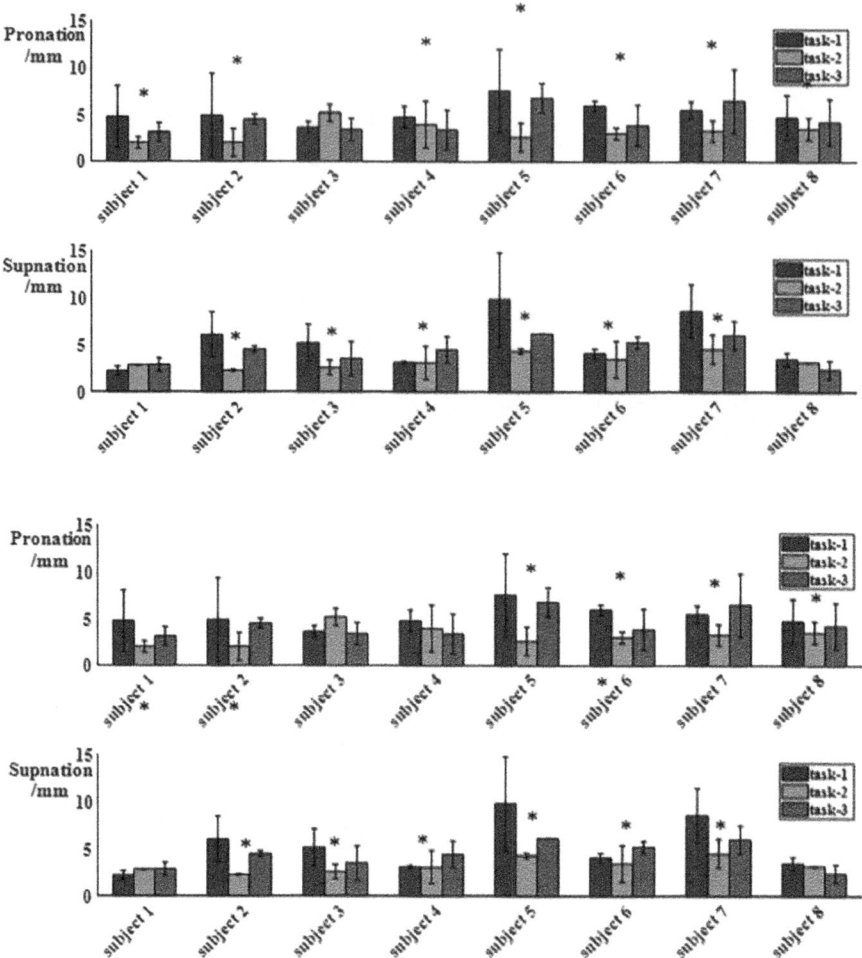

Fig. 6. Filtered results of manipulation for three tasks, the horizontal axis represents eight subjects (**A**) P.D. during pronation, (**B**) P.E. during Supination. (adapted from [10]).

These results indicate that the co-contraction index influences performance within a certain range. Variations in load generally lead to a decrease in performance accuracy, but there exists an optimal CCI range where performance is maximized. This finding highlights the importance of muscle synergy in motor tasks, particularly through the adjustment of muscle co-contraction to optimize performance [17]. Individuals can enhance motor control by adjusting the level of muscle co-contraction when performing complex motor tasks, thereby maintaining high performance accuracy under different load conditions [64].

Table 4. Pearson correlation between similarity and results of manipulation in the cluster.

	Task	P.A.-L				P.A.-R			
		W_1	W_2	W_3	W_4	W_1	W_2	W_3	W_4
Subject1	1	0.223	0.255	0.022	0.36	−0.47*	−0.512*	**−0.04**	**0.213**
Subject1	2	0.341	0.345	0.33	−0.093	0.208	0.294	0.053	−0.502*
Subject1	3	0.343	0.254	−0.229	−0.197	−0.076	0.045	−0.356	0.05
Subject2	1	0.318	−0.133	0.093	−0.026	0.017	0.057	−0.215	−0.811***
Subject2	2	−0.245	0.137	−0.587**	−0.362	−0.279	−0.158	0.136	0.089
Subject2	3	0.036	−0.267	0.195	−0.038	0.452*	0.279	0.322	−0.337
Subject3	1	0.057	0.383	−0.25	−0.525**	−0.033	0.042	0.289	−0.491*
Subject3	2	−0.13	0.083	−0.219	−0.423	−0.288	0.395	0.232	0.235
Subject3	3	0.16	0.038	−0.253	0.403	−0.06	0.141	0.089	0.433
Subject4	1	−0.025	0.094	0.229	0.245	0.097	−0.186	0.229	0.295
Subject4	2	−0.33	−0.285	0.344	0.314	−0.015	0.091	0.17	−0.192
Subject4	3	0.371	0.284	0.018	−0.002	0.189	0.031	0.029	−0.379
Subject5	1	0.242	−0.083	0.024	−0.198	−0.128	−0.325	0.421	0.108
Subject5	2	**−0.332**	0.425	−0.314	0.059	−0.609**	−0.22	0.043	−0.028
Subject5	3	−0.15	0.072	−0.279	−0.039	0.298	0.242	−0.186	−0.125
Subject6	1	−0.046	0.197	0.166	−0.033	0.073	−0.495*	−0.429*	−0.108
Subject6	2	−0.221	−0.014	−0.539**	−0.356	0.102	−0.228	0.292	−0.573**
Subject6	3	0.072	0.434	−0.424	0.386	0.149	0.242	−0.006	−0.165
Subject7	1	0.159	0.322	0.371	−0.225	0.265	0.097	−0.282	0.36
Subject7	2	0.093	−0.017	0.061	0.336	−0.373	−0.332	0.156	0.016
Subject7	3	0.42	−0.482**	0.228	−0.2	0.121	0.209	−0.302	−0.461*
Subject8	1	−0.127	−0.161	−0.113	−0.507**	0.16	−0.258	0.185	0.335
Subject8	2	0.104	−0.484**	−0.369	−0.056	−0.185	0.139	0.2	−0.004
Subject8	3	0.278	0.368	0.175	0.169	0.058	−0.182	0.424	0.366

***$p \leq 0.01$, **$p \leq 0.05$, *$p \leq 0.1$

5.3 Manipulation Performance and the Structure Similarity of Muscle Synergy

Numerous studies have indicated that for the same motor task, individuals often have various muscle compensation strategies, and these different strategies can accomplish the same movement effectively [31,40]. In our study, all three tasks were isometric, and the position distribution at the end of the exercise varied with the load, aligning with findings from a previous study [30]. We observed that among the three tasks, the manipulation error in task 2 was smaller than in the other two tasks. This trend became more evident when the experimental data was filtered using the quartile method, indicating that manipulation performance is not linearly related to loading. According to the results shown in Figs. 5 and 6, variations in load lead to a decrease in manipulation accuracy, but there is an optimal value within a certain range.

We hypothesize that motion accuracy is related not only to loading, co-contraction index, and impedance [51], but also to muscle synergy similarity [14, 36]. This hypothesis is supported by our macroscopic experimental results. As shown in Table 3, the intragroup correlation coefficient of W_4 was significantly negatively correlated with P.E.-L ($r = -0.48$, $p < 0.05$). In the pronation action, PD, TM, INF, TRLA, and TRIL within the W_4 synergy are antagonistic muscles. This finding suggests that the CNS activates antagonistic muscles to adjust motor impedance, minimizing load-induced interference and improving movement accuracy [54, 63].

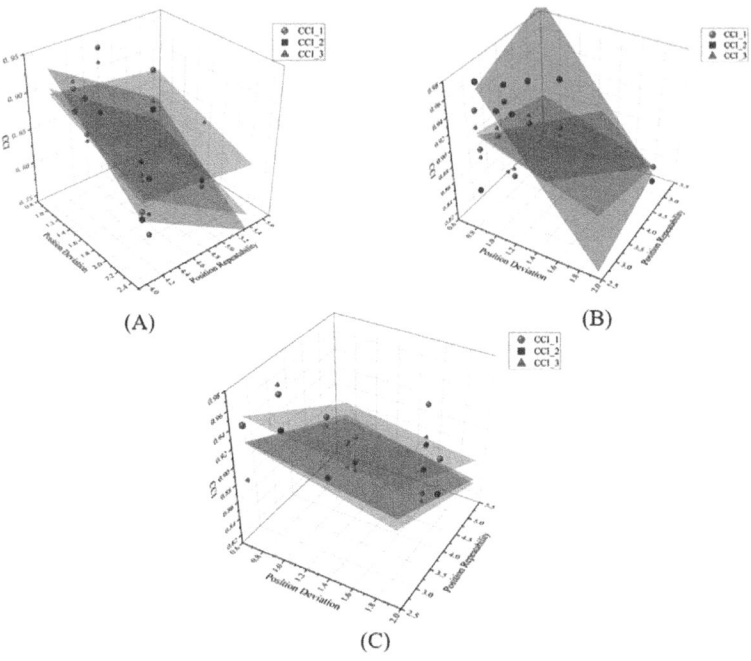

Fig. 7. P.D. and P.R. vs. the co-contraction index in three tasks, **(A)** Task 1, **(B)** Task 2, **(C)** Task 3.

Further research on individual manipulations was conducted to observe the correlation between their accuracy and the average similarity with other manipulations, as shown in Fig. 8. No apparent statistical law was found, but W_2 and W_4 showed more significant correlations than the other two synergies. From the analysis of the results with significant correlations, W_4 was negatively correlated with bilateral manipulation errors, similar to the previous results, and W_2 was also negatively correlated with bilateral manipulation outcomes. This proves the role of antagonistic muscles in performing precision-targeted movements. The manipulation error decreased as the synergistic similarity of the antagonistic muscle groups increased.

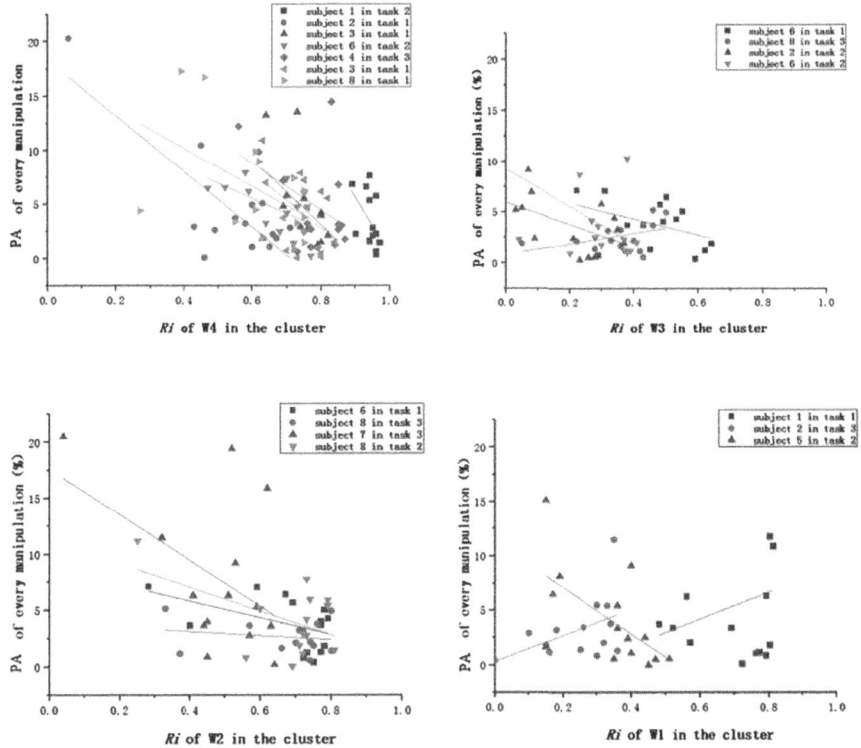

Fig. 8. P.A. vs. the R_i of muscle synergy in the cluster **A** (W_4), **B** (W_3), **C** (W_2), **D** (W_1). (adapted from [10]).

6   Conclusion

Our experiments and data analysis showed that synergistic muscle structure did not change with load level when healthy subjects performed rocker manipulations. The similarity of muscle synergy was negatively correlated with load level, which we interpret as the body's ability to adapt to different loading levels by altering biomechanical strategies. We also observed that joystick manipulation performance was negatively correlated with the similarity of certain muscle synergies. These results supported the alternative hypothesis that the human body increased the activation of antagonistic muscle groups to achieve better manipulation outcomes.

Additionally, our study highlighted the critical role of the co-contraction index (CCI) in manipulation performance. Significant negative correlations were found between CCI and performance error (P.E.), particularly in tasks two and three, involving muscle pairs such as the posterior deltoid (PD) and anterior deltoid (AD), infraspinatus (INF) and pectoralis major (PM), and the triceps brachii (TRIL and TRLA). These findings underscore the importance of muscle co-contraction in maintaining high performance accuracy under varying load conditions.

Our results provide valuable insights for the ergonomic design of flight joysticks and the development of training protocols to enhance pilots' upper limb manipulation skills.

Acknowledgements. The authors gratefully acknowledge the financial support of "National Key R&D Program of China" (No. 2020YFC2007402, No.2020YFC2007401, No. 2020YFC2007404, No. 2020YFC2007403, No. 2020YFC2007405, No. 2020YFC2007400), Basic Research Program of Suzhou (SJC2022011), and Special project of basic research on frontier leading technology in Jiangsu Province (BK20192004C).

References

1. Scano, A., Dardari, L., Molteni, F., Giberti, H., Tosatti, L.M., d'Avella, A.: A comprehensive spatial mapping of muscle synergies in highly variable upper-limb movements of healthy subjects. Front. Physiol. **10**, 1231 (2019). https://doi.org/10.3389/fphys.2019.01231

2. Alnajjar, F., Shimoda, S.: Muscle synergies indices to quantify the skilled behavior in human. In: Converging Clinical And Engineering Research On Neurorehabilitation II, Vols. 1 and 2, vol. 15, pp. 959–963 (2017). https://doi.org/10.1007/978-3-319-46669-9_155

3. Asaka, T., Yahata, K., Mani, H., Wang, Y.: Modulations of muscle modes in automatic postural responses induced by external surface translations. J. Motor Behav. **43**(2), 165 (2011). https://doi.org/10.1080/00222895.2011.552079

4. Barnamehei, H., et al.: Identification and quantification of modular control during Roundhouse kick executed by elite Taekwondo players. Department of Biomedical Engineering, Islamic Azad University (2018)

5. Barnamehei, H., Tabatabai Ghomsheh, F., Safar Cherati, A., Pouladian, M.: Upper limb neuromuscular activities and synergies comparison between elite and nonelite athletics in badminton overhead forehand smash. Appl. Bionics Biomech. **2018**, 1–10 (2018). https://doi.org/10.1155/2018/6067807

6. Bizzi, E., Cheung, V.C.K., d'Avella, A., Saltiel, P., Tresch, M.: Combining modules for movement. Brain Res. Rev. **57**(1), 125–133 (2008). https://doi.org/10.1016/j.brainresrev.2007.08.004

7. Bizzi, E., Cheung, V.: The neural origin of muscle synergies. Front. Comput. Neurosci. **7**(1), 51 (2013). https://doi.org/10.3389/fncom.2013.00051

8. Burdet, E., Osu, R., Franklin, D.W., Milner, T.E., Kawato, M.: The central nervous system stabilizes unstable dynamics by learning optimal impedance. Nature **414**(6862), 446 (2001). https://doi.org/10.1038/35106566

9. Wang, C., Zhang, S., Hu, J., Huang, Z., Shi, C.: Upper-limb muscle synergy features in human-robot interaction with circle-drawing movements. Appl. Bionics Biomech. **2021**, 8850785 (2021). https://doi.org/10.1155/2021/8850785

10. Cai, L., et al.: Associating endpoint accuracy and similarity of muscle synergies. In: Proceedings of the 17th International Joint Conference on Biomedical Engineering Systems and Technologies, vol. 1, pp. 683–694 (2024). https://doi.org/10.5220/0012586800003657

11. Cai, L.M., et al.: Muscle synergies in joystick manipulation. Front. Physiol. **14** (2023). https://doi.org/10.3389/fphys.2023.1282295. Go to ISI://WOS:001088201500001

12. Cai, L., et al.: Evaluation method and experimental study of pilot fine handling ability under different loads. J. Xi'an Jiaotong Univ. **57**(06), 39–46 (2023). https://link.cnki.net/urlid/61.1069.T.20230203.1107.001

13. Cheung, V.C.K., et al.: Plasticity of muscle synergies through fractionation and merging during development and training of human runners. Nat. Commun. **11**(1) (2020). https://doi.org/10.1038/s41467-020-18210-4
14. Choi, Y., Kim, Y., Kim, M., Yoon, B.: Muscle synergies for turning during human walking. J. Motor Behav. **51**(1), 1–9 (2019). https://doi.org/10.1080/00222895.2017.1408558
15. Coscia, M., et al.: The effect of arm weight support on upper limb muscle synergies during reaching movements. J. Neuroeng. Rehabil. **11**(1), 22 (2014). https://doi.org/10.1186/1743-0003-11-22
16. Curado, M.R., et al.: Residual upper arm motor function primes innervation of paretic forearm muscles in chronic stroke after brain-machine interface (BMI) training. PLoS ONE **10**(10), e0140161 (2015). https://doi.org/10.1371/journal.pone.0140161
17. Dai, C., Cao, Y., Hu, X.: Prediction of individual finger forces based on decoded motoneuron activities. Ann. Biomed. Eng. **47**(6), 1357–1368 (2019). https://doi.org/10.1007/s10439-019-02240-1
18. d'Avella, A., Saltiel, P., Bizzi, E.: Combinations of muscle synergies in the construction of a natural motor behavior. Nat. Neurosci. **6**(3), 300–308 (2003). https://doi.org/10.1038/nn1010
19. Durandau, G., Farina, D., Sartori, M.: Robust real-time musculoskeletal modeling driven by electromyograms. IEEE Trans. Biomed. Eng. **65**(3), 556–564 (2018). https://doi.org/10.1109/TBME.2017.2704085
20. Esmaeili, J., Maleki, A.: Muscle coordination analysis by time-varying muscle synergy extraction during cycling across various mechanical conditions. Biocybern. Biomed. Eng. **40**(1), 90–99 (2020). https://doi.org/10.1016/j.bbe.2019.10.005
21. Ettema, G.J.C., Taylor, E., North, J.D., Kippers, V.: Muscle synergies at the elbow in static and oscillating isometric torque tasks with dual degrees of freedom. Mot. Control **9**(1), 59–74 (2005). https://doi.org/10.1123/mcj.9.1.59
22. Feldman, A.G., Levin, M.F.: The origin and use of positional frames of reference in motor control. Behav. Brain Sci. **18**(4), 723–806 (1995). https://doi.org/10.1017/s0140525x0004070x
23. Franklin, D.W., Osu, R., Burdet, E., Kawato, M., Milner, T.E.: Adaptation to stable and unstable dynamics achieved by combined impedance control and inverse dynamics model. J. Neurophysiol. **90**(5), 3270–3282 (2003). https://doi.org/10.1152/jn.01112.2002
24. Franklin, D.W., Theodore, E., et al.: Endpoint stiffness of the arm is directionally tuned to instability in the environment. J. Neurosci. **27**(29), 7705–7716 (2007). https://doi.org/10.1523/jneurosci0968-07
25. Hartmann, Y., Liu, H., Lahrberg, S., Schultz, T.: Interpretable high-level features for human activity recognition. In: Proceedings of the 15th International Joint Conference on Biomedical Engineering Systems and Technologies (BIOSTEC 2022) - Volume 4: BIOSIGNALS, pp. 40–49 (2022). https://doi.org/10.5220/0010840500003123
26. Hartmann, Y., Liu, H., Schultz, T.: High-level features for human activity recognition and modeling. In: Roque, A.C.A., et al. (eds.) BIOSTEC 2022. CCIS, vol. 1814, pp. 141–163. Springer, Cham (2023). https://doi.org/10.1007/978-3-031-38854-5_8
27. Hermens, H.J., Freriks, B., Disselhorst-Klug, C., Rau, G.: Development of recommendations for SEMG sensors and sensor placement procedures. J. Electromyogr. Kinesiol. **10**(5), 361–374 (2000). https://doi.org/10.1016/s1050-6411(00)00027-4
28. Zhao, K., Zhang, Z., Wen, H., Scano, A.: Intra-subject and inter-subject movement variability quantified with muscle synergies in upper-limb reaching movements. Biomimetics **6**(4), 63 (2021). https://doi.org/10.3390/biomimetics6040063
29. Kieliba, P., Tropea, P., Pirondini, E., Coscia, M., Micera, S., Artoni, F.: How are muscle synergies affected by electromyography pre-processing? IEEE Trans. Neural Syst. Rehabil. Eng. **26**(4), 882–893 (2018). https://doi.org/10.1109/tnsre.2018.2810859

30. Kojima, S., Takeda, M., Nambu, I., Wada, Y.: Relations between required accuracy and muscle synergy in isometric contraction tasks. In: 2017 IEEE International Conference on Systems, Man, and Cybernetics (SMC), pp. 1191–1195 (2017)

31. Ting, L.H., Macpherson, J.M.: A limited set of muscle synergies for force control during a postural task. J. Neurophysiol. **93**(1), 609–613 (2004). https://doi.org/10.1152/jn.00681.2004

32. Latash, M.L., Scholz, J.P., Schöner, G.: Motor control strategies revealed in the structure of motor variability. Exerc. Sport Sci. Rev. **30**(1), 26–31 (2002). https://doi.org/10.1097/00003677-200201000-00006

33. Lee, D.D., Seung, H.S.: Learning the parts of objects by non-negative matrix factorization. Nature **401**(6755), 788 (1999). https://doi.org/10.1038/44565

34. Liming, C., Chenli, Jun, Z., YunChao, Z., Xin, M.: Design and research of a fine operation capability evaluation system based on Fitts. In: 2021 International Conference on Machine Learning and Intelligent Systems Engineering (MLISE), pp. 239–242 (2021). https://doi.org/10.1109/MLISE54096.2021.00050

35. Liming, C., Qian, Y., Jun, Z., YunChao, Z., YinXiao, L., Xin, M.: Design and research of the clutch device in knee joint exoskeleton drive. In: 2021 4th International Conference on Electron Device and Mechanical Engineering (ICEDME), pp. 1–4 (2021). https://doi.org/10.1109/ICEDME52809.2021.00008

36. Liming, C., Shuhao, Y., Jun, Z., Li, C., Xin, M.: Muscle synergies in joystick manipulate task: evaluation of inter-group variability. SSRN (2022). https://doi.org/10.1287/mnsc.1.2.187

37. Liu, H., Schultz, T.: How long are various types of daily activities? Statistical analysis of a multimodal wearable sensor-based human activity dataset. In: Proceedings of the 15th International Joint Conference on Biomedical Engineering Systems and Technologies (BIOSTEC 2022) - Volume 5: HEALTHINF, pp. 680–688 (2022). https://doi.org/10.5220/0010896400003123

38. Liu, H., Xue, T., Schultz, T.: On a real real-time wearable human activity recognition system. In: Proceedings of the 16th International Joint Conference on Biomedical Engineering Systems and Technologies (BIOSTEC 2023) - WHC, pp. 711–720 (2023). https://doi.org/10.5220/0011927700003414

39. McGraw, K.O., Wong, S.P.: Forming inferences about some intraclass correlation coefficients. Psychol. Methods **1**(1), 30–46 (1996). https://doi.org/10.1037/1082-989x.1.1.30

40. McKay, J.L., Ting, L.H.: Functional muscle synergies constrain force production during postural tasks. J. Biomech. **41**(2), 299–306 (2008). https://doi.org/10.1016/j.jbiomech.2007.09.012

41. Mira, R.M., Tosatti, L.M., Sacco, M., Scano, A.: Detailed characterization of physiological EMG activations and directional tuning of upper-limb and trunk muscles in point-to-point reaching movements. Curr. Res. Physiol. **4**, 60–72 (2021). https://doi.org/10.1016/j.crphys.2021.02.005

42. Miyazaki, H.T.K.H.: Extraction and implementation of muscle synergies in hand-force control. Department of Mechanical Science and Bioengineering, Graduate School of Engineering Science, Osaka University, Japan (2011)

43. Nicolas, A.T., Romain, M., Mickael, B.: Shoulder muscle activation strategies differ when lifting or lowering a load. Eur. J. Appl. Physiol. **120**(11), 2417–2429 (2020). https://doi.org/10.1007/s00421-020-04464-9

44. Osu, R., Kamimura, N., Nakano, E., Harris, C.M., Wada, Y.: Optimal impedance control for task achievement in the presence of signal-dependent noise. J. Neurophysiol. **92**(2), 1199–1215 (2004). https://doi.org/10.1152/jn.00519.2003

45. Ouyang, C.Y., Cai, L.M., Liu, B., Zhang, T.X.: An improved wavelet threshold denoising approach for surface electromyography signal. Eurasip J. Adv. Signal Process. **2023**(1) (2023). https://doi.org/10.1186/s13634-023-01066-3. Go to ISI://WOS:001086830700001

46. Robert, T., Latash, M.: Time evolution of the organization of multi-muscle postural responses to sudden changes in the external force applied at the trunk level(article). Neurosci. Lett. **438**(2), 238–241 (2008). https://doi.org/10.1016/j.neulet.2008.04.052

47. Roh, J., Rymer, W., Beer, R.: Robustness of muscle synergies underlying three-dimensional force generation at the hand in healthy humans (article). J. Neurophysiol. **107**(8), 2123–2142 (2012). https://doi.org/10.1152/jn.00173.2011

48. Roh, J., Rymer, W., Perreault, E., Yoo, S., Beer, R.: Alterations in upper limb muscle synergy structure in chronic stroke survivors (article). J. Neurophysiol. **109**(3), 768–781 (2013). https://doi.org/10.1152/jn.00670.2012

49. Salman, B., Vahdat, S., Lambercy, O., Dovat, L., Burdet, E., Milner, T.: Changes in muscle activation patterns following robot-assisted training of hand function after stroke. Sion Frser Universiy, Burnby, BC CndMcGi Universiy, Monre, QC CndETH Zurich, Zurich, Swizernd-Goech, SwizerndIeri Coege of Science, Technoogy nd Medicine, London UKMcGi Universiy (2010)

50. Sanger, T.D., Delgado, M.R., Gaebler-Spira, D., Hallett, M., Mink, J.W., Task Force Childhood Motor, D.: Classification and definition of disorders causing hypertonia in childhood. Pediatrics **111**(1) (2003). https://doi.org/10.1542/peds.111.1.e89

51. Sangwan, S., Green, R.A., Taylor, N.F.: Stabilizing characteristics of rotator cuff muscles: a systematic review. Disabil. Rehabil. **37**(12), 1033–1043 (2015). https://doi.org/10.3109/09638288.2014.949357

52. Santos, A.D.-D., Poston, B., Jesunathadas, M., Bobich, L., Hamm, T.M.M.C.: Influence of fatigue on hand muscle coordination and EMG-EMG coherence during three-digit grasping. J. Neurophysiol. **104**(6), 3576–3587 (2010). https://doi.org/10.1152/jn.00583.2010

53. Sepehrikia, M., Abedanzadeh, R., Saemi, E.: Brain gym exercises improve eye-hand coordination in elderly males. Somatosens. Motor Res. 1–6 (2023). https://doi.org/10.1080/08990220.2023.2191706

54. Serres, S.J.D., Milner, T.E.: Wrist muscle activation patterns and stiffness associated with stable and unstable mechanical loads. Exp. Brain Res. **86**(2), 451–458 (1991). https://doi.org/10.1007/bf00228972

55. Taborri, J., Palermo, E., Masiello, D., Rossi, S.: Factorization of EMG via muscle synergies in walking task: evaluation of intra-subject and inter-subject variability. University of Tuscia, Viterbo, Italy (2017)

56. Tang, L., Chen, X., Cao, S., Wu, D., Zhao, G., Zhang, X.: Assessment of upper limb motor dysfunction for children with cerebral palsy based on muscle synergy analysis. Front. Hum. Neurosci. **11**, 130 (2017). https://doi.org/10.3389/fnhum.2017.00130

57. Todorov, E., Li, W., Pan, X.: From task parameters to motor synergies: A hierarchical framework for approximately-optimal control of redundant manipulators. J. Robot. Syst. **22**(11), 691–710 (2005). https://doi.org/10.1002/rob.20093

58. Torres-Oviedo, G.W.H., Ting, L.H.: Muscle synergies characterizing human postural responses. J. Neurophysiol. **98**(4), 2144–2156 (2007). https://doi.org/10.1152/jn.01360.2006

59. Tsubasa, Sano and Misaki, T., Isao, N., Yasuhiro, W.: Relations between speed-accuracy trade-off and muscle synergy in isometric contraction tasks. In: Annual International Conference of the IEEE Engineering in Medicine and Biology Society, vol. 2020, pp. 4803–4806 (2020). https://doi.org/10.1109/embc44109.2020.9176540

60. Veldanda, A., Liu, H., Koschke, R., Schultz, T., Küster, D.: Can electromyography alone reveal facial action units? A pilot EMG-based action unit recognition study with real-time validation. In: BIODEVICES 2024—7th International Conference on Biomedical Electronics and Devices. INSTICC, SciTePress (2024)

61. Velden, L.L.V.D., et al.: Reliability and validity of a new diagnostic device for quantifying hemiparetic arm impairments: an exploratory study. J. Rehabil. Med. **54**, jrm00283 (2022). https://doi.org/10.2340/jrm.v54.12

62. Wang, T., Okada, S., Guo, A., Makikawa, M., Shiozawa, N.: Effect of assist robot on muscle synergy during sit-to-stand movement. In: IEEE International Conference on Intelligence and Safety for Robotics (2021)

63. Wong, J., Wilson, E.T., Malfait, N., Gribble, P.L.: Limb stiffness is modulated with spatial accuracy requirements during movement in the absence of destabilizing forces. J. Neurophysiol. **101**(3), 1542–1549 (2009). https://doi.org/10.1152/jn.91188.2008

64. Yeoh, W.L., Choi, J., Loh, P.Y., Fukuda, O., Muraki, S.: Motor characteristics of human adaptations to external assistive forces. J. Robot. Mechatron. **35**(3), 547–555 (2023). https://doi.org/10.20965/jrm.2023.p0547

65. Zhang, S., Kolensnikov, S., Rennspieß, T., Porzel, R., Schultz, T., Liu, H.: Really can't hold on anymore? Physiological indicators versus self-reported motivation drop during jogging. In: BIOSIGNALS 2024—17th International Conference on Bio-Inspired Systems and Signal Processing. INSTICC, SciTePress (2024)

66. Zhao, K., Zhang, Z., Wen, H., Wang, Z., Wu, J.: Modular organization of muscle synergies to achieve movement behaviors. J. Healthc. Eng. **2019**, 8130297 (2019). https://doi.org/10.1155/2019/8130297

Health Informatics

Application of Formal Concept Analysis to Characterize Social Behaviors

Diogo Miranda, Diogo Castro, Heleny Bessa, Luis Zarate, and Mark Song[✉]

Instituto de Ciencias Exatas e Informática, Pontifícia Universidade Catolica de Minas Gerais,
Belo Horizonte, Brazil
{damiranda,heleny}@sga.pucminas.br, {zarate,song}@pucminas.br

Abstract. In this article, we propose a methodology for investigating social behavior databases using Formal Concept Analysis and we present two case studies. One addresses the global concern for road safety, where frequent accidents on roads and streets result in loss of human lives, severe injuries, and significant material damage, impacting not only the direct victims but also their families and society at large. To tackle this challenge, it is crucial to analyze the factors contributing to these accidents, particularly driver behaviors. The other case study uses a longitudinal database of students on exchange programs. It has 3 waves and allows for studies to better comprehend how the geographical mobility affects factors related to the health of the exchange students. We aim to discover patterns related to the consumption of alcohol within exchange students. The objective is the understanding of how the change in environment affects the habits and aggravates the states of these individuals which certainly would prove useful in the prevention of alcohol abuse.

Keywords: Formal concept analysis · Triadic concept analysis · Driving behaviors · Exchange students · Alcohol consumption

1 Introduction

Traffic accidents pose a global issue, leading to fatalities, severe injuries, and substantial economic losses worldwide. They occur daily on roads and streets globally, ranking among the primary causes of death. Beyond affecting victims directly, these incidents also impact their families and society overall. To effectively address and reduce this problem, it is essential to analyze and comprehend the contributing factors to these accidents.

Studying traffic behaviors offers valuable insights into identifying and addressing factors that contribute to accidents, ultimately aiming to reduce fatalities. This aspect is crucial for a country's developmental progress. Moreover, such studies can uncover nuanced aspects, like the interplay of personality traits and socio-cultural factors, which increase risks and contribute to accidents, as highlighted in [22].

Reckless driving is a significant contributing factor to traffic accidents, encompassing behaviors such as speeding, dangerous overtaking, ignoring traffic regulations, and

M. P. Guarino et al. (Eds.): BIOSTEC 2024, CCIS 2546, pp. 295–313, 2026.
https://doi.org/10.1007/978-3-031-96899-0_17

using electronic devices while driving. Additionally, socio-cultural and educational factors play a crucial role in road safety, as discussed in [9].

Therefore, one objective of this study is to expand upon the findings presented in [16] by examining the socio-cultural influences on drivers, as well as external influences from friends and/or family. This will involve applying Formal Concept Analysis (FCA) to a database containing information about Chinese drivers, utilizing the data processing methods outlined in [11].

Many studies in the field rely on cross-sectional data, treating it akin to a snapshot in time, as noted in [2,20]. However, this approach can be likened to trying to determine the speed of a moving vehicle using only its location data captured in a single moment— it freezes the object and fails to capture its movement dynamics. For certain research questions, particularly those involving variables that change over time, a cross-sectional approach may be insufficient. Analyzing these changes over time can provide valuable insights that enhance the overall study.

In contrast to cross-sectional methods, longitudinal research involves collecting data across multiple time points, often referred to as waves. This approach offers several advantages: it enables the study of dynamic relationships and allows for the examination of heterogeneity among the subjects being studied. By following objects over time, researchers can analyze how their attributes change and compare these changes across different objects.

This methodological approach, focusing on correlations between observations made at various moments, facilitates the discovery of hidden patterns within the data, as outlined in [7]. This longitudinal perspective not only provides insights into temporal dynamics but also enhances the depth of understanding in research contexts where change and development are critical factors.

We utilize a longitudinal database as described in [1], focusing on exchange students' data collected over 3 waves. This dataset enables a comprehensive exploration of how geographical mobility impacts various health-related factors among exchange students. According to the authors, analyzing this data can significantly enhance initiatives aimed at promoting health actions tailored to this demographic. It also supports the development of regulations by institutions, leaders, professionals, student associations, and other stakeholders involved in student mobility and health management efforts.

In this study, we aim to uncover patterns related to alcohol consumption among exchange students. The primary objective is to understand how changes in environment influence their habits and exacerbate their conditions, which is crucial for preventing alcohol abuse.

To achieve this, we will analyze data from the Brief Young Adult Alcohol Consequences Questionnaire (BYAACQ), developed by Kahler, Strong, and Read [12]. This questionnaire consists of 24 items that assess the negative consequences experienced by students due to alcohol consumption, ordered by severity. The goal is to measure these consequences to detect early signs of alcoholic behavior among university students.

By identifying patterns in the data collected over multiple waves from the longitudinal study described earlier, we aim to contribute valuable insights into the factors influencing alcohol consumption among exchange students. This knowledge can inform targeted interventions and policies aimed at promoting healthier behaviors and reducing the risk of alcohol-related harm in this population.

The technique used to uncover these patterns is Triadic Concept Analysis (TCA), an extension of Formal Concept Analysis (FCA). TCA identifies the relationships between objects, attributes, and conditions, characterizing and describing them through implication rules known as triadic rules.

The TCA approach was validated by comparing the model created with the rules obtained, as their inferences between items produced approximately the same answers. Furthermore, triadic rules proved advantageous over the Rasch model due to the easier understanding of the triadic approach.

When compared to Rasch Modelling, TCA has proven to be a simpler and more direct method for extracting relationships between factors, without requiring advanced statistical knowledge for its use and interpretation. Additionally, there is a scarcity of practical applications utilizing triadic rules for information discovery in recent works.

2 Background

2.1 Formal Concept Analysis

Formal Concept Analysis (FCA) can be used to recognize patterns with the help of association rules and their implications. It consists of a set of objects in a formal context, formal concepts, and rules. A formal context can be represented as a triple $K = (G, M, I)$, consisting of a set G of objects, a set M of attributes, and an incidence relation $I \subseteq G \times M$, with $(g, m) \in I$ meaning that *object g has attribute m.*. For a set of objects $A \subseteq G$, the set of *common attributes for the objects* of A is denoted by $A' := \{m \in M | \forall g \in A : (g, m) \in I\}$, similarly, the set of *common attributes for the objects* of B is denoted by $B' := \{g \in G | \forall m \in B : (g, m) \in I\}$.

A formal concept of a formal context $K = (G, M, I)$ is defined by pair (A, B) where A is called *extension* and B is called *intention*. For a pair (A, B) to be considered a concept, one needs to follow the condition where $(A = B')$ and $(B = A')$. The set of formal concepts of a context K is said to be $\beta(K)$.

Association rules are dependencies between elements of a formal context. The rule $A \rightarrow B$ is valid only if for every object containing attributes B, it also contains attributes from C. Given a rule r and parameters s and c, one can denote [5]:

$s = \text{suppr}(r) = \frac{|A' \cap B'|}{|G'|}$ - called the support of rule r, and

$c = \text{conf}(r) = \frac{|A' \cap B'|}{|A'|}$ - called confidence.

When $\text{conf}(r) = 100\%$ the rule is referred to as an implication. Studies that explore domains that can be represented as a binary tabular base of objects and attributes can often apply FCA. Longitudinal study approaches aim to investigate a sample of individuals with certain characteristics over consecutive time periods, referred to as waves. On the other hand, FCA is an approach in formal set theory that focuses on the representation and analysis of the semantic structure of data at a single point in time, without considering evolution or changes over time.

FCA is based on the idea that concepts can be defined based on the relationships between objects and attributes, enabling the creation of conceptual hierarchies and the understanding of associations between meaningful terms. It is a useful technique for organizing and extracting information from data sets.

2.2 Triadic Concept Analysis

Developed by Lehmann and Wille [13], Triadic Concept Analysis is an augment to Formal Concept Analysis, boasting a third dimension not present in its dyadic counterpart, conditions. It is formally defined as a quadruple, $\mathbb{K} := (K_1, K_2, K_3, Y)$, whose elements are respectively defined as objects (K_1), attributes (K_2), conditions (K_3) and the relations between them (Y).

It is possible to discern from Table 1 that $(o_1, o_2, o_3, o_4) \in K_1$, $(a_1, a_2, a_3) \in K_2$ and $(c_1, c_2, c_3) \in K_3$. The first line of this table shows that object o_1 has attribute a_2 in condition c_1, meaning there is a relationship between these three elements, defined as $(o_1, a_2, c_1) \in Y$.

Table 1. Representation of a Triadic Context.

K	c_1			c_2			c_3		
	a_1	a_2	a_3	a_1	a_2	a_3	a_1	a_2	a_3
o_1		×			×		×		
o_2	×		×	×	×	×			×
o_3		×			×		×	×	
o_4			×				×	×	

The triadic concept is defined as (A, B, C). As in dyadic concepts, $A \subseteq K_1$ (extent) and $B \subseteq K_2$ (Intent) exist, however, there is also the addition of a third component, $C \subseteq K_3$ (modus). From this concept, it is possible to extract triadic rules, that are in the scope of this paper.

Biedermann [4] defines a triadic implication as $(A \rightarrow B)_C$, meaning A implies B given condition C. The subsets of attributes A and B are shared by the same objects given condition C. In [8] different types of implications were explored in a hypothetical triadic situation, such as: attribution condition, conditional attribute and attributional condition. Such rules are synthesized as such:

- **BCAAR** (Biedermann Conditional Attribute Association Rule). $(A_1 \rightarrow A_2)_C$(sup = X%, conf = Y%), in which A_1, $A_2 \in K_2$ and $C \in K_3$, meaning when attributes in A_1 happen in every condition C, attributes in A_2 also occur in all conditions C.
- **BACAR** (Biedermann Attribution Condition Association Rule). $(C_1 \rightarrow C_2)_A$(sup = X%, conf = Y%), in which C_1, $C_2 \in K_3$ and $A \in K_2$, meaning when conditions C_1 happen in every attribute A, conditions in C_2 also occur in all attributes A.

The introduction of a third dimension allows for a better characterization and representation of data. Bi-dimensional data may receive the dimension time to monitor the evolution of objects in relation to attributes and discovery of hidden patterns in the database [17], and this is exactly the shape of longitudinal studies, such as the database used in this study.

2.3   Aggressive Behaviors in Traffic

Traffic behaviors that can lead to accidents are categorized into three main areas: 1) aggressive behaviors in traffic, 2) influence of friends and close acquaintances, and 3) family influence. These categories include a fourth category used as a threshold for analysis, which is socio-cultural information about the drivers. The data involves 1039 Chinese drivers, whose sociocultural factors were linked to these behaviors. This database was collected through an online survey and is publicly available in the Data in Brief journal. The study, published in August 2023, used the Bayesian Mindsponge Framework (BMF) as a validation index. It specifically demonstrated how safe driving behaviors are influenced by information promoting safe driving, which is actively absorbed with support from friends, colleagues, and/or the driver's family.

A fundamental concept of the Mindsponge Theory is that the human mind tends to be influenced by information absorbed from external sources. As analyzed in [11], the factors contributing to safe driving may be related to external influences from family, friends, and colleagues. These external factors, along with socio-cultural factors, offer valuable insights for analysis on this issue.

The application of FCA to the dataset in question can provide important insights into the behavior of drivers in traffic leading to accidents. Rules of the form A → B take into account that when drivers exhibit a certain aggressive behavior A, it implies B.

3   Related Works

This work utilizes Formal Concept Analysis and the approach is justified through a relationship between theoretical and practical knowledge of this subject. Related works are presented as follows.

[21] analyzes the triadic approach of formal concept analysis in four aspects: (i) the basic approach of triadic concept analysis, (ii) triadic implications and rules, (iii) the triadic factor of analysis, and (iv) the analysis of fuzzy triadic concepts.

[4] systematically demonstrates the application of triadic formal concept analysis in databases to represent complex concepts that are difficult to visualize. It also explains the generation of rules and implications from an analyzed dataset.

In our work, triadic rules are used to describe a longitudinal study based on alcohol consumption. Waves and their relationships over time were analysed.

Mendes et al. [15] has done a similar work, extracting triadic rules from a database with records of patients afflicted by Parkinsons disease. With the obtained rules, it was possible to profile the patients and the reactions triggered in any given moment, adding value to the clinical analysis and therefore decisions in relation to the efficiency in treating this group in particular. In [18] the triadic concept was applied in the database ELSA-UK (English Longitudinal Study of Aging) to discover which factors collected showed larger impact on the longevity of the study partakers and which are the patterns within those factors. The results were corroborated by existing literature about longevity, which proposes that social, economical and familiar environments have an impact on it. Both studies had results that are supported by bibliographical material in the social sciences, corroborating that the knowledge found with the triadic rules has theoretical support and that new knowledge may be obtained from the use of this technique.

Within the longitudinal research field about alcohol consumption in university students, the Triadic Concept Analysis approach has not yet been utilized even if many other perspectives on how to deal with this data have been applied to visualize changes and discover their causes. This information may be used in early detection of alcoholism and in development of policies in universities.

For that purpose, surveys such as the Young Adult Alcohol Problems Screening Test (YAAPST) [10], Young Adult Alcohol Consequences Questionnaire (YAACQ) [19] and Brief Young Adult Alcohol Consequences (BYAACQ) [12].

In [3], the alcohol consumption of British university students was monitored from the first to third year of their courses with an original questionnaire, which contained questions about weekly alcohol consumption in units of 10ml and negative impacts the students believed they suffered because of its use. The data was analysed using Variance Analysis (ANOVA), to investigate the change in consumption over time and reasons that could predict consumption in different years. While there was a drop in consumption over time, the analysis revealed the negative consequences of alcohol consumption. However, relationship between factors that could have aided in the review of the results and relevant insights were not extracted, as opposed to our work.

4 Case Study: Aggressive Behaviors of Chinese Drivers in Traffic

This article explores the application of formal concept analysis to human behavior aiming to investigate aggressive behaviors of Chinese drivers in traffic. The process involves data collection, exploration, attribute selection, and transformation, as well as the extraction of contexts and rules.

4.1 Materials

The dyadic database used in this study is available in [11]. It contains records from 1039 Chinese drivers who responded to a questionnaire consisting of 37 variables, including responses from various perspectives. Following, we present some example of the attributes extracted from these questionnaires, displaying only the first three attributes from each category for simplification. The study was divided into groups, each focusing on analyzed subcategories, with each subcategory having a specific number of attributes.

1. **Driving and Insurance Purchasing Information**
   - A1: Commercial insurance for vehicle
   - A2: Frequency of driving for work
   - A3: Confidence in driving skills
2. **Aggressive Driving Behaviors**
   - B1: Speed limit - rarely exceed
   - B2: Normal speed, avoid weaving, reckless overtaking

 – B3: Safe distance, no tailgating
3. **Friend/Peer Influence**
 – C1: Supportive friends
 – C2: Advocating safe driving
 – C3: Caution against driving under the influence
4. **Family Influence**
 – D1: Planned driving
 – D2: Follow traffic rules
 – D3: Praise safe driving
5. **Socio-Demographic Factors**
 – E1: Gender
 – E2: Education level
 – E3: Monthly salary

4.2   Methods

Preprocessing. The first step is to collect the necessary data and its description. Validated data is available in the Data in Brief journal data repository [11]. The data includes objects and attributes related to Chinese drivers, with attribute types being either categorical or numerical. The database has been pre-processed to remove irrelevant attributes and filter outliers. Data balancing was not performed, as all data in the database pertains to the class that the study aims to characterize.

It was necessary to create categories for the analysis of the objects at hand. To do this, sub-categories were created, and the selection of which attributes would be present in them was made. Initially, the analysis to be conducted is about the influence of external factors on the behavior of drivers in traffic. For this purpose, a Cartesian product of general categories into sub-categories was performed. The attributes in the categories related to *driving and insurance purchase information* (A), *socio-demographic factors* (E), and *aggressive behaviors* (B) were considered general attributes, meaning they are present in all other sub-categories. The sub-categories analyzed pertain to external factors that influence driver behavior and/or attention.

Discretization. Next, to achieve the objectives of this article, it will be necessary to transform the data into a formal context, using the database as input for concept extraction algorithms. For this purpose, the data should correspond to binary attributes. Not all attributes have this characteristic, as some are of a numeric and/or categorical type, within the range $[1, 5]$, where the variation pertains to how much a driver agrees with a statement. We present the numeric Values and thrie meaning: 1 - Strongly Disagree; 2 - Disagree; 3 - Neutral; 4 - Agree; 5 - Strongly Agree.

To transform this data into a formal context, an algorithm was used that considers value ranges and separates them into two binary groups, indicating whether the data agrees or disagrees with the question. A slight modification to the algorithm is made when it is necessary to invert the values 0 and 1. In some cases, an attribute may yield an interesting rule if it is marked as 1, not necessarily because it belongs to the group containing values corresponding to 0.

After binarizing the values using the algorithm, a formal context is obtained, enabling the extraction of rules and implications from the database (Table 2). This formal context was varied according to the attributes of interest, separating them into different analyses. This approach was necessary due to the limitation on the number of attributes that FCA algorithms can handle. In each analysis, the maximum number of attributes was 13, considering the Cartesian product of attributes from different general categories with sub-categories.

Table 2. Part of the formal context - obtained from [16].

less than 5 years of driver's license	exceeds speed limit	drives under the influence of friends	drinks while driving	less than 40 years of age	has a college degree	drives carefully when with family	trusts driving skills
X	X			X		X	X
	X	X	X		X	X	
			X	X			X
X				X		X	
	X	X					X

4.3   Results and Discussion

When AFC was used, support values were set above 40% and confidence values above 60% in the Chinese drivers' scenario. The first analysis was performed using sociocultural factors (age, educational factor, and income) along with driving factors (time spent driving, confidence in driving skills, driving frequency, etc.), and aggressive driving behavior factors (exceeding speed limits, maintaining safe distances, etc.), generating two hundred and forty (240) rules.

It is possible to collect these results in XML format and analyze the rules in the form of A → B. Assuming that B is a consequence, generating support (sup) and confidence (conf) generates implication rules pointing to attributes.

Following are rules extracted considering only aggressive behaviors:

1. **IF** a driver has less than 5 years of driving and tends to drive cautiously
   THEN he will not exceed the speed limit of the road (sup = 49% conf = 88%)
2. **IF** a driver has less than 5 years of driving and is under 40 years old
   THEN he will yield the right of way to other drivers (sup = 40% conf = 90%)
3. **IF** the driver trusts his skills and has more than 5 years of driving experience
   THEN he will use his turn signal when changing lanes (sup = 44% conf = 80%)

These rules show an interesting characteristic of the database, leading to the understanding that around 60% of the drivers present drive better and more cautiously when accompanied by of friends and/or close individuals, with a confidence level of approximately 88%.

Following are rules extracted considering the influence of friends and/or close individuals:

1. **IF** the driver has friends who influence not drinking
   THEN they will not exhibit aggressive behavior (sup = 60% conf = 90%)
2. **IF** the driver, even in a hurry, has friends who encourage safe driving
   THEN they will yield in traffic (sup = 61% conf = 87%)
3. **IF** the driver has friends who recommend slowing down at the yellow signal
   THEN they will slow down at the yellow signal (sup = 60% conf = 87%)

In the Chinese socio-cultural context, the three primary rules emphasize the significance of external factors in decision-making and suggest that a notable portion of drivers exhibiting aggressive behavior do not attribute this behavior to external influences while driving.

On the other hand, an analysis focused on the category of family influence during driving. This analysis integrated socio-cultural aspects along with factors related to family members present in the car with the driver. It resulted in the extraction of one hundred and five (105) rules, with the primary ones documented. Following are rules extracted considering family influence:

1. **IF** the driver has their family in the car
   THEN he will not exhibit aggressive behavior (sup = 60% conf = 86%)
2. **IF** the driver is criticized by the family for irresponsible driving
   THEN he will not exceed the speed limit of the road (sup = 8% conf = 88%)
3. **IF** the driver's traffic behavior is monitored by the family
   THEN he will not run yellow signals (sup = 59% conf = 88%)

In this way, the main extracted rules show that around 59% of drivers tend not to have aggressive behaviors influenced by the family, with a confidence level of approximately 87%. With these rules, it can be affirmed that drivers who have family influence are generally less prone to exhibiting aggressive behavior on the road.

5   Case Study: Exchange Program

The database chosen contains information related to the health habits of students from 200 cities of 40 European countries that have participated in exchange programs in other European countries gathered during the 2015 and 2016's academical years. Originally it had 908 instances and 252 attributes, divided in 3 waves. The first one, right after arriving in the country (T1), to serve as the control of the students behaviour; the second, 4 months after and still during the exchange programs duration (T2); and the third 4 months past their return home (T3).

During preprocessing, some refinements to standardize the database and culling of irrelevant attributes were done. Firstly, attributes that were BYAACQ affirmations were excluded. Students that did not select an European country of origin or destination were excluded to reduce cultural differences alongside those that did not answer all BYAACQ in the 3 waves. Secondly, the attributes were renamed to include the domain of the questions, as defined by the creators of the questionnaire [17]. At the end of the process, 263 objects and 72 attributes, 24 per wave, remained.

The low support value comes mostly from the high number of participants who had reported little to no consequences of alcohol abuse, which resulted in a sparse context.

5.1 Scenarios Description

The triadic rules may be categorized in situations that describe the inference relation of a given consequence in different time periods (BCAAR) and the inference relation between consequences in the same wave (BACAR).

Scenarios 1 to 4 are based on BCAAR rules and scenarios 5 to 6 on BACAR rules. A, B, C are attributes (consequences) and T1, T2, T3 refer to the waves 1 to 3. Scenario 5 illustrates the profile of a student who has just arrived, before any change. Scenario 6 does so for the student that is in the process of change, during the exchange program.

- **Scenario 1:** Relationship between the consequences selected on host country arrival as well as during the exchange program.

$$(T1 \rightarrow T2)_C \tag{1}$$

$$(T2 \rightarrow T1)_C \tag{2}$$

- **Scenario 2:** Relationship between the selected consequences during the exchange program as well as after returning.

$$(T2 \rightarrow T3)_C \tag{3}$$

$$(T3 \rightarrow T2)_C \tag{4}$$

- **Scenario 3:** Relationship between the selected consequences on host country arrival as well as after returning.

$$(T1 \rightarrow T3)_C \tag{5}$$

$$(T3 \rightarrow T1)_C \tag{6}$$

- **Scenario 4:** Relationship between the selected consequences in all three waves, on host country arrival , during the exchange program and after returning.

$$(T1 \rightarrow T2)_C \tag{7}$$

$$(T2 \rightarrow T3)_C \tag{8}$$

$$(T1 \rightarrow T3)_C \tag{9}$$

- **Scenario 5:** Relationship between the selected consequences on host country arrival. (Behavior prior to exchange program)

$$(A \rightarrow B)_{T1} \tag{10}$$

$$(B \rightarrow A)_{T1} \tag{11}$$

– **Scenario 6:** Relationship between the selected consequences during program duration. (Behavior during the exchange program)

$$(A \rightarrow B)_{T2} \tag{12}$$

$$(B \rightarrow A)_{T2} \tag{13}$$

Using these scenarios to group up found triadic rules, it is possible to discover the impact exchange programs have on alcohol consumption habits from the reported consequences. As such, it is possible to visualize the initial state of the student, their state during the exchange program and the temporal relations of their reported consequences.

5.2   Experiments and Results

The generated rules were observed in multiple distinct scenarios. All the found attributes have been described in Table 3, as well as the meaning of each category (Table 4). In scenarios 5 and 6, rules with higher confidence were selected (Table 5).

Table 3. Variables seen in extracted rules.

Waves	
T1	Before exchange program
T2	During exchange program
T3	After exchange program
Attributes	
BLK1	I've gotten hungover (headaches, nausea) in the morning after having consumed alcohol in excessive amounts
BLK2	I wasn't capable of remembering my actions, during long time periods after excess consumption
BLK3	I've felt very nauseated or vomited after having consumed alcohol in excessive amounts
CON1	I've drunk excessively on nights I didn't plan on drinking
RISK1	I've taken stupid risks when drinking excessively
SELFC1	I've felt low on energy or tired after drinking excessively
SOC1	When drinking excessively, I've said or done embarrassing things

In every scenario, the attribute that refers to getting hungover (BLK1) had the largest support, which leads to the conclusion that it is the most common consequence within the students who consumed alcohol during the whole study.

Table 4. Meaning of each category.

Category	Frequency in the last 30 days
1	0
2	1–2
3	3–5
4	6–9
5	10–19
6	20–39
7	40+

Table 5. Generated rules.

Scenario	Rules
1	6
2	2
3	2
4	3
5	12
6	19

Scenario 1.

$$(T1 \to T2)_{BLK1} [sup = 50.4\%, conf = 84.1\%] \tag{14}$$

$$(T2 \to T1)_{BLK1} [sup = 50.4\%, conf = 75.8\%] \tag{15}$$

$$(T1 \to T2)_{SELFC1} [sup = 35.1\%, conf = 75.9\%] \tag{16}$$

$$(T2 \to T1)_{SELFC1} [sup = 35.1\%, conf = 67.5\%] \tag{17}$$

$$(T1 \to T2)_{SOC1} [sup = 20.2\%, conf = 67.1\%] \tag{18}$$

$$(T2 \to T1)_{SOC1} [sup = 20.2\%, conf = 64.5\%] \tag{19}$$

Being hungover (BLK1), reported before (T1) and during (T2) the exchange program was the rule with the most support and with a drop in confidence from T1 $\to$ T2 (14) to T2 $\to$ T1 (15). This shows that there was a higher number of students who had gotten hungover during the exchange program that had not before, suggesting an increase of this consequence during the stay in the host country. The other consequences follow the same pattern. We can conclude there was an overall increase in the alcohol consumption between the period before and during the exchange program.

Scenario 2.

$$(T3 \rightarrow T2)_{BLK1}[sup = 29.8\%, conf = 58.5\%] \tag{20}$$

$$(T2 \rightarrow T3)_{BLK1}[sup = 29.8\%, conf = 44.7\%] \tag{21}$$

Scenario 3.

$$(T3 \rightarrow T1)_{BLK1}[sup = 28.5\%, conf = 56.1\%] \tag{22}$$

$$(T1 \rightarrow T3)_{BLK1}[sup = 28.5\%, conf = 47.6\%] \tag{23}$$

Scenarios 2 and 3 had similar rules, with the former rules showing that people got hungover more frequently during the exchange program than after it (T3) (20), this reaffirms the finding of scenario 1 about the increase in alcohol consumption during the exchange program, and suggests that this increase was temporary, as the amount of alcohol consumed went down after going back to their home countries. Scenario 3 reinforces this by showing that most students who suffered consequences of alcohol abuse after the exchange program, already suffered from the same consequences prior to it, indicating their habits already existed before the program.

Scenario 4.

$$(T3, T1 \rightarrow T2)_{BLK1}[sup = 23.1\%, conf = 81.2\%] \tag{24}$$

$$(T2, T3 \rightarrow T1)_{BLK1}[sup = 23.1\%, conf = 77.8\%] \tag{25}$$

$$(T2, T1 \rightarrow T3)_{BLK1}[sup = 23.1\%, conf = 45.9\%] \tag{26}$$

Almost one fourth of the students got hungover in the three waves and each of the rules brings one important information, (7) suggests that alcohol consumption for 81.2% of students that got hungover in the 3 waves were not affected by the exchange program, (8) shows that for 22.2% of the students, the exchange program has stimulated a new habit and finally (9) demonstrates that 54.1% of the students who got hungover did not after the exchange program, reaffirming the decline in drinking habits.

Scenario 5.

$$(SELFC1 \rightarrow BLK1)_{T1}[sup = 38.8\%, conf = 93.9\%] \tag{27}$$

$$(SOC1 \rightarrow BLK1)_{T1}[sup = 24.8\%, conf = 82.2\%] \tag{28}$$

$$(CON1 \rightarrow BLK1)_{T1}[sup = 24.4\%, conf = 75.6\%] \tag{29}$$

$$(T2 \rightarrow BLK1)_{T1}[sup = 20.7\%, conf = 90.9\%] \tag{30}$$

$$(SOC1 \rightarrow SELFC1)_{T1}[sup = 20.2\%, conf = 67.1\%] \tag{31}$$

$$(CON1 \rightarrow SELFC1)_{T1}[sup = 20.2\%, conf = 62.8\%] \tag{32}$$

These rules indicate that getting hungover is the most common consequence in this scenario, since it is already included in rules with the largest support and its confidence is around 83%. Tiredness or lack of energy (SELFC1) comes in second place and had a drop of approximately 18% in confidence.

Getting hungover, tiredness, lack of energy, social humiliation (SOC1), drinking outside planned occasions (CON1) and nausea or vomiting (BLK3) were the most common consequences prior to the exchange program. Their relationships are represented in Fig. 1, with arrows being the stronger incidents and the dotted arrows the weaker ones.

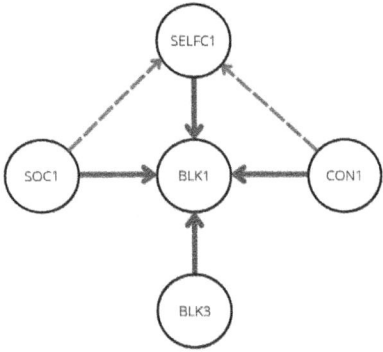

Fig. 1. Representation of Scenario 5.

Scenario 6.

$$(SELFC1 \rightarrow BLK1)_{T2}[sup = 44.6\%, conf = 85.7\%] \tag{33}$$

$$(CON1 \rightarrow BLK1)_{T2}[sup = 33.1\%, conf = 85.1\%] \tag{34}$$

$$(BLK3 \rightarrow BLK1)_{T2}[sup = 27.3\%, conf = 94.3\%] \tag{35}$$

$$(SOC1 \rightarrow BLK1)_{T2}[sup = 27.3\%, conf = 86.8\%] \tag{36}$$

$$(CON1 \rightarrow SELFC1)_{T2}[sup = 26.9\%, conf = 69.1\%] \tag{37}$$

$$(\text{SELFC1}, \text{CON1} \rightarrow \text{BLK1})_{T2}[\sup = 24.0\%, \text{conf} = 89.2\%] \qquad (38)$$

$$(\text{BLK2} \rightarrow \text{BLK1})_{T2}[\sup = 23.6\%, \text{conf} = 95.0\%] \qquad (39)$$

$$(\text{SOC1} \rightarrow \text{SELFC1})_{T2}[\sup = 22.3\%, \text{conf} = 71.1\%] \qquad (40)$$

$$(\text{RISK1} \rightarrow \text{BLK1})_{T2}[\sup = 21.9\%, \text{conf} = 89.8\%] \qquad (41)$$

In scenario 6, there was an increase of rules and larger variety of consequences reported, which indicates a general increase in alcohol consumption by the students. Getting hungover, tiredness or lack of energy have maintained themselves as the most common and the inference relation between them still is the strongest of these rules (12), reaffirming the consensus that getting hungover may cause lack of energy. The consequences of the period before the exchange program reappeared (including their relations) and there was an increase of two more incidences: memory loss (BLK2) (39) and "stupid" risk taking (RISK1) (41). Approximately one fourth of the students got hungover, drank too much unexpectedly and has felt tired (38). Note that there is a closer relationship between these three items as shown in Fig. 2.

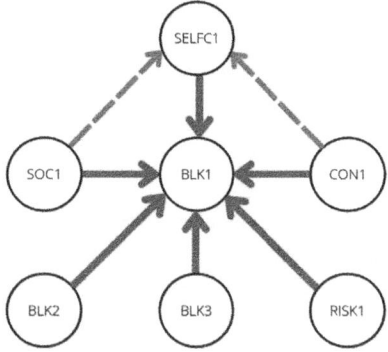

Fig. 2. Representation of Scenario 6.

Using the data from the database, the BYAACQ score was calculated per wave. BYAACQ scores each reported item as worth a point and the total score goes from 0 to 24. Figure 3 represents the amount students as the y-axis, their respective scores as the x-axis and their waves as colors. Note that during the exchange program there was a smaller number of students with 0 consequences of alcohol use, a significant increase in the 4 and 9 scores and was the only wave with a score larger than 20 consequences suffered (22 score). We can also observe that while the waves had their scores concentrated in the lower half of the total score, the consumption of alcohol during the program made this wave get many scores above the half mark.

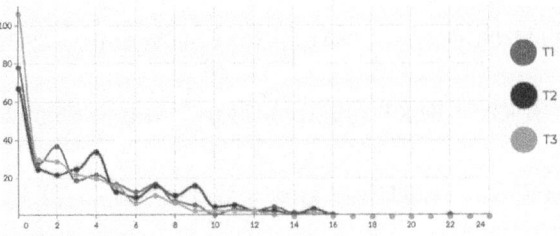

Fig. 3. BYAAC score distribution in the three waves.

This increase in alcohol usage may also be seen analysing other attributes chosen from the database after preprocessing, with the exception of the exclusion of columns that were not BYAACQ. The data referring to binge drinking in the last 30 days was restored and also the occasion in which the students were drunk. Immoderate consumption was defined as 5 or more cups in a row for men and 4 cups or more in a row for women. Drunkenness was defined as, for example, stumbling while walking, forgetting how to speak or of situations that had happened and vomiting. Figure 4 has students in the y-axis, binge drinking frequency (per the last 30 days) as the x-axis and waves as colors, respecting the same coloring scheme as Fig. 3. Alongside it, Fig. 5 also has students in the y-axis, with drunkeness frequency (per the last 30 days) as the x-axis and waves as colors, the same coloring scheme as the previous graphs.

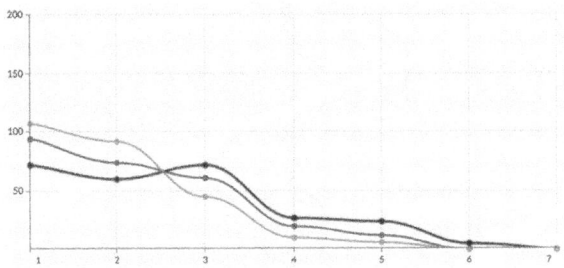

Fig. 4. Binge drinking frequency.

There was an inversion in binge drinking. In drunkenness, there was different in behaviour during the exchange program (T2) when compared to prior (T2) and after (T3) it, whose behavior was both similar to each other.

Finally, to validate the discoveries, Rasch models and their respective Wright Maps [6] were generated. Attributes such as infit and outfits outside the 0 to 60 range and 1 to 40 range were removed [14], resulting in some models having more attributes than others.

Rasch analysis generated a severity scale of which question based on the data it receives. In this study, the severity scale indicated which consequences are considered

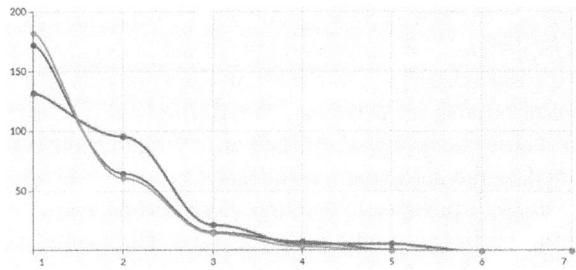

Fig. 5. Drunkenness frequency.

light and which are considered severe based on the idea that if a person reported a grave consequence (G), they also reported light ones (L). The contrary does not necessarily happen. The IF-THEN expression results in (G → L).

This correlation inter items is not explicitly given. The items are mapped alongside the scale in a way that every consequence with severity x has great probability of being reported alongside others with lower severity than x. As an example, people who drank outside planning (CON1) are very likely to have also suffered from tiredness (SELFC1) and an even larger chance that they got hungover (BLK1).

The information obtained by the Rasch models is explicitly verified by the triadic rules generated. Observing the confidence scores of rules in Scenario 6, in (34) and (37), it is possible to observe that both bring the same information, but TCA allowed for a higher precision in probability and a easier to interpret format than the Wright Maps, possibly being more accessible to people without statistical knowledge.

6   Conclusions

This paper employs FCA, a novel method for examining driving behaviors from a large database, with features that allow the application of this method grounded in the theoretical framework of the "Mindsponge Theory". This approach is not commonly utilized in the field of intelligent transportation and road safety research.

The association of rules demonstrates characteristics of aggressive behaviors associated with external factors such as family and friends. It can be inferred that this is an important factor in a driver's decision-making and may be a crucial factor in whether or not accidents occur. These rules can be generalized to the Chinese socio-cultural context, and efforts can be made to understand the primary reasons why this problem occurs.

On the other hand, it becomes difficult to accurately characterize more specific individual aspects due to subjectivity and bias involved in self-reported survey data.

We had a geographical scope limitation as the dataset only includes data from Chinese drivers which may limit the generalizability of our research findings. So, for future work, it will be necessary to explore different scenarios and use different tools to expand this analysis from the Chinese socio-cultural context to a more general context, seeking implications that can lead to better understanding of the causes of traffic accidents.

This article also shown one use for triadic rules in the field of early alcoholism detection in university students with focus on the effect of exchange programs on pre-existing habits. Using the extracted triadic rules, it was a possible to define relevant scenarios for observation of changes between prior, during and posterior behavior in the exchange program. These changes were tracked observing the consequences of alcohol consumption reported by the participating students.

The rules have made it possible to see that there was an increase in consumption of alcohol during the exchange program, but it did not last after returning to home country. These hypothesis were confirmed from other collected variables. Therefore, a monitoring program to check on students in these situations may be beneficial, as the change may be a reflection of deeper issues, such as decline in mental health (depression or stress for example), social pressure or simply hedonism from the student, who may pose risk to themselves and others around them.

In future works, it would be possible for TCA to be applied on measurement and efficacy of such a project in practice.

The results have shown the potential of triadic rules to extract knowledge in longitudinal studies, in the social sciences field. The explicable nature of the rules make it more friendly to people without extensive statistical knowledge, as it is not necessary to interpret the rules. However, it is necessary that the rules and metrics are understood, there is still a need to preprocess the data, and the choice of minimum acceptable value and attributes must be made carefully in the process of inference creation, since the rules may lead to hasty, meaningless conclusions.

Acknowledgements. The present work was carried out with the support of Fundação de Amparo á Pesquisa do Estado de Minas Gerais (FAPEMIG) under grant number APQ-01929-22. The authors thank CNPq, the Pontifícia Universidade Católica de Minas Gerais – PUC-Minas and Coordenação de Aperfeiçoamento de Pessoal de Nível Superior – CAPES – (Grant PROAP 88887.842889/2023-00 – PUC/MG, Grant PDPG 88887.708960/2022-00 – PUC/MG - INFORMÁTICA and Finance Code 001).

References

1. Aresi, G., Moore, S., Marta, E.: The health behaviours of European study abroad students sampled from forty-two countries: data from a three-wave longitudinal study. Data Brief **38**, 107285 (2021). https://doi.org/10.1016/j.dib.2021.107285
2. Babbie, E.: The Practice of Social Research, 14th edn. CENGAGE Learning Custom Publishing, Mason (2014)
3. Bewick, B.M., Mulhern, B., Barkham, M., Trusler, K., Hill, A.J., Stiles, W.B.: Changes in undergraduate student alcohol consumption as they progress through university. BMC Public Health **8**, 163 (2008)
4. Biedermann, K.: How triadic diagrams represent conceptual structures. In: Lukose, D., Delugach, H., Keeler, M., Searle, L., Sowa, J. (eds.) ICCS-ConceptStruct 1997. LNCS, vol. 1257, pp. 304–317. Springer, Heidelberg (1997). https://doi.org/10.1007/BFb0027879
5. Felde, M., Stumme, G.: Triadic exploration and exploration with multiple experts. Knowledge & Data Engineering Group, University of Kassel, Germany (2023)
6. Florentino, P.I.A., et al.: Modelo rasch: introdução, simulação e estimaaçãoo (2017). https://editorarealize.com.br/artigo/visualizar/28624. Accessed 18 Feb 2024

7. Frees, E.W.: Longitudinal and Panel Data. Cambridge University Press, Cambridge (2004)
8. Ganter, B., Obiedkov, S.: Implications in triadic formal contexts. In: Wolff, K.E., Pfeiffer, H.D., Delugach, H.S. (eds.) ICCS-ConceptStruct 2004. LNCS (LNAI), vol. 3127, pp. 186–195. Springer, Heidelberg (2004). https://doi.org/10.1007/978-3-540-27769-9_12
9. Houston, J.M., Harris, P.B., Norman, M.: The aggressive driving behavior scale: developing a self-report measure of unsafe driving practices. N. Am. J. Psychol. **5**, 193–202 (2003). https://doi.org/10.0000/0000-0002-3734-788X
10. Hurlbut, S.C., Sher, K.J.: Assessing alcohol problems in college students. J. Am. Coll. Health **41**(2), 49–58 (1992)
11. Jin, R., Wang, X., Nguyen, M.H., La, V.P., Le, T.T., Vuong, Q.H.: A dataset of Chinese drivers' driving behaviors and socio-cultural factors related to driving. Data Brief **49**, 109337 (2023). https://doi.org/10.1016/j.dib.2023.109337, https://www.sciencedirect.com/science/article/pii/S2352340923004559
12. Kahler, C., Strong, D., Read, J.: Toward efficient and comprehensive measurement of the alcohol problems continuum in college students: the brief young adult alcohol consequences questionnaire. Alcohol. Clin. Exp. Res. **29**, 1180–1189 (2005). https://doi.org/10.1097/01.ALC.0000171940.95813.A5
13. Lehmann, F.,Wille, R.: A triadic approach to formal concept analysis. In: International Conference on Conceptual Structures (1995). https://api.semanticscholar.org/CorpusID:5577535
14. Linacre, J.M., Heinemann, A.W., Wright, B.D., Granger, C.V., Hamilton, B.B.: The structure and stability of the functional independence measure. Arch. Phys. Med. Rehabil. **75**(2), 127–132 (1994)
15. Mendes, H.F.V., Nobre, C.N., Song, M.A.J., Zárate, L.E.: Analisando um estudo longitudinal para tratamento do parkinson via regras triádicas. J. Health Inform. **14**(Especial) (2022). https://jhi.sbis.org.br/index.php/jhi-sbis/article/view/969
16. Miranda, D., Zárate, L., Song, M.: Application of formal concept analysis to characterize driving behaviors and socio-cultural factors related to driving (2024). https://doi.org/10.5220/0012335000003657
17. Neves, J., Ananias, K., Nobre, C., Zárate, L., Song, M.: Applying binary decision diagram to extract concepts from triadic formal context, pp. 466–469 (2020). https://doi.org/10.1145/3341105.3374086
18. Noronha, M.D.M., Nobre, C.N., Song, M.A.J., Zárate, L.E.: Interpreting the human longevity profile through triadic rules - a case study based on the ELSA-UK longitudinal study. Stud. Health Technol. Inform. **290**, 782–786 (2022)
19. Read, J.P., Kahler, C.W., Strong, D.R., Colder, C.R.: Development and preliminary validation of the young adult alcohol consequences questionnaire. J. Stud. Alcohol **67**(1), 169–177 (2006)
20. Stidham, M., Olsen, C., Toman, E., Frederick, S., Mccaffrey, S., Shindler, B.: Longitudinal social science research in natural resource communities: lessons and considerations. Soc. Nat. Resour. **27** (2014). https://doi.org/10.1080/08941920.2014.905895
21. Wei, L., Qian, T., Wan, Q., Qi, J.: A research summary about triadic concept analysis. Int. J. Mach. Learn. Cybern. **9**(4), 699–712 (2016). https://doi.org/10.1007/s13042-016-0599-7
22. Yang, J., Du, F., Qu, W., Gong, Z., Sun, X.: Effects of personality on risky driving behavior and accident involvement for Chinese drivers. Traffic Inj. Prev. **14**(6), 565–571 (2013). https://doi.org/10.1080/15389588.2012.748903

Combining Languages to Set a PACS on FHIR

Sébastien Jodogne[(⊠)][iD]

Computer Science and Engineering Department (INGI), Institute of Information
and Communication Technologies, Electronics and Applied Mathematics (ICTEAM),
UCLouvain, 1348 Louvain-la-Neuve, Belgium
`sebastien.jodogne@uclouvain.be`
`https://perso.uclouvain.be/sebastien.jodogne/`

Abstract. FHIR has quickly emerged as a crucial standard for the interoperability of clinical data. While FHIR supports medical imaging through its `ImagingStudy` resource, the absence of openly available software combining FHIR with DICOM limits the development of applications linking clinical and imaging data. On another front, deep learning applied to medical imaging is becoming increasingly popular, and it is essential to educate a broad audience about its possibilities. However, the current lack of open, easy-to-use environments capable of executing a library of open-access models directly on DICOM images and on a standard computer poses an issue from a pedagogical perspective. In this paper, the Orthanc server is presented as a promising solution to both challenges. Plugins are developed to enable Orthanc to call software libraries written in the Java and Python programming languages. These plugins are then used to turn Orthanc into a FHIR server using the HAPI framework, as well as into a platform for running the inference of a deep learning model for breast imaging using either PyTorch or Deep Java Library. The resulting source code is released as free and open-source software, aiming to promote support for medical imaging in FHIR, to share technological knowledge about medical interoperability and deep learning, and to provide a test environment for the integration of imaging data into clinical workflows.

Keywords: Medical imaging · FHIR · DICOM · Java · Python · Deep learning

1 Introduction

Healthcare interoperability refers to the ability of different medical systems, software, and devices to communicate and exchange data effectively and efficiently [4]. Healthcare interoperability is critical for patient-centered care and for continuity of care because patient information is typically spread over multiple software entities, such as electronic health records, hospital information system, laboratory information system, or pharmacy information system, possibly across different hospitals and different general practitioners. Healthcare interoperability is also becoming increasingly important because of the growing interest in telemedicine, in tele-expertise, in patient empowerment, and in artificial intelligence.

© The Author(s), under exclusive license to Springer Nature Switzerland AG 2026
M. P. Guarino et al. (Eds.): BIOSTEC 2024, CCIS 2546, pp. 314–334, 2026.
https://doi.org/10.1007/978-3-031-96899-0_18

Many healthcare interoperability standards have emerged over the years. In the context of medical imaging, DICOM (*Digital Imaging and Communications in Medicine*) has been the *de facto* international standard for the encoding, transmission, storage, and sharing of digital images since 1985 [21]. In the typical clinical workflow, imaging modalities create DICOM instances that are collected on a central PACS server (*Picture Archiving and Communication System*), which in turn provides features for the viewing and distribution of the collected medical images. DICOM is adopted by any hospital in the world for the management of digital images, and its recent DICOMweb extensions have progressively introduced REST APIs (*Representational State Transfer Application Programming Interfaces*) for medical imaging since the 2010s.

Thanks to the availability of DICOM as an open standard, many free and open-source software libraries dedicated to medical imaging have been created. When developing a desktop or a back-end application, the choice of a software library is primarily guided by the programming language used by the development team. Java developers will typically choose dcm4che [28], Python developers will use pydicom [19], while C++ developers will rely on DCMTK [9]. Beyond these general-purpose libraries that handle the DICOM file format and network protocol, specialized libraries focused on the rendering and processing of medical images have also been developed. For instance, the C++ libraries VTK [24] and ITK [20] are commonly used in software applications that display and analyze medical images. The alignment of medical images is a specific field of research, which has led to the development of Plastimatch, also written in C++ [25]. In radiation therapy and nuclear medicine, the Python library dicompyler offers a research platform dedicated to processing the DICOM RT substandard [22]. Finally, developers of deep learning applications for medical imaging commonly rely on libraries written in Python, such as TensorFlow [1] and PyTorch [15].

Besides DICOM, another healthcare interoperability standard is currently attracting increasingly more attention. FHIR (*Fast Healthcare Interoperability Resources*) is an international, modern standard for exchanging clinical information electronically [3]. FHIR is actively developed as an open specification by the HL7 International organization and is released in the public domain under the Creative Commons CC0 license. The original proposal for FHIR was released in 2011, its first draft version (referred to as DSTU1, which stands for *First Draft Standard for Trial Use*) was published in 2014, and its first normative content (called R4—*Release 4*) appeared in 2019. At the time of writing, the current version of FHIR is R5 (*Release 5*), which was issued in March 2023.

FHIR is based on a set of standardized resources, which represent discrete pieces of healthcare data, such as patients, medications, allergies, or observations. These resources act as building blocks that can be combined to represent complex clinical concepts and workflows. FHIR employs REST APIs to access and manipulate these resources. The fact that REST APIs are widely used for the development of Web and mobile applications explains the growing popularity of FHIR among software engineers. FHIR also fully embraces existing medical terminologies such as SNOMED-CT and LOINC, which enables semantic interoperability, ensuring that healthcare data is understood consistently across different systems and organizations. The most complete implementation of the FHIR standard is the HAPI framework [2]. HAPI closely follows the release cycle of the FHIR standard. It can be used as a building block to design both FHIR clients and FHIR servers. HAPI is free and open-source software that is written in the Java programming language.

Due to the universal adoption of DICOM by hospitals, researchers, and vendors, FHIR does not attempt to introduce a new competing standard for medical imaging. Instead, FHIR defines the ImagingStudy resource as its official method for connecting clinical and imaging data. The ImagingStudy resource does not store all the DICOM tag values or pixel data. Instead, it uses the DICOMweb API to reference DICOM entities stored on a separate PACS server. Unfortunately, there is currently a lack of open, reference implementation combining FHIR with DICOM. While public implementations of ImagingStudy do exist, such as those found in HAPI and available in public FHIR test sandboxes, their content is not linked to an actual DICOMweb endpoint. The availability of a DICOM server implementing both the DICOMweb and the FHIR REST APIs could hopefully promote the support of medical imaging in FHIR, while providing a testing environment for the development of new applications combining clinical with imaging data.

In addition, as discussed above, a complex application that processes medical images according to standard-compliant workflows will presumably integrate multiple programming languages to benefit from different software libraries. For instance, adding FHIR support to a medical imaging application will likely involve using Java, while deploying an artificial intelligence algorithm will likely involve using Python. The typical software architecture therefore consists in implementing multiple microservices written in different languages that operate alongside each other, each dedicated to the handling of a part of the processing pipeline. These services can then be encapsulated as containers and orchestrated using technologies like Docker Swarm or Kubernetes. This approach is perfectly adapted if creating a proprietary platform with a professional team dedicated to its administration and maintenance. It is less suitable if developing a desktop or back-end application that needs to be deployed in a less controlled environment or where users have less expertise in system administration.

The contributions of this paper are threefold. Firstly, a free and open-source PACS server supporting DICOMweb and written in C++ is extended to incorporate the capability of invoking plugins written in Java or Python. This allows software integrators to choose the programming language (C++, Java, or Python) that is best suited for calling an existing software library for medical imaging. Python plugins are especially adapted to automate imaging workflows. Secondly, it is demonstrated how a Java plugin can be created to integrate with HAPI, allowing the PACS server to serve the parts of the REST API of FHIR related to medical imaging in addition to the DICOMweb endpoint. Because these software modules are running in the same process, the FHIR resources are guaranteed to remain continuously synchronized with the DICOM instances. Thirdly, it is shown how both Java and Python plugins can execute deep learning inference directly on the DICOM instances stored by the PACS server. The Java plugin is proven to be particularly well-suited for simplifying the deployment of deep learning models by distributing the deep learning inference engine as a single .jar archive. The preliminary version of this paper that appeared in the Proceedings of the 17th International Joint Conference on Biomedical Engineering Systems and Technologies (BIOSTEC 2024) introduced the Java plugin together with the FHIR server [14]. This extended version introduces the Python plugin and the deep learning applications.

2   Background

This section reviews the various building blocks that will be combined to introduce a PACS server compatible with multiple programming languages. It successively describes the Orthanc server, the DICOM model of the real world, the `ImagingStudy` resource of the FHIR standard, and the HAPI framework.

2.1   Orthanc Server

In the context of medical imaging, multiple free and open-source PACS servers are available, such as dcm4chee [28] and Dicoogle [8]. This work is focused on the Orthanc PACS server, which is licensed under the GPLv3 license and is developed in the C++ programming language [12]. Besides its native DICOM primitives, Orthanc comes with a REST API that can be used to script imaging workflows, which is widely used to set up auto-routing between local DICOM servers or between remote sites. This REST API can be used to search the content of the DICOM database and to retrieve the content of individual DICOM resources, which will be used in this work. Orthanc has the advantage of being lightweight, cross-platform, and extensible: Multiple Orthanc servers can run on any computer at low cost, without necessitating any complex configuration.

Very importantly, Orthanc proposes a plugin mechanism that can be used to extend its core features using the C language. An Orthanc plugin takes the form of a shared library (i.e., a `.so` file under GNU/Linux distributions or a DLL under Microsoft Windows). Plugins notably have full access to the REST API of Orthanc and can add new routes to this REST API. The fact that Orthanc plugins can extend the REST API of Orthanc has already been used to provide an implementation of the DICOMweb standard [12], as well as to integrate popular Web viewers such as OHIF [30] and Kitware VolView [29]. In this work, the extensibility of Orthanc will be utilized to seamlessly integrate it with the Java and Python computer languages, providing a way to efficiently design processing pipelines that can be deployed on any computer by leveraging the small footprint of Orthanc.

2.2   DICOM Model of the Real World

To understand the connection between DICOM and FHIR, it is essential to comprehend how the DICOM specification organizes the medical imaging resources. In this so-called "DICOM model of the real world", a patient benefits from a sequence of imaging studies during his or her life. Each of these studies consists of a set of series. In turn, each series is made of a set of DICOM instances that are created by the same imaging device. An isolated DICOM instance can often (but not always) be thought of as one 2D image slice that is associated with a dataset providing patient-related and acquisition-related information that enriches the pixel data. This dataset is a tree-like structure that associates values to standardized DICOM tags, identified by a pair of hexadecimal numbers. For instance, a DICOM study generated by a PET-CT-scanner would typically correspond to a set of two DICOM series (representing the PET volume and the CT volume), with the two series encoded as a set of DICOM instances that contain the individual 2D axial slices of the parent 3D volume.

Each resource in the patient/study/series/instance hierarchy is identified by one specific DICOM tag. The patient level is identified by the value of the "*Patient ID*" (0x0010, 0x0020) DICOM tag, the study level by the "*Study Instance UID*" (0x0020, 0x000d) tag, the series level by the "*Series Instance UID*" (0x0020, 0x000e) tag, and finally the instance level by the "*SOP Instance UID*" (0x0008, 0x0018) tag. While the UIDs (*Unique IDentifiers*) at the study, series, and instance levels are assumed to be globally unique, the "*Patient ID*" tag is only locally unique within an institution, which necessitates reconciliation in multi-centric contexts. PACS systems typically use the values of these four important DICOM tags to index the DICOM resources in a relational database. The basic structure of the REST API of Orthanc is directly mapped on this four-level DICOM model of the real world. The DICOMweb substandard, for its part, organizes its REST API using only the globally unique identifiers at the study, series, and instance levels.

2.3   FHIR for Medical Imaging

FHIR brings support for medical imaging through its ImagingStudy resource. The ImagingStudy resource includes the globally unique identifiers of DICOM resources, along with minimal information about their content. This allows linking patient data stored in the FHIR server to a separate DICOMweb server that is responsible for the actual storage of the medical images. Consequently, the ImagingStudy resource can be thought of as a higher-level service on the top of DICOMweb. ImagingStudy is associated with maturity level 4 in FHIR R5. This maturity level indicates that ImagingStudy has been implemented in multiple prototype projects, hereby showing a certain level of stability. Nonetheless, this also means that the resource has been implemented in less than five independent production systems, or in no more than one country yet. This fact reinforces the interest in developing an open implementation of ImagingStudy to raise the maturity level of the associated part of the FHIR standard.

The main content of the ImagingStudy resource is depicted in Fig. 1. One instance of this FHIR resource corresponds to one DICOM study. To create the link between the ImagingStudy resource and its associated DICOM study, the identifier field of the FHIR resource must contain the value of the "*Study Instance UID*" DICOM tag. This is because FHIR does not store the images, but rather pointers to DICOM resources. The DICOM resources themselves must be stored in a separate DICOMweb-compliant server, the address of which must be provided in the endpoint field. The latter field contains a reference to a separate Endpoint FHIR resource that specifies the connection parameters to the DICOMweb server, including its URL. If needed, the referenced DICOM instances can be retrieved or ren-

Name	Flags	Card.	Type	Description & Constraints
ImagingStudy	TU		DomainResource	A set of images produced in single study (one or more series of references images)
				Elements defined in Ancestors: id, meta, implicitRules, language, text, contained, extension, modifierExtension
identifier	Σ	0..*	Identifier	Identifiers for the whole study
status	?! Σ	1..1	code	registered | available | cancelled | entered-in-error | unknown Binding: Imaging Study Status (Required)
modality	Σ	0..*	CodeableConcept	All of the distinct values for series' modalities Binding: Modality ⬀ (Extensible)
subject	Σ	1..1	Reference(Patient | Device | Group)	Who or what is the subject of the study
referrer	Σ	0..1	Reference(Practitioner | PractitionerRole)	Referring physician
endpoint	Σ	0..*	Reference(Endpoint)	Study access endpoint
numberOfSeries	Σ	0..1	unsignedInt	Number of Study Related Series
numberOfInstances	Σ	0..1	unsignedInt	Number of Study Related Instances
description	Σ	0..1	string	Institution-generated description

Fig. 1. Excerpt of the main structure of the `ImagingStudy` resource in FHIR R5 (Figure from [14]). For each field in the resource, the "Card." column indicates its cardinality, and the "Type" column indicates the data type of its values. Fields whose minimum cardinality is 1 are mandatory. This is a screenshot of the official specification of FHIR available at: https://hl7.org/fhir/R5/ImagingStudy.html.

dered using the DICOMweb WADO-RS[1] service offered by the DICOMweb endpoint. Most existing public sandboxes for FHIR do not contain a working `endpoint` field, which prevents access to the content of the DICOM studies that are indexed by the `ImagingStudy` resources.

As can be seen in Fig. 1, besides the `Endpoint` and `ImagingStudy` resources, a FHIR server for medical imaging must also support the `Patient` resource, because the `subject` field is mandatory and must contain a reference to the patient who is associated with the DICOM study. Consequently, similarly to the one-to-one relation that exists between a FHIR `ImagingStudy` and a DICOM study, there exists a mapping between a `Patient` FHIR resource and a DICOM patient.

In addition to the patients and to the studies, FHIR for medical imaging also provides pointers to both the DICOM series and the DICOM instances. To this end, the `ImagingStudy` resource contains a field named `series`, as shown in Fig. 2. This field stores an array, each item of which declares one DICOM series whose "*Series Instance UID*" DICOM tag is contained in the `uid` subfield. In turn, each item in the `series` field contains a subarray called `instance` that provides the list of the DICOM instances of the parent series, in which the `uid` subfield indicates the "*SOP Instance UID*" DICOM tag of the individual instances. This means that, contrary to DICOM studies that are mapped as separate `ImagingStudy` resources, FHIR does not encode DICOM series and DICOM instances as standalone resources: The series or instance information can only be retrieved by accessing their parent study.

---

[1] The WADO acronym stands for "*Web Access to DICOM Objects,*" while RS stands for "*RESTful Service.*".

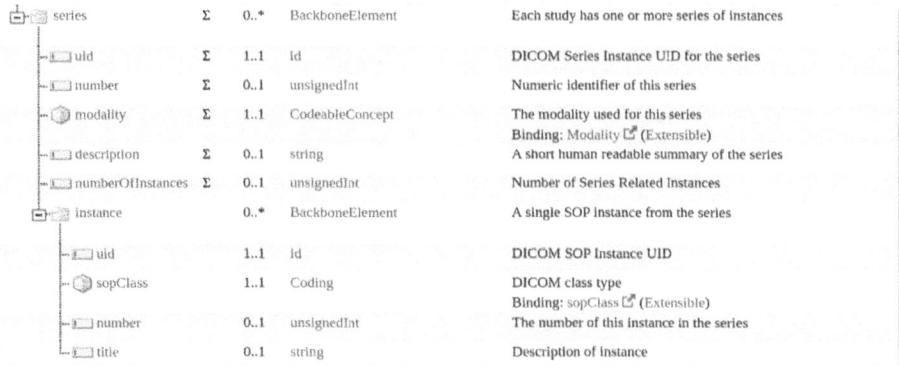

Fig. 2. Excerpt of the information to be provided in the `ImagingStudy` for each of its associated DICOM series (Figure from [14]). This screenshot is the continuation of Fig. 1 in the FHIR standard.

Figure 3 summarizes the relations between the DICOM and FHIR models of the real world. As can be observed in this figure, careful attention must be given to continuously updating FHIR resources, as the content of the FHIR server needs to be updated each time a new instance is added to or deleted from the DICOMweb server. This requires robust communication mechanisms between these two servers. In this work, we will adopt an approach where the `ImagingStudy` FHIR resources are not explicitly stored but are generated on-the-fly as needed by querying the content of the Orthanc server.

Previous research work about the `ImagingStudy` resource has consisted in providing static databases as pedagogical resources to learn FHIR for medical imaging [11], in deploying a multi-site infrastructure dedicated to pediatric scoliosis [26], in collecting radiation dose information [5], and in implementing complex clinical imaging workflows [27]. However, to the best of our knowledge, no free and open-source PACS server can currently act as a standalone FHIR server that transparently, automatically synchronizes with the DICOM resources it publishes using DICOMweb.

2.4 HAPI Framework

As explained in the Introduction, the HAPI framework proposes an implementation of the FHIR standard in the Java programming language. The HAPI framework can be used either as a software library for creating FHIR clients and servers, or as a fully-fledged FHIR server. Importantly, HAPI supports the `ImagingStudy` resource that is needed to implement medical imaging in FHIR. HAPI is licensed under the Apache Software License 2.0.

More precisely, when it comes to designing a FHIR server, the HAPI framework can be used in two distinct ways. On the one hand, the HAPI project provides the so-called "HAPI Plain Server" as a software library that can be used to create custom FHIR endpoints against arbitrary data sources. On the other hand, the "HAPI JPA Server" is a fully standalone application that incorporates JPA (*Java Persistence API*) to store and

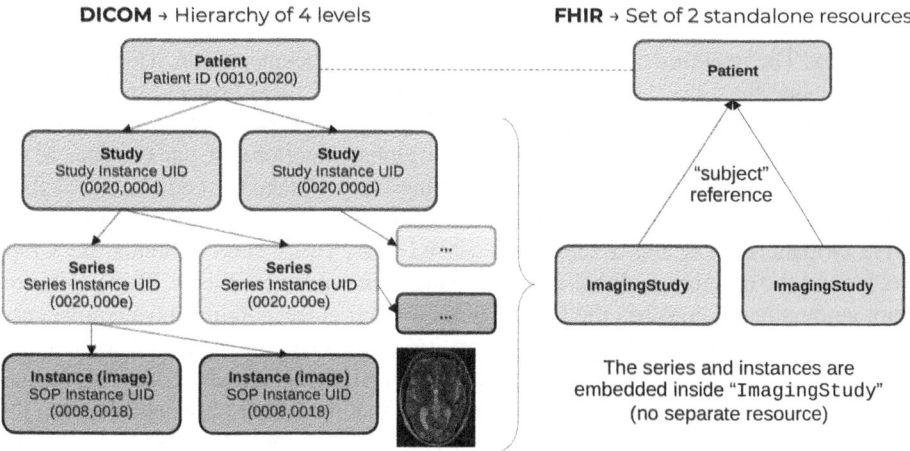

Fig. 3. Comparison between the DICOM and FHIR models of the real world.

retrieve FHIR resources in a relational database such as PostgreSQL. This paper will focus on the combination of the HAPI framework with the Orthanc server to provide a tight integration between FHIR and DICOM.

3   Methods

In this section, the software architecture that is used to create Java and Python plugins for Orthanc is first introduced. Then, the integration between Orthanc and HAPI is described.

3.1   Wrapping the Orthanc SDK in Java and Python

The Orthanc plugin SDK (*Software Development Kit*) proposes a large library of functions declared in a plain C header that can be used to invoke the various primitives implemented by the Orthanc core. For instance, the Orthanc plugin SDK allows registering callbacks to process incoming HTTP requests, which can be used to extend the built-in REST API of Orthanc. The SDK can also make internal calls to the built-in REST API, enabling a wide variety of operations. Consequently, it is essential for the Java and Python plugins to be able to call these native functions implemented by the Orthanc runtime.

To this end, this work introduces different Python scripts to automatically wrap the Orthanc plugin SDK as a collection of Java and Python classes. The first Python script analyzes the content of the `OrthancCPlugin.h` header that defines the Orthanc plugin SDK, then creates a code model that is saved in the JSON file format. This script detects all the global functions that are part of the Orthanc SDK and analyzes their signature. In addition, it automatically discovers the native objects that are published by the Orthanc core (such as DICOM instances, images, or responses to REST requests) and that are managed through C global functions defining their methods, constructors, and destructors. The resulting code model also contains the documentation. This analysis is achieved using the `libclang` library that is part of the LLVM project [16].

Once the code model is extracted, additional Python scripts are used to generate language-specific wrappers around the native global functions of the Orthanc SDK. These Python scripts depend upon the target language and take the code model as their input. If targeting Java, one separate `.java` class file is generated to encapsulate each native Orthanc object, and a separate `Functions.java` class contains the wrappers around the remaining global functions that do not manage objects. The generation script automatically converts the C data types to their corresponding Java equivalents. Each generated Java class belongs to the `be.uclouvain.orthanc` package and is enriched with a Javadoc-compliant documentation. All the wrapped methods are tagged using the `native` Java keyword, which indicates that the actual implementation of the method is not provided in Java. A separate Python script generates a single, large C++ source file called `NativeSDK.cpp` that contains the implementation of each of those `native` methods. This C++ code is responsible for first reading the content of the Java objects passed as arguments through JNI (*Java Native Interface*), then calling the concrete implementation provided by the Orthanc plugin SDK, and finally converting the possibly resulting C value as a Java data type (which may involve the creation of a Java wrapper around an object managed by Orthanc).

Another Python script has been developed based on the same principle if targeting the Python language. In the case of Python, there is no equivalent to the `native` keyword and it is not necessary to explicitly create standalone `.py` files. Indeed, the Python C API library (often referred to as `libpython`) provides the functionality for defining new Python classes and modules directly from C or C++ code. Therefore, our generation script takes the code model and produces a single C++ source file. This file first registers all the classes, methods, and global functions in a Python module named `orthanc`, and then associates each of them with a C++ native function. As in the case of Java, these native functions are in charge of reading the content of the Python objects passed as arguments through `libpython`, of calling the corresponding C primitives in the Orthanc SDK, and possibly of creating a result value as a Python object using `libpython` (again, this last step may involve the creation of a Python wrapper around an Orthanc object). One separate Python file called `orthanc.pyi` is also generated, which is a Python interface providing documentation and type hints for static type checking and auto-completion in an IDE (*Integrated Development Environment*).

The global generation process is represented in Fig. 4. Thanks to this automated mechanism, 122 functions from the Orthanc plugin SDK are automatically wrapped in the Java and Python languages, out of a total of 165 primitives available in Orthanc 1.10.0. This represents a coverage of about 74%. No human intervention is required, which would have been highly time-consuming and error-prone, especially when keeping up with new releases of the Orthanc SDK. Note that the extracted code model could be used to wrap the Orthanc plugin SDK in other programming languages beyond Java and Python.

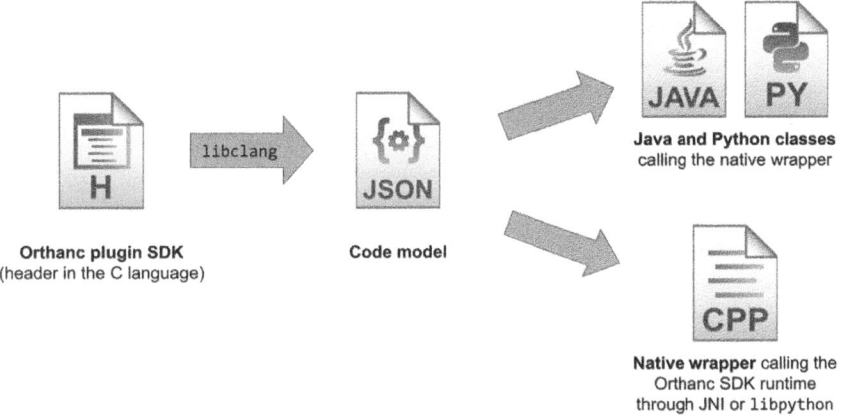

Fig. 4. Mapping the Orthanc SDK in the Java and Python languages. Python classes are not explicitly stored as standalone files but are directly registered using `libpython`.

The primitives that are not automatically wrapped mostly correspond to the registration of callbacks, which requires a manual implementation due to their language-specific nature. The most important example of a callback corresponds to the handling of HTTP requests received by the Web server of Orthanc, which can be used to add new routes in the REST API. Another example is the callback that is triggered when specific events occur in the Orthanc server, for instance when Orthanc starts or stops, or when a new DICOM instance is received. To deal with such situations, the Java and Python plugins register internal C functions as native callbacks using the Orthanc plugin SDK. Once one of these callback functions is invoked by the core of Orthanc, it uses either the JNI or `libpython` to call the corresponding Java callable or Python handler that were registered by the user.

The C++ code that is generated either for Java or Python is linked as a shared library that can be loaded as a plugin for Orthanc, as explained in Sect. 2.1. This shared library also contains code for configuring the plugin and for starting either a Java virtual machine (using JNI) or an embedded Python interpreter (using `libpython`). In the case of Java, the configuration specifies a user-defined Java class that is included in the Java classpath, enabling this class to install the Java callables that will handle the various events processed by Orthanc. Likewise, in Python, the configuration provides the filesystem path to a user-defined Python script that is responsible for registering handlers.

3.2   Integrating Orthanc and HAPI

This section describes how FHIR support can be added to Orthanc by integrating HAPI. Figure 5 depicts three possible high-level architectures to combine HAPI with Orthanc. The first architecture consists in executing the standalone HAPI JPA Server next to the Orthanc server, in two separate processes. In this architecture, a third process is used to continuously synchronize the content of the HAPI JPA server with Orthanc. To this end,

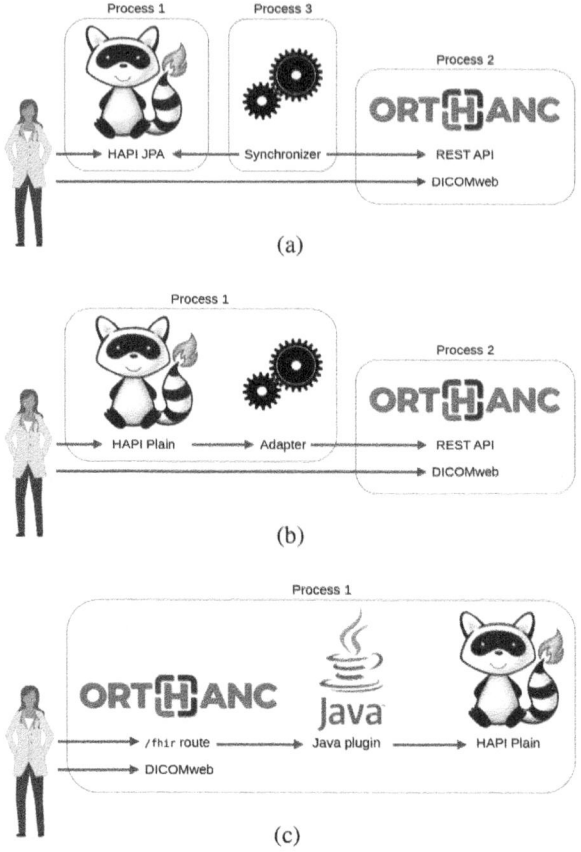

Fig. 5. Three possible architectures to integrate the Orthanc server with the HAPI framework: (a) continuous synchronization between Orthanc and the HAPI JPA Server, (b) custom HAPI Plain Server with a data source corresponding to Orthanc, or (c) branching HAPI Plain Server as a plugin to Orthanc (Figure from [14]).

the synchronization process monitors the addition and removal of DICOM resources using the REST API of Orthanc, and replicates the detected modifications in the HAPI JPA Server. In this architecture, the FHIR and DICOM databases are kept separate, which results in a substantial risk of de-synchronization between the two servers, and which requires a specific infrastructure dedicated to the execution of the JPA-compliant database.

The second possible architecture consists in replacing the standalone HAPI JPA Server by the HAPI Plain Server software library. In this architecture, a custom HAPI Plain Server is deployed in a standalone Java servlet container and acts as a facade in front of the Orthanc server. This facade is responsible for generating the `ImagingStudy` and `Patient` FHIR resources after querying the REST API of Orthanc. This solution has the great advantage of using a single database that is shared by the FHIR and DICOM servers. However, this architecture implies the deployment of

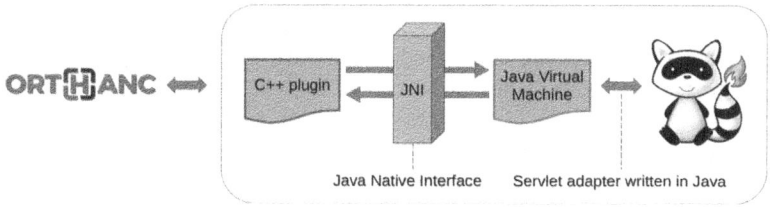

Fig. 6. Integration between Orthanc and HAPI Plain Server. The arrow pointing to the right (resp. to the left) in the servlet adapter corresponds to Java objects of the class `MockHttpServletRequest` (resp. `MockHttpServletResponse`) of the Spring framework.

two distinct processes and two distinct Web servers (one for the servlet container, and one for Orthanc), which keeps the setup slightly complex, especially when it comes to the mapping of the DICOMweb API.

Consequently, this work focuses on a third architecture, in which a HAPI Plain Server is directly branched into the Web server of Orthanc. In this architecture, Orthanc acts similarly to a Java servlet container, by redirecting all the FHIR requests to the HAPI framework. This architecture offers the advantage of requiring a single database and a single process, which further simplifies the setup, and of providing consistent access to both FHIR resources and DICOMweb routes, as only a single Web server is involved. The technical challenge with this third architecture is that Orthanc is developed in C++, while HAPI is written in Java, necessitating the creation of a bridge between these two languages. The solution is to utilize the Java plugin presented in Sect. 3.1 to enable the use of the HAPI Plain Server library directly within Orthanc.

Nonetheless, the HAPI Plain Server library is based on the Java servlets API, which does not directly align with the primitives offered by the Orthanc plugin SDK. This compatibility issue is addressed by utilizing the two standard classes `MockHttpServletRequest` and `MockHttpServletResponse` provided by the Spring Framework. These two classes can be used to turn the Web server of Orthanc into a servlet container: Whenever an HTTP request must be handled by the Java callable, an instance of the `MockHttpServletRequest` class is filled with the parameters of the HTTP request and is sent to the Java servlet. In return, the Java servlet fills a `MockHttpServletResponse` whose content can be unwrapped and sent back to the client through the Orthanc Web server. By default, the HAPI Plain Server servlet is branched at the root path `/fhir/` in the REST API of Orthanc. This integration is depicted on Fig. 6. It will be referred to as the "FHIR plugin for Orthanc", although it is a slight misuse of language, as this integration actually involves executing user-defined Java code that utilizes the HAPI Plain Server library within the environment provided by the Java plugin for Orthanc.

The last step to bring FHIR to Orthanc consists in implementing read-only HAPI providers that are responsible to retrieve and search the `ImagingStudy`, `Patient`, and `Endpoint` FHIR resources. To retrieve resources, the FHIR plugin implements the `IResourceProvider` interface, as defined by the HAPI Plain Server library, for each of those categories of resources. The `Endpoint` resource simply declares the address of the DICOMweb plugin, which is a purely static behavior that does not require querying the content of the Orthanc database. As far as the `ImagingStudy` (resp. `Patient`) resources are concerned, the content of an individual DICOM study (resp. DICOM patient) with identifier `id` can be retrieved by issuing a GET request to the `/studies/{id}` (resp. `/patients/{id}`) route in the built-in REST API of Orthanc. This route returns a JSON object whose content can easily be converted as an `ImagingStudy` (resp. `Patient`) Java object, as expected by the HAPI framework.

Searching over the `ImagingStudy` and `Patient` FHIR resources is implemented by issuing POST requests to the `/tools/find` route of the built-in REST API of Orthanc. This route executes a lookup operation on the Orthanc database, which can be filtered by specifying values for selected DICOM tags. These constraints can directly be derived from the parameters of the FHIR query. The route answers with a JSON array that contains the matching resources, which are converted into the `List<ImagingStudy>` and `List<Patient>` Java objects that are expected by the HAPI framework.

4   Results

Section 3.2 explained how the HAPI framework can be integrated as a plugin to Orthanc, which provides a working, free and open-source implementation of a FHIR server for medical imaging that is tightly coupled with a PACS server. This integration leverages another key deliverable of this research work described in Sect. 3.1, namely the ability to create plugins for Orthanc that can use the Java and Python programming languages. Some examples of Java and Python plugins, as well as an interaction with the FHIR server plugin for Orthanc, are now discussed. This section concludes with an application of the Java and Python plugins to deep learning for breast imaging.

4.1   Using `Dcm4che` in Orthanc

The `dcm4che` project was previously mentioned as a highly popular software library that provides an implementation of the DICOM standard in Java. This contrasts with Orthanc that internally uses the DCMTK library written in C++. The new Java plugin for Orthanc can be used to complement DCMTK with `dcm4che`, allowing it to benefit from the respective strengths of these two software libraries inside the Orthanc ecosystem. Depending on their technical background, a software developer might also find it easier to develop a DICOM pipeline as a Java plugin rather than as a C++ plugin.

As an illustration, Fig. 7 shows a sample Java plugin that uses the `dcm4che` library. The configuration file of Orthanc must specify both the classpath for the Java virtual machine (which must contain the `.jar` archive providing `dcm4che` and the bytecode of the user-defined `Main` class), and the name of the main Java class whose `static` method will be executed during the initialization of the plugin (in this case, `Main`). In this sample plugin, the `static` method registers a new route in the REST API of Orthanc using the method `Callbacks.register()` that is manually implemented in the Java plugin. Whenever an HTTP request is triggered against the `/dcm4che-parse` route, the custom Java callable is invoked. Inside the Java callable, the body of incoming HTTP POST requests is parsed as a DICOM instance using `dcm4che`. On success, the client receives the dump of the DICOM dataset, as generated by `dcm4che`.

4.2 FHIR Server in Orthanc

Starting the FHIR server plugin for Orthanc simply consists in writing a configuration file that loads the Java classes of the FHIR plugin for Orthanc together with the Java classes of the HAPI framework. A single precompiled .jar archive that bundles all the required dependencies is freely available for download on the Orthanc official homepage. This package is generated by Maven and its maven-assembly-plugin plugin. As soon as Orthanc is running, its FHIR server is accessible at default URL: http://localhost:8042/fhir/. FHIR clients can access the content of Orthanc using this URL. The Endpoint resource of the FHIR server is automatically mapped to the route of the DICOMweb server of Orthanc, whose default location corresponds to: http://localhost:8042/dicom-web/studies. This means that only one single Web server is running at any time, with this Web server being shared by the REST API of Orthanc, by the DICOMweb endpoint, and by a HAPI Plain Server.

As an illustration, Fig. 8 shows an interactive session in which the FHIR server plugin for Orthanc answers queries issued by the FHIRPACK client. Importantly, the

```
/**
 * This plugin can be triggered from the command line as follows:
 * $ curl http://localhost:8042/dcm4che-parse -X POST --data-binary @sample.dcm
 **/

import org.dcm4che3.data.Attributes;
import org.dcm4che3.io.DicomInputStream;

public class Main {
    static {
        Callbacks.register("/dcm4che-parse", new Callbacks.OnRestRequest() {
            @Override
            public void call(RestOutput output,
                             HttpMethod method,
                             String uri,
                             String[] regularExpressionGroups,
                             Map<String, String> headers,
                             Map<String, String> getParameters,
                             byte[] body) {
                if (method != HttpMethod.POST) {
                    output.sendMethodNotAllowed("POST");  // Answer with HTTP status 405
                } else {
                    ByteArrayInputStream stream = new ByteArrayInputStream(body);

                    try (DicomInputStream din = new DicomInputStream(stream)) {
                        Attributes dataset = din.readDataset();
                        output.answerBuffer(dataset.toString().getBytes(), "text/plain");
                    } catch (IOException e) {
                        output.sendHttpStatus((short) 400, "Cannot parse DICOM
                            file\n".getBytes());
                    }
                }
            }
        });
    }
}
```

Fig. 7. Example of a Java plugin for Orthanc that uses dcm4che to dump the content of a DICOM file provided in the body of a POST request (Figure adapted from [14]).

```
$ fp -s http://localhost:8042/fhir -o "getPatients" -p all -o "gatherSimplePaths id name.family birthDate"

0      fYET5.0    [COMUNIX]    1941-09-01
1      5Yp0E      [BRAINIX]    1949-03-01
2      Vafk,T,6   [PHENIX]     1991-01-01
3      SOtNwu     [INCISIX]         None
4  ozp00SjY2xG    [KNIX]            None
5      vAD7q3     [VIX]             None


$ fp -s http://localhost:8042/fhir -o "getImagingStudies" -p all -o \
  "gatherSimplePaths identifier.value subject.reference description numberOfSeries numberOfInstances"

                  identifier.value    subject.reference            description numberOfSeries numberOfInstances
0  [urn:oid:2.16.840.1.113669.632.20...    Patient/vAD7q3  Pied_cheville_UHR (Adulte)           1            250
1  [urn:oid:2.16.840.1.113669.632.20...    Patient/5Yp0E   IRM cérébrale, neuro-crâne          7            232
2  [urn:oid:2.16.840.1.113669.632.20...    Patient/Vafk,T,6      CT2 tête, face, sinus          3            723
3  [urn:oid:1.2.840.113745.101000.10...    Patient/fYET5.0      Neck^1HEAD_NECK_PETCT           2            166
4  [urn:oid:1.2.840.113619.2.176.202...  Patient/ozp00SjY2xG                 Knee (R)           6            135
5  [urn:oid:2.16.840.1.113669.632.20...    Patient/SOtNwu        Tête^Dental (Adulte)           1            166
```

Fig. 8. Sample interactive session of the FHIRPACK client against an Orthanc server that contains sample DICOM studies provided by the OsiriX project [23] (Figure adapted from [14]). The first request lists the `Patient` FHIR resources, while the second lists the `ImagingStudy` FHIR resources.

reported FHIR resources (i.e., `Patient` and `ImagingStudy`) are generated on-the-fly using a HAPI Plain Server, directly from the DICOM resources that are stored by Orthanc: No separate database dedicated to FHIR resources is used, and all the information is extracted from the Orthanc database. This ensures that the DICOMweb and the FHIR views of the content of the Orthanc server are always perfectly synchronized.

4.3   Using `Pydicom` in Orthanc

```python
# This plugin can be triggered from the command line as follows:
# $ curl http://localhost:8042/pydicom-parse -X POST --data-binary @sample.dcm

import io
import orthanc
import pydicom

def ParseInstance(output: orthanc.HttpMethod, uri: str, **request):
    if request['method'] != 'POST':
        output.SendMethodNotAllowed('POST')   # Answer with HTTP status 405
    else:
        stream = io.BytesIO(request['body'])
        dicom = pydicom.dcmread(stream)
        output.AnswerBuffer(str(dicom), 'text/plain')

orthanc.RegisterRestCallback('/pydicom-parse', ParseInstance)
```

Fig. 9. Example of a Python plugin for Orthanc that uses `pydicom` to dump the content of a DICOM file. This offers the same functionality as the Java sample code of Fig. 7.

The `pydicom` library is the Python equivalent to `dcm4che` and DCMTK. Just like `dcm4che` can be accessed from Orthanc through the Java plugin, `pydicom` is readily available through the Python plugin. Many end users will find it natural to implement custom pipelines as Python plugins for Orthanc, since this approach does not require the use of a compiler, which contrasts with the C, C++, and Java plugins for Orthanc. The Python source code in Fig. 9 implements the same behavior as the Java source code of Fig. 7, substituting dcm4che by pydicom. Moreover, the Python source code can access any module that is installed in the Python environment. For instance, the sample code of Fig. 10 shows how to combine Orthanc with PIL (*Python Imaging Library*) to generate thumbnails of DICOM instances stored in the Orthanc database.

```python
# This plugin can be triggered from the command line as follows:
# $ curl http://localhost:8042/thumbnail/19816330-cb02e1cf-df3a8fe8-bf510623-ccefe9f5

import PIL.Image
import io
import orthanc

def CreateThumbnail(output: orthanc.HttpMethod, uri: str, **request):
    if request['method'] == 'GET':
        # Retrieve the instance ID from the regular expression (*)
        instanceId = request['groups'][0]

        # Render the instance, then open it in Python using PIL/Pillow
        png = orthanc.RestApiGet('/instances/%s/rendered' % instanceId)
        image = PIL.Image.open(io.BytesIO(png))

        # Downsize the image as a 64x64 thumbnail
        image.thumbnail((64, 64), PIL.Image.ANTIALIAS)

        # Save the thumbnail as a JPEG image, then send the buffer to the caller
        jpeg = io.BytesIO()
        image.save(jpeg, format = 'JPEG', quality = 80)
        jpeg.seek(0)
        output.AnswerBuffer(jpeg.read(), 'image/jpeg')

    else:
        output.SendMethodNotAllowed('GET')

orthanc.RegisterRestCallback('/thumbnail/(.*)', CreateThumbnail)  # (*)
```

Fig. 10. Sample Python plugin that generates the thumbnail of a DICOM instance stored in the Orthanc database using the PIL module. The identifier of the DICOM instance of interest must be part of the URL.

4.4 Deep Learning for Breast Imaging

The previous section has indicated that any Python library can be invoked from Orthanc through the Python plugin. This evidently includes Python libraries for deep learning such as TensorFlow and PyTorch. This capability has very recently been exploited to create a platform integrated into Orthanc for the automated detection of masses on mammograms [7]. A RetinaNet model [18] based on a ResNet-50 backbone [10] was trained on the CBIS-DDSM (*Curated Breast Imaging Subset*) dataset [17] to detect the bounding boxes of breast masses. The trained model offers detection performance in line with the state-of-the-art on the CBIS-DDSM dataset. The Python plugin for Orthanc described in Sect. 3.1 of this work was then used to invoke PyTorch for performing inference with the trained model on the DICOM instances stored in the Orthanc database. The output bounding boxes were then encoded as standard-compliant DICOM-SR (*Structured Report*) instances using the `highdicom` Python library [6]. These DICOM-SR instances were stored into Orthanc next to the input DICOM mammograms. Finally, the Stone Web viewer [13] was specifically extended to render such DICOM-SR instances on the top of the mammograms.

Even though this workflow using the Python plugin for Orthanc is perfectly functional, it requires the installation of a heavyweight Python virtual environment that includes numerous third-party dependencies and whose proper setup may pose challenges for end users. But the Java ecosystem includes the Deep Java Library (DJL), a free and open-source deep learning framework that simplifies the development and deployment of machine learning models in Java applications. Moreover, unlike Python virtual environments, Java allows the bundling of all the third-party dependencies into a single, durable, cross-platform `.jar` archive, which enhances the portability of the runtime environment for deep learning inference. These elements position Java as an interesting alternative to Python when deep learning models need to be integrated into Orthanc and deployed for inference to a broad audience.

In this work, the same RetinaNet model that was trained using Python was exported as a TorchScript, a serialization format for PyTorch models suitable for various runtime environments. Models serialized with TorchScript can readily be imported by the Deep Java Library. Thanks to this approach, the Java plugin for Orthanc can in theory immediately replace the Python plugin to perform inference of the exported RetinaNet model on DICOM instances managed by Orthanc. However, certain components of the RetinaNet architecture, such as the non-maximum suppression step, cannot be exported as a TorchScript. This posed a significant technical challenge, necessitating a manual re-implementation of these components to fully restore the functionality of the RetinaNet model in Java. Furthermore, given the absence of a Java library that offers features like `highdicom`, the generation of the DICOM-SR instances had to be re-implemented from scratch in the Java language.

Figure 11 depicts the resulting user interface, which is identical to that of the original Python plugin [7]. However, the deployment of the Java plugin is now straightforward for the end user: It is sufficient to download one single `.jar` archive and to load it using the Java plugin for Orthanc. Thanks to the lightness of Orthanc, this shows that deep learning models can easily be executed on any computer equipped with a Java virtual machine.

4.5   Software Availability

All the contributions of this paper are released as free and open-source software. The source code of the Java plugin for Orthanc and of its sample codes is available under the GPLv3 license, which matches the license of the Orthanc server, at: https://orthanc. uclouvain.be/hg/orthanc-java/. This amounts to more than 10,000 lines of code, as reported by the `cloc` command-line tool, indicating its complexity. Technical documentation and additional examples are available in the Orthanc Book, the official doc-

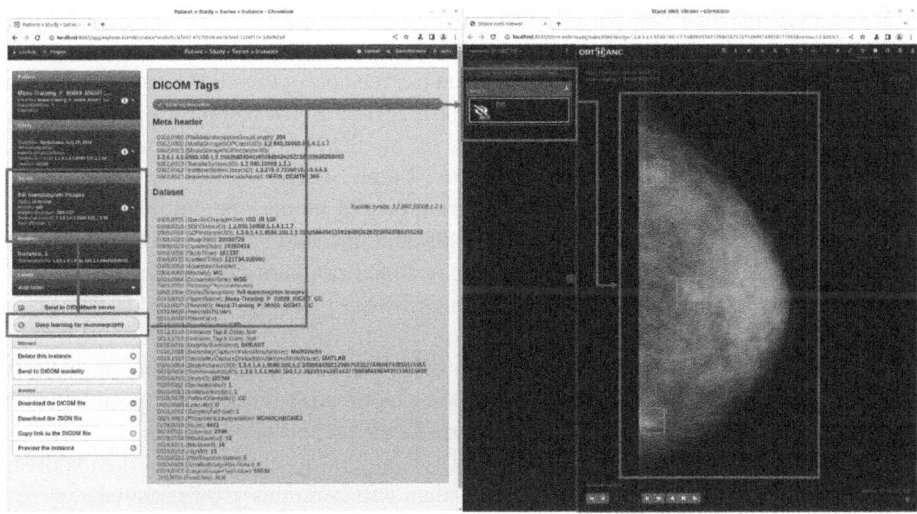

Fig. 11. Mammography inference integrated within the Orthanc ecosystem using the Java plugin. *Left:* The user selects a DICOM instance in the built-in user interface of Orthanc, and executes the inference by clicking on a button. *Right:* This operation generates a standard DICOM-SR instance that can be displayed using the Stone Web viewer. This figure is identical to the one presented in the recent paper that executed inference of the RetinaNet model using the Python plugin [7], as both the Python and Java plugins share equivalent features.

umentation of the Orthanc project. The weights of the deep learning model for the detection of masses on mammograms are available as open data as well. The source code of the Python plugin for Orthanc and its sample codes, which also contains more than 10,000 lines of code, is available under the AGPLv3 license at: https://orthanc. uclouvain.be/hg/orthanc-python/. Extensive technical documentation and examples can be found in the Orthanc Book. Finally, note that the official download site of the Orthanc project provides precompiled binaries and installers for both the Java plugin and the Python plugin.

5 Conclusions

This paper presents several technical contributions. Firstly, it explains how plugins extending the core features of the Orthanc server can be developed using the Java and Python programming languages. These languages enable users unfamiliar with C++ to create Orthanc plugins implementing specific DICOM pipelines and leveraging popular libraries for medical imaging and image processing. Secondly, a framework to deploy a FHIR server for medical imaging alongside a DICOMweb server is introduced by integrating Orthanc with HAPI through the Java plugin. The resulting architecture is lightweight, easy to deploy, and robust, ensuring the continuous synchronization of FHIR and DICOM resources. Thirdly, this paper demonstrates that the Java plugin for

Orthanc represents an attractive solution to deploy pre-trained deep learning models for medical imaging to a broad audience.

All contributions in this paper are released as free and open-source software, in the hope to raise the maturity level of the `ImagingStudy` FHIR resource and to promote the deployment of open deep learning models for medical imaging that could be used in academic contexts and in emerging economies. Future work includes the development of a pedagogical platform for teaching the principles of modern health interoperability in medical imaging. Thanks to the code model that encapsulates the primitives of the Orthanc plugin SDK, plugins could also be developed for additional programming languages like C#, Go, or Rust. Moreover, the main limitation of the designed FHIR server is that it currently only implements the `ImagingStudy`, `Patient`, and `Endpoint` FHIR resources in a read-only mode. From this perspective, it would be particularly interesting to enrich the FHIR plugin for Orthanc by creating a bridge between DICOM worklists and FHIR using the `Task` and `ServiceRequest` resources. Finally, the value of FHIR for artificial intelligence and for integrating multi-modal data sources including clinical, imaging, and multi-omics data will continue to be explored.

References

1. Abadi, M., et al.: TensorFlow: a system for Large-Scale machine learning. In: 12th USENIX Symposium on Operating Systems Design and Implementation (OSDI 2016), pp. 265–283. USENIX Association, Savannah, GA (2016)
2. Ayaz, M., Pasha, M.F., Alzahrani, M.Y., Budiarto, R., Stiawan, D.: The Fast Health Interoperability Resources (FHIR) standard: systematic literature review of implementations, applications, challenges and opportunities. JMIR Med. Inform. **9**(7), e21929 (2021). https://doi.org/10.2196/21929
3. Bender, D., Sartipi, K.: HL7 FHIR: an agile and RESTful approach to healthcare information exchange. In: Proceedings of the 26th IEEE International Symposium on Computer-Based Medical Systems. IEEE (2013). https://doi.org/10.1109/cbms.2013.6627810
4. Benson, T., Grieve, G.: Principles of Health Interoperability. Springer, Cham (2021). https://doi.org/10.1007/978-3-030-56883-2
5. Boufahja, A., Nichols, S., Pangon, V.: Custom FHIR resources definition of detailed radiation information for dose management systems. In: Pesquita, C., Fred, A.L.N., Gamboa, H. (eds.) Proceedings of the 14th International Joint Conference on Biomedical Engineering Systems and Technologies, BIOSTEC 2021, Volume 5: HEALTHINF, Online Streaming, 11–13 February 2021, pp. 467–474. SCITEPRESS (2021). https://doi.org/10.5220/0010251104670474
6. Bridge, C.P., Gorman, C., Pieper, S., Doyle, S.W., Lennerz, J.K., et al.: Highdicom: a Python library for standardized encoding of image annotations and machine learning model outputs in pathology and radiology. J. Digit. Imaging **35**(6), 1719–1737 (2022). https://doi.org/10.1007/s10278-022-00683-y
7. Chatzopoulos, E., Jodogne, S.: Integrated and interoperable platform for detecting masses on mammograms. In: Proceedings of the 34th Medical Informatics Europe Conference (MIE 2024) (2024)
8. Costa, C., Ferreira, C., Bastião, L., Ribeiro, L., Silva, A., Oliveira, J.L.: Dicoogle: an open-source peer-to-peer PACS. J. Digit. Imaging **24**(5), 848–856 (2010). https://doi.org/10.1007/s10278-010-9347-9

9. Eichelberg, M., Riesmeier, J., Wilkens, T., Hewett, A.J., Barth, A., Jensch, P.: Ten years of medical imaging standardization and prototypical implementation: the DICOM standard and the OFFIS DICOM toolkit (DCMTK). In: Ratib, O.M., Huang, H.K. (eds.) SPIE Proceedings. SPIE (2004). https://doi.org/10.1117/12.534853

10. He, K., Zhang, X., Ren, S., Sun, J.: Deep residual learning for image recognition. In: Conference on Computer Vision and Pattern Recognition (CVPR), pp. 770–778. IEEE (2016). https://doi.org/10.1109/cvpr.2016.90

11. Hussain, M.A., Langer, S.G., Kohli, M.: Learning HL7 FHIR using the HAPI FHIR server and its use in medical imaging with the SIIM dataset. J. Digit. Imaging **31**(3), 334–340 (2018). https://doi.org/10.1007/s10278-018-0090-y

12. Jodogne, S.: The Orthanc ecosystem for medical imaging. J. Digit. Imaging **31**(3), 341–352 (2018). https://doi.org/10.1007/s10278-018-0082-y

13. Jodogne, S.: On the use of WebAssembly for rendering and segmenting medical images. Commun. Comput. Inf. Sci. **1814**(1), 393–414 (2023). https://doi.org/10.1007/978-3-031-38854-5_20

14. Jodogne, S.: Setting a PACS on FHIR. In: Proceedings of the 17th International Joint Conference on Biomedical Engineering Systems and Technologies (HEALTHINF), vol. 2, pp. 123–131. SCITEPRESS (2024). https://doi.org/10.5220/0012384600003657

15. Ketkar, N.: Introduction to PyTorch. In: Deep Learning with Python, pp. 195–208. Apress (2017). https://doi.org/10.1007/978-1-4842-2766-4_12

16. Lattner, C., Adve, V.: LLVM: a compilation framework for lifelong program analysis & transformation. In: Proceedings of the 2004 International Symposium on Code Generation and Optimization (CGO 2004), Palo Alto, California (2004)

17. Lee, R., Gimenez, F., Hoogi, A., Miyake, K., Gorovoy, M., Rubin, D.: A curated mammography data set for use in computer-aided detection and diagnosis research. Sci. Data **4**(1) (2017). https://doi.org/10.1038/sdata.2017.177

18. Lin, T., Goyal, P., Girshick, R., He, K., Dollar, P.: Focal loss for dense object detection. In: Proceedings of the 2017 IEEE International Conference on Computer Vision (ICCV), pp. 2999–3007. IEEE Computer Society, Los Alamitos, CA, USA (2017). https://doi.org/10.1109/ICCV.2017.324

19. Mason, D.: SU-e-t-33: pydicom: an open source DICOM library. Med. Phys. **38**(6Part10), 3493 (2011). https://doi.org/10.1118/1.3611983

20. McCormick, M., Liu, X., Jomier, J., Marion, C., Ibanez, L.: ITK: enabling reproducible research and open science. Front. Neuroinform. **8** (2014). https://doi.org/10.3389/fninf.2014.00013

21. NEMA: National Electrical Manufacturers Association PS3/ISO 12052, Digital Imaging and Communications in Medicine (DICOM) Standard (2024). http://www.dicomstandard.org/

22. Panchal, A., Keyes, R.: SU-GG-t-260: dicompyler: an open source radiation therapy research platform with a plugin architecture. Med. Phys. **37**(6Part19), 3245 (2010). https://doi.org/10.1118/1.3468652

23. Rosset, A., Spadola, L., Ratib, O.: OsiriX: an open-source software for navigating in multidimensional DICOM images. J. Digit. Imaging **17**(3), 205–216 (2004). https://doi.org/10.1007/s10278-004-1014-6

24. Schroeder, W., Martin, K., Lorensen, B.: The Visualization Toolkit, 4th edn. Kitware, New York (2006)

25. Shackleford, J., Kandasamy, N., Sharp, G.: Plastimatch: an open-source software for radiotherapy imaging. In: High Performance Deformable Image Registration Algorithms for Manycore Processors, pp. 107–114. Elsevier (2013). https://doi.org/10.1016/b978-0-12-407741-6.00006-2

26. Shi, W., et al.: A FHIR-compliant application for multi-site and multi-modality pediatric scoliosis patient rehabilitation. In: Huang, Y., et al. (eds.) IEEE International Conference on Bioinformatics and Biomedicine, BIBM 2021, Houston, TX, USA, 9–12 December 2021, pp. 1524–1527. IEEE (2021). https://doi.org/10.1109/BIBM52615.2021.9669649
27. Tang, S.T., et al.: Creating a medical imaging workflow based on FHIR, DICOMweb, and SVG. J. Digit. Imaging **36**(3), 794–803 (2023). https://doi.org/10.1007/s10278-021-00522-6
28. Warnock, M., Toland, C., Evans, D., Wallace, B., Nagy, P.: Benefits of using the DCM4CHE DICOM archive. J. Digit. Imaging **20**(S1), 125–129 (2007). https://doi.org/10.1007/s10278-007-9064-1
29. Xu, J., et al.: Interactive, in-browser cinematic volume rendering of medical images. Comput. Methods Biomech. Biomed. Eng. Imaging Visualization **11**(4), 1019–1026 (2022). https://doi.org/10.1080/21681163.2022.2145239
30. Ziegler, E., et al.: Open health imaging foundation viewer: an extensible open-source framework for building web-based imaging applications to support cancer research. JCO Clin. Cancer Inform. **4**, 336–345 (2020). https://doi.org/10.1200/cci.19.00131

Evaluating the Viability of Neural Networks for Analyzing Electromyography Data in Home Rehabilitation: Estimating Load on the Leg

Finn Siegel[1]([⊠]) [iD], Christian Buj[1] [iD], Ricarda Merfort[2], Andreas Hein[1],
and Frerk Müller-von Aschwege[1]

[1] OFFIS E.V.- Institute for Information Technology, Escherweg 2, Oldenburg, Germany
Finn.siegel@offis.de
[2] Experimental Orthopaedics and Trauma Surgery, University Hospital RWTH Aachen,
Aachen, Germany

Abstract. Intramedullary (IM) nailing is a widely accepted treatment for femoral shaft fractures due to its good healing rate and rapid return to full weight bearing. However, a significant number of patients experience impairments years after treatment. To enhance individual outcomes, a personalized rehabilitation protocol based on impairment monitoring is essential. We propose a continuous surface electromyography (EMG) measurement system worn on vastus lateralis (VL) and vastus medialis (VM) in combination with a convolutional neural network (CNN) to monitor the load put on the treated leg, as this is an indicator of impairments and healing progress. To test the feasibility of such an approach, a study was conducted with healthy participants (N = 8) simulating a reduced load on the leg. Our study showed promising results, as the CNN could on average achieve a validation accuracy of 91.6% in classifying steps with normal and reduced load on the leg. These results demonstrate the potential of using EMG measurements from VL and VM to monitor changes in leg loading during rehabilitation and offer the opportunity to improve individual rehabilitation after IM nailing.

Keyword: Electromyography · Neural network · Deep learning · Rehabilitation · Intramedullary nailing · Femur shaft fracture · Load on the leg · Weigh bearing

1 Introduction

1.1 Medical Background

The established gold standard for the treatment of femoral shaft fractures is the use of an intramedullary (IM) nail. The widespread adoption of this method is attributed to its compelling properties, including a high likelihood of fracture union (99%) [1], a low risk of infection [2] and a rapid weight bearing [3].

M. P. Guarino et al. (Eds.): BIOSTEC 2024, CCIS 2546, pp. 335–353, 2026.
https://doi.org/10.1007/978-3-031-96899-0_19

Despite the relatively low risk associated with IM nailing, approximately 20% of patients subjected to this procedure suffer from long-term residual impairments. These complications can include chronic pain, hip ossification, altered gait patterns or restricted mobility in hip and knee [2, 4, 5]. The cause of these complications remains a topic of ongoing debate.

Irrespective of an identified cause, long-term residual impairments pose a substantial burden to the affected patient. One possible solution to reduce or even eliminate long-term impairments is appropriate rehabilitation with individual adapted exercises [6–10]. Hayden et al. [6] concluded in a review, that specific exercise treatment is probably more effective than standard care in reducing pain intensity. Rudin [8] describes exercises to restore flexibility, and strengthening of muscles and joints as one key aspect to fight chronic pain. The teams around Sherrington et al. [9] and Mangione et al. [7] have shown that home exercise has a positive impact on long term mobility. Taraldsen et al. [10] found that gait recovery can be improved by home exercise.

In order to provide appropriate rehabilitation with individually adapted exercises, it is necessary to accurately identify and monitor the limitations of the patient. This can be challenging, particularly in the context of home rehabilitation, as monitoring is often based on subjective self-assessments, which tend to be inaccurate [11]. In addition, short sessions with experts only provide a snapshot of the patient's status, failing to provide a comprehensive overview [12, 13].

Previous research by Siegel et al. [14] suggests the use of wearable home devices as a strategy to improve the accuracy of rehabilitation monitoring. This allows for the identification of long-term impairments, providing a basis for the treating specialist to take adapted countermeasures and potentially improving patient outcomes while reducing the workload of the treating specialist.

An important parameter to monitor during the rehabilitation process is the load on the fractured leg. This is because weight bearing after a fracture is generally considered to be an indicator of the healing process. For example:

- Weight bearing on the leg can indicate the level of inflammation. An increase in tolerable load, may indicate that the inflammation is decreasing and the fracture is stabilizing [15]. In addition, weight bearing on the leg is an indicator of soft tissue healing. Increased weight bearing indicates that tissues such as muscles, ligaments and tendons have healed or adapted sufficiently to support the affected area [16].
- Weight bearing is an important parameter to monitor as insufficient or no weight bearing on the leg, contrary to prescribed guidelines, can potentially prolong the healing process. Flanagan et al. [17] demonstrated that non-weight bearing was associated with delayed healing. If reduced weight bearing is identified, clinicians can encourage the patient to increase it in order to improve healing.
- Changes in weight loading may indicate pain [18] and if changes are registered, targeted training of the supporting muscles can be implemented as a countermeasure [8].
- Monitoring the instantaneous load on the leg is a crucial parameter for patients. In Germany, patients are given a maximum load that they are allowed to place on the fractured leg (weight scale method). Research has shown that this method often leads to significant uncertainty, as many patients struggle to differentiate between various

percentages of weight bearing on the leg [19]. Real-time information about the load on the leg and alerts in the event of overloading can help patients more effectively adhere to the prescribed maximum load.

- Finally, return to full weight bearing can be used as a measure for the success of the treatment method. Stryker is developing a new tool to restore the original length and rotation of the femur during surgery. This Length Alignment Rotation (LAR) system has significant potential to improve individual patient outcomes [14]. However, verifying its success compared to the traditional method is challenging and requires a way to evaluate the outcome after treatment with an IM nail. One indicator of treatment success could be to compare the time it takes for patients after different treatments to return to full weight bearing on the leg.

In conclusion, a reliable way of measuring the load on the leg is needed. One approach is the use of insoles, as these are a practical method of monitoring the weight load on the leg. Various research teams have demonstrated that these reliably measure the pressure under the foot during walking [20–22]. However, for optimal usability, insoles should ideally be worn throughout the day. This is a challenge because many people do not wear the same shoes indoors as outdoors. As a result, data is not recorded while shoes are not worn, or patients have to change their insoles frequently. Not only is each replacement a burden on the patient, especially in the immediate post-operative period, but there is also a risk that the insole will be incorrectly placed, leading to potential data inaccuracies. Consequently, either information is lost when the footwear is not worn, or the patient is subjected to additional burden [23]. In order to obtain a more comprehensive overview without increasing the burden on the patient, it is necessary to consider alternative measurement systems.

An alternative would be to record EMG data from the lower limb and derive information about the load on the leg. An EMG measurement records biopotentials when an electrochemical stimulus triggers muscle fiber [25]. The possibility of using EMG measurements to draw conclusions about load on the leg is based on the premise that alterations in movement are accompanied by a corresponding change in the measurable EMG signal [26].

In order to detect these alterations in muscle activity, a surface EMG measurement should ideally record the electrical activity of uniformly active motor units within one muscle. However, the resulting EMG signal is subject to many influences, including fatigue, quantity of active motor units, firing rates, firing amplitudes, superposition from surrounding muscles, low-pass characteristics of surrounding tissue, sensor properties and extraneous signals such as ambient noise. This complexity makes it difficult to reliably classify EMG recordings using basic filter algorithms or feature extraction methodologies. As a possible answer to this challenge, deep learning has proven to be a successful tool [27]. Especially the usage of Convolutional Neural Networks (CNNs) has been proven reliable [28–30]. CNNs are particularly suitable for detecting patterns in one-dimensional or multi-dimensional data due to a high degree of invariance to translation, scaling, skewing or distortion. This is possible because each neuron receives its input from a local receptive field from the previous layer. Thus, the position of features becomes less important as long as they maintain their relative position to each other [31], enabling a classification of variant time series [32]. I.e. Bakircioğlu and Öskurt

[33] used a CNN to classify EMG recordings of movements made while gripping six different objects and achieved 95.9% accuracy. Olsson et al. [28] used a CNN, classifying 16 independent states of the hand recorded using an EMG system and achieved 78.7% accuracy.

2 Research Question

In a previous paper, the concept of using a wearable device, positioned above the knee and equipped with EMG sensors to monitor the patient's rehabilitation progress was introduced. A first feasibility study to classify the foot progression angle (FPA) with a CNN, was conducted [24]. It was found that a CNN can be used to classify different FPAs with a validation accuracy of 75%. The next step in advancing the concept of using EMG sensors as a measurement system as a basis for individualized rehabilitation is to extend it to include the classification of loads on the leg. Therefore, **the viability of using EMG sensors to assess the load on the leg needs to be evaluated.**

3 Aim of This Study

The aim of this study is to evaluate the potential usefulness of EMG sensors for monitoring the weight bearing of the leg during home rehabilitation - as this is a crucial aspect of the healing process.

As of now, EMG measurements have been successfully used in numerous rehabilitation applications:

- In neuromuscular rehabilitation, EMG measurements have been used to quantitatively assess spasticity as well as monitor treatment progress [34].
- In post-stroke rehabilitation, EMG measurements have been used to monitor the healing process [35] or to control an exoskeleton aimed to reactivate paralyzed limbs [36].
- In orthopedic rehabilitation, EMG measurements were used to evaluate muscle function, to detect abnormalities or to manage pain-inducing syndromes during sessions with specialists [37, 38].
- In monitoring FPAs, it was found that EMG measurements can be used to classify FPAs [24].

However, until now, EMG measurements have not been used to monitor a patient's load on the leg while walking on crutches.

Since this study is intended to provide an initial overview of the usability of lower limb EMG measurements to monitor the load on the leg during walking with crutches, it was decided to conduct the study with a healthy cohort rather than patients. The study will evaluate the following hypotheses:

Hypothesis A: A CNN can classify the load on the leg of unknown steps for a single participant, after training on EMG data obtained from the same participant.

If a CNN is capable to discriminate EMG signals from different weight bearings (normal and reduced) within a single participant, this knowledge holds potential to monitor changes during rehabilitation. However, this is limited, since the participant would need to simulate different loads on the leg in order to train such neural network. In practical clinical scenarios, this data aggregation may not be feasible, due to the recently treated femur shaft fracture. Therefore, it is important to investigate, whether a neural network can be trained using data from diverse patients and enabling it to classify EMG signal of different loads without prior subject specific training. To test this the following hypotheses is formulated:

Hypothesis B: A CNN can classify the load on the leg for an unknown participant, after training on EMG data obtained by different participant.

To test hypotheses A and B, EMG signals of several participants simulating different loads on the leg while walking on crutches are recorded and analyzed using a CNN.

4 Material and Methods

4.1 Study Design

A study is conducted to evaluate the usability of a CNN in classifying different loads on the leg. Healthy participants are asked to wear EMG sensors on the lower limb while walking on crutches over a gait mat. Walks are performed with normal and reduced load on one leg. The gait mat is used to label each step recorded by the EGM Sensors with the applied load. This data is used to train and validate a CNN that classifies reduced and normal load on the leg.

5 Study Protocol

The study design for evaluating the usability of CNNs in classifying different loads on the leg is outlined in Fig. 1. First participants were informed about study protocol, data protection and potential risks. The risks were relatively low as data is recorded anonymously, participants are healthy thus have a low potential of falling, the EMG system records noninvasively and is CE certified. Furthermore, participants can stop participating at any time. After consent was obtained, the first step of the protocol, was to determine the side, on which the load on the leg is varied. The side to be varied could be chosen freely, but had to remain consistent throughout the study. Prior to data collection, walking on crutches with reduced and normal load on the leg was practiced. This was done to ensure similar walks and prevents the neural network to learn cues that are not related to weight bearing, but to different gait styles. Training also included walking to the beat of a metronome standardizing stride pace across different tasks. The pace of the metronome was adjusted for each participant to achieve a comfortable walking speed. During data collection, each participant had to complete a total of 16 walks on the gait mate. Eight normal walks and eight walks with reduced load on the leg.

Ten volunteers were recruited for this study. Exclusion criteria were adhesive tape and silver allergy (due to the type of electrodes), implanted electrical devices and known lower limb deformities. Two participants were excluded from the study. One was unable to coordinate walking with crutches in rhythm of the metronome. Another reported shoulder pain when walking with crutches. Ultimately, eight participants successful completed the walks. The gender distribution was 50% male to 50% female with an average age of 36.5 years ($\pm$14.3 years).

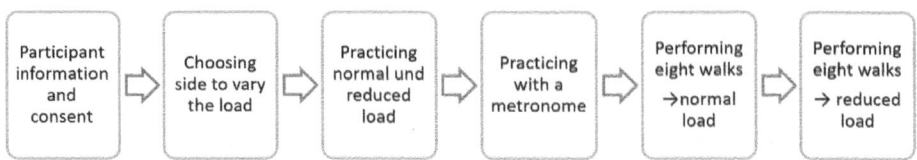

Fig. 1. The different phases participant performed in the course of the study

6   Sensor Placement

The optimal sensor placement, aligned to answer the hypotheses (A and B), is based on previous research and verified by literature [39–42]. In a previous study the EMG signal was recorded from Vastus Lateralis (VL) and Vastus Medialis (VM) to detect changes in FPAs, suggesting that these measurement points are suitable for monitoring changes in gait. As part of the quadriceps, VL and VM help to straighten the leg during gait and they are essential in supporting the body weight during stance [39] suggesting that a change in the load on the leg is visible in the muscle activity of VL and VM. This is in line with findings from other research teams. Kristiansen et al. [40] could show that the EMG signal amplitude significantly decreases for VL and VM when walking on a Lower Body Positive Pressure Treadmill. Tm et al. [41] showed that the activation of the VL changes during walking when comparing an ergonomically designed walking aid with crutches and different loads. Stastny et al. [42] found that the activity ratio of VL and VM changes significantly with increasing load over body mass.

In conclusion it was decided to place the EMG sensors on VL and VM (Fig. 2). The European recommendations for sensors and sensor placement for EMG [43] was used as a guide to ensure optimal placement of the sensors on VL and VM, minimizing superposing of signals by surrounding muscles. To further improve signal quality, skin was shaved and cleaned prior to sensor placement.

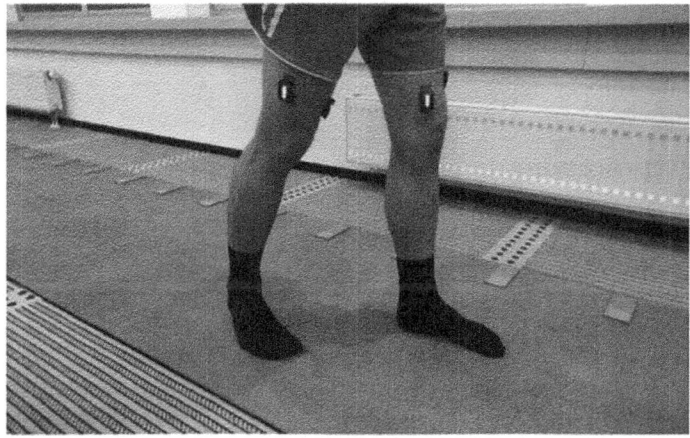

Fig. 2. Exemplary image from the study, displaying the GAITRite mat, used for load verification and the placement of EMG sensors on VL and VM. Picture by Siegel et al. [33]

7 Data Acquisition

The EMG signal was recorded using the Delsys Trigno-Wireless-Biofeedback System [44]. This system consists of a base station that wirelessly collects data from individual sensors. Each sensor is capable of collecting data at a frequency of 4 kHz with a bandwidth of 20–450 Hz and an input range of 11 mV. The sensor contact material is made from 99.9% silver.

For the purpose of supervised learning, it is necessary to label EMG data recordings. Consequently, a GAITRite mat was used to record each step taken. The mat is manufactured by CIR Systems and represents a gold standard in gait analysis. 36 864 pressure sensors evenly distributed over a length of 793 cm and a width of 61 cm allow steps to be recorded and a gait profile to be created. This profile contains a representation of the pressure measured by each individual sensor. A section of the mat can be seen in (Fig. 2).

8 Data Preparation

EMG recordings are labeled with the load put on the leg during each step, allowing supervised CNN training. This is done using recordings of the GAITRite mat. For each step taken on the mat, a color-coded heat map of the force per sensor under the foot is generated (Fig. 3). This data is analyzed using a developed Python tool and combined into a percentile load compared to the unchanged side.

EMG data preprocessing is performed according to a general data preparation paradigm [30]. During the study, 16 walks across the GAITRite mat were recorded alongside the corresponding EMG signals (Fig. 1), resulting in eight datasets per class (normal and reduced load on the leg). However, this quantity proved insufficient to train a supervised deep learning algorithm [45]. To increase the size of each class, the walks are divided into individual steps. For this purpose, software was developed that extracts individual steps based on EMG peak detection and assigns them to the appropriate load class. This results in one dataset for each participant, containing the EMG signal for VL and VM and the corresponding load for each step.

9 Data Preprocessing

To extract non-stationary properties from the EMG signal, time windowing is performed [41]. Initially, the EMG signal of one step spans over a duration of one second. This can be contracted, since VL and VM are only active for approximately 20% to 25% of the time during one gait cycle [42]. The average duration of a gait cycle is around one second [43], enabling the EMG signal be to contracted to a duration of 250 ms. As data was collected at 4 kHz, the EMG signal is truncated to a time window of 1000 data points (250 ms). The next step is a bandpass filtering [44]. To filter motion artifacts, a low-pass filter with a cutoff frequency of 20 Hz is used. A high-pass filter with a cutoff frequency of 450 Hz is applied, as not much additional information is available above this frequency [33]. This is followed by a rectification of the data, enhancing the chances of successful training of deep learning algorithms [45]. Next, a

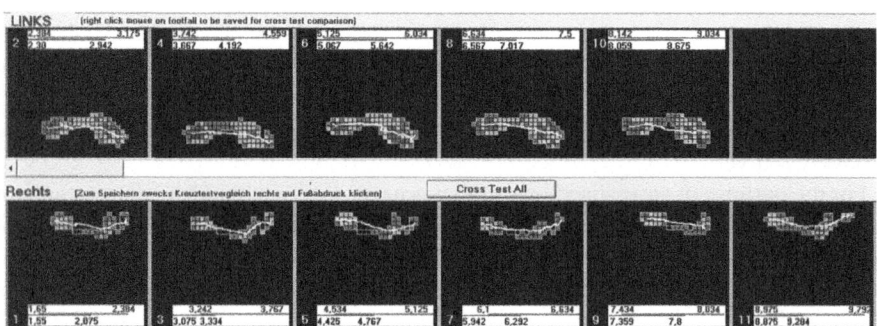

Fig. 3. Illustration of the weight distribution over all pressure sensors that were loaded during one walk. The recorded pressure profile of a normal load is shown in the top row and a reduced load in the bottom row. It can be seen that significantly more sensors recorded a load during the normal load and the average color coding is more intense

Fast Fourier Transformation (FFT) is performed creating additional input features and enhancing information density [29]. Finally, data is normalized using the peak-dynamic method, requiring each data point to be divided by the maximum value. While this method results in a loss of information regarding the degree of muscle activation, it enhances the comparability between participants.

The result is a matrix containing both a time series and a frequency series for each labeled step and each sensor. Combining measurements for VL and VM results in a matrix of four features with 1000 data points times the number of steps. In this study, a total of 57–92 steps were recorded per participant (with 33–45 normal and 31–47 reduced load), resulting in 589 steps available to train the CNN (Table 1). This is a relatively modest dataset size for the application of deep learning [40], but the purpose of this feasibility study is to provide an initial insight into the possibility of discriminating loads on the leg using EMG measurements in conjunction with deep learning evaluations and is therefore acceptable.

The average rate and the standard deviation of the reduced load in comparison to the fully loaded side is displayed in Table 2.

Table 1. Distribution of steps generated in this study across different participants and loads on the leg (normal and reduced) and total class sizes used to train the neural network

Classes	P. 1	P. 2	P. 3	P. 4	P. 5	P. 6	P. 7	P. 8	Total
Normal	40	33	26	35	42	40	30	45	291
Reduced	42	33	31	35	42	38	30	47	298
Total	82	66	57	70	84	78	45	92	589

Table 2. Average percentage and standard deviation for steps with reduced load on the leg. Percentages refer to comparison with steps with normal load on the leg

	P. 1	P. 2	P. 3	P. 4	P. 5	P. 6	P. 7	P. 8
Av	51.92%	42.16%	29.95%	33.21%	33.85%	46.45%	74.39%	59.47%
Std	± 6.79%	± 8.69%	± 8.59%	± 13.78%	± 3.45%	± 6.35%	± 5.69%	± 6.12%

10   Data Processing

The structure of the CNN used to classify normal and reduced load on the leg is shown in Fig. 4. The network is built using TensorFlow [46] and Keras [47] libraries in Python. To validate the CNN the accuracy (ratio of correct predictions divided by total predictions) and the F1-score (measure of symmetry between precision and recall) are used. Additionally, the confusion matrixes of the most and least successful classifications are displayed. To obtain reliable results each run was performed three times and the average accuracy and F1-score is taken as the result.

$$Accuracy = \frac{TP + TN}{TP + TN + FN + FP} \ [48]$$

$$F1 = 2 \times \frac{precision \times recall}{recision + recall} = \frac{2 \times TP}{2 \times TP + FP + FN} \ [49]$$

With TP = True Positive, TN = True Negative, FN = False Negative and FP = False Positive.

11   Data Processing for Testing Hypothesis A

H: A CNN can classify the load on the leg of unknown steps for a single participant, after training on EMG data obtained from the same participant.

To test this hypothesis, data obtained by each participant individually is used to train the CNN. The labeled data is combined, randomly mixed and 85% used for training and the remaining 15% serve as validation data. To ensure a reliable conclusion, each training iteration is performed three times. Firstly, time-domain data from each muscle is tested individually, followed by a combined evaluation of both muscles. The frequency domain data is then analyzed separately before time and frequency domain data are combined for hypothesis testing.

12   Data Processing for Testing Hypothesis B

H: A CNN can classify the load on the leg for an unknown participant, after training on EMG data obtained by different participants.

To test this hypothesis, datasets from all participants excluding one for validation were combined and used to train the CNN. The most successful data combination from testing hypothesis A is used for training (time series data only or in combination with frequency domain data). This process was repeated, ensuring each participant's data was tested against the combined majority. The process is repeated three times and averaged.

Layer	Modules	Configurations	Layer	Modules	Configuration
1	Input	n_steps * 1000 * 4	10	Flatten	
1	Convolution	Filters=512, Kernel=4, Padding=same, Activation=ReLu (α=0.001)	11	Dense	Units=64, Activation=ReLu(α=0.001)
2	Max Pooling	Pool size=2, Strides=2, Padding=same	12	Dropout	0.3
3	Dropout	0.2	13	Dense	Units=32, Activation=ReLu(α=0.001)
4	Convolution	Filters=256, Kernel=3, Padding=same, Activation=ReLu (α=0.001)	14	Dropout	0.2
5	Max Pooling	Pool size=3, Strides=2, Padding=same	Final	Dense	Units=1, Activation=Sigmoid
6	Dropout	0.2			
7	Convolution	Filters=64, Kernel=2, Padding=same, Activation=ReLu (α=0.001)			
8	Max Pooling	Pool size=3, Strides=2, Padding=same			
9	Dropout	0.2			

Fig. 4. The structure of the CNN used. The *adam* optimizer and the *binary crossentropy* loss function were used for training. Batch sizes of four and 30 epochs were used

13 Results

In the following, the results gained from the analysis of the study data are presented in relation to the tested hypothesis.

13.1 Results for Testing Hypothesis A

H: A CNN can classify the load on the leg of unknown steps for a single participant, after training on EMG data obtained from the same participant.

To test this hypothesis, data obtained by each participant individually was used to train the CNN. Steps are classified into two load classes (normal and reduced load), the results are shown in Table 3. The best average accuracy of 91.6% ($\pm$7.8%) with an average F1-score of 0.9 was archived using the combined times series of VM and VL. This performance exceeds chance level of 50%. The accuracy for each individual participant, when training the CNN on time series data of VM and VL is shown in Table 4. Additionally, a confusion matrix is displayed, for the most successful and the least successful classification for a single participant, see Fig. 5.

The result suggests that a CNN can learn and discriminate features within the EMG signal allowing conclusions to be drawn about applied load on the leg. However, the high variance of 7.8% indicates inconsistency in the quality of features identified by the CNN between participants.

Table 3. Average classification accuracy and standard deviation for different combinations of time domain data and frequency domain data of VM and VL

Muscle	Domaine	Average accuracy	Standard deviation
VL	Time	90.5%	$\pm$ 9.9%
VL	Frequency	87.5%	$\pm$ 11.9%
VM	Time	85.1%	$\pm$ 12.8%
VM	Frequency	83.0%	$\pm$ 13.4%
VM + VL	Time	82.3%	$\pm$ 12.7%
VM + VL	Frequency	70.6%	$\pm$ 9.9%
VM + VL	Time + Frequency	91.6%	$\pm$ 7.8%

13.2 Results for Testing Hypothesis B

H: A CNN can classify the load on the leg for an unknown participant, after training on EMG data obtained by different participants.

To test this hypothesis, datasets of all participants excluding one for validation were combined and used to train a CNN. This process was repeated, ensuring each participant's data was tested against the combined majority. The results are shown in Table 5. It can

Table 4. Most successful classification accuracy, standard deviation and F1-Score for training a CNN to classify normal and reduced loads on the leg for individual participants (combination of time and frequency domain data of VL and VM)

Participant	P.1	P.2	P.3	P.4	P.5	P.6	P.7	P.8	Av	Std
Accuracy [%]	100	100	92	92	80	80	89	100	91.63	7.8
F1-Score	1	1	0.86	0.9	0.75	0.82	0.92	1	0.9	0.08

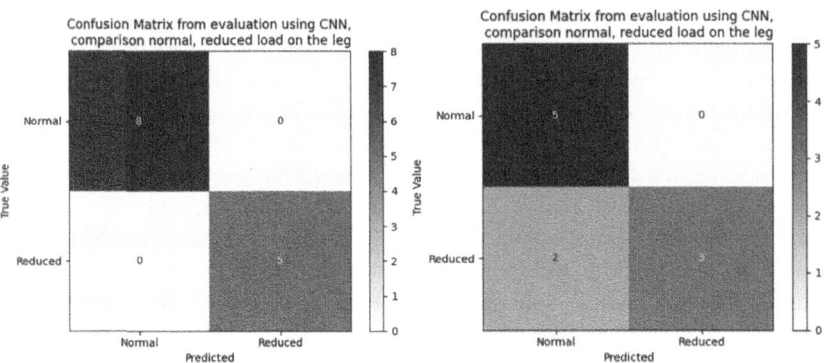

Fig. 5. Confusion matrix from evaluating the CNN for classification of normal, reduced load on the leg (combination of time and frequency domain data of VL and VM). Left: For participant 2, the CNN archived 100% accuracy in classifying normal and reduced load on the leg. Right: For participant 5, the CNN archived 80% accuracy in classifying normal and reduced load on the leg

be seen that a CNN, trained on a whole population, can distinguish validation steps of an unknown participant with an average accuracy of 75.4% ± 10% across normal and reduced load on the leg. The results indicate a limited reliability for a classification of EMG data recorded from unknown participants.

Table 5. Classification accuracy, standard deviation and F1-Score for testing an unknown participant on a CNN trained on data obtained by different participants

Participant	P.1	P.2	P.3	P.4	P.5	P.6	P.7	P.8	Av	Std
Accuracy [%]	85.4	78.9	61.2	89.8	72.6	69.4	58.1	88.0	75.43	10.0
F1-Score	0.87	0.73	0.54	0.86	0.59	0.74	0.52	0.90	0.72	0.14

14   Discussion

In this study, all classes (normal and reduced load) contain 1178 trials (for VL and VM combined), which, in the context of deep learning, accounts for a relatively small dataset [40]. However, when working with EMG measurements, the availability of data is limited by the number of times a person can repeat a specific movement. This limitation restricts the size of available datasets, which needs to be considered when working with deep neural networks. Nevertheless, researchers have shown that small datasets can be used successfully, i.e. Garg et al. [50] used three classes of EMG recordings and a total of 1575 trials while achieving an accuracy of 85.44%.

The inclusion of eight participants in an EMG study is in line with the approach of other researchers. I.e. Rehman et al. [30] collected data from seven healthy participants and Bakircioğlu and Öskurt [33] had five participants enrolled in their study.

A limitation of this study is that it was conducted in a clinical setting. Further research is needed to confirm whether the results are applicable to real-world scenarios. In addition, the sensors were fixated by an expert, which is not feasible in a home setting. Therefore, further development is needed to adapt this technology for use in home rehabilitation. In addition, the sensors have to be attached daily in the home environment, and even minimal displacements can lead to significant changes in the recorded EMG signal. This makes it necessary to pursue further research in the area of sensor placement-independent measurements.

An important aspect to be considered is that only healthy participants were recruited, and some of them had no prior experience in walking with crutches, which may contribute to the found results.

14.1   Discussion of Hypothesis A

H: A CNN can classify the load on the leg of unknown steps for a single participant, after training on EMG data obtained from the same participant.

This study has shown, a CNN can learn features from EMG recordings of VL and VM to distinguish between normal and reduced load on the leg with an average success rate of 91.6%. The standard deviation of 7.8% reflects the high variance of the EMG signal, which has also been reported by other researchers [51]. The variability of the EMG signal can be attributed to its inherent nature, which is non-stationary, non-linear, stochastic and unpredictable [52]. At the same time, the characteristics of the sensor play a role, as the signal varies depending on the position relative to the muscle and the quality of the contact with the skin. In addition, the signal is prone to noise, including instrument noise, ambient noise, motion artefacts, and signal instability [53].

The accuracy result in our findings are in line with findings by other researchers. Jain and Greg could reach an accuracy of up to 92.4% when classifying normal and painful movements using Machine Learning approaches [54]. Uwisengeyimana and Ibrikci [55] could reach an accuracy of 91.3% using Deep Neural Networks to discriminate between EMG signals recorded from a healthy person or one with osteoarthritis.

The results show that a change in load leads to an altered EMG signal, thus the CNN can learn features to classify steps with unknown loads, which is also in line with observations by other researchers, e.g. Kristiansen et al. [40] were able to show that the

EMG signal amplitude for VL and VM significantly decreases when walking on a lower body positive pressure treadmill.

The next steps will be to increase the classification accuracy, which can be done by using CNNs in combination with other deep learning algorithms. For example, by connecting CNNs to bidirectional Long Short-Term Memory (LSTM) networks. Karnam et al. [57] were able to improve the accuracy of classifying EMG recordings of hand gestures by up to 18.7% compared to state-of-the-art models.

Another way to improve the accuracy of the CNN is to use transfer learning. This involves pre-training the network on subjects with comparable data recorded followed by training on target data. Soroushmojdehi et al. [58] showed that this methodology can improve the accuracy of a CNN, when predicting hand movements based on EMG data, up to 10%.

14.2 Discussion of Hypothesis B

H: A CNN can classify the load on the leg for an unknown participant, after training on EMG data obtained by different participants.

The result of this hypothesis testing shows an average accuracy of 75.4% ± 10%, surpassing chance level (50%). A major contributing factor is the high interpatient variability. This high variability has already been reported by Anders et al. [59], who demonstrated substantial interindividual variability and Guidetti et al. [60] found significant variation between subjects.

Furthermore, the interpatient comparison results are consistent with findings in existing literature. In this study, two classes of load on the leg were classified with up to 75.4% validation accuracy (Table 5). This is in line with findings by Nazmi et al. [61] who achieved an accuracy of 77% for classifying two gait events when using an unlearned dataset.

The next steps will be to increase the classification accuracy. This can be done by using the normal gait pattern of a subject under investigation as calibration followed by detecting changes in load with the help of a trained CNN. Cano et al. [62] showed, that the accuracy of predicting high blood pressure in unknown subjects could be increased by up to 30% this way.

15 Conclusion

The aim of this study was to provide initial insights into the potential utility of EMG sensors in improving the reliability of weight bearing monitoring during home rehabilitation. It is shown that EMG measurements, evaluated by a CNN trained on a single participant, can be used to classify between normal and reduced load on the leg with an average validation accuracy of 91.6%. This can be used to determine when a patient returned to a full weight bearing on the treated leg, indicating reduced inflammation, increased fracture stabilization, reduced pain and overall treatment success. However, for clinical use interpatient accuracy needs to be increased, as a freshly treated patient will not be able to record different loads on the leg to train a CNN. Additionally, an

EMG system needs to classify load gradations in order to generate rehabilitation support comparable to a pressure insole. In conclusion, while the results show that such a system is not yet ready for use as a medical device, they do highlight the potential and need for further research.

The results are also consistent with our previous research. We have shown that EMG measurements, can be used to classify between inward, outward and normal FPAs with an average validation accuracy of 70.4% [24]. This highlighted the potential use of EMG sensors in monitoring the rehabilitation phase. Our recent findings can further support this assumption, as EMG measurements can be used to classify normal and reduced load on the leg with an average validation accuracy of 91.6%. This combination brings us a step further towards the development of an EMG system that can monitor the rehabilitation phase and thus support individualized treatment, leading to improved outcomes and reduced workload of treating experts.

Further research will include the use of an EMG sensor array, as this allows the density of information recorded from one muscle to be increased. In addition, increasing the size of the dataset is a crucial factor in improving the classification accuracy of neural networks. The ability to integrate more steps could significantly increase the accuracy of a neural network. Other optimization approaches include combining different deep learning algorithms and testing the applicability of transfer learning.

Acknowledgements. This work is a proceeding of the earlier paper: Evaluating the Viability of Neural Networks for Analysing Electromyography Data in Home Rehabilitation: Estimating Foot Progression Angle.

This work is founded by the German Federal Ministry of Education and Research (BMBF) (FKZ: 01IS21085) and is part of the ITEA Secure-e-Health project.

To the best of our knowledge, this study represents the first instance of utilizing EMG measurements in combination with CNNs to provide insight into the load on the leg during walking on crutches.

Disclosure of Interest. The authors have no competing interests to declare that are relevant to the content of this article.

References

1. Mavrogenis, A.F., et al.: Complications after hip nailing for fractures. Orthopedics **39**(1) (2016). https://doi.org/10.3928/01477447-20151222-11
2. El Moumni, M., Voogd, E.H., Ten Duis, H.J., Wendt, K.W.: Long-term functional outcome following intramedullary nailing of femoral shaft fractures. Injury **43**(7), 1154–1158 (2012). https://doi.org/10.1016/j.injury.2012.03.011
3. Rommens, P.M., Hessmann, M.H., Eds.: Intramedullary Nailing. Springer, London (2015). https://doi.org/10.1007/978-1-4471-6612-2.
4. Hamahashi, K., Uchiyama, Y., Kobayashi, Y., Ebihara, G., Ukai, T., Watanabe, M.: Clinical outcomes of intramedullary nailing of femoral shaft fractures with third fragments: a retrospective analysis of risk factors for delayed union. Trauma Surg Acute Care Open **4**(1), e000203 (2019). https://doi.org/10.1136/tsaco-2018-000203
5. Jaarsma, R.L., van Kampen, A.: Rotational malalignment after fractures of the femur. J. Bone Joint Surg. Br. **86-B**(8), 1100–1104 (2004). https://doi.org/10.1302/0301-620X.86B8.15663

6. Hayden, J.A., Ellis, J., Ogilvie, R., Malmivaara, A., van Tulder, M.W.: Exercise therapy for chronic low back pain. Cochrane Database Syst. Rev. **9**(9), CD009790 (2021). https://doi.org/10.1002/14651858.CD009790.pub2.

7. Mangione, K.K., Craik, R.L., Palombaro, K.M., Tomlinson, S.S., Hofmann, M.T.: Home-based leg-strengthening exercise improves function 1 year after hip fracture: a randomized controlled study. J. Am. Geriatr. Soc. **58**(10), 1911–1917 (2010). https://doi.org/10.1111/j.1532-5415.2010.03076.x

8. Rudin, N.: Chronic pain rehabilitation: principles and practice. WMJ: Official Publication of the State Medical Society of Wisconsin **100**, 36–43, 66 (2001)

9. Sherrington, C., et al.: Exercise to reduce mobility disability and prevent falls after fall-related leg or pelvic fracture: RESTORE randomized controlled trial. J. Gen. Intern. Med. **35**(10), 2907–2916 (2020). https://doi.org/10.1007/s11606-020-05666-9

10. Taraldsen, K., et al.: 'Short and long-term clinical effectiveness and cost-effectiveness of a late-phase community-based balance and gait exercise program following hip fracture. The EVA-Hip Randomised Controlled Trial', PLoS ONE **14**(11), e0224971 (2019). https://doi.org/10.1371/journal.pone.0224971

11. Toogood, P.A., Abdel, M.P., Spear, J.A., Cook, S.M., Cook, D.J., Taunton, M.J.: The monitoring of activity at home after total hip arthroplasty. The Bone & Joint J. 98-B, no. 11, pp. 1450–1454 (2016), https://doi.org/10.1302/0301-620X.98B11.BJJ-2016-0194.R1.

12. Latham, N.K., Bean, J.F., Jette, A.M.: Home-based exercise and hip fracture rehabilitation—reply. JAMA **311**(23), 2440 (2014). https://doi.org/10.1001/jama.2014.5173

13. Pidani, A.S., Sabzwari, S., Ahmad, K., Mohammed, A., Noordin, S.: Effectiveness of home-based rehabilitation program in minimizing disability and secondary falls after a hip fracture: protocol for a randomized controlled trial. Int. J. Surg. Protoc. **22**, 24–28 (2020). https://doi.org/10.1016/j.isjp.2020.06.002

14. Siegel, F., et al.: Concept for general improvements in the treatment of femoral shaft fractures with an intramedullary nail. In: Proceedings of the 16th International Joint Conference on Biomedical Engineering Systems and Technologies, Lisbon, Portugal: SCITEPRESS - Science and Technology Publications, pp. 360–367 (2023). https://doi.org/10.5220/001167910 0003414.

15. Maruyama, M., et al.: Modulation of the inflammatory response and bone healing. Front. Endocrinol. **11**, 386 (2020). https://doi.org/10.3389/fendo.2020.00386

16. Loi, F., Córdova, L.A., Pajarinen, J., Lin, T., Yao, Z., Goodman, S.B.: Inflammation, fracture and bone repair. Bone **86**, 119–130 (2016). https://doi.org/10.1016/j.bone.2016.02.020

17. Flanagan, C.D., Joseph, N.M., Copp, J., Romeo, N., Alfonso, N., Hirschfeld, A.: Weight-bearing status may influence rates of radiographic healing following reamed, intramedullary fixation of diaphyseal femur fractures. OTA Int. Open Access J. Orthop. Trauma **4**(4), e154 (2021). https://doi.org/10.1097/OI9.0000000000000154

18. Aoyagi, K., et al.: Does weight-bearing versus non-weight-bearing pain reflect different pain mechanisms in knee osteoarthritis?: The Multicenter Osteoarthritis Study (MOST). Osteoarthritis Cartilage **30**(4), 545–550 (2022). https://doi.org/10.1016/j.joca.2021.10.014

19. Walczyk, D.F., Bartlet, J.P.: An inexpensive weight bearing indicator used for rehabilitation of patients with lower extremity injuries. J. Med. Devices **1**(1), 38–46 (2007). https://doi.org/10.1115/1.2355690

20. Acharya, I., Van Tuyl, J.T., De Lange, J., Quenneville, C.E.: A force-sensing insole to quantify impact loading to the foot. J. Biomechanical Eng. **141**(2), 024501 (2019). https://doi.org/10.1115/1.4041902

21. Melia, G., Siegkas, P., Levick, J., Apps, C.: Insoles of uniform softer material reduced plantar pressure compared to dual-material insoles during regular and loaded gait. Appl. Ergon. **91**, 103298 (2021). https://doi.org/10.1016/j.apergo.2020.103298

22. Peebles, A.T., Maguire, L.A., Renner, K.E., Queen, R.M.: Validity and repeatability of single-sensor loadsol insoles during landing. Sensors **18**(12), 4082 (2018). https://doi.org/10.3390/s18124082

23. Subramaniam, S., Majumder, S., Faisal, A.I., Deen, M.J.: Insole-based systems for health monitoring: current solutions and research challenges. Sensors **22**(2), 438 (2022). https://doi.org/10.3390/s22020438

24. Al-Ayyad, M., Owida, H.A., De Fazio, R., Al-Naami, B., Visconti, P.: Electromyography monitoring systems in rehabilitation: a review of clinical applications. Wearable Devices Signal Acquisition Methodol. Electron. **12**(7), 1520 (2023). https://doi.org/10.3390/electronics12071520

25. Akuzawa, H., Imai, A., Iizuka, S., Matsunaga, N., Kaneoka, K.: The influence of foot position on lower leg muscle activity during a heel raise exercise measured with fine-wire and surface EMG. Phys. Therapy Sport **28**, 23–28 (2017). https://doi.org/10.1016/j.ptsp.2017.08.077

26. Faust, O., Hagiwara, Y., Hong, T.J., Lih, O.S., Acharya, U.R.: Deep learning for healthcare applications based on physiological signals: a review. Comput. Methods Programs Biomedicine **161**, 1–13 (2018). https://doi.org/10.1016/j.cmpb.2018.04.005

27. Olsson, A.E., Sager, P., Andersson, E., Björkman, A., Malešević, N., Antfolk, C.: Extraction of multi-labelled movement information from the raw HD-sEMG image with time-domain depth. Sci. Rep. **9**(1), 7244 (2019). https://doi.org/10.1038/s41598-019-43676-8

28. Yang, W., Yang, D., Liu, Y., Liu, H.: EMG pattern recognition using convolutional neural network with different scale signal/spectra input. Int. J. Human. Robot. **16**(04), 1950013 (2019). https://doi.org/10.1142/S0219843619500130

29. Zia Ur Rehman, M., et al.: Multiday EMG-based classification of hand motions with deep learning techniques. Sensors **18**(8), 2497 (2018). https://doi.org/10.3390/s18082497

30. Al-Jabery, Kd., Obafemi-Ajayi, T., Olbricht, G., Wunsch, D.: Computational Learning Approaches to Data Analytics in Biomedical Applications. Academic Press, London (2020)

31. Zhao, B., Lu, H., Chen, S., Liu, J., Wu, D.: Convolutional neural networks for time series classification. JSEE **28**(1), 162–169 (2017). https://doi.org/10.21629/JSEE.2017.01.18

32. Bakircioğlu, K., Özkurt, N.: Classification of EMG signals using convolution neural network. Int. J. Appl. Math. Electron. Comput. **8**(4), 115–119 (2020). https://doi.org/10.18100/ijamec.795227

33. Siegel, F., Buj, C., Merfort, R., Hein, A., Aschwege, F.: Evaluating the viability of neural networks for analysing electromyography data in home rehabilitation: estimating foot progression angle. In: Proceedings of the 17th International Joint Conference on Biomedical Engineering Systems and Technologies, Rome, Italy: SCITEPRESS - Science and Technology Publications, pp. 132–141 (2024). https://doi.org/10.5220/0012385100003657.

34. Campanini, I., Disselhorst-Klug, C., Rymer, W.Z., Merletti, R.: Surface EMG in clinical assessment and neurorehabilitation: barriers limiting its use. Front. Neurol. **11**, 934 (2020). https://doi.org/10.3389/fneur.2020.00934

35. Simpson, K.M., Munro, B.J., Steele, J.R.: Backpack load affects lower limb muscle activity patterns of female hikers during prolonged load carriage. J. Electromyography Kinesiol. **21**(5), 782–788 (2011). https://doi.org/10.1016/j.jelekin.2011.05.012

36. Nam, C., et al.: An exoneuromusculoskeleton for self-help upper limb rehabilitation after stroke. Soft Robot. **9**(1), 14–35 (2022). https://doi.org/10.1089/soro.2020.0090

37. Barton, C.J., Lack, S., Malliaras, P., Morrissey, D.: Gluteal muscle activity and patellofemoral pain syndrome: a systematic review. Br. J. Sports Med. **47**(4), 207–214 (2013). https://doi.org/10.1136/bjsports-2012-090953

38. Benedetti, M.G., Catani, F., Bilotta, T.W., Marcacci, M., Mariani, E., Giannini, S.: Muscle activation pattern and gait biomechanics after total knee replacement. Clin. Biomech. **18**(9), 871–876 (2003). https://doi.org/10.1016/S0268-0033(03)00146-3

39. Vakula, M.N., Garcia, S.A., Holmes, S.C., Pamukoff, D.N.: Association between quadriceps function, joint kinetics, and spatiotemporal gait parameters in young adults with and without obesity. Gait Posture **92**, 421–427 (2022). https://doi.org/10.1016/j.gaitpost.2021.12.019

40. Kristiansen, M., Odderskær, N., Kristensen, D.H.: Effect of body weight support on muscle activation during walking on a lower body positive pressure treadmill. J. Electromyography Kinesiol. **48**, 9–16 (2019). https://doi.org/10.1016/j.jelekin.2019.05.021

41. Tm, M., Ordway, N., Ploutz-Snyder, L.: An EMG and force comparision for walking with crutches and an ergonomically designed walker. Med. Sci. Sports Exerc. **34**(5), S247 (2002). https://doi.org/10.1097/00005768-200205001-01380

42. Stastny, P., Lehnert, M., Zaatar, A., Svoboda, Z., Xaverova, Z., Jelen, K.: Knee joint muscles neuromuscular activity during load-carrying walking. Neuro Endocrinol. Lett. **35**(7), 633–639 (2014)

43. Hermens, F., Merletti, R., Disselhorst-Klug, Stegeman: SENIAM (Surface ElectroMyoGraphy for the Non-Invasive Assessment of Muscles) project. http://www.seniam.org/

44. Delsys, Trigno Wireless Biofeedback System. https://www.delsys.com/downloads/USERSG UIDE/trigno/wireless-biofeedback-system.pdf

45. Alwosheel, A., Van Cranenburgh, S., Chorus, C.G.: Is your dataset big enough? Sample size requirements when using artificial neural networks for discrete choice analysis. J. Choice Model. **28**, 167–182 (2018). https://doi.org/10.1016/j.jocm.2018.07.002

46. Zha, X., et al.: A deep learning model for automated classification of intraoperative continuous EMG. IEEE Trans. Med. Robot. Bionics **3**(1), 44–52 (2021). https://doi.org/10.1109/TMRB.2020.3048255

47. Howard, R.: The application of data analysis methods for surface electromyography in shot putting and sprinting (2017). https://doi.org/10.13140/RG.2.2.15907.04640.

48. Murray, M.P., Drought, A.B., Kory, R.C.: Walking patterns of normal men. J. Bone Joint Surg. Am. **46**, 335–360 (1964)

49. Morbidoni, C., Cucchiarelli, A., Fioretti, S., Di Nardo, F.: A deep learning approach to EMG-based classification of gait phases during level ground walking. Electronics **8**(8), 894 (2019). https://doi.org/10.3390/electronics8080894

50. Li, G., Li, Y., Yu, L., Geng, Y.: Conditioning and sampling issues of EMG signals in motion recognition of multifunctional myoelectric prostheses. Ann. Biomed. Eng. **39**(6), 1779–1787 (2011). https://doi.org/10.1007/s10439-011-0265-x

51. Abadi, M., et al.: TensorFlow: large-scale machine learning on heterogeneous systems (2015). https://www.tensorflow.org/

52. Chollet, F., others, 'Keras' (2015). https://keras.io

53. Wani, M.A., Bhat, F.A., Afzal, S., Khan, A.I.: Advances in deep learning. In: Studies in Big Data, vol. 57. Springer Singapore, Singapore (2020). https://doi.org/10.1007/978-981-13-6794-6

54. Hicks, S.A., et al.: On evaluation metrics for medical applications of artificial intelligence. Sci. Rep. **12**(1), 5979 (2022). https://doi.org/10.1038/s41598-022-09954-8

55. Garg, N., Balafrej, I., Beilliard, Y., Drouin, D., Alibart, F., Rouat, J.: Signals to spikes for neuromorphic regulated reservoir computing and EMG hand gesture recognition. In: International Conference on Neuromorphic Systems 2021, Knoxville, TN, USA, pp. 1–8. ACM (2021). https://doi.org/10.1145/3477145.3477267.

56. Rane, L., Ding, Z., McGregor, A.H., Bull, A.M.J.: Deep learning for musculoskeletal force prediction. Ann. Biomed. Eng. **47**(3), 778–789 (2019). https://doi.org/10.1007/s10439-018-02190-0

57. Geng, W., Du, Y., Jin, W., Wei, W., Hu, Y., Li, J.: Gesture recognition by instantaneous surface EMG images. Sci. Rep. **6**(1), 36571 (2016). https://doi.org/10.1038/srep36571

58. Reaz, M.B.I., Hussain, M.S., Mohd-Yasin, F.: Techniques of EMG signal analysis: detection, processing, classification and applications. Biol. Proced. Online **8**(1), 11–35 (2006). https://doi.org/10.1251/bpo115

59. Jain, R., Garg, V.K.: EMG signal feature extraction, normalization and classification for pain and normal muscles using genetic algorithm and support vector machine. RIA **34**(5), 653–661 (2020). https://doi.org/10.18280/ria.340517

60. Uwisengeyimana, J.D., Ibrikci, T.: diagnosing knee osteoarthritis using artificial neural networks and deep learning. Biomed. Stat. Inform. **2**(3), 95–102 (2017). https://doi.org/10.11648/j.bsi.20170203.11

61. Karnam, N.K., Dubey, S.R., Turlapaty, A.C., Gokaraju, B.: EMGHandNet: a hybrid CNN and Bi-LSTM architecture for hand activity classification using surface EMG signals. Biocybern. Biomed. Eng. **42**(1), 325–340 (2022). https://doi.org/10.1016/j.bbe.2022.02.005

62. Soroushmojdehi, R., Javadzadeh, S., Pedrocchi, A., Gandolla, M.: Transfer learning in hand movement intention detection based on surface electromyography signals. Front. Neurosci. **16**, 977328 (2022). https://doi.org/10.3389/fnins.2022.977328

63. Anders, J.P.V., et al.: Inter- and Intra-Individual differences in EMG and MMG during maximal bilateral, dynamic leg extensions. Sports **7**(7), 175 (2019). https://doi.org/10.3390/sports7070175

64. Guidetti, L., Rivellini, G., Figura, F.: EMG patterns during running: Intra- and inter-individual variability. J. Electromyography Kinesiol. **6**(1), 37–48 (1996). https://doi.org/10.1016/1050-6411(95)00015-1

65. Nazmi, N., Abdul Rahman, M.A., Yamamoto, S.-I., Ahmad, S.A.: Walking gait event detection based on electromyography signals using artificial neural network. Biomed. Signal Process. Control **47**, 334–343 (2019). https://doi.org/10.1016/j.bspc.2018.08.030.

66. Cano, J., Fácila, L., Gracia-Baena, J.M., Zangróniz, R., Alcaraz, R., Rieta, J.J.: The relevance of calibration in machine learning-based hypertension risk assessment combining photoplethysmography and electrocardiography. Biosensors **12**(5), 289 (2022). https://doi.org/10.3390/bios12050289

Enhancing Emotional Well-Being Through Virtual Reality: The 2ViTA-B Cognitive System

Nicoletta Balletti[1,3], Antonella Cascitelli[2], Patrizia Gabrieli[2], Emanuela Guglielmi[3], Aldo Lazich[1], Gianluca Marcilli[4], Marco Notarantonio[1], Rocco Oliveto[3,5(✉)], and Daniela Scognamiglio[2]

[1] Defense Veteran Center, Ministry of Defense, Rome, Italy
[2] Atlantica Digital spa, Rome, Italy
`{antonella.cascitelli,patrizia.gabrieli,`
`daniela.scognamiglio}@atlantica.it`
[3] University of Molise, Pesche, IS, Italy
`{emanuela.guglielmi,rocco.oliveto}@unimol.it`
[4] National Armaments Directorate (NAVARM), Ministry of Defense, Rome, Italy
`gianlucam.marcilli@marina.difesa.it`
[5] Datasound srl, Spin-Off of the University of Molise, Pesche, IS, Italy

Abstract. The growing interest in treating emotional disorders has led to the exploration of virtual reality (VR) as a tool for cognitive rehabilitation. This paper present an extensive evaluation of the 2ViTA-B Cognitive system, an innovative software and hardware system designed to enhance psychological and emotional engagement through customizable stimuli sequences in both standard and VR modes. A controlled study with 16 participants was conducted to assess the effectiveness of the system in enhancing emotional well-being and cognitive function, as well as its impact on self-assessed affectivity using well-established questionnaires. Additionally, the study evaluated the system usability, a critical factor for its overall effectiveness. Results indicate that 2ViTA-B Cognitive significantly enhances mood and cognitive performance, with VR providing a particularly immersive and impactful experience. These findings suggest promising directions for the use of VR in therapeutic practices aimed at improving mental well-being. The paper also discusses the potential benefits and limitations of VR as a therapeutic tool and highlights areas for future research.

Keywords: Cognitive rehabilitation · Medical support · Home rehabilitation · Virtual reality · Meta quest 2 · EEG

1 Introduction

Affectivity, which includes emotions, moods, attitudes, and interpersonal relationships, plays a vital role in shaping behavior, well-being, and cognitive processes [42]. Affective cognition refers to the mental processes involved in interpreting and responding to emotionally significant stimuli [40]. There is a growing

M. P. Guarino et al. (Eds.): BIOSTEC 2024, CCIS 2546, pp. 354–375, 2026.
https://doi.org/10.1007/978-3-031-96899-0_20

body of research focused on treating emotional disorders to enhance affective function and mitigate symptoms, particularly by understanding how various stimuli influence emotions and mood.

Both traditional and digital platforms are used to deliver these stimuli, with virtual reality (VR) emerging as a particularly compelling medium in recent years [45,49,54]. Numerous studies have investigated the potential of VR and related technologies to improve mental health [14,34,36]. These endeavors often align with the principles of positive psychology, a field of clinical psychology that focuses on promoting mental well-being and happiness [22]. VR has shown promise in enhancing mood, reducing symptoms associated with fear, stress, depression, and anxiety [12,15,29,31,37,53], and inducing positive emotional experiences [2,13,20].

Moreover, VR has been effectively employed in the treatment of various anxiety disorders, such as phobias, generalized anxiety, social anxiety, post-traumatic stress disorder, and obsessive-compulsive disorder [16,34,35,39,46]. The influence of VR on emotions is largely due to its immersive 360-degree environments, which provide a level of emotional engagement that is difficult to achieve with other methods [6]. However, the use of VR is not without limitations, as it can lead to side effects such as nausea, dizziness, and discomfort, which may vary depending on individual sensitivity.

In line with this growing interest in VR for emotional and cognitive therapy, this paper extends our previous work [1] by extensively evaluate 2ViTA-B Cognitive, a comprehensive software and hardware system designed to foster psychological and emotional engagement. 2ViTA-B Cognitive allows therapists to personalize sequences of stimuli—such as images, sounds, and videos—in both standard and VR modes for use in cognitive rehabilitation. A controlled study with 16 participants demonstrated the system effectiveness of the system, particularly in leveraging VR to enhance emotional well-being and cognitive functioning.

This paper introduces several new contributions beyond our earlier work [1]. In addition to utilizing the Positive and Negative Affect Schedule (PANAS) questionnaire [51] to assess both positive and negative affectivity, we expanded our evaluation by including the Global Vigor-Affect Scale (GVAS) [33], which measures mood and vigor indices. Furthermore, we assessed self-evaluative affectivity using the Self-Assessment Manikin (SAM) scale [4], which evaluates participants' valence, activation, and dominance.

We also conducted a comprehensive usability evaluation of the 2ViTA-B Cognitive system, through a questionnaire in which participants rated the system's ease of use, comfort, and learnability. Usability is a critical factor for the effectiveness of such systems, as it directly influences user engagement and the overall success of the intervention. Ensuring that the system is intuitive, comfortable, and easy to learn is essential for encouraging consistent use, particularly in therapeutic and rehabilitation contexts where user experience can significantly impact outcomes.

The rest of the paper is organized as follows. Section 2 discusses the related literature. Section 3 presents in details 2ViTA-B Cognitive system. Section 4 describes the empirical study that we conducted to evaluate the capability of

2ViTA-B Cognitive VR to enanche self-assessment affectiveness, improve participants' attention, and the usability of the system. We present the results of the study in Sect. 5. Section 6 concludes the paper and highlights future research directions.

2   Related Work

Emotional responses triggered by visual stimuli are closely linked to various physical and physiological parameters, including facial expressions [11], heart rate, and body temperature [9]. The valence (positive or negative quality) and activation (level of arousal) of these images can be quantitatively assessed through methods such as facial electromyography, electrocardiography, and skin conductance [3,28]. In the scientific literature, several image sets have been rigorously validated for their effectiveness in evoking specific emotional responses [27,32].

However, static images often have a limited emotional impact compared to dynamic stimuli, such as videos or music, which can evoke more intense and complex emotional reactions [52]. As a result, many studies have explored the psychological and neurological effects of auditory stimuli, including music, speech, noise, and soundscapes, on human emotions and mood [38,50]. These auditory stimuli have been shown to induce measurable physiological changes, such as variations in skin conductance and heart rate [10,23].

Despite the importance of sound in emotional research, there are relatively few validated sound collections available. Nonetheless, some studies have developed specific sound stimuli or curated internet-based sound samples that have been validated according to user preferences and physiological responses [17,25]. Among these, two widely used sound libraries have been validated using physiological measures, providing reliable tools for affective research [18,26].

Videos, due to their multimodal, dynamic, and immersive nature, have been found to elicit stronger emotional responses compared to static images or sound alone [19,47]. This heightened impact is largely because videos can engage multiple senses simultaneously, creating a richer emotional experience. Commonly used video stimuli include carefully selected film clips and amateur online videos, both of which are designed to evoke a broad spectrum of emotions, from basic feelings like anger and disgust to more complex emotions such as joy and amusement [24,41]. Established video libraries often categorize films to target specific emotional states, facilitating their use in experimental settings [43].

In addition to these traditional forms of stimuli, virtual reality (VR) has emerged as a powerful tool for inducing emotional responses. Ulrich and colleagues [48] pioneered the use of natural environments as stimuli within VR, drawing on the Stress Reduction Theory. This theory suggests that exposure to natural settings can activate the parasympathetic nervous system, which is associated with relaxation and the reduction of stress, fear, and anger. The immersive quality of VR allows for the creation of highly controlled and realistic environments, making it an effective medium for studying emotional responses and their physiological correlates.

While the existing body of research has made significant strides in utilizing static images, auditory stimuli, and video clips to elicit emotional responses, these methods often lack the personalized and interactive elements necessary for effective cognitive rehabilitation. Moreover, while virtual reality has been explored as a tool for emotional engagement, there remains a gap in systems that integrate customizable, multimodal stimuli tailored to individual therapeutic needs. In our previous work [1], we address these limitations by offering a versatile platform, the 2Vita-B Cognitive system, that allows therapists to design and deliver individualized sequences of stimuli—ranging from images and sounds to immersive VR experiences. This system not only leverages the immersive capabilities of VR to enhance emotional engagement but also incorporates real-time feedback mechanisms, enabling a more dynamic and responsive therapeutic process.

To substantiate the efficacy of 2ViTA-B Cognitive, in this paper we extended the evaluation of the 2Vita-B Cognitive system in order to evaluate (i) the impact of the system on emotional well-being and cognitive function; (ii) its influence on self-evaluative affectivity, measured through standardized questionnaires; (iii) the usability of the system. These findings not only validate the practical utility of 2ViTA-B Cognitive but also highlight its potential to advance therapeutic practices by bridging the gap between traditional affective stimuli and cutting-edge VR technologies.

3   System Overview and Workflow of 2ViTA-B Cognitive

2ViTA-B Cognitive is a comprehensive hardware and software platform designed to enhance mental well-being and alleviate stress through the use of multimedia sequences in both standard and VR modes. These sequences are tailored to evoke specific emotional responses and include daily cognitive training activities. The system integrates physiological data collection from wearable devices and utilizes artificial intelligence to assist therapists in decision-making. Gamification elements are embedded to boost user engagement, creating a more interactive and effective therapeutic experience.

3.1   User Roles and Content Management

The system supports three distinct user roles:

- administrators, who manage content;
- specialists, who oversee rehabilitation plans;
- patients, who participate in training activities.

Administrators are responsible for enrolling patients into the system, during which patients complete a medical history questionnaire. This information is crucial for therapists to assess the patient's current and past health status.

Administrators also curate multimedia content, which psychologists then use to create personalized, multisensory stimulus sequences. These sequences may include images, sounds, videos, and immersive VR scenes. Additionally, patients can upload their own multimedia content, which can be integrated into the sequences following validation by the therapist.

As shown in Fig. 1, the process of creating a sequence is supported by the 2ViTA-B Cognitive virtual assistant, which suggests additional elements that align with the chosen ones in terms of valence and arousal. However, the psychologist has full discretion to accept or reject these suggestions, ensuring the final sequence is tailored to the patient's specific needs.

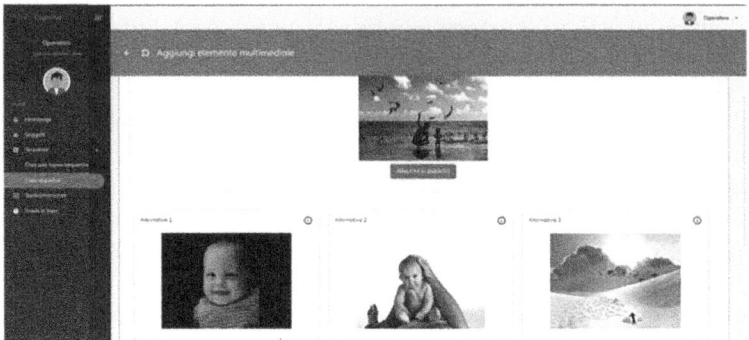

Fig. 1. Definition of a sequence for an administration [1].

3.2   Typical Session Workflow

A typical session with 2ViTA-B Cognitive involves three key steps:

1. **Preliminary Screening**: Patients complete the Perceived Stress Scale (PSS-10) questionnaire, which measures perceived stress levels [8].
2. **Self-Assessment Questionnaires**: Patients fill out three questionnaires: the Positive and Negative Affect Scale (PANAS) to assess affective state [51], the Self-Assessment Manikins (SAM) to measure emotional reactions to stimuli [4], and the Global Vigor-Affect Scale (GVAS) to gauge mood and energy levels.
3. **Multimedia Sequence Presentation**: A sequence of media items created by the psychologist is presented to the patient.

The multimedia sequences are categorized into two groups: standard and virtual reality. The standard sequence comprises images, sounds, and videos with positive valence from validated sources. The current system library includes 32 images from the International Affective Picture System (IAPS) catalog [27], 20 sounds from the International Affective Digital Sounds (IADS) [5], and 5 videos validated by Maffei et al. [30]. These stimuli are presented randomly, with images and sounds displayed for six seconds each, and videos lasting approximately two minutes. The entire sequence, including intervals of two-second black screens between stimuli, runs for around twelve minutes.

Alternatively, sessions can be conducted using virtual reality, which requires a VR headset. The current implementation of 2ViTA-B Cognitive utilizes the Meta Quest 2. The virtual sequences include two immersive scenes: a realistic natural landscape (Fig. 2) and an interactive space exploration environment (Fig. 3). These settings were chosen based on research demonstrating the positive effects of natural environments on emotional states [6, 21, 48]. The first scene, referred to as the "static scene", focuses on high realism and environmental quality. The second scene, the "dynamic scene," allows patients to navigate within a spacecraft, interact with objects, and engage in a virtual space exploration journey.

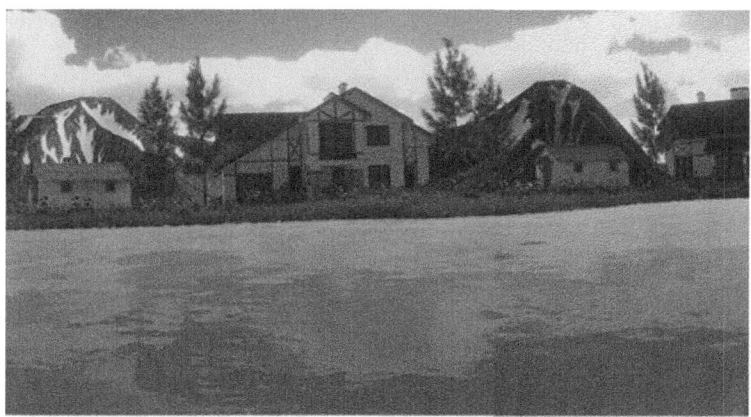

Fig. 2. The first virtual scene: static scene [1].

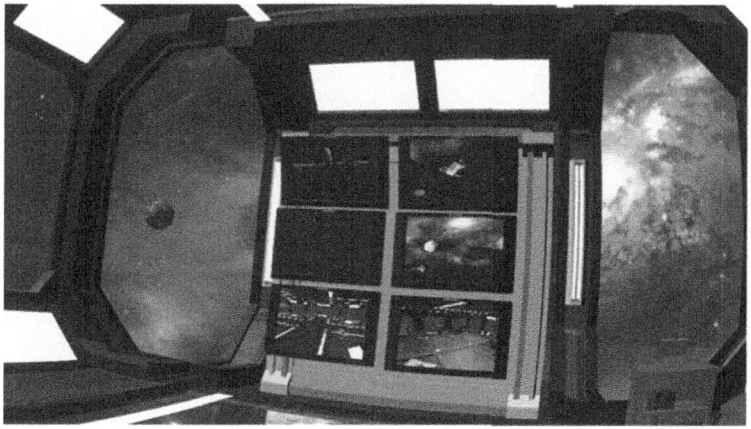

Fig. 3. The second virtual scene: dynamic scene [1].

3.3 Real-Time Monitoring and Data Analysis

The system notifies therapists when a new session begins, providing them the option to monitor the patient's progress in real-time or review it later. A comprehensive dashboard displays the patient's profile, history, responses, and the administered multimedia sequences (see Fig. 4) as well as the vital signs monitored during the administration (see Fig. 5).

After each session, therapists can provide numerical assessments and feedback. They can evaluate a patient's progress by comparing multiple sessions, aided by an AI algorithm that identifies trends in the data. The system also offers optional blockchain verification to ensure the integrity of patient data.

Patients, on the other hand, can access their session history, including dates, times, and therapist evaluations, and track their progress visually through an avatar-based path in their profile.

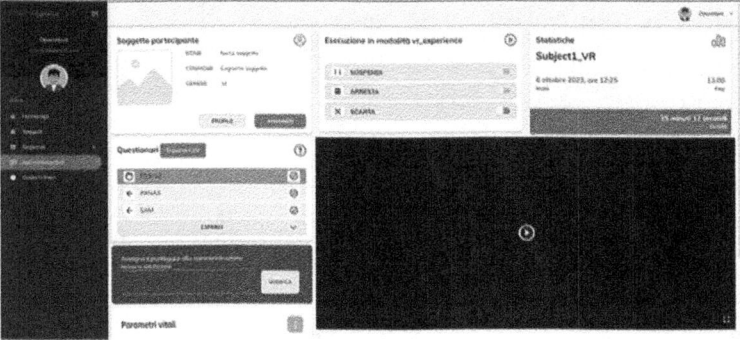

Fig. 4. Patient's profile visualization during the execution of administration [1].

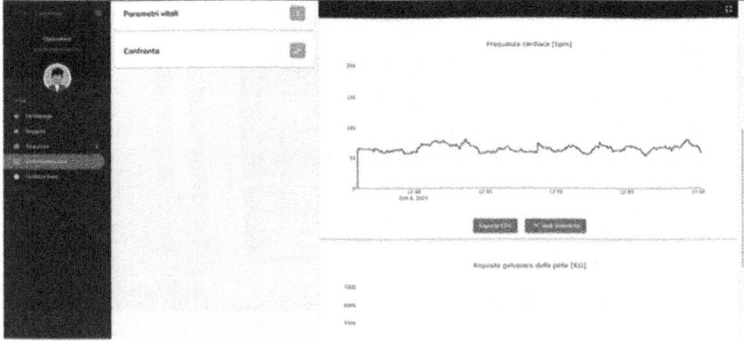

Fig. 5. Patient's vital parameters monitoring during an administration [1].

3.4   Extension of Immersive Reality and Customization Capabilities

A significant innovation within the 2ViTA-B Cognitive system is the development of a versatile VR plugin, designed to simplify the creation and customization of immersive environments. The VR plugin provides standardized components that developers can utilize to build new scenes with minimal effort. By simply replacing graphical assets, developers can create entirely new immersive environments tailored to specific therapeutic needs.

This adaptability ensures that the VR component of 2ViTA-B Cognitive is not limited to the two initial scenes but can be expanded into a wide variety of customized virtual experiences. The plugin architecture is designed to be highly extensible, supporting the development of a broad range of therapeutic VR environments. This makes 2ViTA-B Cognitive a powerful and flexible tool, capable of evolving to meet diverse therapeutic requirements and advancing the field of emotional and cognitive rehabilitation.

4   Empirical Evaluation of the 2Vita-B Cognite System

We conducted an experiment to evaluate the effects of hematogenic stimulation on cognitive attention functions. In the following we present the design of the experiment we conducted to validate the 2ViTA-B Cognitive system, particularly focusing on the effectiveness of incorporating virtual reality (VR) during cognitive rehabilitation sessions.

4.1   Study Definition and Context

The primary objective of this study was to explore the potential benefits of virtual reality (VR) in cognitive rehabilitation activities, specifically its impact on emotional well-being and affectivity. To assess the advantages of employing VR, we conducted a controlled experiment where participants interacted with two versions of the 2ViTA-B Cognitive virtual assistant. In the first version, participants engaged in cognitive rehabilitation sessions using multimedia content designed to modulate affect and reduce negative emotional states [7]. In the second version, participants were immersed in VR sessions to enhance affectivity and cognitive functions.

The experiment involved 16 healthy participants (13 males and 3 females), aged between 22 and 63, recruited through *convenience sampling*. Participants were divided into two groups. Each group completed two sessions using both versions of the 2ViTA-B Cognitive system: one with the standard multimedia content and the other with immersive VR experiences. The Meta Quest 2[1] headset was used for the VR sessions, while all participants, regardless of the session type, wore the Muse S (Gen 2) headband[2] to monitor brain activity and assess selective attention.

---

[1] https://www.meta.com/quest/products/quest-2/ [Verified on August 14th, 2024].

[2] https://choosemuse.com/products/muse-s-gen-2 [Verified on August 14th, 2024].

4.2   Experimental Design

The controlled experiment aimed to determine whether the integration of VR into cognitive rehabilitation activities improves participants' affectivity and cognitive functions. Additionally, the study sought to identify effective methods for measuring the positive impact of this technology on therapeutic practices and overall user well-being.

This study was guided by the following research questions:

– RQ$_1$: *Does the use of 2ViTA-B Cognitive VR improve self-assessment of affectivity?* This question examined whether immersive VR experiences provided by 2ViTA-B Cognitive VR enhance participants' self-assessment of their affective states.
– RQ$_2$: *Does the use of 2ViTA-B Cognitive VR improve participants' attention?* This question aimed to evaluate whether the 2ViTA-B Cognitive VR system enhances participants' attention during cognitive tasks.
– RQ$_3$: *How do participants perceive the usability and overall experience of using the 2ViTA-B Cognitive VR system?* This question sought to understand whether the 2ViTA-B Cognitive VR system is intuitive and provides a satisfying user experience.

To address RQ$_1$ and RQ$_2$, we defined independent variables and observed dependent variables. The independent variables included the *type of treatment*: (i) the conventional version of 2ViTA-B Cognitive (referred to as "Standard"), which uses a web browser to access multimedia content, and (ii) the new 2ViTA-B Cognitive VR version (referred to as "VR"), which provides immersive experiences through VR. Additionally, the experiment involved two administration sessions, labeled as "S1" and "S2".

The dependent variables monitored were *affectivity self-assessments* and *attention*. The former was gauged through standardized questionnaires administered before and after the multimedia or VR sessions, allowing us to measure the impact of the stimuli on participants' emotions. The latter was measured using the cognitive Stroop test [44] and by analyzing electroencephalography (EEG) biosignals recorded during the sessions.

The experiment design, shown in Table 1, involved Group A starting with a VR session followed by a Standard session, while Group B experienced the reverse order. A substantial temporal gap (one to two days) was introduced between the two sessions to mitigate potential carryover effects.

Table 1. Experiment design [1].

	Group A	Group B
S1	VR	Standard
S2	Standard	VR

This design allowed us to compare the effectiveness of Standard and VR treatments while accounting for the order of administration. By systematically analyzing these combinations, we aimed to isolate the impact of VR on cognitive and affective outcomes.

To address RQ_3, we conducted a usability survey at the end of the experiment to evaluate the ease of use, intuitiveness, and overall user experience of the 2ViTA-B Cognitive VR system.

4.3   Preparation

Participants were recruited through direct acquaintance and personal contact by the researchers involved in the study. Those who voluntarily expressed interest in participating, without any form of compensation, were required to complete a medical history questionnaire and the PSS-10 stress assessment. All participants confirmed they had no existing medical conditions, history of psychological disorders, medication use, excessive alcohol consumption, or recreational drug use. Before the study, participants provided informed consent, and the study received approval from the Ethics Committee of the Policlinico Militare "Celio".

The experiment was conducted in the laboratories of the "Veterans Defence Centre" in Rome, Italy. Before the experiment, volunteers were briefed on the administration process, the use of devices (including the VR headset), and the rationale behind the Stroop test.

4.4   Experiment Material and Execution

As previously mentioned, participants engaged in two experimental sessions: one involving cognitive rehabilitation in the Standard version and the other in VR. Participants were evenly distributed between Group A and Group B (as shown in Table 1).

The experimental protocol included three successive phases:

– **PRE Phase**: Participants completed the PANAS, GVAS, and SAM questionnaires, followed by wearing the EEG device for a brief calibration. After calibration, participants undertook the Stroop cognitive test, which was administered either in real or virtual reality depending on the treatment condition.
– **STIM Phase**: Participants viewed the sequence of multimedia elements or immersive VR scenes, depending on their assigned treatment.
– **POST Phase**: This phase mirrored the PRE phase, with participants filling out the PANAS, GVAS, and SAM questionnaires again, and repeating the Stroop test. During VR sessions, participants briefly removed the headset for questionnaire completion before re-engaging with the VR environment for the Stroop test.

After the experiment, we collected data from (i) the self-assessment questionnaires to evaluate affectivity (PANAS, GVAS, and SAM) and (ii) the Stroop test to assess selective attention. The Stroop test scoring system awarded 1 point for correct answers, -1 point for incorrect answers, and 0 points for unanswered questions. Additionally, EEG data focusing on Beta wave activity, associated with attention and cognitive processes, was collected for comparative evaluation.

4.5 Analysis Procedure

To address RQ_1 and RQ_2, we analyzed PANAS, GVAS, and SAM questionnaires:

- **PANAS**. The Positive and Negative Affect Schedule (PANAS) questionnaire [51] measures both positive and negative affectivity. Developed by Watson *et al.* [51], it is one of the most widely used questionnaires in clinical and non-clinical studies. The questionnaire consists of 20 words describing both positive and negative emotions and feelings, using a 5-point Likert scale for rating (*i.e.*, not at all, slightly, moderately, very much, extremely). Participants are asked to indicate how strongly they feel each of the emotions described at the time. In the context of our study, the PANAS results were used to calculate differences in affectivity before and after stimulus administration for both VR and Standard treatments.
- **GVAS**. The Global Vigor-Affect Scale (GVAS) [33] is a self-assessment tool that measures mood and vigor using a visual analog scale. The questionnaire assesses eight dimensions, with four related to mood and four to alertness. Participants respond by placing a mark on a 100 mm horizontal line, where the endpoints represent "not at all" and "very much". Each response is then scored on a scale from 0 to 100, based on the position of the mark. In this study, we analyzed the changes in scores before and after the stimulus presentation, focusing on both the Negative Mood Index (NMI) and the Alertness Index (AI). The NMI is derived by summing the scores for responses related to feelings of sadness, tension, happiness, and calmness, while the AI is calculated by summing the scores for alertness, tiredness, sleepiness, and the effort required to perform tasks.
- **SAM**. The Self-Assessment Manikin (SAM) scale [4] is a widely used tool for assessing emotional responses along three key dimensions: valence, activation, and dominance. The questionnaire comprises three scales, each with nine levels depicted by figures representing different emotional states—ranging from sad to happy, calm to excited, and in control to out of control. Participants are asked to select the figure that best corresponds to their current emotional state, with options ranging from 0 to 9. In this study, the SAM questionnaire was utilized to measure changes in participants' affectivity by comparing their self-assessments of valence, activation, and dominance before and after treatment.

The data collected through the aforementioned questionnaires were analyzed to quantify the differences between the two different treatments: VR and standard administration. Descriptive statistics, including mean, median, and standard deviation, were examined for each treatment. The differences between the two treatments were then analyzed using the Wilcoxon test [55], to test the following null hypotheses:

- H_{01a} *The use of 2ViTA-B Cognitive VR does not lead to an improvement in self-assessed affectivity, in terms of positive and negative emotional states.*
- H_{01b} *The use of 2ViTA-B Cognitive VR does not result in an improvement in self-assessed affectivity, in terms of mood, vigor, and alertness.*
- H_{01c} *The use of 2ViTA-B Cognitive VR does not result in an improvement in self-assessed affectivity, in terms of valence, activation, and dominance.*

A null hypothesis was rejected if the p-value was less than 0.05. This threshold suggests that there is less than a 5% probability that the observed results are due to random chance alone. If the p-value falls below this level, we concluded that the evidence is strong enough to reject the null hypothesis in favor of the alternative hypothesis, which supports the positive effect of 2ViTA-B Cognitive VR on the dependent variable.

To assess the effectiveness of 2ViTA-B Cognitive VR in enhancing participants' attention, we collected the results of the Stroop test and biological signals recorded by the wearable EEG device, with a particular focus on Beta wave activity. The Beta score, provided by the EEG device vendor, is a normalized value ranging from 0 to 1, enabling a straightforward comparison of results across participants. To analyze the impact of the treatment, we calculated the difference between pre- and post-stimulus scores for each participant under both the VR and Standard conditions. Additionally, we computed the mean, median, and standard deviation to compare the effects of the two treatments. Finally, a statistical test, *i.e.*, Wilcoxon Signed-Rank test [55], was employed to evaluate the following null hypothesis:

H_{02} *The use of 2ViTA-B Cognitive VR does not lead to improvements in participants' attention.*

Similarly to H_{01}, H_{02} will also be rejected if the p-value is less than 0.05

Finally, to address RQ_3, we conducted a usability survey (reported in Table 2) to evaluate the ease of use, comfort, and overall user experience of the 2ViTA-B Cognitive VR system. Participants rated their experience on a 5-point Likert scale, and the results were summarized using boxplots to visualize the distribution and trends in usability ratings.

Table 2. Usability questionnaire.

ID	Question
1	Do you find the 2Vita-B Cognitive system easy to use?
2	How comfortable did you feel using the 2Vita-B Cognitive system?
3	Do you think most people can learn to use the 2Vita-B Cognitive system easily?

4.6   Limitations and Threats to Validity

The primary threat to the validity of this study relates to the representativeness of the results. Our test sample consisted of only 16 individuals, which raises concerns about the robustness and generalizability of the findings. Such a small sample size may not accurately reflect the broader population, potentially compromising the reliability of our conclusions. This is a common challenge in human-subject research, but it was particularly pronounced in our study due to the difficulty of recruiting participants willing to undergo double experimental sessions without compensation.

Additionally, the gender distribution of our participants was heavily skewed toward males, introducing a potential bias in the data. Research suggests that emotional responses can vary significantly by gender, and this imbalance may have influenced our results, limiting their applicability across a more diverse population.

Finally, it is crucial to note that the proposed system is still in the early stages of testing and has not yet been certified as a medical device. Consequently, our experiments were limited to healthy individuals, further restricting the generalizability of the results to broader populations, including those with medical conditions.

5   Analysis of the Results

In this section, we present the analysis of results for the three research questions (RQs) of our study.

5.1   RQ$_1$: Impact on Self-assessment Affectivity

Table 3 provides descriptive statistics from the PANAS questionnaire scores for both treatments (VR and Standard). The scores represent the difference between the POST and PRE administration for both sessions (S1 and S2).

Table 3. Results of RQ$_1$. Descriptive statistics of PANAS questionnaire. A high score suggests a positive emotional state, while a low score suggests a less positive or more neutral emotional state.

	VR	Standard
Mean	39.37	−12.50
Median	35.00	−10.00
Std. dev	57.90	56.74

The results from the affectivity self-assessment questionnaire show that immersive virtual reality experiences provided by 2ViTA-B Cognitive VR significantly outperformed the standard administration in enhancing participants' perceived affectivity. The mean score for the VR treatment was 39.37, while the standard treatment had a much lower mean score of -12.50. Notably, one participant in the VR group reported a low score of -50, likely due to nausea experienced during the VR session.

The difference between the two treatments is both substantial and statistically significant, as indicated by the Wilcoxon Signed-Rank test, which returned a p-value of 0.006 ($z = -2.54$, $W = 12$). Consequently, we can confidently reject the null hypothesis H_{01a} and conclude that *the use of 2ViTA-B Cognitive VR leads to a significant improvement in self-assessment affectivity, in terms of positive and negative emotional states.*

Table 4 presents the descriptive statistics of the scores from the GVAS questionnaires for both treatments (VR and Standard). The scores reflect the difference between POST and PRE administrations for two specific indices: the Negative Mood Index (NMI) and the Alertness Index (AI).

Table 4. Results of RQ_1. Descriptive statistics of GVAS questionnaire. A high NMI score reflects more negative emotional states. A high AI score reflects increased levels of alertness.

	NMI		AI	
	VR	Standard	VR	Standard
Mean	−4.25	9.94	22.25	−21.81
Median	−5.00	−2.50	12.00	−4.00
Std. dev	43.91	65.16	56.92	81.40

The results from the GVAS questionnaire illustrate the effects of immersive virtual reality (VR) compared to Standard treatments on participants' mood and alertness. For the Negative Mood Index (NMI), the mean score for the VR treatment was -4.25, indicating a slight reduction in negative mood, whereas the Standard treatment had a mean score of 9.94, suggesting an increase in negative mood. In contrast, the mean Alertness Index (AI) score for the VR treatment was 22.25, significantly higher than the mean score of -21.81 for the Standard treatment.

The difference in NMI scores between the VR and Standard treatments suggests that VR generally led to a lower negative mood than the Standard treatment. However, this difference is not statistically significant, as indicated by the Wilcoxon Signed-Rank test, which returned a p-value of 0.3225 ($z = -2.04$, $W = 48.00$). Therefore, we cannot definitively conclude that VR significantly reduces negative mood compared to the Standard treatment.

On the other hand, the difference in AI scores is statistically significant, with the Wilcoxon Signed-Rank test yielding a p-value of 0.0443 ($z = -2.04$, $W = 28.50$). These findings suggest that *VR significantly enhances participants' alertness compared to the Standard treatment.*

The improvement in alertness with the VR treatment indicates that immersive virtual environments can effectively engage participants and enhance their cognitive state of alertness. However, the lack of a statistically significant difference in NMI scores suggests that while VR may improve alertness, its effect on reducing negative mood remains unclear.

Based on these results, we cannot reject the null hypothesis H_{01b} for the Negative Mood Index due to the lack of statistical significance. However, we can reject the null hypothesis H_{01b} for the Alertness Index, as the difference is statistically significant.

Table 5 presents the descriptive statistics of the scores obtained from the SAM questionnaires for both the VR and Standard treatments. The scores reflect the differences between POST and PRE assessments across three dimensions: (i) *Valence*, (ii) *Activation*, and (iii) *Dominance*.

Table 5. Results of RQ_1. Descriptive statistics of SAM questionnaire. A high score on Valence suggests a positive emotional state. A high Activation score suggests that the person feels excited. A high value of Dominance suggests that the person feels powerless.

	Valence		Activation		Dominance	
	VR	Standard	VR	Standard	VR	Standard
Mean	0.44	0.13	0.13	−0.81	−0.38	−0.44
Median	0.00	0.00	0.00	0.00	0.00	0.00
Std. dev	0.89	1.63	1.59	1.33	1.71	1.21

This analysis allows us to discern the varying impacts of the treatments on these three emotional measures. For *Valence*, the mean score for the VR treatment was 0.44, slightly higher than the 0.13 mean score for the Standard treatment. However, the variability in responses, as indicated by the standard deviations (0.89 for VR and 1.63 for Standard), suggests that this difference is not statistically significant, with a p-value of 0.565 ($z = -2.77$, $W = 22$).

In contrast, *Activation* showed a significant difference between the two treatments. The mean score for VR was 0.13, compared to −0.81 for the Standard treatment. This substantial difference indicates that VR significantly enhances participants' activation levels, supported by a p-value of 0.0418 ($z = -3.48$, $W = 5.5$). This finding underscores *the effectiveness of VR in increasing cognitive and emotional arousal*.

For *Dominance*, the mean score was −0.38 for VR and −0.44 for the Standard treatment, with standard deviations of 1.71 and 1.21, respectively. Such a difference suggests a slight increase in the sense of control for VR participants. However, this difference is not statistically significant, as indicated by the p-value of 0.8096 ($z = -1.65$, $W = 36$).

Based on this analysis, we cannot reject the null hypothesis H_{01c} for *Valence* and *Dominance*, as the differences are not statistically significant. However, we can reject the null hypothesis H_{01c} for *Activation*, given the statistically significant enhancement observed with VR.

> **Answer to RQ_1.** The use of 2ViTA-B Cognitive VR significantly improves participants' self-assessed activation levels and alertness, demonstrating its effectiveness in enhancing cognitive and emotional engagement. However, it does not show a statistically significant impact on reducing negative mood (NMI) or altering feelings of valence and dominance when compared to the standard treatment.

5.2 RQ_2: Impact on Attention

Table 6 presents the descriptive statistics for the Stroop test scores, detailing the results for both treatment groups.

Table 6. Results of RQ_2. Descriptive statistics of the Stroop test score differences, calculated by comparing the scores before and after each administration.

	VR	Standard
Mean	2.86	0.50
Median	2.00	0.50
Std. dev	3.56	2.45

A higher number of correct answers was observed during the VR administration, indicating a notable increase in participants benefiting from the immersive experience. However, despite this apparent difference, it is not statistically significant. The Wilcoxon Signed-Rank test returned a p-value of 0.05 ($z = -1.61$, $W = 22.5$), suggesting that we cannot reject the null hypothesis H_{02}. Therefore, we cannot conclude that the use of 2ViTA-B Cognitive VR improves participants' attention as measured by the Stroop test.

Similar findings were observed in the EEG analysis. Table 7 shows that VR administration did not lead to an improvement in participants' attention, as indicated by the EEG Beta scores. After VR administration, participants' attention slightly decreased, while the standard treatment resulted in minimal change in beta scores. The Wilcoxon Signed-Rank test returned a p-value of 0.12 ($z = -1.18$, $W = 24$), indicating that while VR may effectively elicit positive emotions, it could also increase cognitive workload, potentially diminishing attention.

Table 7. Results of RQ$_2$. Descriptive statistics of EEG Beta score differences, calculated by comparing the Beta scores before and after each administration.

	VR	Standard
Mean	−0.11	0.02
Median	−0.40	0.01
Std. dev	0.27	0.23

Based on the results, we cannot reject the null hypothesis H$_{02}$ when considering the EEG Beta scores. Consequently, we cannot conclude that the use of 2ViTA-B Cognitive VR leads to an improvement in participants' attention as measured by EEG Beta scores.

> **Answer to RQ$_2$.** The use of 2ViTA-B Cognitive VR did not significantly improve participants' attention. While VR showed a higher number of correct answers on the Stroop test, the difference was not statistically significant, and EEG Beta scores also showed no improvement.

5.3   RQ$_3$: Usability Evaluation

Figure 6 presents a summary of the usability data collected from participants who used the 2ViTA-B Cognitive VR system.

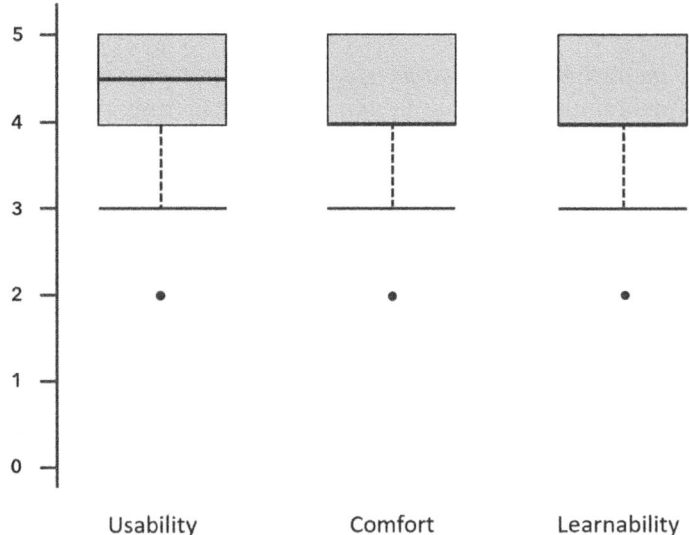

Fig. 6. Results of RQ$_3$. Usability evaluation.

Usability. The majority of participants (82.1%) reported that they found the system easy to use, with a median score of 4. The low variability in responses suggests a strong consensus among participants regarding the system's user-friendliness.

Comfort. In terms of comfort, 76% of participants indicated that they felt comfortable using the 2ViTA-B Cognitive VR system, with a median score of 4. While most participants found the system comfortable, the variability in responses likely reflects individual differences in sensitivity, particularly among those who experienced discomfort during rapid VR movements.

Learnability. Participants also responded positively about the ease of learning to use the 2ViTA-B Cognitive system, with a median score of 4. However, the presence of a few outliers with scores below 3 indicates that a small number of participants found the system more challenging to learn.

Answer to RQ$_3$. Participants generally found the 2ViTA-B Cognitive VR system easy to use and comfortable, though some encountered challenges with learning the system and comfort during rapid VR movements. This indicates that individual or contextual factors may affect the user experience for certain participants.

---

6   Conclusion

We introduced 2ViTA-B Cognitive, a virtual assistant designed to positively influence human emotions. To assess its effectiveness in cognitive rehabilitation using virtual reality (VR), we performed a controlled experiment with 16 participants. The results showed that the use of 2ViTA-B Cognitive VR significantly improves participants' self-assessed activation levels and alertness, demonstrating its effectiveness in enhancing cognitive and emotional engagement. However, it does not have a statistically significant impact on reducing negative mood (NMI) or altering feelings of valence and dominance compared to the standard treatment. Additionally, 2ViTA-B Cognitive VR did not lead to significant improvements in participants' attention, as evidenced by the lack of statistically significant differences in Stroop test results and EEG Beta scores. Regarding the usability of the system, we observed that while the system was generally perceived as easy to use and comfortable, some participants encountered difficulties with learning the system and experienced discomfort during rapid VR movements, indicating that individual or contextual factors may influence the overall user experience.

Future research should aim to replicate the study with a larger sample size and explore the integration of electroencephalogram (EEG) data with biofeedback techniques in VR environments. This integration could enhance participants' awareness of their cognitive state, potentially leading to more effective rehabilitation outcomes.

Acknowledgements. The 2ViTA-B project was developed under the National Plan of Military Research (PNRM), with funding provided by the Ministry of Defence. We would like to extend our gratitude to the 16 participants who took part in our experiments, whose contributions were invaluable to the success of this study.

References

1. Balletti, N., et al.: 2vita-b cognitive: a virtual assistant for cognitive rehabilitation. In: BIOSTEC (2), pp. 545–553 (2024)
2. Baños, R.M., Etchemendy, E., Farfallini, L., García-Palacios, A., Quero, S., Botella, C.: Earth of well-being system: a pilot study of an information and communication technology-based positive psychology intervention. J. Posit. Psychol. **9**(6), 482–488 (2014)
3. Bradley, M.M., Codispoti, M., Sabatinelli, D., Lang, P.J.: Emotion and motivation II: sex differences in picture processing. Emotion **1**(3), 300 (2001)
4. Bradley, M.M., Lang, P.J.: Measuring emotion: the self-assessment manikin and the semantic differential. J. Behav. Ther. Exp. Psychiatry **25**(1), 49–59 (1994)
5. Bradley, M.M., Lang, P.J.: International affective digitized sounds (IADS): stimuli, instruction manual and affective ratings (Technical report no. b-2). The Center for Research in Psychophysiology, University of Florida, Gainesville (1999)
6. Browning, M.H., Mimnaugh, K.J., Van Riper, C.J., Laurent, H.K., LaValle, S.M.: Can simulated nature support mental health? Comparing short, single-doses of 360-degree nature videos in virtual reality with the outdoors. Front. Psychol. **10**, 2667 (2020)
7. Burattini, C., et al.: Managing human stress level: a multimedia sequence approach. In: 2021 IEEE International Conference on Environment and Electrical Engineering and 2021 IEEE Industrial and Commercial Power Systems Europe (EEEIC/I&CPS Europe), pp. 1–5. IEEE (2021)
8. Cohen, S., Kamarck, T., Mermelstein, R.: A global measure of perceived stress. J. Health Soc. Behav. 385–396 (1983)
9. Davidson, R.J., Sherer, K.R., Goldsmith, H.H.: Handbook of Affective Sciences. Oxford University Press (2009)
10. Dillman Carpentier, F.R., Potter, R.F.: Effects of music on physiological arousal: explorations into tempo and genre. Media Psychol. **10**(3), 339–363 (2007)
11. Ekman, P.: Facial expression and emotion. Am. Psychol. **48**(4), 384 (1993)
12. Felnhofer, A., Hlavacs, H., Beutl, L., Kryspin-Exner, I., Kothgassner, O.D.: Physical presence, social presence, and anxiety in participants with social anxiety disorder during virtual cue exposure. Cyberpsychol. Behav. Soc. Netw. **22**(1), 46–50 (2019)
13. Felnhofer, A., et al.: Is virtual reality emotionally arousing? Investigating five emotion inducing virtual park scenarios. Int. J. Hum. Comput. Stud. **82**, 48–56 (2015)
14. Gaggioli, A., et al.: Experiential virtual scenarios with real-time monitoring (inter-reality) for the management of psychological stress: a block randomized controlled trial. J. Med. Internet Res. **16**(7), e3235 (2014)
15. Garrett, B., Taverner, T., McDade, P., et al.: Virtual reality as an adjunct home therapy in chronic pain management: an exploratory study. JMIR Med. Inform. **5**(2), e7271 (2017)

16. Gerardi, M., Rothbaum, B.O., Ressler, K., Heekin, M., Rizzo, A.: Virtual reality exposure therapy using a virtual Iraq: case report. J. Traumatic Stress: Official Publication Int. Soc. Traumatic Stress Stud. **21**(2), 209–213 (2008)
17. Greer, T., Ma, B., Sachs, M., Habibi, A., Narayanan, S.: A multimodal view into music's effect on human neural, physiological, and emotional experience. In: Proceedings of the 27th ACM International Conference on Multimedia, pp. 167–175 (2019)
18. Grewe, O., Katzur, B., Kopiez, R., Altenmüller, E.: Chills in different sensory domains: frisson elicited by acoustical, visual, tactile and gustatory stimuli. Psychol. Music **39**(2), 220–239 (2011)
19. Gross, J.J., Levenson, R.W.: Emotion elicitation using films. Cogn. Emotion **9**(1), 87–108 (1995)
20. Herrero, R., García-Palacios, A., Castilla, D., Molinari, G., Botella, C.: Virtual reality for the induction of positive emotions in the treatment of fibromyalgia: a pilot study over acceptability, satisfaction, and the effect of virtual reality on mood. Cyberpsychol. Behav. Soc. Netw. **17**(6), 379–384 (2014)
21. Huang, Q., Yang, M., Jane, H., Li, S., Bauer, N.: Trees, grass, or concrete? The effects of different types of environments on stress reduction. Landscape Urban Plan. **193**, 103654 (2020)
22. Huppert, F.A., So, T.T.: Flourishing across Europe: application of a new conceptual framework for defining well-being. Soc. Indic. Res. **110**, 837–861 (2013)
23. Khalfa, S., Isabelle, P., Jean-Pierre, B., Manon, R.: Event-related skin conductance responses to musical emotions in humans. Neurosci. Lett. **328**(2), 145–149 (2002)
24. Knautz, K., Stock, W.G.: Collective indexing of emotions in videos. J. Documentation **67**(6), 975–994 (2011)
25. Koelsch, S., Bashevkin, T., Kristensen, J., Tvedt, J., Jentschke, S.: Heroic music stimulates empowering thoughts during mind-wandering. Sci. Rep. **9**(1), 10317 (2019)
26. Koelstra, S., et al.: Deap: a database for emotion analysis; using physiological signals. IEEE Trans. Affect. Comput. **3**(1), 18–31 (2011)
27. Lang, P.J.: International affective picture system (IAPS): technical manual and affective ratings. The Center for Research in Psychophysiology, University of Florida (1995)
28. Lang, P.J., Greenwald, M.K., Bradley, M.M., Hamm, A.O.: Looking at pictures: affective, facial, visceral, and behavioral reactions. Psychophysiology **30**(3), 261–273 (1993)
29. Liu, C., Liu, W., Liu, T., Lu, T., Fang, H., Liu, L.: Application of virtual reality in the treatment of anxiety and autism. J. Syst. Simul. **27**, 2233–2238 (2015)
30. Maffei, A., Angrilli, A.: E-movie-experimental movies for induction of emotions in neuroscience: an innovative film database with normative data and sex differences. PLoS ONE **14**(10), e0223124 (2019)
31. Malloy, K.M., Milling, L.S.: The effectiveness of virtual reality distraction for pain reduction: a systematic review. Clin. Psychol. Rev. **30**(8), 1011–1018 (2010)
32. Marchewka, A., Żurawski, Ł, Jednoróg, K., Grabowska, A.: The nencki affective picture system (naps): introduction to a novel, standardized, wide-range, high-quality, realistic picture database. Behav. Res. Methods **46**, 596–610 (2014)
33. Monk, T.H.: A visual analogue scale technique to measure global vigor and affect. Psychiatry Res. **27**(1), 89–99 (1989)
34. Oing, T., Prescott, J., et al.: Implementations of virtual reality for anxiety-related disorders: systematic review. JMIR Serious Games **6**(4), e10965 (2018)

35. Pallavicini, F., Algeri, D., Repetto, C., Gorini, A., Riva, G., et al.: Biofeedback, virtual reality and mobile phones in the treatment of generalized anxiety disorder (gad): a phase-2 controlled clinical trial. J. Cyberther. Rehabil. **2**(4), 315–327 (2009)
36. Pallavicini, F., Argenton, L., Toniazzi, N., Aceti, L., Mantovani, F.: Virtual reality applications for stress management training in the military. Aerosp. Med. Hum. Perform. **87**(12), 1021–1030 (2016)
37. Pizzoli, S.F.M., Mazzocco, K., Triberti, S., Monzani, D., Alcañiz Raya, M.L., Pravettoni, G.: User-centered virtual reality for promoting relaxation: an innovative approach. Front. Psychol. **10**, 479 (2019)
38. Rauscher, F.H., et al.: Music and spatial task performance: a causal relationship (1994)
39. Rizzo, A.S., et al.: Development and early evaluation of the virtual Iraq/Afghanistan exposure therapy system for combat-related PTSD. Ann. N. Y. Acad. Sci. **1208**(1), 114–125 (2010)
40. Roiser, J.P., Sahakian, B.J.: Hot and cold cognition in depression. CNS Spectr. **18**(3), 139–149 (2013)
41. Samson, A.C., Kreibig, S.D., Soderstrom, B., Wade, A.A., Gross, J.J.: Eliciting positive, negative and mixed emotional states: a film library for affective scientists. Cogn. Emot. **30**(5), 827–856 (2016)
42. Sander, D., Scherer, K.: Oxford Companion to Emotion and the Affective Sciences. OUP Oxford (2014)
43. Schaefer, A., Nils, F., Sanchez, X., Philippot, P.: Assessing the effectiveness of a large database of emotion-eliciting films: a new tool for emotion researchers. Cogn. Emot. **24**(7), 1153–1172 (2010)
44. Stroop, J.R.: Studies of interference in serial verbal reactions. J. Exp. Psychol. **18**(6), 643 (1935)
45. Tageldeen, M.K., Elamvazuthi, I., Perumal, N., Ganesan, T.: A virtual reality based serious games for rehabilitation of arm. In: 2017 IEEE 3rd International Symposium in Robotics and Manufacturing Automation (ROMA), pp. 1–6. IEEE (2017)
46. Takac, M., Collett, J., Blom, K.J., Conduit, R., Rehm, I., De Foe, A.: Public speaking anxiety decreases within repeated virtual reality training sessions. PLoS ONE **14**(5), e0216288 (2019)
47. Tempesta, D., Socci, V., Dello Ioio, G., De Gennaro, L., Ferrara, M.: The effect of sleep deprivation on retrieval of emotional memory: a behavioural study using film stimuli. Exp. Brain Res. **235**(10), 3059–3067 (2017). https://doi.org/10.1007/s00221-017-5043-z
48. Ulrich, R.: Stress recovery during exposure to natural and urban environments. J. Environ. Psychol. **36**, 729–742 (1993)
49. Vargas-Orjuela, M., Uribe-Quevedo, A., Rojas, D., Kapralos, B., Perez-Gutierrez, B.: A mobile immersive virtual reality cardiac auscultation app. In: 2017 IEEE 6th Global Conference on Consumer Electronics (GCCE), pp. 1–2. IEEE (2017)
50. Wang, H.L., Cheong, L.F.: Affective understanding in film. IEEE Trans. Circuits Syst. Video Technol. **16**(6), 689–704 (2006)
51. Watson, D., Clark, L.A., Tellegen, A.: Development and validation of brief measures of positive and negative affect: the PANAS scales. J. Pers. Soc. Psychol. **54**(6), 1063 (1988)
52. Westermann, R., Spies, K., Stahl, G., Hesse, F.W.: Relative effectiveness and validity of mood induction procedures: a meta-analysis. Eur. J. Soc. Psychol. **26**(4), 557–580 (1996)

53. Wiederhold, B.K., Gao, K., Sulea, C., Wiederhold, M.D.: Virtual reality as a distraction technique in chronic pain patients. Cyberpsychol. Behav. Soc. Netw. **17**(6), 346–352 (2014)
54. Wiederhold, B.K., Miller, I.T., Wiederhold, M.D.: Using virtual reality to mobilize health care: mobile virtual reality technology for attenuation of anxiety and pain. IEEE Consum. Electron. Mag. **7**(1), 106–109 (2017)
55. Wilcoxon, F., Katti, S., Wilcox, R.A., et al.: Critical values and probability levels for the Wilcoxon rank sum test and the Wilcoxon signed rank test. Selected Tables Math. Stat. **1**, 171–259 (1970)

Predicting the Bed Occupancy in a Hospital

Simon Schiff[1]([✉]) [iD], Natalie Kohler[2] [iD], Sebastian Wolfrum[3] [iD], Ralf Möller[1] [iD],
and Mattis Hartwig[1,2] [iD]

[1] German Research Center for Artificial Intelligence, Ratzeburger Allee 160,
23562 Lübeck, Germany
{robert_simon.schiff,hartwig}@dfki.de
[2] singularIT GmbH, Inselstraße 27, 04103 Leipzig, Germany
[3] University Medical Center Schleswig-Holstein Campus Lübeck,
Ratzeburger Allee 160, 23538 Lübeck, Germany

Abstract. More and more people are choosing hospitals as their first place of admission when they fall ill. This trend has continued to increase over the years, resulting in overcrowded hospitals. Many solutions to hospital overcrowding have been proposed. These include trying to discharge patients as early as possible and reduce their length of stay (LoS), which is achievable through precise planning without compromising the quality of treatment. In this paper, we simplify planning by automatically predicting hospital occupancy both in the emergency room and later, when patients stay on the ward. This approach relieves hospital staff of planning tasks, allowing them more time to care for patients. The prediction is done by aggregating the predicted LoS with an estimate of how many patients will arrive in the future and their expected LoS to determine occupancy. We demonstrate how the accuracy of LoS predictions affects the accuracy of occupancy predictions. We evaluate our approach using the anonymized MIMIC-IV EHR (electronic health record) database and successfully apply it to a real-world scenario at another hospital in Germany.

Keywords: Bed occupancy prediction · Emergency department · CatBoost architecture · MIMIC-IV

1 Introduction

For decades, overcrowding in hospitals has been a worldwide issue, particularly in the (ED) [20]. This problem is further intensified by the increasing number of patients choosing the ED as their first point of admission and staff shortages.

Thereby, patients seeking help in an overcrowded ED are likely to experience multiple problems, ranging from delays in assessment, treatment or admission after treatment (exit stop), up to a full stop of patient admission for the whole ED [17]. It is non-surprising that overcrowding was shown to be connected to

M. P. Guarino et al. (Eds.): BIOSTEC 2024, CCIS 2546, pp. 376–403, 2026.
https://doi.org/10.1007/978-3-031-96899-0_21

increased stress, yet, in addition, it can lead to an increase of violence and inpatient mortality [17]. Therefore, the efficient planning of hospital occupancy, especially in the ED, is crucial to ensure timely patient care and resource allocation in order to reduce the risk of overcrowding and exit stop. One time-consuming aspect of the ED-process involves bed-occupancy management, as it is still performed manually, which requires a high amount of communication, often with several different wards. Automatizing the management of bed occupancy may reduce overcrowding by allowing practitioners to focus more of their time on their core-task: patient treatment. The current study therefore aimed to identify approaches allowing for automatizing hospital-, and especially ED-occupancy management on the basis of predictive models.

Hospital bed occupancy is primarily influenced by two factors: the number of patients admitted and their respective length of stay (LoS) [5,15]. While previous research involved machine learning to predict patients' LoS with promising results [1,3,6,13,16,19,22,23], accurately forecasting the number of patients admitted is hardly, or not predictable at all. The complexity of admission-prediction arises from the dynamic interplay between individual factors tracked in ED-data (e.g. admission due to a concussion) and environmental factors that are usually not tracked (e.g. the traffic jam that caused the accident).

To address this issue, we previously introduced a scheme for translating LoS predictions of individual patients into a prediction of bed occupancy across the whole clinic in Hartwig et al. [9]. To this end, we utilized the anonymized (including a time-shift) MIMIC-IV EHR (electronic health record) database that presents data acquired at a US-American hospital, specifically curated for research purposes [11].

In the current paper, we extend our previous work in two ways. First, in addition to utilizing the pre-curated MIMIC-IV EHR database, we evaluated our approach with real-life data from a hospital in Germany. Second, next to predictive modelling of daily hospital bed occupancy (from now on referred to as *bed occupancy*), we were able to investigate hourly ED-occupancy, on the basis of the realistic and precise timestamps contained in the additional real-life dataset. Due to their precision, these real-life data further allowed for hourly ED-LoS predictions, related to differences in ED-occupancy levels throughout a day. By comparing the predicted LoS with actual occupancy data, we demonstrate how the accuracy of LoS predictions directly impacts the reliability of occupancy forecasts. Our results indicate that automated occupancy prediction can significantly enhance hospital management, particularly in resource-constrained settings.

The remainder of this paper is structured as follows. Section 2 covers the related work on LoS prediction and bed occupancy in hospitals. Section 3 presents the datasets and the methodology used to calculate occupancy. This is followed by Sect. 4, which explains how the LoS of a patient is predicted, given the information available at the time of the patient's admission. In the main part, we demonstrate in Sect. 5 and Sect. 6 how to calculate occupancy under different settings. Finally, results are discussed in Sect. 7, and we conclude in Sect. 8.

2 Related Work

The body of research relevant to this study investigated the prediction of either LoS or bed occupancy in hospitals, mainly on the basis of machine learning algorithms. The two main related studies are those of our previous work in Hartwig et al. in [9], which was based on Winter et al. in [21,23]. As described in the introduction, the current paper extends our findings in Hartwig et al. in [9], where we introduced a translation scheme from (H)-LoS prediction to bed occupancy. More specifically, in Hartwig et al. [9], we compared actual bed occupancy against predictions derived from machine learning-based H-LoS estimates. We further employed simulations to evaluate the impact of different error margins and patterns in H-LoS predictions on the accuracy of bed occupancy forecasts, ultimately translating individual patient H-LoS predictions into comprehensive bed occupancy forecasts for the entire hospital. The state-of-the-art machine learning models used in our previous study [9] where provided by Winter et al. in [23]. Both studies used the MIMIC-IV data set, comprising US-based EHR data [11]. Furthermore our aim in [21], is to improve the LoS for specific patient cohorts, using synthetic data.

Similar to our approach, other previous studies used machine learning to predict patients' LoS in a variety of clinical scenarios. Gentimis et al.in [6] developed models to predict H-LoS following a patient's discharge from the intensive care unit (ICU). Rocheteau et al. in [19] concentrated on forecasting the remaining days in the ICU.

The prediction of bed occupancy combines a more complex composition of relevant factors, hence, several streams of research can be related to our work. One approach is to model patient admission and bed assignment as a queuing problem. Gorunescu et al. in [7] formulated a queuing model aimed at optimizing patient scheduling to minimize delays, and Belciug and Gorunescu in [2] extended this by incorporating evolutionary optimization techniques. Another approach employs compartment models to describe patient flow through different hospital compartments, as demonstrated by Harrison in [8] and Mackay and Lee in [14]. These models offer a structured way to understand patient distribution and movement within the hospital.

A third approach comprises classical time-series forecasting methods to predict bed occupancy. Early work by Farmer and Emami in [4] utilized autoregressive movingaverage (ARMA) models, while more recent efforts by Kutafina et al. in [12] employed Recurrent Neural Networks (RNNs). Mackay and Lee in [14] critiqued the use of the mean H-LoS for bed occupancy calculations, advocating instead for compartment modeling to provide more accurate predictions.

In our previous study [9], we could bridge a critical conceptual gap by combining insights from early occupancy research with the advanced capabilities of machine learning for individual patient predictions. In the current paper, we evaluate our previous approach on the basis of real-life data and additionally investigate ED-occupancy on a more fine-grained (hourly) level. By doing so, we seek to enhance the accuracy and utility of bed occupancy forecasts, ultimately contributing to more efficient hospital management and patient care.

3 Datasets

In this work, we transfer our previous approach from Hartwig et al. in [9] using the MIMIC-IV EHR dataset [10,11] to the UKSH (Universitätsklinikum Schleswig-Hol stein), located near our campus in Germany. At UKSH (Universitätsklinikum Schleswig- Holstein), we extend our predictions to include not only daily bed occupancy in the wards but also hourly occupancy in the ED.

3.1 MIMIC-IV

The MIMIC-IV dataset is extracted from the Beth Israel Deaconess Medical Center (BIDMC) located in Boston [10,11], containing high-quality records from 2008 to 2019. It includes data on 180k different patients, resulting in 430k distinct hospital admissions. The dataset is organized into several modules: *hosp*, *ICU*, *notes*, and *ED*. Data is anonymized in accordance with the HIPAA (Health Insurance Portability and Accountability Act) to protect patient privacy. While maintaining privacy is the highest priority, this anonymization introduces certain limitations. For instance, all dates are consistently shifted by a fixed offset for each stay. Although a patient's age at the time of admission can still be determined, it is impossible to calculate the actual hospital occupancy between 2008 and 2019. In the anonymized dataset, the minimum and maximum timestamps span 107 years. To align with the real recording period, we consistently shift all timestamps to span 11 years instead, reflecting the actual data collection period.

As in Winter et al. [23], we extract the following features to predict the H-LoS for a patient after being admitted from the ED to the hospital. All extracted features originate from the ED, ensuring that data leakage is avoided prior to training.

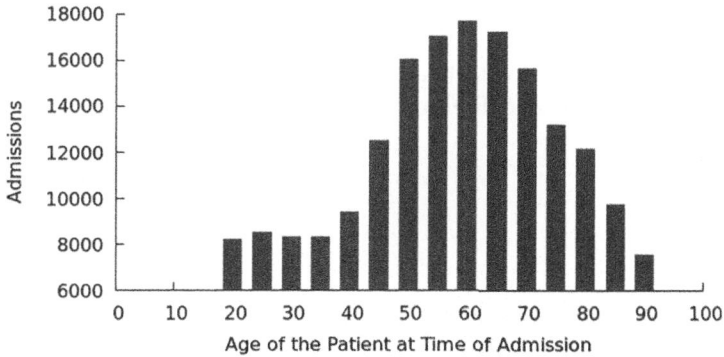

Fig. 1. Patients age at when they where admitted to the hospital ED at MIMIC-IV [9].

Age. The age of the patient at the time of admission. The distribution of ages is depicted in Fig. 1.

Gender. The patient's gender is recorded as either Female or Male, with no further distinctions made. Approximately 49% of the patients are male, while 51% are female.

Insurance. Whether the patient has insurance or not. In 9% of all cases, the patient has Medicaid, 38% have Medicare, and in the remaining of 53% cases, the type of insurance is not further specified.

Ethnicity. The patient's ethnicity.

Admission Location. The location from which the patient was prior to being admitted to the hospital. This could include, for example, the emergency room or a physician referral.

ICD-code The primary diagnosis of a patient is recorded in the form of an ICD (International Statistical Classification of Diseases and Related Health Problems) code. Approximately half of these ICD codes are from version 9, while the other half are from version 10.

Respiratory Rate. The respiratory rate of the patient during the triage.

SBP. The systolic blood pressure of the patient during triage.

Pain. Patients are asked to rate their pain on a scale from 1 to 10.

Diagnosis Count. The number of diagnoses made during the patient's stay in the ED of the hospital.

Medication Count. Patients are asked about the medications they are taking during triage. We extract the number of these medications as a feature from the database.

Mean LoS of Previous Admissions. If a patient has previously been to the ED, we extract the mean duration of all previous stays as a feature from the database.

LoS. The actual feature we aim to predict: The stationary H-LoS of a patient at the hospital.

All patients younger than 18 years old and those with a H-LoS longer than 50 days are filtered out prior to training. The distribution of H-LoS in the final dataset is depicted in Fig. 2. Please note that all graphs containing MIMIC-IV data are depicted in purple.

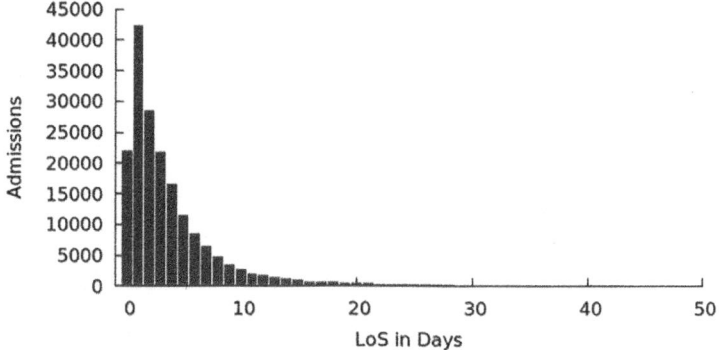

Fig. 2. H-LoS distribution for all patient admissions extracted from the MIMIC-IV database with a mean of 3.87 and standard deviation (SD) of 4.95 [9]. (Color figure online)

3.2 UKSH

The second anonymized data source comes from the UKSH hospital located adjacent to our campus in Germany. The UKSH data set contains only patients who entered the hospital via the ED. Unlike the MIMIC-IV dataset, the timestamps in the UKSH data are unchanged, allowing us to accurately determine the occupancy at the ED and other hospital units after patients are transferred from the ED and remain hospitalized for a specific duration.

The ED-LoS distribution from UKSH is depicted in Fig. 3. All 1290 out of roughly 140k patients with an ED-LoS longer than 40 h where filtered out. For all patients admitted to the hospital after the ED, the H-LoS distribution is depicted in Fig. 4. All 634 out of approximately 140k patients with a ED-LoS longer than 50 days were filtered out. Please note that all graphs containing UKSH data are depicted in green, with a darker shade depicting H-data and a brighter shade depicting ED-data.

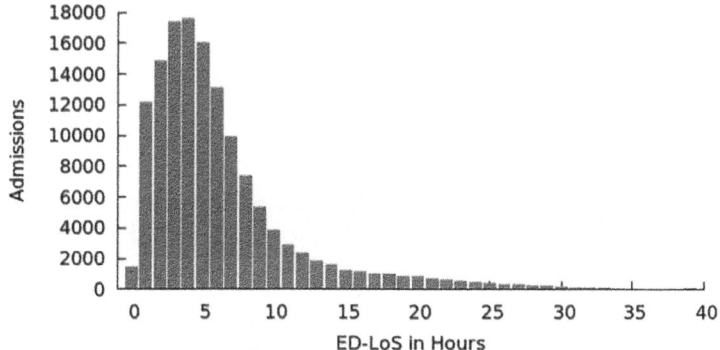

Fig. 3. ED-LoS distribution at the UKSH with a mean of 6.28 and SD of 5.41. (Color figure online)

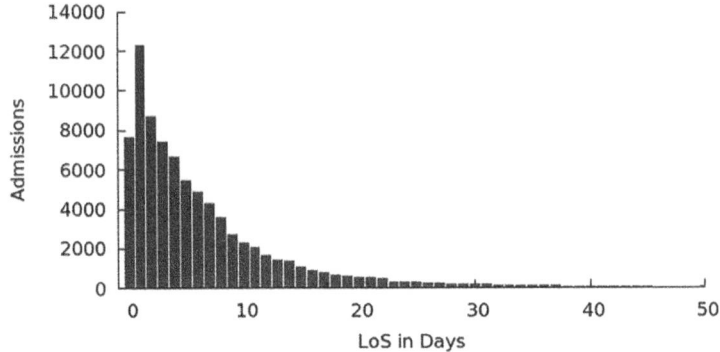

Fig. 4. H-LoS distribution at the UKSH with a mean of 6.60 and SD of 7.47. (Color figure online)

3.3 Occupancy

As we have shown in Sect. 2, predicting the H-LoS for each patient admitted to a hospital has been an area of research for decades, with promising results. However, the predicted H-LoS does not directly aid in the decision-making and planning processes for hospital practitioners. To assess bed occupancy at a specific future point in time, it is necessary to aggregate the H-LoS of all patients currently in the hospital. Additionally, one must consider all patients who will be admitted in the future and are expected to remain in the hospital at least until the target point in time for which bed occupancy is being predicted. Therefore, the goal of this paper is to predict bed occupancy in a hospital. Before we can predict bed occupancy, we need to calculate it prior to evaluation.

As already mentioned, MIMIC-IV is an anonymized database, and the dates for each patient's admission are shifted by a randomly selected offset. Consequently, it is impossible to predict the actual bed occupancy of the hospital. To address this, we consistently shift all dates for all patients so that the admission dates span 11 years instead. The bed occupancy for such an artificial year (after shifting the dates as described) is depicted in Fig. 5. And aggregated over the year in Fig. 6.

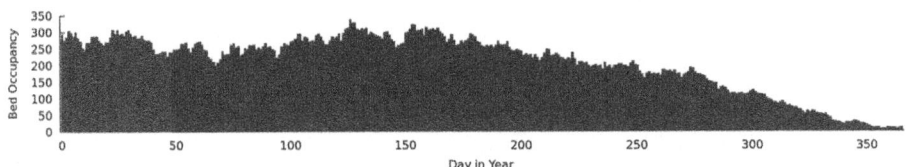

Fig. 5. Bed occupancy distribution for an example year at the MIMIC-IV database [9].

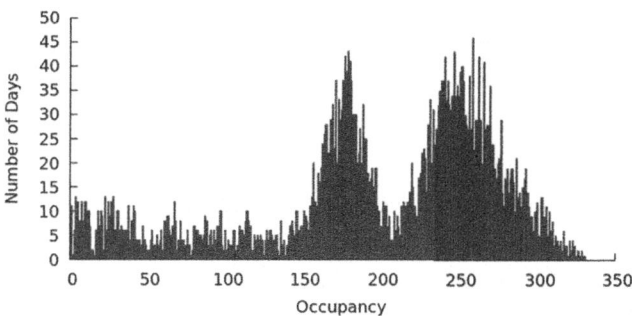

Fig. 6. Aggregated bed occupancy at the MIMIC-IV database when dates are shifted [9].

It can be seen that the bed occupancy is spread relatively evenly throughout the year. The number of patients in the hospital on the same day ranges from 8 to 338, with a mean of 208.6 and a SD of 88.54 throughout the year.

At the UKSH, data is anonymized, but the dates are not shifted and therefore reflect the actual timeline. The bed occupancy at the UKSH is depicted in Fig. 7.

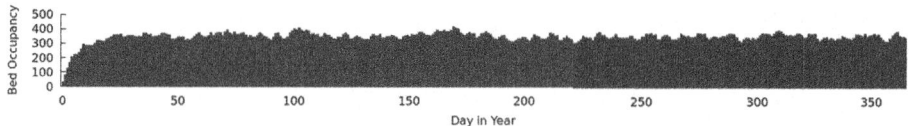

Fig. 7. Bed occupancy at the UKSH for the year 2023 with a mean of 348.99 and SD of 36.67, for patients with a LoS under 50 days after being discharged from the ED.

It can be observed that the bed occupancy is relatively evenly distributed throughout the year, with a mean of 348.99 and a SD of 36.67. Note that the depicted occupancy does not reflect the real overall occupancy at the hospital, because we only look at patients who have been given a bed after the emergency room. However, patients can also come from elsewhere and get a bed. In reality, the hospital has a total bed capacity of 800 beds. In addition to predicting daily bed occupancy at the hospital, we also aim to predict occupancy in the ED. However, in the ED, time is much more critical, so we focus on predicting ED-occupancy on an hourly basis rather than daily. Figure 8 shows the ED-occupancy for two consecutive days.

One can clearly see a repeating pattern each day, where the highest ED-occupancy occurs around $3PM$. Having access to the actual dates allows for further optimizations in predicting ED-occupancy, as we will demonstrate later in the evaluation.

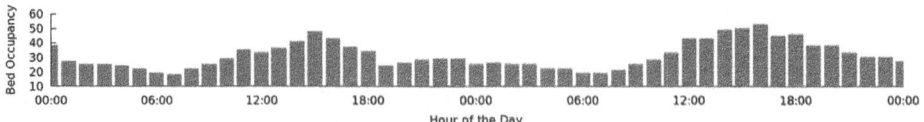

Fig. 8. Actual ED-occupancy at the UKSH for two consecutive days with a mean of 29.68 and SD of 7.66, for patients with an ED-LoS under 40 h.

4   Generating LoS Predictions

In this section, we present how we train the models for predicting the (i) H-LoS at the MIMIC-IV database, (ii) H-LoS at the UKSH, (iii) and ED-LoS at the UKSH, using CatBoost [18].

4.1   MIMIC-IV

As described by Winter et al. in [23], we use CatBoost to predict the H-LoS of patients after leaving the ED at MIMIC-IV. CatBoost is a gradient boosting algorithm specifically designed to handle numerical, categorical, and textual data as input. For training, most hyperparameters are kept at their default settings with the most commonly adjusted ones listed in Table 1. We use all the features described in Sect. 3.1 he dataset into a 60% training and a 40% test set. We create four scenarios, namely the (i) basis one, where we use the model's predictions as they are, (ii) symmetric one, where we modify the error distribution of the predictor to have a symmetric shape, (iii) narrowed one, where the distribution of the error is narrowed, (iv) and finally where the distribution is symmetric as well as narrowed for calculating the bed occupancy. While we use the original predictor in the former scenario, the latter three are simulations to examine how each respective error distribution affects the calculation of bed occupancy.

Table 1. Hyperparameter selection of the final CatBoost model, after the grid search has been performed [23].

Hyperparameter	Value	Default
Learning rate	0.1	no
Tree depth	6	no
L2 regularization	50	no
Random strength	1	yes
Bagging temperature	1	yes
Border count	128	yes
Internal dataset order	False	yes
Tree growing policy	Symmetric	yes

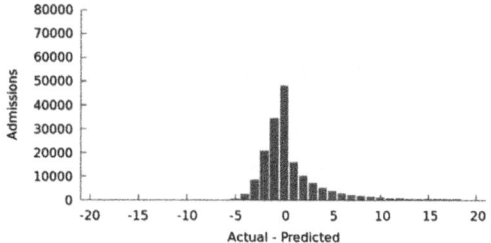

(a) H-LoS prediction error in the basis scenario [23]
with mean = 0.98 and deviation = 4.51

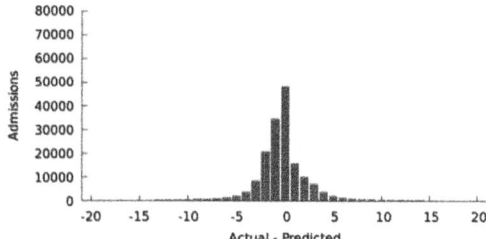

(b) Symmetric H-LoS prediction error with mean =
−0.25 and deviation = 4.61

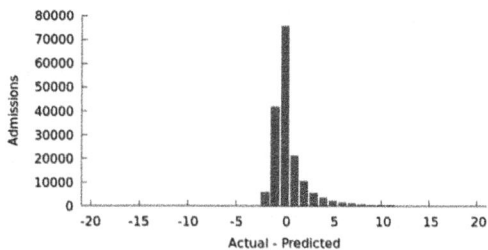

(c) Narrowed H-LoS prediction error distribution with
mean = 0.49 and deviation = 2.25

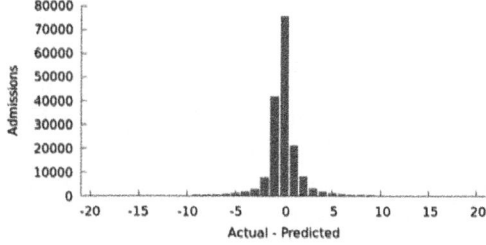

(d) Symmetric and then narrowed H-LoS prediction
error with mean = −0.12 and deviation = 2.31

Fig. 9. H-LoS error distribution for all four scenarios in MIMIC-IV.

Scenario 1 (Basis). In this scenario, we use the predictions of the trained model to determine the hospital's bed occupancy on a daily basis. The error distribution of the predictor is depicted in Fig. 9a. One can observe that the error distribution has a positive skew, which affects the calculated bed occupancy, as we will demonstrate later in the evaluation. The MAE (mean absolute error) is 2.36, the mean is 0.98, and the SD is 4.51 days. Although 2.36 might seem high at first glance, it is important to consider that the mean H-LoS is 3.87 days.

Scenario 2 (Simulation, Symmetric). The error distribution in the baseline scenario has a positive skew, caused by patients with a high H-LoS that the predictor fails to accurately predict. In this scenario, we simulate a predictor that predicts H-LoS such that the error distribution is symmetric, as depicted in Fig. 9b. We achieve this symmetry by calculating the difference between all positive error buckets greater than 3 (e.g., 5) and their counterparts (e.g., −5), and then shifting half of the difference from all admissions into the negative bucket by overriding the prediction with the corresponding value. The center of all admissions with an absolute error of 3 or less is already mostly symmetric and is therefore not altered. For each admission, the absolute error remains unchanged, so the MAE of 2.36 stays the same.

Scenario 3 (Simulation, Narrow). In both the baseline and symmetric scenarios, the error distributions of the H-LoS have a large SD, which we reduce by narrowing the distribution. The resulting narrowed error distribution is depicted in Fig. 9c. In this case, the mean changes to 0.49 and the SD, changes to 2.25.

Scenario 4 (Simulation, Narrow, Symmetric). Finally, in the fourth and last scenario, we combine the second and third scenarios to achieve a symmetric and narrowed H-LoS error distribution. It is expected that the calculated bed occupancy using this predicted H-LoS will have the lowest error rate among all four scenarios.

4.2   UKSH

The patient-flow in the emergency department is as depicted in Fig. 10. In the first step, a patient is administratively recorded. Subsequently, during triage, the urgency of their treatment is assessed, and after all evaluations by practitioners, it is decided whether the patient needs to remain in the hospital or can be discharged. The distribution of the time between the first encounter and the administrative recording is depicted in Fig. 11. It is evident that most patients are administratively recorded within 5 min, with a mean time of 2.36 min (Fig. 11).

After administrative admission, patients are prioritized during triage and consulted about their case. On average, triage takes place after 10.94 min, and much of the information needed for predicting ED-LoS is already available at that point. We use all available information between the administrative recording and

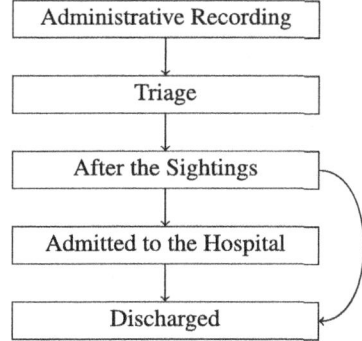

Fig. 10. Rough ED-process diagram of all patient stays that we have extracted from the UKSH database.

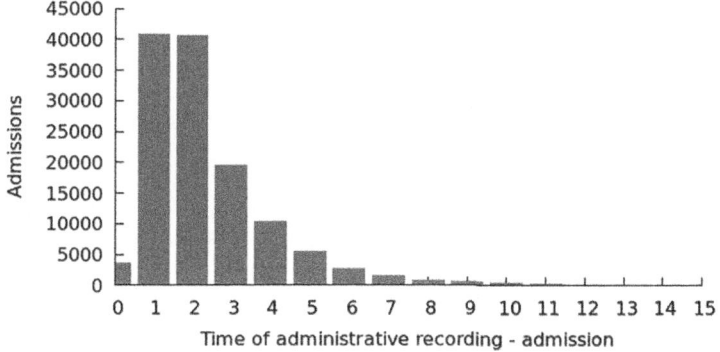

Fig. 11. Time between admission and administrative recording in minutes with a mean of 2.36 min at UKSH.

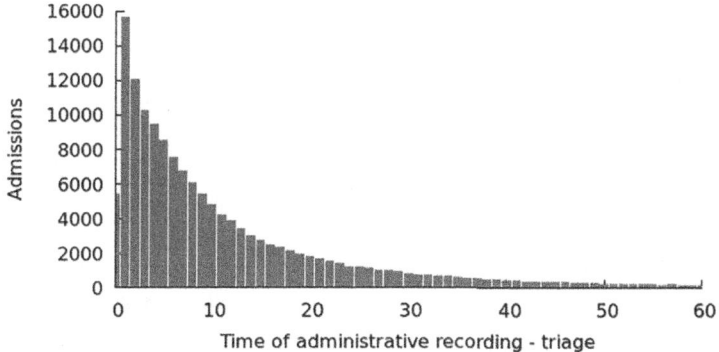

Fig. 12. Time between admission and triage in minutes with a mean of 10.94 min at UKSH.

the triage for predicting the ED-LoS. The resulting ED-LoS error distribution is depicted in Fig. 13. Note that the error is measured in hours, not days.

Similarly to the baseline scenario with the MIMIC-IV database, the error distribution in this case also has a positive skew. Patients with an ED-LoS greater than 9 h are difficult to predict, as they are rare and their ED-LoS often depends more on hospital shortages than on the actual treatment.

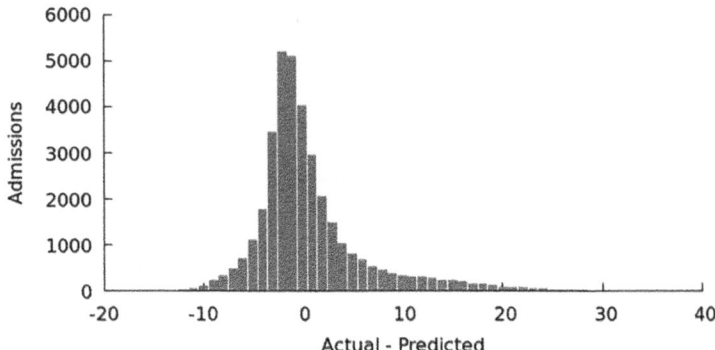

Fig. 13. ED-LoS prediction error at UKSH with mean = 0.75, MAE = 3.73 and SD = 5.70.

Furthermore, we predict the H-LoS of all patients leaving the ED and being admitted to any ward in the hospital. For these patients, all information collected during their stay in the ED can be used to predict the H-LoS. The resulting H-LoS error distribution is depicted in Fig. 14.

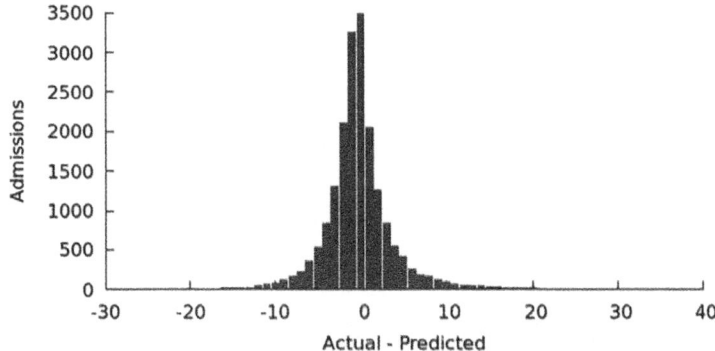

Fig. 14. Stationary H-LoS at the UKSH with mean = −0.17, MAE = 2.68 and SD = 4.11.

It is evident that the error distribution is almost symmetric, with very few admissions where the predictor underestimates the H-LoS.

5   Overarching View

To create an overarching view, we calculate the bed occupancy error distribution by first separately aggregating the predicted LoS as depicted in Fig. 15, and the actual LoS, as depicted in Fig. 8 over time.

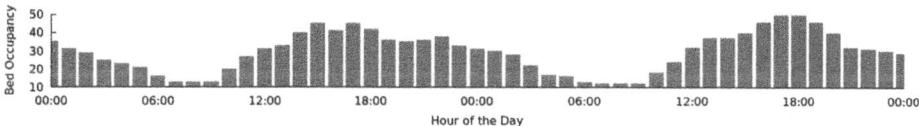

Fig. 15. Predicted ED-occupancy at the UKSH for two consecutive days with a mean of 30.08 and SD of 9.89.

We then substracted the aggregated predicted LoS from the aggregated actual LoS to return the error distribution. Please note that the H-LoS was aggregated per day, while ED-LoS was aggregated per hour. While this method does not reflect how a real hospital provider would calculate occupancy, it effectively demonstrates how the LoS error distribution impacts occupancy calculations. In reality, a hospital provider would need to know the occupancy at a specific point in the future based on the current information available. For example, on Monday, one might want to know the expected occupancy three days later. However, in contrast to our overarching view, the provider cannot know how many patients will be admitted on Tuesday and stay for at least two days, or on Wednesday and stay for one day, or on Thursday. In the overarching view, we assume that this information is known.

5.1   Stationary Bed Occupancy at MIMIC-IV

The bed occupancy error distributions in the overarching view for all four scenarios are depicted in Fig. 16. Errors on the left-hand side of zero along the horizontal axis indicate that bed occupancy is overestimated, while errors on the right-hand side indicate that bed occupancy is underestimated.

For a more intuitive visualization of the overestimation and underestimation of bed occupancy, we plotted the error throughout the year in Fig. 17.

It is evident that in scenario 1, depicted in Fig. 16a, bed occupancy is underestimated. This outcome was expected, as the predictor for H-LoS tends to underestimate patients' H-LoS as well. The mean error is 42.05, and the MAE is 42.1.

In scenario 2, the bed occupancy error distribution is shown in Fig. 16b, resulting from a simulated H-LoS predictor with a symmetric error distribution. As depicted in Fig. 17b, the bed occupancy is now slightly overestimated. However, the MAE decreased from 42.1 in the baseline scenario to 9.82, and the mean error changed from 42.05 to -7.53.

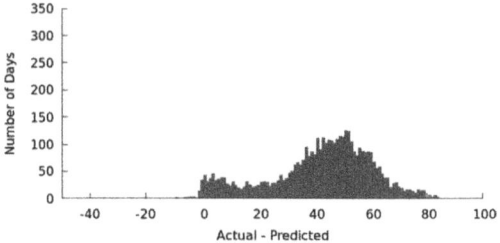

(a) Bed occupancy error from H-LoS distribution with mean = 42.05, MAE = 42.1

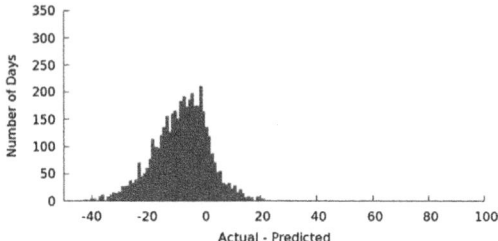

(b) Bed occupancy error from symmetric H-LoS distribution with mean = −7.53, MAE = 9.82

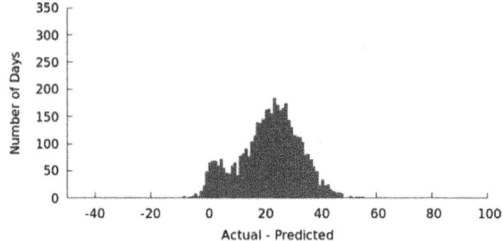

(c) Bed occupancy error from narrowed H-LoS distribution with mean = 22.13, MAE = 22.2

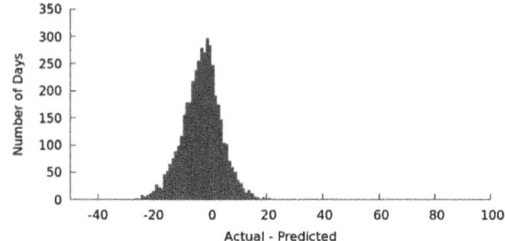

(d) Bed occupancy error from symmetric and then narrowed H-LoS distribution with mean = −2.68, MAE = 5.78

Fig. 16. Bed occupancy error distributions for all four scenarios (MIMIC-IV).

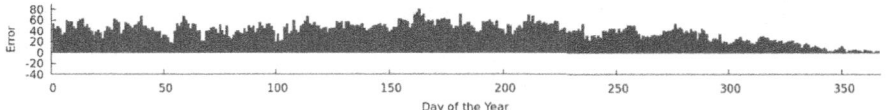

(a) Bed occupancy error from H-LoS distribution over the year 2010

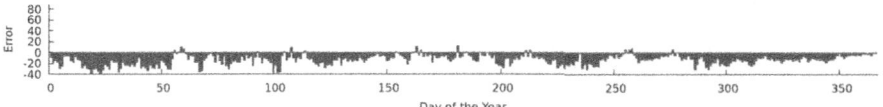

(b) Bed occupancy error from symmetric H-LoS distribution over the year 2010

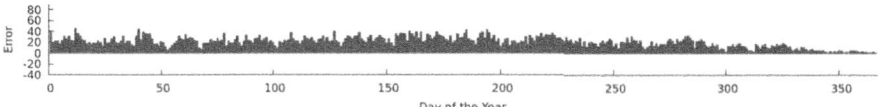

(c) Bed occupancy error from narrowed H-LoS distribution over the year 2010

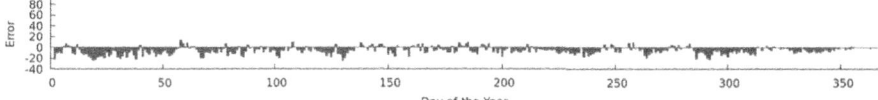

(d) Bed occupancy error from symmetric and then narrowed H-LoS distribution over the year 2010

Fig. 17. Bed occupancy error within an example year all four scenarios (MIMIC-IV).

In scenario 3, the H-LoS predictor was simulated such that its corresponding error distribution is narrowed. The resulting bed occupancy error is visualized in Fig. 16c, and as shown in Fig. 17c, the bed occupancy is also narrowed. The mean of 22.13 and the MAE of 22.2 have been halved, but the occupancy, as in the baseline scenario, is still underestimated.

Finally, we combined scenarios 2 and 3 by simulating a H-LoS predictor that has a symmetric and narrowed error distribution compared to the predictor from the baseline scenario. Now, the bed occupancy is only slightly over- or underestimated, with a mean of just -2.68 and a MAE of 5.78.

To conclude, if the error distribution of the LoS predictor has a positive skew, it is more important to reduce the skew rather than its deviation.

5.2 Stationary Bed Occupancy at the UKSH

We transferred the calculation of bed occupancy, given the predicted H-LoS, to the UKSH hospital located near our campus in Germany. In contrast to the MIMIC-IV EHR dataset, all dates are kept as they are, allowing for a realistic analysis of bed occupancy at the hospital. The H-LoS of the predictor is depicted in Fig. 14. One can see that the H-LoS error distribution, with a mean of -0.17, is almost similar to the simulated predictor in scenario 2, which also has a symmetric error distribution. As expected, Fig. 18 and Fig. 19 show that the occupancy error distribution, with a mean of −10.38, is mostly symmetrical with a tendency to overestimate bed occupancy.

5.3   ED-Occupancy at the UKSH

Access to the UKSH's future ED-occupancy would drastically simplify planning. Instead, on a daily basis, we aim to predict the occupancy on the hour, as time is most critical compared to any other station at the hospital. The ED-LoS error distribution of the predictor is depicted at Fig. 13 and one can see that the predictor tends to underestimate the ED-LoS of patient admissions. As expected, the ED-occupancy is slightly underestimated at the UKSH, as can be seen in Fig. 20 with a mean of 3.07 and MAE of 5.94. However, the mean of 3.07 is not that high and one can see in Fig. 21, that the ED-occupancy is only slightly over- and underestimated over the year 2023.

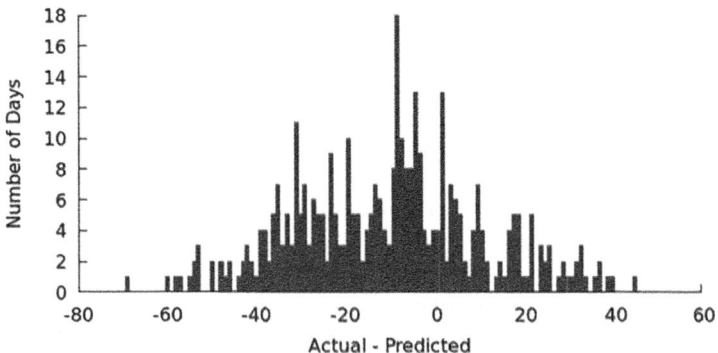

Fig. 18. Bed occupancy error at the UKSH with an overarching view with mean = −10.38, MAE = 18.91.

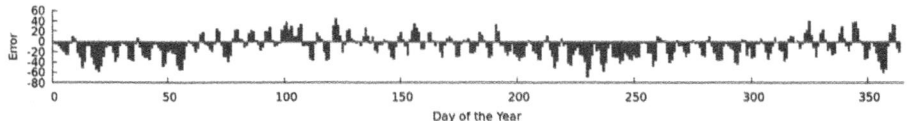

Fig. 19. Bed occupancy error within the year 2023 at UKSH.

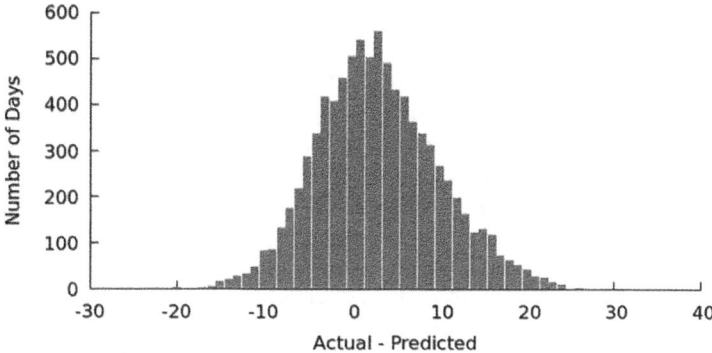

Fig. 20. ED-occupancy error at the UKSH with an overarching view with mean = 3.07 and MAE = 5.94.

6   Time Dependent View

A more realistic scenario, compared to the overarching view we presented in Sect. 5, is a time-dependent view. At any point in time t_n, a hospital administrator would like to know the occupancy for a certain point in the future t_{n+i}, i days ahead. The administrator can only use the predictor to estimate the LoS of patients admitted to the hospital before t_n and then sum up all those patients who have a LoS long enough that they will still be in the hospital at t_{n+i}. Predicting occupancy in this way would likely result in an underestimation, as many patients might be admitted between t_n and t_{n+i} and stay in the hospital at least until t_{n+i}. However, this would require predicting the future admission rate at the hospital, which is nearly impossible. Instead, one can add, for each time step t_j within $(t_n, t_{n+i}]$, the mean number of patients admitted to the hospital with a LoS equal to or greater than $t_{n+i} - t_j$. At t_{n+i}, this would be equal to the mean number of patients admitted daily to the hospital, as they technically have at least a LoS of zero. Again, we investigate the H-LoS per day and the ED-LoS per hour.

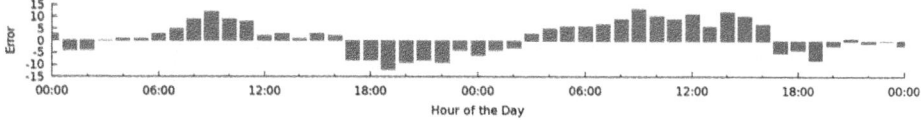

Fig. 21. ED-occupancy error within the year 2023 at the UKSH.

6.1   Stationary Bed Occupancy at MIMIC-IV

In case of MIMIC-IV, where all timestamps for each patient's admission are shifted by a randomly selected fixed offset, we add to the prediction the mean numbers of patients being admitted daily after t_n at the hospital staying long enough until t_{n+i} at the hospital.

In this scenario, the hospital administrator wants to predict the bed occupancy for three days from now, t_{n+3} from t_{n+0}. In addition to those patients who are in the hospital at t_{n+0} with a H-LoS long enough to stay until at least t_{n+3}, we also need to account for those patients who will be admitted within the time span $(t_{n+0}, t_{n+3}]$, as depicted in Fig. 22. On average, 22.05 patients are admitted daily to the hospital and stay for more than two days. Therefore, we add 22.05 patients for day t_{n+1} to the bed occupancy prediction for day t_{n+3}. The same applies for day t_{n+2} with a mean of 29.00 patients staying one day in the hospital, and for t_{n+3} with a mean of 40.85 patients being admitted to the hospital during the day.

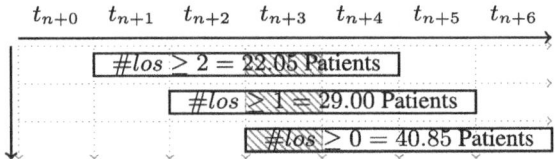

Fig. 22. Occupancy filling at t_0 for predicting bed occupancy at t_3 with $22.05 + 29.00 + 40.85 \approx 92$ additional patients on average at the hospital at t_3.

The resulting bed occupancy error distributions for all four scenarios we presented in Sect. 4.1 are depicted in Fig. 23. All four error distributions are almost identical, as expected. The error curves resemble the aggregated bed occupancy depicted in Fig. 6 and the number of patients admitted post t_n and present at t_{n+3} is assumed to be a constant, estimated at 92.

In Scenario 1, depicted in Fig. 23a, the MAE is 29.87, and the bed occupancy is slightly overestimated, with a mean of -5.99. With a more symmetric H-LoS error distribution, the MAE improves slightly to 28.3, but the mean worsens to -13.44. In Scenarios 3 and 4, shown in Fig. 23c and Fig. 23d, respectively, the mean is improved, but the MAE is slightly worse than in Scenarios 1 and 2.

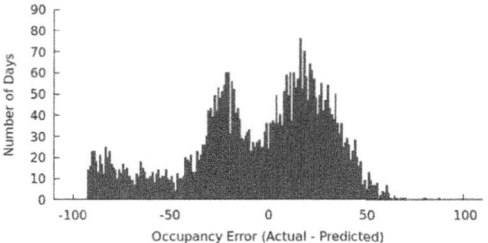

(a) With the baseline H-LoS distribution, the mean is −5.99 and MAE is 29.87

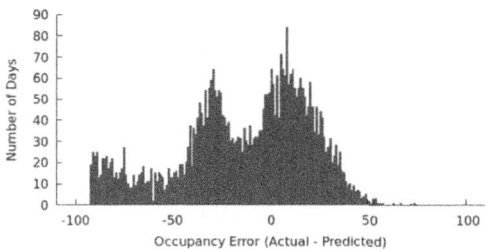

(b) With the symmetric H-LoS distribution, the mean is −13.44 and MAE is 28.30

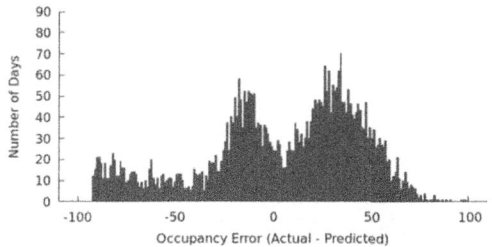

(c) With the narrowed H-LoS distribution, the mean is 4.13 and the MAE is 34.08

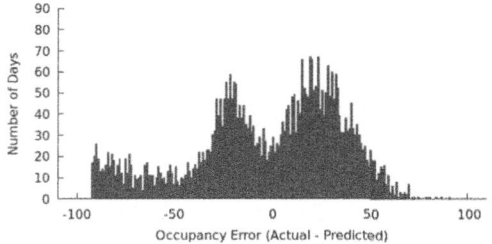

(d) With the symmetric and then narrowed H-LoS distribution, the mean is −2.74 and the MAE is 31.57

Fig. 23. Time dependent bed occupancy error distribution with a forecast of three days.

6.2   Stationary Bed Occupancy at the UKSH

This scenario is identical to that presented in Sect. 6.2, except that we apply it to the UKSH data. At UKSH, the mean number of admissions with a H-LoS greater than i differs from that of MIMIC-IV, as depicted in Fig. 24.

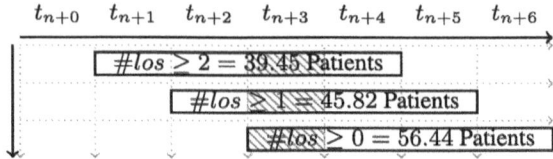

Fig. 24. Occupancy filling at t_0 for predicting bed occupancy at t_3 with $39.45 + 45.82 + 56.44 \approx 142$ additional patients on average at the UKSH at t_3.

On average, 56.44 patients are admitted to the hospital per day. Of those, 45.82 have a H-LoS greater than one day, including 39.45 with a H-LoS greater than two days. The resulting bed occupancy error distribution with filling is depicted in Fig. 25.

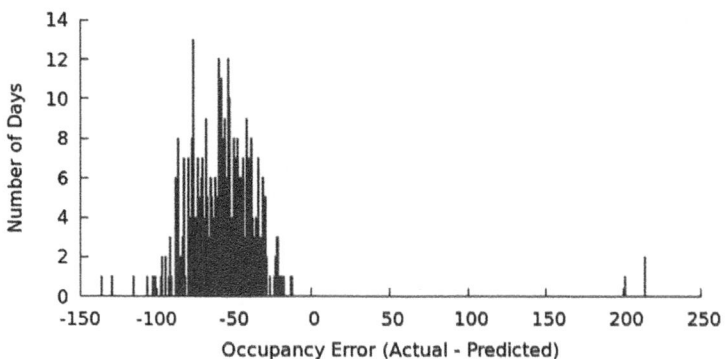

Fig. 25. Bed occupancy error with a forecast of three days with filling from H-LoS distribution with mean $= -52.50$, MAE $= 56.00$ and SD $= 18.00$.

One can see that the bed occupancy is overestimated with a mean of -52.50.

6.3   ED-Occupancy at the UKSH

In this scenario, the hospital administrator would like to know the ED-occupancy at the UKSH hospital in six hours t_{n+6} from any given time t_n. As before, we predict the ED-LoS of any patient currently in the ED and check whether their remaining ED-LoS is at least six hours. The resulting occupancy error distribution is depicted in Fig. 26.

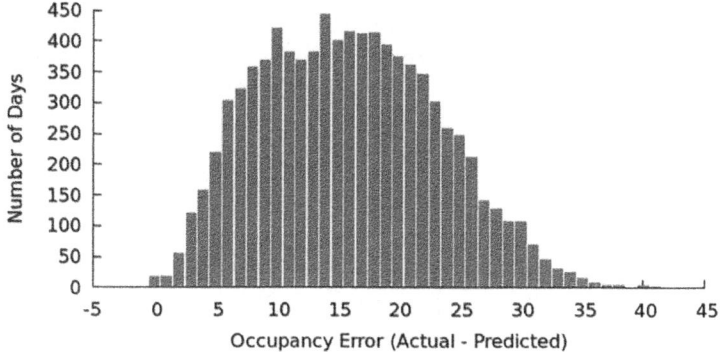

Fig. 26. Time dependent ED-occupancy error with a forecast of six hours at the UKSH without filling with a mean of 15.89, MAE of 15.89 and SD of 7.29.

As one can see in the figure, and as expected, the ED-occupancy is significantly underestimated because all patients admitted within $(t_n, t_{n+6}]$ who stay at the hospital at least until t_{n+6} are completely ignored. Since we have access to real admission times at the UKSH, we can estimate the mean number of patients admitted at each hour of the day, as depicted in Fig. 27. Most patients, approximately seven, are admitted daily on average at 11:00, while the fewest are admitted at 05:00 in the morning.

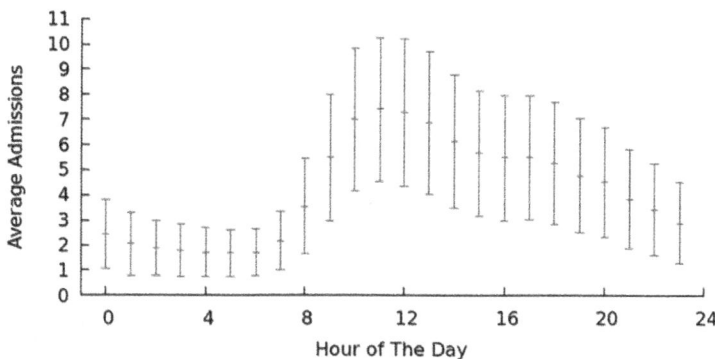

Fig. 27. Mean number of admissions at the UKSH-ED aggregated by the hour of the day with standard deviation.

Not only the mean number of daily admissions depends on the hour of the day. Additionally, the ED-LoS depends on the hour of the day as well, as illustrated in Fig. 28.

For instance, one can see in the figure that patients admitted to the ED at 12:00 with an ED-LoS shorter than 6 h have a mean ED-LoS of 3.52. This is higher than the mean ED-LoS of 2.87 for those admitted to the hospital at 03:00

with a ED-LoS shorter than 6 h. Therefore, the number of patients added to the
ED-occupancy prediction for a more accurate forecast strongly depends on the
hour of the day. The resulting ED-occupancy error distribution is depicted in
Fig. 29.

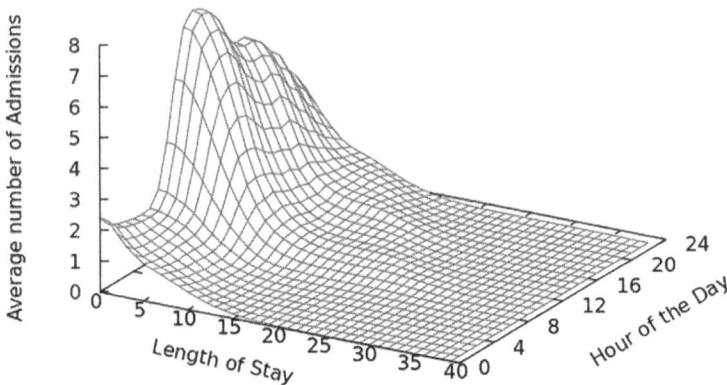

Fig. 28. Mean number of admissions at the UKSH-ED over time, aggregated by the
hour of the day.

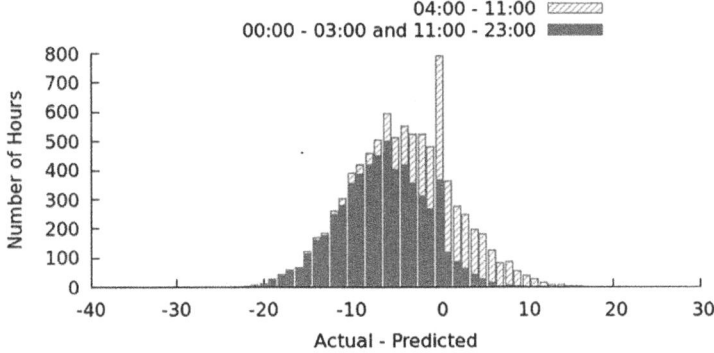

Fig. 29. Time dependent ED-occupancy error with a forecast of six hours at the UKSH
with filling with a mean of -4.15, MAE of 5.81, and SD of 6.04.

One can see that, in contrast to the ED-occupancy depicted in Fig. 26, the
ED-occupancy prediction has greatly improved by filling the prediction with
patients admitted to the hospital during $(t_n, t_{n+6}]$, depending on the hour of the
day. The error distribution clearly corresponds to that of a normal distribution,
with one major exception. The error of 0 occurs unusually frequently, which is
good for the results, however requires further investigations.

As listed in Table 2, one can see, that the accuracy of the prediction at t_{n+6}
strongly depends on the hour of the day.

Table 2. ED-occupancy error distribution metrics with a forecast of six hours at the UKSH, with filling aggregated by two different time ranges.

Point of Time t_{n+6}	Distribution	Mean	MAE	SD
04:00–11:00	Actual	22.97	22.97	6.87
	Predicted	21.98	21.98	6.85
	Occ Error	0.46	3.78	5.03
00:00–03:00 & 04:00–23:00	Actual	32.07	32.07	8.75
	Predicted	38.44	38.44	8.75
	Occ Error	−6.46	6.83	5.03

If one predicts the ED-occupancy only for the hours between 04:00 and 11:00 in the morning, the ED-occupancy error has a mean of 0.46 and an MAE of 3.78, and its error distribution is depicted in Fig. 30.

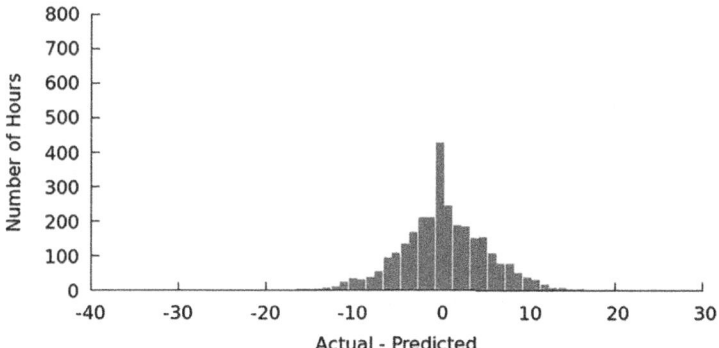

Fig. 30. Time dependent ED-occupancy error with a forecast of six hours at the UKSH with filling for t_{n+6} between 04:00 and 11:00.

On the other hand, if one predicts the ED-occupancy for the hours between 00:00 and 03:00, 12:00 and 23:00, the ED-occupancy error has a mean of −6.46 and MAE of 6.83, and its error distribution is depicted in Fig. 31.

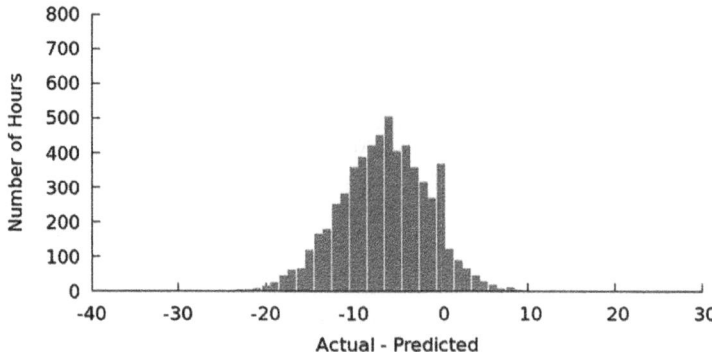

Fig. 31. Time dependent ED-occupancy error with a forecast of six hours at the UKSH with filling for t_{n+6} between 04:00 and 11:00, and 12:00 and 23:00.

One can see, that the error distribution depicted in Fig. 29, is a combination of Fig. 30, and Fig. 31.

7   Discussion of the Results

As we already discovered using the MIMIC-IV dataset, a simulated H-LoS predictor with a symmetric H-LoS error distribution leads to a bed occupancy error with a relatively small mean and MAE. The H-LoS error distribution for the UKSH is also symmetric, and the resulting bed occupancy error distributions, in both the overarching and time-dependent views, also have relatively small errors. Hence, simulating the LoS error distribution is quite effective to analyze how it affects the occupancy calculation.

Access to real time points at when patients are admitted and discharged from the hospital allows for further optimizations, as we have shown in Sect. 5.3 at where we added patients to the ED-occupancy prediction depending on the current time. That has reduced the ED-occupancy error with a mean of 15.89 to −4.15, the MAE from 15.89 to 5.81 and the SD from 7.29 to 6.04. These results are promising, if one considers that the mean ED-occupancy has a mean of 29.68 and SD of 7.66.

Finally, all our results can be found in Table 3.

Table 3. Overview of all four scenarios including the overarching as well as the time dependent view at MIMIC-IV at all scenarios at UKSH (*actual LoS of 0 left out).

	Scenario	LoS Error			Occupancy Error		
		Mean	MAE	MAPE	Mean	MAE	MAPE
Overarching	Scenario 1	0.98	2.34	134.25	42.05	42.10	21.80
	Scenario 2	−0.25	2.35	134.28	−7.53	9.82	7.40*
	Scenario 3	0.49	1.17	67.12	22.13	22.20	11.95
	Scenario 4	−0.12	1.17	67.14	−2.68	5.78	4.04
	UKSH LoS	−0.17	2.68	89.00	−10.38	18.91	6.00
	UKSH ED-LoS	0.75	3.73	96.00	3.07	5.94	23.00
Dependent	Scenario 1	0.98	2.34	134.25	−5.99	29.87	88.58
	Scenario 2	−0.25	2.35	134.28	−13.44	28.30	89.01
	Scenario 3	0.49	1.17	67.12	4.13	34.08	89.08
	Scenario 4	−0.12	1.17	67.14	−2.74	31.57	89.01
	UKSH LoS	−0.17	2.68	89.00	−52.50	56.00	18.00
	UKSH ED-LoS	0.75	3.73	96.00	−4.15	5.81	26.77

The mean value as a metric is an indication of how asymmetric/symmetric the respective error distribution is.

8 Conclusion

We extended our previous work by successfully transferring the calculation of occupancy from predicted LoS using the MIMIC-IV dataset to the UKSH hospital located in Germany. In addition to calculating bed occupancy at the UKSH hospital, we also calculate the occupancy for patients admitted to the ED on an hourly basis. Calculated occupancy error margins are low enough to support quick decision making at the hospital, thereby reducing stress and costs. Access to real-time data points at the ED of the UKSH helps reduce occupancy errors, with the mean error decreasing from 15.89 to −4.15 closer to 0, the MAE decreasing from 15.89 to 5.81, and the SD decreasing from 7.29 to 6.04.

In this work, we predict the LoS for each individual patient's admission exactly once and then use the predictions for all currently hospitalized patients to calculate the overall bed occupancy. In a more realistic scenario, if one wants to know the bed occupancy at a specific point in the future t_{n+i}, one would predict the LoS at t_n for all currently hospitalized patients, as more information is available about the patients' stay at t_n. For example, a patient could be connected to a monitor where their vital signs are continuously measured, examination results could be available, medication may have been adjusted, or the doctor may have created new notes about the patient's health status. All this information is continuously generated, can be aggregated over time, and then used at t_n to predict the bed occupancy at t_{n+i}. We assume that with more information, the accuracy of predicting the LoS and therefore the occupancy is higher.

As we have shown in Fig. 9a, the error distribution for predicting the LoS of patients admitted from the ED to the hospital in MIMIC-IV has a high positive skew. Using that predicted LoS to calculate bed occupancy lead to an error with a mean of 42.05 and MAE of 42.1. The simulated LoS error distribution in Fig. 9b is symmetrical and resulted in a bed occupancy error with a mean of only −7.53 and MAE of 9.82. Narrowing the LoSerror distribution reduced the mean and MAE to 22.13 and 22.2 respectively. Therefore, in future work, we aim to reduce the positive skew of the LoS predictor. One potential solution to this problem could be to synthesize patient admissions to balance the LoS distribution, as depicted in Fig. 2, such that the distribution has not such a high skew.

Acknowledgments. The research for the current paper was funded as part of the APONA project, by the state of Schleswig-Holstein, project no. 220 23 020.

Disclosure of Interests. The authors have no competing interests to declare that are relevant to the content of this article.

References

1. Baek, H., Cho, M., Kim, S., Hwang, H., Song, M., Yoo, S.: Analysis of length of hospital stay using electronic health records: a statistical and data mining approach. PLoS ONE **13**(4), e0195901 (2018). https://doi.org/10.1371/journal.pone.0195901
2. Belciug, S., Gorunescu, F.: Improving hospital bed occupancy and resource utilization through queuing modeling and evolutionary computation. J. Biomed. Inform. **53**, 261–269 (2015)
3. Buttigieg, S.C., Abela, L., Pace, A.: Variables affecting hospital length of stay: a scoping review. J. Health Organ. Manag. **32**(3), 463–493 (2018). https://doi.org/10.1108/jhom-10-2017-0275
4. Farmer, R., Emami, J.: Models for forecasting hospital bed requirements in the acute sector. J. Epidemiol. Commun. Health **44**(4), 307–312 (1990)
5. Forster, A.J., Stiell, I., Wells, G., Lee, A.J., Van Walraven, C.: The effect of hospital occupancy on emergency department length of stay and patient disposition. Acad. Emerg. Med. **10**(2), 127–133 (2003)
6. Gentimis, T., Alnaser, A.J., Durante, A., Cook, K., Steele, R.: Predicting hospital length of stay using neural networks on mimic III data. In: 2017 IEEE 15th International Conference on Dependable, Autonomic and Secure Computing, 15th International Conference on Pervasive Intelligence and Computing, 3rd International Conference on Big Data Intelligence and Computing and Cyber Science and Technology Congress (DASC/PiCom/DataCom/CyberSciTech). IEEE (2017). https://doi.org/10.1109/dasc-picom-datacom-cyberscitec.2017.191
7. Gorunescu, F., McClean, S.I., Millard, P.H.: A queueing model for bed-occupancy management and planning of hospitals. J. Oper. Res. Soc. **53**(1), 19–24 (2002)
8. Harrison, G.: Compartmental models of hospital patient occupancy patterns. In: Modelling Hospital Resource Use: A Different Approach to the Planning and Control of Health Care Systems, pp. 53–61 (1994)

9. Hartwig, M., Schiff, R.S., Wolfrum, S., Möller, R.: Aggregating predicted individual hospital length of stay to predict bed occupancy for hospitals. In: Proceedings of the 17th International Joint Conference on Biomedical Engineering Systems and Technologies. International Joint Conference on Biomedical Engineering Systems and Technologies (BIOSTEC-2024), Rome, Italy, 21–23 February, vol. 2, pp. 175–184. SciTePress (2024)
10. Johnson, A., Bulgarelli, L., Pollard, T., Horng, S., Celi, L.A., Mark, R.: Mimic-IV (2023). https://doi.org/10.13026/6MM1-EK67
11. Johnson, A.E.W., et al.: Mimic-IV, a freely accessible electronic health record dataset. Sci. Data 10(1) (2023). https://doi.org/10.1038/s41597-022-01899-x
12. Kutafina, E., Bechtold, I., Kabino, K., Jonas, S.M.: Recursive neural networks in hospital bed occupancy forecasting. BMC Med. Inform. Decis. Mak. 19, 1–10 (2019)
13. Lequertier, V., Wang, T., Fondrevelle, J., Augusto, V., Duclos, A.: Hospital length of stay prediction methods: a systematic review. Med. Care 59(10), 929–938 (2021). https://doi.org/10.1097/mlr.0000000000001596
14. Mackay, M., Lee, M.: Choice of models for the analysis and forecasting of hospital beds. Health Care Manag. Sci. 8, 221–230 (2005)
15. Majeed, M.U., et al.: Delay in discharge and its impact on unnecessary hospital bed occupancy. BMC Health Serv. Res. 12(1) (2012). https://doi.org/10.1186/1472-6963-12-410
16. Mak, G., Grant, W.D., McKenzie, J.C., McCabe, J.B.: Physicians' ability to predict hospital length of stay for patients admitted to the hospital from the emergency department. Emerg. Med. Int. 2012, 1–4 (2012). https://doi.org/10.1155/2012/824674
17. Morley, C., Unwin, M., Peterson, G.M., Stankovich, J., Kinsman, L.: Emergency department crowding: a systematic review of causes, consequences and solutions. PLoS ONE 13(8), e0203316 (2018). https://doi.org/10.1371/journal.pone.0203316
18. Prokhorenkova, L., Gusev, G., Vorobev, A., Dorogush, A.V., Gulin, A.: Catboost: unbiased boosting with categorical features. In: Advances in neural Information Processing Systems, vol. 31 (2018)
19. Rocheteau, E., Liò, P., Hyland, S.: Temporal pointwise convolutional networks for length of stay prediction in the intensive care unit. In: Proceedings of the Conference on Health, Inference, and Learning, ACM CHIL 2021. ACM (2021). https://doi.org/10.1145/3450439.3451860
20. Savioli, G., et al.: Emergency department overcrowding: understanding the factors to find corresponding solutions. J. Personalized Med. 12(2), 279 (2022). https://doi.org/10.3390/jpm12020279
21. Schiff, S., Wolfrum, S., Möller, R., Hartwig, M.: Using data synthesis to improve length of stay predictions for patients with rare diagnoses. In: The International FLAIRS Conference Proceedings, vol. 37 (2024). https://doi.org/10.32473/flairs.37.1.135651
22. Stone, K., Zwiggelaar, R., Jones, P., Mac Parthaláin, N.: A systematic review of the prediction of hospital length of stay: towards a unified framework. PLOS Digit. Health 1(4), e0000017 (2022). https://doi.org/10.1371/journal.pdig.0000017
23. Winter, A., Hartwig, M., Kirsten, T.: Predicting hospital length of stay of patients leaving the emergency department. In: Proceedings of the 16th International Joint Conference on Biomedical Engineering Systems and Technologies. SCITEPRESS - Science and Technology Publications (2023). https://doi.org/10.5220/0011671700003414

Markov Chain Analysis of Interpersonal Attachment Measured by a Digital Application: An Observational Study

Sebastian Unger$^{(\boxtimes)}$ (iD) and Thomas Ostermann

Witten/Herdecke University, 58448 Witten, Germany
`sebastian.unger@uni-wh.de`

Abstract. Dealing with relational data is an important and challenging topic not only in life science, as in the characterization of dynamics of living systems, but also in psychology and social sciences, as in the examination of interpersonal behavior. In this context, stochastic process models are often used for the mathematical description of system dynamics and transition processes. In this observational study, interpersonal attachment of 96 participants (74 females and 22 males, mean age of 23.94 ± 4.16 years) measured by a digital application was represented and analyzed as Discrete Time Markov Chains (DTMCs) after the participants formed 48 dyads. For each participant, 100 DTMCs were formed based on a single measurement by continuously increasing the interval between two states and tested for Markov property as well as for homogeneity with their counterpart within a dyad. The results show, firstly, that the majority of the DTMCs satisfy the Markov property and can therefore actually be interpreted as DTMCs and, secondly, that the DTMCs of a dyad can be both homogeneous and heterogeneous, with the middle intervals appearing to be the most suitable in the two tests. Nonetheless, the results should be further investigated by either optimizing the methodology itself or supporting it with additional measures of interpersonal behavior, e.g., by observing interpersonal interactions or by eye-tracking measurements.

Keywords: Interpersonal attachment · Mental processes · Mental health care · Digital application · Observation · Time series analysis

1 Introduction

1.1 General Background

In life science, the analysis of relational data from living organisms is one of the most important and challenging topics to understand how life is organized. In particular, states and state transitions play an important role, as they characterize the dynamics of living systems. A simple example is the inheritance of dominant and recessive traits over time in a population, the theoretical basis of which was first described in detail by Mendel in the 19th century [1] and then led to a mathematical description in the well-known Hardy-Weinberg law (see [2] for an extensive historical analysis).

But also outside of biology, the analysis of relational data is also an important field of research. In psychology and social science, for example, the study of interpersonal behavior has a long tradition, e.g., in the field of social dynamics [3], group interactions [4], romantic relationships [5], or client-therapist alliances [6]. The last two examples are representatives of a special relationship between two people, the so-called interpersonal attachment.

An interpersonal attachment may occur solely between two people (e.g., in one-to-one therapy sessions [6]) or in larger group contexts (e.g., in school classes, when several students are supposed to work on a task together [7], or in families between siblings [8] or a mother and her child [9]). Thus, methods and models have been developed in psychology and social sciences to approach the relationships between these constellations empirically and theoretically. In this context, the paradigm of "attachment" was established in terms of a quantifiable measure.

One of the most popular methods for the quantification of attachment is the Adult Attachment Interview (AAI), a tool for classifying attachment patterns of adults based on childhood experiences with parents and the influence of these experiences on personality development [10], which was later adapted for children as the Child Attachment Interview (CAI) [11]. Even though both tools have been proven to deliver reliable results [12–14], they should not be underestimated in terms of their workload.

Because of the shared drawback of the AAI and CAI, new and innovative measurement methods were developed. On of which is the Adult Attachment Projective (AAP), an art-based tool designed to measure attachment via drawings [15]. Other methods use, for example, eye movements or facial expressions to draw conclusions about the attachment [16–18]. Taken together, attachment seems to express itself in a variety of ways.

1.2 Stochastic Modelling

Apart from classical study designs, stochastic process models are often used for the mathematical description of system dynamics and transition processes [19–21]. Within the context of attachment and dyadic interactions, almost half a century ago, Benjamin [22] recommended a special class of stochastic processes, the so-called Markov chains. A Markov chain is a stochastic process with finite state space in which the future state of the process is only determined by the current state. Thus, Markov chains are often used for modeling random state transitions of a system if there is reason to assume that the state transitions are memoryless. Although, this is a very strong assumption, Markov chains are nevertheless used to analyze attachment and dyadic dynamics.

Koulomzin et al. [23], for example, analyzed the head orientation towards their mother in 4-month-old infants. Using 12-stage Markov chains consisting of two horizontal head positions, three vertical head positions, and two gaze states, they showed that secure infants at this age already convey face-to-face interaction differently than avoidant infants. In another study on the dyadic interaction between mothers and their 4- to 6-month-old infants [24], a three-stage Markov chain was used to analyze the time series of Respiratory Sinus Arrhythmia: "positive" if $p < .001$ and the regression coefficient beta for infants and mothers was positive, "negative" if $p < .001$ and the regression beta for infants and mothers was negative, and "no change" if $p > .001$. Using a time-sliding window technique, it was shown that this approach made it possible to measure both positive and negative physiological synchrony in infant-mother dyads.

In a behavioral study of eight starlings caught in the wild [25], the birds' location in the cage was investigated as a state variable. Again, a Markov chain analysis was used, but this time to categorize normal and abnormal behavior (e.g., staying on the walls and ceiling). The analysis indicated a high correlation in the behavioral patterns of the caged starlings. In particular, the method showed that it can be used to quantify differences in animals' use of space.

These examples show impressively that movement data in dyads and groups can be analyzed by using Markov chains if the stages and intervals between them are well defined. This approach is also followed in this observational study, which is based on the preliminary study presented in 2024 [26]. As before, data from a drawing app in a dyadic setting is represented and analyzed as Discrete Time Markov Chains (DTMCs) [27].

2   Material and Methods

2.1   Participants

A total of 96 participants (74 females and 22 males) with a mean age of 23.94 $\pm$ 4.16 years were recruited via Witten/Herdecke University. The channels of recruitment were social media, verbal communication, and the university's internal bulletin board. All participants stated that they were able to operate a tablet independently and had no acute disorders that could affect their use of the tablet. If female, they also had to confirm that they were not pregnant, as the effects of the study procedure on stress levels were unknown at the time of execution. Finally, after being informed about the study and the use of data, all participants signed an informed consent form. For successful participation, the participants received compensation for their spent time.

2.2   Hard and Software

As hardware, a dyad received two ASUS Transformer Mini T102HA tablets on which Windows 10 was installed. Each of these tablets was not only equipped with a high-resolution display (1280 x 800 pixels) and sufficient random-access memory (4 gigabytes) for adequate image quality and system performance but also with a pressure-sensitive stylus (1024 level) for a natural drawing experience.

The software used for the measurement was an innovative, self-developed tablet application (app) introduced in 2020 [28]. It was developed with the Windows Presentation Foundation (WPF) framework using C# (.NET framework 4.5.2) as the programming language for the backend. Features of the app include acquiring and storing data as well as handling any events on the user interface. The app's main feature can be found in its name "IU", which is derived from the sounds of the personal pronouns "I" and "you" and represents two of the mental states to be measured. Figure 1 shows that these two states are the first level states, whereby the "I"-state means that the thoughts are with oneself and the "U"-state that the thoughts are with the partner. The app uses the bottom half of the screen to depict the "I"-state and the top half to depict the "U"-state. With the second level states, information about whether a thought is positive or negative can be provided. For this reason, the screen is furthermore divided into a left half to depict negative thoughts (−) and a right half to depict positive thoughts (+). In total, this results in four visualized quadrants that represent the mental states "thinking positively about the partner" (+U), "thinking negatively about the partner" (−U), "thinking positively thinking positively about oneself" (+I), and "thinking negatively about yourself" (−I).

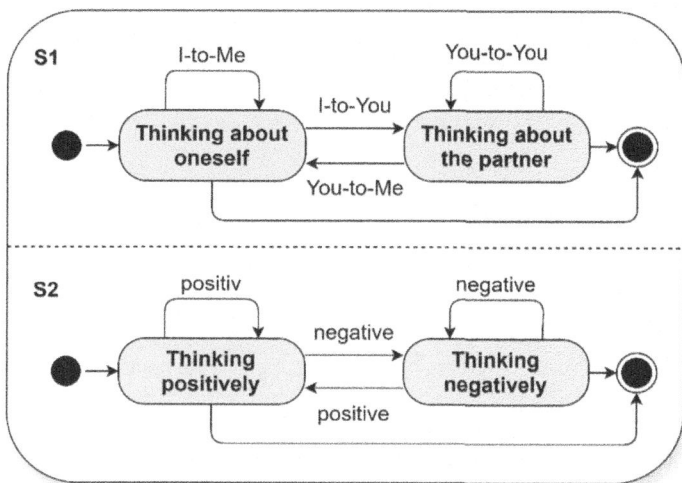

Fig. 1. State diagram taken from [26]. It illustrates the transitions between the two first level states (the thought is with the partner or with oneself) and the two second level states (the thought is positive or negative).

2.3 Study Procedure

Apart from the initial and final step, i.e., the recruitment of the participants and the allocation of their compensation, the study procedure (Fig. 2) consisted of the following three parts: firstly, the formation of the dyads; secondly, the appearance of the dyads at the prepared test location; and thirdly, the digital measurement of the interpersonal attachment.

For the formation of the dyads, there were two options. Participants either registered with a partner that they are comfortable with or registered alone to be assigned to a random partner. These two options are intended to result in a mixed number of dyadic constellations, i.e., different levels of familiarity.

Once the dyads were formed, the participants were asked to appear at the test location in their assigned dyad. A person in charge was waiting at this location to check the participants' eligibility. The person in charge then informed the participants about the study and explained the measurement. For the three-minute-long measurement, the participants were asked to sit opposite their partner at a table. They were then each given a tablet and a stylus with which to perform the measurement.

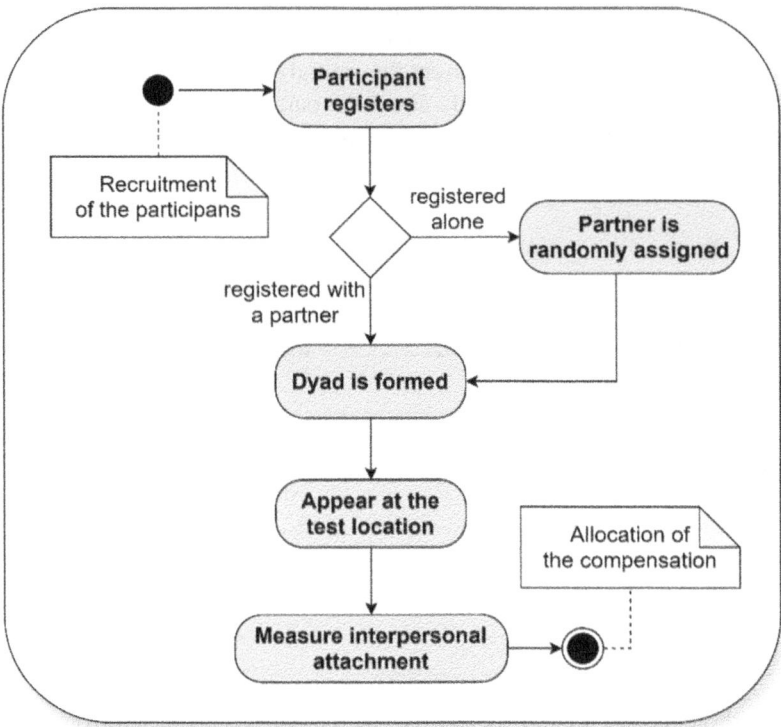

Fig. 2. Study procedure, starting with the first step of participant recruitment through to the allocation of the compensation.

With the app that ran on each of the tablets, participants were asked to enter demographic data (e.g., age and gender) and the identification number (ID) of their dyad. Then, participants switched to the measurement view, in which the screen is divided into the four quadrants that represent the mental states. With these quadrants, participants could express their thoughts that occurred to them throughout the measurement while looking into their partner's eyes. The task was to move the stylus into that quadrant that best corresponds to a thought. The stylus should be kept there as long as this thought did not change. If a thought changed, the stylus had to be moved into the next best corresponding quadrant. This process was repeated until a sound signaled the end of the measurement.

2.4   Output Measures

The drawing process that happened while a participant $j_k(k = A, B)$ of a dyad j looked into its partner's eyes was continuously tracked at 100 ms (ms) intervals (t_i). To be precise, the pixel coordinates of the screen (x_i, y_i) that were touched by the stylus during the curse of the measurement were tracked, resulting in three-dimensional time series $(x_i, y_i, t_i)_{jk}$, consisting of two spatial and one temporal dimension. Each time series was saved in a raw data file together with the y-coordinate of the horizontal screen center line and the x-coordinate of the vertical screen center line. This was necessary in order to reconstruct the mental states retrospectively using the coordinates of the time series.

2.5 Statistical Analysis

First, the chronological sequence of the mental states was reconstructed using the three-dimensional time series $(x_i, y_i, t_i)_{jk}$ and the coordinates of the two screen center lines. Each state was determined via the spatial dimension $(x_i, y_i)_{jk}$, whereas its place in the sequence was determined via the temporal dimension $(t_i)_{jk}$. By default, the interval between the individual states was 100 ms. This interval was repeatedly increased by 100 ms. The maximum interval chosen was 10,000 ms, resulting in a total of 100 chronologically sorted chains of mental states per participant.

Each chain consisted of four potential mental states (+U, −U, +I and −I), depending on how the participant's thoughts proceeded and how precisely the stylus was moved over the screen. For that, each "U" or "I"-state was determined by its spatial dimension $(y_i)_{jk}$. This coordinate was checked whether it is above the horizontal screen centerline, resulting in a "U"-state, otherwise in an "I"-state. Afterwards, each state was defined more precisely by its spatial dimension $(x_i)_{jk}$. This coordinate was checked whether it is to the left of the vertical center line of the screen, resulting in the state being marked as negative (−U or −I), otherwise as positive (+U or +I).

Second, the chains of mental states were to be considered as DTMCs. Therefore, each had to be tested whether it satisfies the Markov property. If the chains of a dyad satisfied this property and thus were classified as DTMCs, homogeneity of a dyad was tested next. Homogeneity in this context means that the chains and thus the thoughts within a dyad are identical. Consequently, the thoughts within the dyad, which did not satisfy homogeneity, were classified as heterogeneous.

Both Markov property and homogeneity was tested using the R package "markovchain" (version 0.9.1) [29]. For these tests, which are based on a chi-square test in this package, $\alpha = 0.05$ was set as the level of significance, i.e., Markov property and homogeneity were assumed if the p-value of a test exceeded α.

3 Results

3.1 Demographic Data

For the analysis, the data from six dyads (12 participants) had to be removed. This was because the gaps in the time series were so large for at least one participant in these dyads that not all intervals could be applied to the data. Demographic data of the 84 remaining participants (64 females and 20 males) is shown in Table 1.

The 42 corresponding dyads were mainly formed by colleagues and friends (15 and 18, respectively). The less frequent dyadic constellations included love couples and strangers (3 and 6, respectively). Table 2 contains the demographic data of all these dyads.

Table 1. Demographic data of the remaining participants.

Gender	Number	Age [years]		
		Mean	Minimum	Maximum
All	84	23.88 ± 4.01	19	39
Females	64 (76.2%)	23.67 ± 4.2	19	39
Males	20 (23.8%)	24.55 ± 3.33	21	32

Table 2. Demographic data of the remaining dyads.

Constellation	Number	Knowing since [years]		
		Mean	Minimum	Maximum
All	42	1.99 ± 1.08	0.25	5
Colleagues	15 (35.7%)	1.69 ± 1	0.25	3
Friends	18 (42.9%)	2.16 ± 0.94	0.3	3.5
Love Couples	3 (7.1%)	2.5 ± 2.18	1	5
Strangers	6 (14.3%)	-	-	-

3.2 Markov Property

Of 8,400 time series, the Markov property was satisfied in 7,776 cases (92.6%). The remaining 624 (7.4%) time series consequently did not satisfy the Markov property. As seen in Fig. 3, the time series that exhibit an unsatisfied Markov property are mostly in smaller intervals, with the 200 ms interval performing the worst. Only 57 out of 84 time series (67.9%) were able to satisfy the Markov property at this interval. Thereafter, the number of such time series increases rapidly with larger intervals. Already at an interval of 2,000 ms, there were 78 out of 84 (92.9%). From then on, however, there is no longer a clear increase of time series that satisfy the Markov property. Instead, the frequency distribution begins to fluctuate. The reason for this is that a time series can satisfy the property with one interval, but not with the next. Although this back and forth can be found over all intervals, the fluctuating frequency distribution of satisfied and unsatisfied Markov properties is particularly visible from 2,000 ms onwards.

3.3 Homogeneity

The total of 4,200 dyadic combinations formed by the 8,400 time series resulted in homogeneity 2,282 times (54.3%) and heterogeneity 1,331 times (31.7%). For the remaining 587 dyadic combinations (14%), no homogeneity test was performed because at least one time series of a combination did not satisfy the Markov property in the preliminary analysis. The frequency distribution (top diagram of Fig. 4) of these three possibilities is not random, but depends on the specific interval as in the Markov property test. This time, however, it appears that increasing the interval has a steady effect on the test.

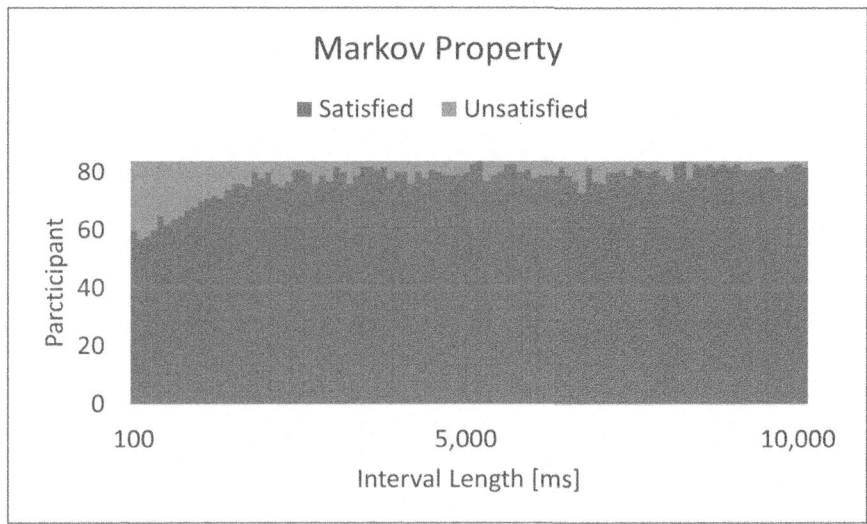

Fig. 3. Frequency distribution, including the data from [26], whether the Markov property of the time series was satisfied as a function of the intervals.

Whereas the number of homogeneous combinations (satisfied homogeneity) increases as the interval increases, the number of both heterogeneous combinations (unsatisfied homogeneity) and non-testable combinations decreases steadily.

The separation of the dyadic combinations into the four constellations of colleagues, friends, love couples, and strangers reveals that the effect caused by the increase in the interval continues in all constellations. However, there are also minor differences in the associated frequency distributions (bottom four diagrams of Fig. 4). Of particular interest here is the consideration of the counterparts, i.e., knowing someone fleetingly vs. being friends (colleagues vs. friends) and not knowing someone vs. being in love (strangers vs. love couples). In comparison to the friends, one of the biggest differences is that the heterogeneous combinations decrease earlier among the colleagues, but occur more frequently in the larger intervals. Both colleagues and friends nevertheless have almost the same number of homogeneous (55% and 52%, respectively), heterogeneous (30.9% and 35.2%, respectively), and non-testable combinations (14.1% and 12.8%, respectively). The most obvious difference between the strangers and the love couples is that the strangers only show heterogeneous and non-testable combinations in the smaller intervals, which in addition are even less frequent in these intervals. This difference between strangers and love couples is even more noticeable in the number of homogeneous (91.2% and 52.3%, respectively), heterogeneous (5.6% and 25.7%, respectively), and non-testable combinations (3.2% and 22%, respectively).

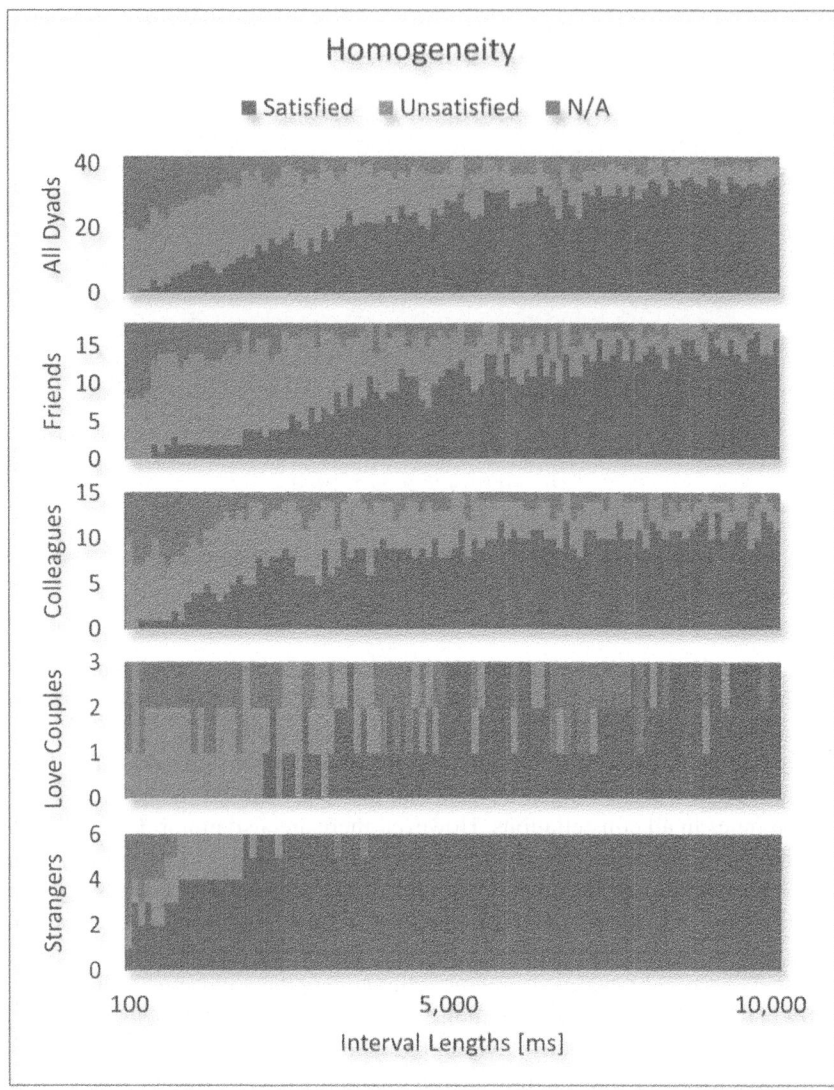

Fig. 4. Frequency distributions, including the data from [26], whether homogeneity exists between the time series of a dyad as a function of the intervals. For a better layout, the y-axes have a uniform size despite the different numbers of dyads.

4   Discussion

4.1   Key Results

With regard to the Markov property test, the results are consistent with those of the preliminary analysis [26], which used only 5,600 (66.7%) of the 8,400 time series analyzed here. This strengthens the statement that thoughts, when represented as chains of mental states, can overall be modeled as Markov chains, especially when the interval between two states exceeds 2,000 ms. However, an increase in the interval length does not automatically lead to a satisfied Markov property. In addition, as before, there is not a single interval that only leads to satisfied properties, i.e., the previous statement should be treated with care.

There is essentially one reason for the increase in satisfied properties as the interval increases: the chains of mental states become smaller, i.e., fewer states are considered in the test. On the one hand, this leads to a change in the transition probabilities, such as the probability of one state transitioning to another, which rarely occurs in the lower intervals due to the mechanics of measuring mental state changes (stylus moves into another quadrant of the screen). On the other hand, the shortening of the chains means that states and state transitions can be lost, as, for example, a 2,000 ms long mental state (stylus remains in one quadrant) could be missed with a 10,000 ms interval. Therefore, neither low nor high intervals seem to be suitable for interpreting the chains of mental states measured with this method as Markov chains.

Despite the increased number of dyads, the homogeneity test also produces similar results to the preliminary analysis [26]. In both analyses, there are many non-testable dyadic combinations in the lower intervals, which is due to the fact that many chains in this range were not recognized as Markov chains. In addition, as with the Markov property test, there is an effect that is associated with an increasing interval. In homogeneity tests of both studies, an increase in the interval means that the number of homogeneous dyadic combinations increases, while the number of heterogeneous combinations decreases. This is again caused by the shortening of the chains, meaning that they contain less information overall and sometimes even miss complete mental states, thereby affecting the result test. Here, as well, the use of low or high intervals appears to be unsuitable.

The separation of the dyadic combinations into the four constellations of colleagues, friends, love couples, and strangers did not reveal any significant differences. Both homogeneous and heterogeneous dyadic combinations were evenly distributed across the constellations. This contradicts the assumption that closely familiar dyads tend to have more homogeneous thoughts than unfamiliar dyads [28]. A reason for this could be the social desirability, i.e., presenting oneself in a generally favorable fashion [30] caused by the test situation and the presence of the partner as well as the person in charge. The thoughts could therefore be fallen into similar patterns. A study on social desirability additionally showed that, depending on which gender (male, female, or none) was given for the questionnaire, the answers were related to the gender [31]. This indicates that thoughts depend on the gender of the other and could be fallen into further similar patterns led to the high percentage of dyadic combinations here.

Taken together, the middle intervals seem to be most appropriate for both the Markov property test and the homogeneity test for the chains of mental states. However, this is not a final answer to the question of whether thoughts can be meaningfully interpreted as Markov chains. Rather, it is an observational study whose measurement method needs to be further researched, e.g., in combination with other methods. A possible combination would be with dyadic interactions that are observed during the measurement. Former studies [22, 32] showed the effectiveness of models, serving this purpose by using a

Markov analysis as well. Another possible combination would be with eye tracking. The findings from the research on gaze duration in relation to social desirability [33] could eventually give an indication of the gaze duration between the dyads.

4.2 Limitations

The first limitation is the small sample size. Even though the sample is larger than in the preliminary analysis [26], it is not sufficient to provide meaningful evidence from this observational study. Based on the small sample size, three further limitations can be identified. Firstly, the number of dyads within the four constellations is low and especially the two constellations of love couples and strangers are strongly underrepresented, making the results of their analysis only partially meaningful. Secondly, gender-specific differences (i.e., social characteristics and interaction [31, 34]) may have influenced the results, as the proportion of female participants was significantly higher. And thirdly, the age range is only 19 to 39 years, which might have included social cohort effects (i.e., social behavior due to different environmental conditions [35, 36]) that would not have been found in younger or older generations.

There are also four limitations in terms of methodology and technical implementation. Firstly, there were times when the stylus was not recognized by the tablet. This resulted in gaps in the time series, which led to exclusion from the analysis. A solution could be an acoustic signal that sounds when the stylus is removed from the screen. Secondly, a mental state was only determined by the position of the stylus. Since the thought was first transferred to the tablet, this can lead to delays, which can be larger or smaller depending on how quickly the stylus was moved to the quadrant that corresponds to this thought. To solve this problem, the direction of movement may be taken into account. Thirdly, the screen was visually divided and the two screen center lines had each to be assigned to one of two quadrants, so that the quadrants are not exactly the same size. But as it only affects a few pixels, this limitation can be neglected. And fourthly, the chains of mental states were formed with intervals of 100 to 10,000 ms with a stepwise increase of 100 ms. The optimal interval length may not have been found. Unfortunately, despite a wide range of literature on Markov chains [20–25], there is no literature on this topic at this time, which could be due to the lack of global acceptance of this method in the field of medical research.

5 Conclusion

This observational study investigated interpersonal attachment in dyads by tracking stylus movements with a digital application. These movements, which were performed based on the participants' thoughts, were represented as DTMCs, consisting of four potential mental states. The analysis showed that the app together with this Markov chain approach is able to detect attachment changes in the course of time. Nonetheless, further studies should focus on optimizing the technical aspects of this app or should analyze the applicability of this approach in other settings, e.g., together with the observation of interpersonal interactions or gaze duration identified by an eye-tracking measurement.

Acknowledgments. We would like to express our special thanks to Theresa Frische and Fidan Brand, who carefully supported us in recruiting participants and conducting the study.

Disclosure of Interests. The authors have no competing interests to declare that are relevant to the content of this article.

References

1. Wolf, J.B., Ferguson-Smith, A.C., Lorenz, A.: Mendel's laws of heredity on his 200th birthday: what have we learned by considering exceptions? Heredity **129**(1), 1–3 (2022)
2. Edwards, A.W.F.: G.H. Hardy (1908) and Hardy–Weinberg Equilibrium. Genetics **179**(3), 1143–1150 (2008)
3. Giambiagi Ferrari, C., Pinasco, J.P., Saintier, N.: Coupling epidemiological models with social dynamics. Bull. Math. Biol. **83**(7), 74 (2021)
4. Dong, W., Lepri, B., Pianesi, F., Pentland, A.: Modeling functional roles dynamics in small group interactions. IEEE Trans. Multimedia **15**(1), 83–95 (2012)
5. de la Cruz, J.H., Rey, J.M.: A computational stochastic dynamic model to assess the risk of breakup in a romantic relationship. Math. Methods Appl. Sci., 1–18 (2023)
6. Horvath, A.O., Luborsky, L.: The role of the therapeutic alliance in psychotherapy. J. Consult. Clin. Psychol. **61**(4), 561–573 (1993)
7. Cumming, M.M., Bettini, E., Pham, A.V., Park, J.: School-, classroom-, and dyadic-level experiences: a literature review of their relationship with students' executive functioning development. Rev. Educ. Res. **90**(1), 47–94 (2020)
8. Jensen, A.C., Killoren, S.E., Campione-Barr, N., Padilla, J., Chen, B.B.: Sibling relationships in adolescence and young adulthood in multiple contexts: a critical review. J. Soc. Pers. Relat. **40**(2), 384–419 (2023)
9. Bornstein, M.H., Putnick, D.L.: Dyadic development in the family: stability in mother-child relationship quality from infancy to adolescence. In: Parenting: Selected Writings of Marc H. Bornstein, pp. 519–543. Routledge (2022)
10. Main, M., Hesse, E., Goldwyn, R.: Studying differences in language usage in recounting attachment history: an introduction to the AAI. In: Clinical Applications of the Adult Attachment Interview, pp. 31–68. The Guilford Press (2008)
11. Target, M., Fonagy, P., Shmueli-Goetz, Y.: Attachment representations in school-age children: the development of the child attachment interview (CAI). J. Child Psychother. **29**(2), 171–186 (2003)
12. Hesse, E.: The adult attachment interview: Historical and current perspectives. In: Handbook of Attachment: Theory, Research, and Clinical Applications, pp. 395–433. The Guilford Press (1999)
13. Privizzini, A.: The child attachment interview: a narrative review. Front. Psychol. **8**, 384 (2017)
14. van Ijzendoorn, M.H., Bakermans-Kranenburg, M.J.: The distribution of adult attachment representations in clinical groups: a meta-analytic search for patterns of attachment in 105 AAI studies. In: Clinical Applications of the Adult Attachment Interview, pp. 69–96. The Guilford Press (2008)
15. George, C., West, M.: The adult attachment projective: measuring individual differences in attachment security using projective methodology. In: Comprehensive Handbook of Psychological Assessment, vol. 2, pp. 431–447. John Wiley & Sons (2004)
16. Kammermeier, M., Duran Perez, L., König, L., Paulus, M.: Attachment security and attention to facial emotional expressions in preschoolers: an eye-tracking study. Br. J. Dev. Psychol. **38**(2), 167–185 (2020)
17. Uccula, A., Mercante, B., Barone, L., Enrico, P.: Adult avoidant attachment, attention bias, and emotional regulation patterns: an eye-tracking study. Behav. Sci. **13**(1), 11 (2022)

18. Altmann, U., et al.: Movement and emotional facial expressions during the adult attachment interview: interaction effects of attachment and anxiety disorder. Psychopathology **54**(1), 47–58 (2021)
19. Carbonaro, B., Serra, N.: Towards mathematical models in psychology: a stochastic description of human feelings. Math. Models Methods Appl. Sci. **12**(10), 1453–1490 (2002)
20. Fromion, V., Robert, P., Zaherddine, J.: Stochastic models of regulation of transcription in biological cells. J. Math. Biol. **87**(5), 65 (2023)
21. Ullah, M., Wolkenhauer, O.: Stochastic approaches in systems biology. Wiley Interdisc. Rev. Syst. Biol. Med. **2**(4), 385–397 (2010)
22. Benjamin, L.S.: Use of structural analysis of social behavior (SASB) and Markov chains to study dyadic interactions. J. Abnorm. Psychol. **88**(3), 303–319 (1979)
23. Koulomzin, M., Beebe, B., Anderson, S., Jaffe, J., Feldstein, S., Crown, C.: Infant gaze, head, face and self-touch at 4 months differentiate secure vs. avoidant attachment at 1 year: a microanalytic approach. Attachment Hum. Dev. **4**(1), 3–24 (2002)
24. Abney, D.H., Lewis, G.F., Bertenthal, B.I.: A method for measuring dynamic respiratory sinus arrhythmia (RSA) in infants and mothers. Infant Behav. Dev. **63**, 101569 (2021)
25. Brilot, B.O., Asher, L., Feenders, G., Bateson, M.: Quantification of abnormal repetitive behaviour in captive European starlings (Sturnus vulgaris). Behav. Proc. **82**(3), 256–264 (2009)
26. Unger, S., Ostermann, T.: Observational study of a digital application to detect attachment in dyads using markov chains. In: Proceedings of the 17th International Joint Conference on Biomedical Engineering Systems and Technologies - HEALTHINF, pp. 185–193. SciTePress (2024)
27. Asmussen, S.: Markov chains. In: Applied Probability and Queues, pp. 3–8. Springer, New York (2003).
28. Unger, S., Theis, C., Ostermann, T.: Examination of interpersonal attachment with the help of a digital tablet application: a proof of concept study. In: Proceedings of the 13th International Joint Conference on Biomedical Engineering Systems and Technologies (BIOSTEC 2020) - HEALTHINF, pp. 310–315. SciTePress (2020)
29. Spedicato, G.A., Kang, T.S., Yalamanchi, S.B., Yadav, D., Cordón, I.: The Markov Chain Package: A Package for Easily Handling Discrete Markov Chains in R (2014)
30. Holden, R.R.: Social desirability. In: The Corsini Encyclopedia of Psychology, pp. 1–2. Wiley (2010)
31. Paunonen, S.V.: Sex differences in judgments of social desirability. J. Pers. **84**(4), 423–432 (2016)
32. Bollenrücher, M., Darwiche, J., Antonietti, J.P.: Dyadic pattern analysis using longitudinal actor-partner interdependence model with markov chains for unique case analysis. Quant. Methods Psychol. **19**(3), 230–243 (2023)
33. Kaminska, O., Foulsham, T.: Eye-tracking social desirability bias. Bull. Sociol. Methodol./Bull. Méthodol. Sociol. **130**(1), 73–89 (2016)
34. Eisenberg, N., Martin, C.L., Fabes, R.A.: Gender development and gender effects. In: Handbook of Educational Psychology, pp. 358–396. Macmillan Library Reference USA (1996)
35. Lindström, J., Kokko, H.: Cohort effects and population dynamics. Ecol. Lett. **5**(3), 338–344 (2002)
36. Van Ingen, E.: Social participation revisited: disentangling and explaining period, life-cycle and cohort effects. Acta Sociol. **51**(2), 103–121 (2008)

Elevating Heart Failure Care: Innovations in Remote Patient Monitoring Through the RETENTION Platform

Ourania Manta[1]([✉]) [iD], Nikolaos Vasileiou[1] [iD], Olympia Giannakopoulou[1] [iD],
Konstantinos Bromis[1], Ioannis Kouris[1], Maria Haritou[1] [iD], Lefteris Koumakis[2],
George Spanoudakis[2], Irina E. Nicolae[3] [iD], C. Septimiu Nechifor[3] [iD],
Miltiadis Kokkonidis[4], Michalis Vakalelis[4], Yorgos Goletsis[5], Maria Roumpi[5],
Dimitrios I. Fotiadis[5], Heraklis Galanis[6], Panagiotis Dimitrakopoulos[6],
George K. Matsopoulos[1] [iD], and Dimitrios D. Koutsouris[1] [iD]

[1] Biomedical Engineering Laboratory, Institute of Communication and Computer Systems,
National Technical University of Athens, 15773 Athens, Greece
rmanta@biomed.ntua.gr
[2] Sphynx Technology Solutions AG, 6300 Zug, Switzerland
[3] Data Analytics and Artificial Intelligence, Configuration Technologies, Siemens Technology,
500097 Brașov, Romania
[4] AEGIS IT Research GmbH, 38106 Braunschweig, Germany
[5] Biomedical Research Institute, FORTH, University of Ioannina, Ioannina, Greece
[6] Datamed SA, 15124 Athens, Greece

Abstract. This paper reveals the transformative potential of the RETENTION Project in revolutionising remote patient monitoring for individuals with heart failure (HF). Examining the detailed architectural design of the RETENTION platform, we uncover a complex ecosystem designed to redefine HF management. The platform includes the Global Insights Cloud (GIC), Clinical Site Backend (CSB), and Patient Edge (PE) components, integrating advanced technologies and data analytics methods. From continuous data collection to personalised interventions based on evidence-based insights, the RETENTION platform stands out as an innovation in HF care. With a strong commitment to ethical standards and data privacy, along with a user-centric design, the platform aims to empower both clinicians and patients. This abstract provides a glimpse into the significant impact of the RETENTION Project, set to reshape HF management and lead to a new era of patient-focused healthcare.

Keywords: Clinical site backend · Data analysis · Global insights cloud · Heart failure · Integration · Machine learning · Patient edge · Personalised Interventions · Retention platform · Testing

1 Introduction

Chronic ailments and enduring medical conditions necessitating continuous attention often impose limitations on daily activities [1]. Among these, heart failure (HF) emerges as a prevalent chronic malady and a formidable global health challenge [2]. HF manifests

M. P. Guarino et al. (Eds.): BIOSTEC 2024, CCIS 2546, pp. 417–430, 2026.
https://doi.org/10.1007/978-3-031-96899-0_23

through symptomatic indications and clinical signs stemming from cardiac irregularities, culminating in diminished cardiac output and heightened intracardiac pressures. Despite strides in preventive measures, diagnostic methodologies, and therapeutic interventions, HF persists as a leading cause of debilitation and premature mortality across the globe [3]. Its impact spans a significant segment of the populace, with estimates projecting approximately 15 million Europeans and 5.8 million Americans grappling with HF [4]. Of particular note is the elevated prevalence of HF among the elderly demographic, exceeding 10% among individuals aged 70 years and older [5]. Notably, HF presents a markedly lower five-year survival rate when juxtaposed with conditions such as myocardial infarction and select cancers [5]. Concurrently, the presence of comorbidities, encompassing an array of ailments and psychological disorders, frequently accompanies HF, thereby influencing its clinical management and therapeutic approaches [5–7]. Moreover, the economic ramifications of HF loom large, with considerable healthcare expenditures allocated towards hospitalisations and the burgeoning elderly populace [8].

Initiatives have been undertaken to prognosticate and forestall episodes of HF decompensation, refine medical interventions, and introduce novel devices aimed at curbing hospitalizations [8]. Remote monitoring, exemplified by e-health applications, has emerged as a promising avenue in the post-treatment oversight of HF patients [9–11]. Technological advancements have facilitated the capture of patient data, encompassing vital signs, routine electrocardiograms (ECGs), and sophisticated monitoring parameters, thereby bolstering disease management efforts [12]. Moreover, therapies, devices, and disease management regimens grounded in evidence-based practices have showcased enhanced outcomes for individuals grappling with HF [4].

Nevertheless, notwithstanding these strides, certain patients transition to an advanced stage of HF, necessitating mechanical assist devices or cardiac transplants [6, 7]. Remote monitoring of device metrics and patient data stands poised to detect complications and is imperative for hospital assessment [6]. Recipients of heart transplants frequently necessitate multiple outpatient visits for surveillance and rejection appraisal.

Given these obstacles, the RETENTION project endeavours to institute daily remote monitoring for patients with HF. The objective is to amass diverse clinical, behavioural, and real-world data. The initiative will scrutinise this data using innovative data analytics and artificial intelligence (AI) to refine clinical management, curtail hospitalisations, and enhance patient outcomes. Additionally, it will appraise the viability of remote monitoring, data analysis models, and clinical interventions. This evaluation will encompass various health policy viewpoints, addressing patient safety, quality of care, and the escalating healthcare demand stemming from the ageing populace with intricate conditions [6, 7].

2   Innovations in Remote Patient Monitoring for Heart Failure

RETENTION aims to improve remote patient monitoring for HF by refining existing technology on various fronts. Its goal is to enhance the quality of life, clinical care, and remote monitoring of HF patients. In essence, RETENTION's significant contributions can be summarised as follows:

2.1   Leveraging Artificial Intelligence

Crafting a personalised decision support system capable of enhancing the effective-ness and reliability of diagnosis, prognosis, and therapy for HF patients represents a formidable challenge [13]. AI techniques, including Bayesian networks, machine learn-ing (ML) methods, and supervised learning algorithms such as artificial neural networks (ANN), decision trees (DT), genetic algorithms (GA), and support vector machines (SVM), have been leveraged to formulate risk assessments and mortality predictions using pertinent medical data sources [14]. The application of ML algorithms to individ-ual patient data enables more precise predictions and the elimination of extraneous and inconsequential features. Moreover, the ethical considerations surrounding AI utilization in healthcare, as elucidated in the novel EU framework for trustworthy AI, underscore the imperative of upholding lawful, ethical, and robust decision-making processes [15]. RETENTION is poised to address these imperatives by adhering to GDPR guidelines, ensuring meticulous privacy management, furnishing insights into data analytics, and perpetually assessing security standards and the reliability of machine learning models.

We plan to employ a combination of several advanced ML algorithms, like deep neural networks (DNN), random forests (RF), and the like, for developing precise risk assessments and mortality predictions in HF patients. Also, applying recent evolutionary algorithms like modified particle swarm optimization (MPSO) [16] could speed up the optimal selection of the model's features and/or parameters.

Furthermore, following the guidelines laid out in the EU regulations for AI (https://artificialintelligenceact.eu/), RETENTION will incorporate Explainable AI (XAI) to explain the reasoning behind AI, offering a transparent and trustworthy system. The AI models and transparency are developed with Advanced Notebook (Jupyter Notebooks and MLFlow) [17] in order to better secure, monitor, reproduce, and deploy the ML models. This integration not only streamlines model development and monitoring but also ensures robust privacy management and data security.

2.2   Enhancing Interpretability of Machine Learning Models

Machine learning techniques, encompassing deep learning, have been deployed to scru-tinise extensive datasets in HF research [18]. The interpretability and explainability of ML models have assumed pivotal roles in validating and comprehending the deci-sions formulated by these models [19]. Methods for elucidating and comprehending the acquired models have been devised to illuminate intricate machine learning models [20]. RETENTION will explore model-agnostic approaches for elucidating ML models to refine the interpretability and explainability of the system.

To this end, we plan to utilise mode-agnostic methods like Local Interpretable Model-agnostic Explanations (LIME) and Shapley Additive exPlanations (SHAP). These meth-ods are selected for their versatility and ability to provide insights into complex models like DNN used in HF research. Adding evolutionary algorithms can help enhance the symbolic representation (like decision trees) that approximates the decisions of DNNs, providing an intuitive and transparent view of the model's rationale.

By employing such techniques, RETENTION will facilitate a deeper understanding of the models' decisions, ensuring that clinicians can trust and effectively interpret the AI recommendations.

2.3   Integration of Internet of Things Devices

Smart homes and Internet of Things (IoT) devices stand poised to revolutionise conventional healthcare systems, ushering in a new era of efficiency and personalisation [21]. These technological advancements facilitate the collection of health data, enable real-time self-monitoring, and empower healthcare providers to conduct remote interventions. Wearable sensors, implantable devices, and intelligent information platforms have the capacity to continuously monitor physiological metrics in heart failure patients, enhancing their comfort and amalgamating data from diverse origins [22–24]. RETENTION will harness a broad spectrum of inputs from smart medical apparatuses utilised daily by patients at home, wearable technologies, electronic questionnaires for patient-reported outcome measures, and real-time sensor readings. Coupled with cutting-edge ML models offering tailored prognostications, RETENTION aspires to establish an innovative yet pragmatic IT-enhanced patient monitoring framework. This framework endeavours to assist healthcare practitioners in enhancing patient outcomes, curbing emergency room visits, and mitigating hospitalisations, thereby fostering effective and efficient management of HF patients.

2.4   Harnessing Big Data Analytics

Big data analytics (BDA) platforms have undergone significant evolution to tackle the intricate correlations present in diverse datasets, encompassing heterogeneous, open, public, and private data, in a manner that is both cost-effective and user-friendly [25]. In line with this evolution, RETENTION will embrace a model-driven approach to the design and implementation of big data infrastructures, with a focus on achieving modularity, reusability, and automation. Ensuring the interpretability and explainability of data analytics outcomes will be pivotal for validating results and facilitating evidence-based interventions [26, 27].

2.5   Tailored User Interfaces

Human-Computer Interaction (HCI) assumes a crucial role in the implementation of digital technologies within the healthcare sector [28]. In crafting user interfaces, it is imperative to account for user needs and usability factors, including health literacy, age-related conditions, and the presentation of intricate health data [29, 30]. To this end, RETENTION will embrace a user-centric methodology, engaging users in an iterative design process and creating adaptive visualisations and interfaces tailored to the needs of healthcare practitioners and patients.

2.6   Enhancing Security and Privacy

IoT applications within the healthcare realm encounter significant security and privacy hurdles, encompassing aspects like mutual authentication, encryption, and data integrity [31]. To address these challenges, various cryptographic techniques, including privacy-preserving encryption and differential privacy, have been proposed to uphold data confidentiality. Effective identity and authorisation management, in conjunction with robust access control policies, are indispensable for safeguarding user privacy [32, 33]. In this context, RETENTION will amalgamate innovative and standardised technologies to furnish lightweight and user-friendly mechanisms for authentication, authorisation, privacy preservation, and secure communications. Moreover, the implementation will entail continuous monitoring and evaluation tools to ensure ongoing security and privacy assurance [33].

3 Comprehensive Architecture of the RETENTION System

3.1 Retention Project Overview

The architectural blueprint of the RETENTION project adopts a holistic strategy directed towards bolstering remote patient monitoring for heart failure. In essence, the core aim of the RETENTION endeavour is to forge ahead in creating and deploying an innovative platform that fosters advanced clinical monitoring and interventions to elevate the management of patients afflicted with chronic HF [34]. This endeavour is driven by the dual objective of diminishing mortality and hospitalization rates while concurrently enhancing the overall quality of life, safety, and well-being of these patients.

The RETENTION platform is poised to significantly augment clinical decision-making capabilities and furnish evidence-based personalised interventions for HF patients through the following methodologies:

- Continuously monitoring and consolidating a broad spectrum of medical, clinical, physiological, behavioural, psychosocial, and real-world data relevant to patients with HF.
- Employing state-of-the-art model-driven big data analytics, statistical analysis, artificial intelligence, and machine learning methodologies to scrutinise this data.
- Discerning patterns in the advancement of HF and assessing the quality of life of patients through a meticulous scrutiny of the amassed data.
- Rigorously cross-referencing and validating these discoveries against prevailing clinical literature.
- Cultivating transparent, understandable, and verifiable decision-making capabilities that harness the evidence produced by the underlying data analysis, thereby reinforcing clinical investigations focused on HF and other cardiovascular ailments.

The efficacy of the RETENTION approach and its corresponding platform will undergo rigorous validation via a clinical study encompassing 450 HF patients enlisted from six distinct hospitals across four EU nations. This comprehensive study accounts for the varying approaches to patient management observed within these healthcare facilities.

3.2 Conceptual Framework and Architectural Design of the RETENTION System

The goal of the system architecture was to create a clear and comprehensive solution for the RETENTION platform, based on interconnected principles, concepts, and functions.

This section provides a detailed explanation of the RETENTION system's architecture, describing its conceptual framework and main components. The RETENTION platform emphasises privacy, avoiding the unnecessary aggregation of patients' personal data on external cloud infrastructures beyond the control of patients or hospitals. Instead, it enables machine learning model training using data from various hospital patients. This is achieved through a carefully designed architecture that prioritises privacy while allowing direct access to clinically relevant patient data from clinical sites. RETENTION also enhances patient monitoring beyond hospital settings. The RETENTION Platform aims to achieve high standards of human-machine interaction, making it user-friendly for managing workflows, handling outputs from advanced models, validating these outputs with visualised knowledge, and delivering interventions.

The ensuing diagram offers a comprehensive portrayal of the system's high-level components, predominantly interconnected via REST API interfaces to streamline integration. Notably, the architecture is structured upon a tri-layer model (derived from a structured IoT architecture tailored for the RETENTION initiative):

- the Global Insights Cloud (GIC);
- the Clinical Site Backend (CSB); and
- the Patient Edge (PE)

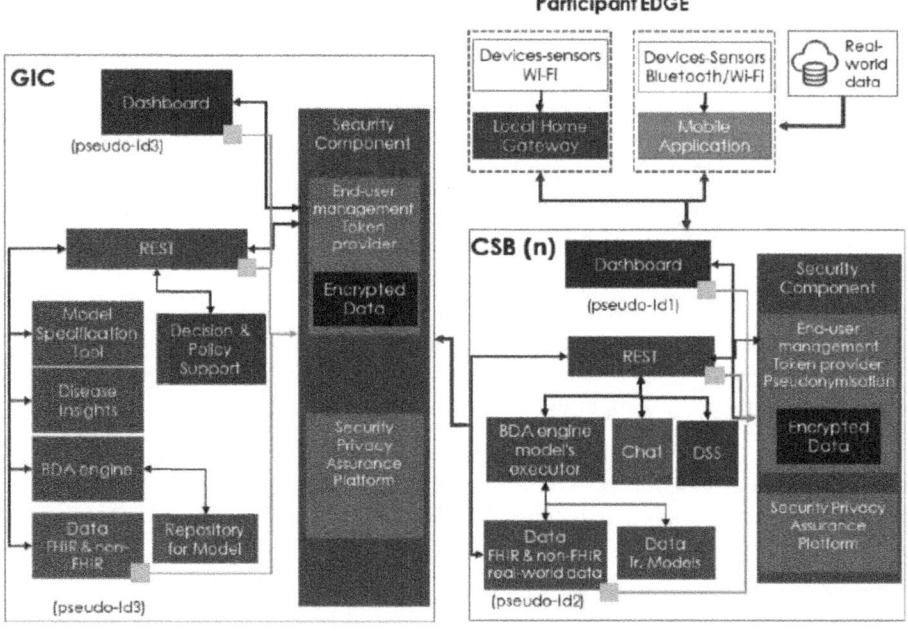

Fig. 1. RETENTION Architecture: (Global Insights Cloud (GIC), Clinical Site Backend (CSB), and Patient Edge (PE)) [34].

These layers synergise to facilitate the processes of data collection, analysis, and personalised interventions. Illustrated in Fig. 1, the diagram furnishes an extensive overview of the RETENTION architecture, elucidating the diverse entities operating within each respective layer.

The Global Insights Cloud (GIC) functions as the central hub for big data analytics within the RETENTION platform. Within the GIC layer, various sub-components operate synergistically, including the GIC Dashboard, Federated RW Data Repository and Repository for Models, BDA Engine, Model Specification Tool, Disease Insights, Decision and Policy Support, Security Component, and GIC Rest API. This infrastructure systematically gathers anonymised patient data from all sources, facilitating comprehensive global data analytics and insight generation. By hosting the analytics engine and offering specialised tools, the GIC empowers data scientists, clinical experts, and healthcare policymakers to make well-informed decisions regarding the management of HF diseases. Furthermore, the GIC supports incremental data analysis and model refinement, ensuring the implementation of evidence-based interventions.

The Clinical Site Backend (CSB) functions as the operational backbone at each clinical site, responsible for patient data management and local analytics. Comprising various sub-components such as the CSB Dashboard, FHIR (Fast Healthcare Interoperability Resources) and Non-FHIR Repository, BDA Engine Models Executor, Decision Support System (DSS), Security Component, and CSB Rest API, it enables clinicians to monitor patients, gather medical and usage data, and make informed decisions. The CSB facilitates the execution of personalised interventions derived from trained machine learning models while ensuring the pseudonymisation of patient data, thus safeguarding privacy while providing clinicians with access to relevant information.

The Patient Edge (PE) encompasses a mobile application and a home gateway, serving as the interface for continuous patient monitoring and real-world data collection. The mobile application allows patients to report symptoms, record medication adherence, and report health metrics in a user-friendly, semi-automated manner. It aggregates data from various smart medical devices used daily by the patient, such as smartwatches, blood pressure metres, oximetres, and weight scales, transmitting it to the CSB for monitoring. The home gateway complements this by aggregating and transmitting data from indoor sensors and external environmental conditions, contributing to comprehensive patient monitoring and management.

To store medical data securely, the RETENTION project leverages a FHIR database, integrating healthcare terminologies and coding systems such as SNOMED CT, LOINC, and ICD-10 into the FHIR standard. This integration ensures the use of standardised codes and terminologies for representing clinical concepts, laboratory observations, and disease classifications. By enhancing interoperability, this approach facilitates the consistent and meaningful exchange of healthcare information across different systems and applications adhering to the FHIR standard.

Security and privacy are paramount considerations within the RETENTION architecture. The security component, a cornerstone of the project, is entrusted with authentication, authorisation, and data protection during both transit and storage phases (see Fig. 1). Compliance with GDPR regulations is rigorously upheld to ensure the secure management of personal data. This component is integral to ensuring that personal data is handled, distributed, and presented securely to authorised users, safeguarding data privacy throughout the process.

Within both the GIC and CSB instances, the security component employs various mechanisms to achieve its objectives. These include API management, role-based access control (RBAC), data encryption, API logs, device management, and RETENTION pseudonymisation. API management ensures the security and protection of exposed APIs, while RBAC restricts access to authorised roles and registered end-users. Data encryption serves to safeguard personal and identifiable information, while API logs monitor activity for potential security threats. Device management enables efficient technical support without compromising sensitive identification.

An essential aspect of the Security Component's strategy is pseudonymisation, which minimises the risk of identifying data subjects. Within the GIC, data is anonymised, further enhancing privacy protection measures and ensuring compliance with data protection regulations.

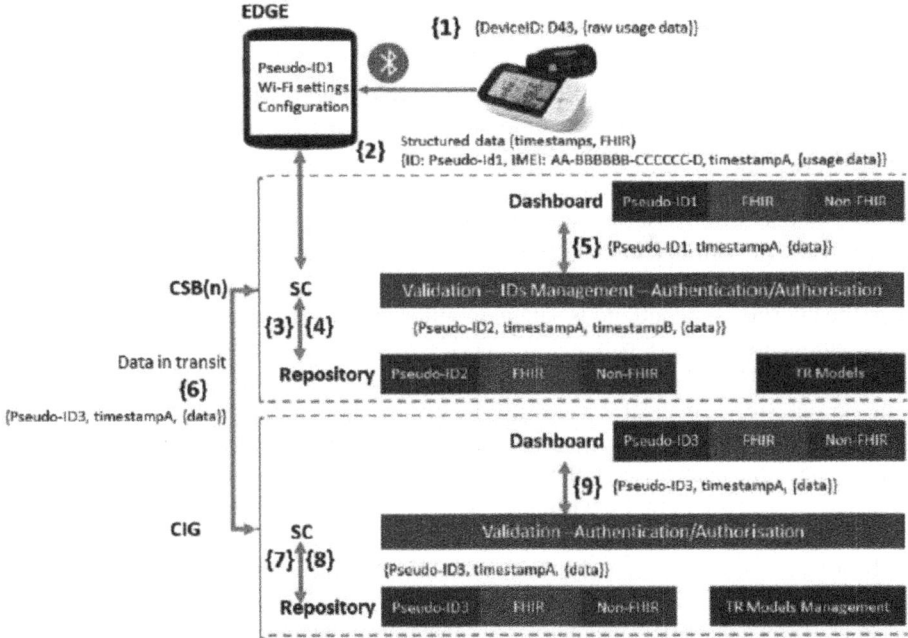

Fig. 2. Transmission of data between Global Insights Cloud (GIC), Clinical Site Backend (CSB), and Patient Edge (PE) [34].

In essence, the architecture of the RETENTION system is poised to empower data-driven decision-making, personalised interventions, and the secure management of data. Catering to various user roles such as system administrators, clinicians, patients, data scientists, and healthcare policymakers, it ensures inclusivity and functionality across diverse stakeholders. Through the synergistic integration of the GIC, CSB, and PE, the architecture is primed to facilitate comprehensive monitoring and management of patients grappling with heart failure. This holistic approach promises to enhance clinical outcomes, ensuring that patients receive tailored interventions and optimal care. Harnessing the collective strengths of its constituent components, the RETENTION system architecture not only empowers healthcare professionals to make informed decisions but also fosters active engagement from patients. By leveraging state-of-the-art technology and adhering to stringent security standards, it sets the stage for a paradigm shift in the management of heart failure, paving the way for improved patient outcomes and enhanced quality of care.

3.3   Rigorous Integration and Testing of the RETENTION System

The integration and testing phases of the RETENTION system played pivotal roles in its development and ultimate completion. These phases encompassed the installation of key components, rigorous software quality assurance measures, and comprehensive evaluations of system functionality and performance.

Software quality assurance efforts entailed the creation of test scenarios, meticulous data entry, and rigorous control procedures to ensure the integrity and robustness of the software product. Integration followed a meticulously staged approach, commencing with the installation and tailoring of software components. Docker containers emerged as instrumental tools for deploying system components, including the dashboard, security module, decision support system (DSS), and data repositories, while seamlessly integrating modules like the GIC, CSB, and PE.

Testing unfolded across multiple stages, spanning unit tests, application tests, integration tests, system tests, and user acceptance tests. Unit testing scrutinised individual subsystems, while application testing delved into the intricacies of business logic. Integration testing focused on verifying seamless communication and system reliability, while system testing ensured alignment with operational requirements. User acceptance tests provided the final validation of system functionality and performance.

The deployment phase will unfold in two distinct stages. Initially, data collection will take precedence, enabling the training of AI models. Subsequently, the system will transition into full operational mode, providing robust support to clinical teams and their respective patients.

Deployment will not only ensure the availability, security, and operational efficacy of the RETENTION system but also ensure compliance with GDPR regulations, safeguarding sensitive data. The meticulous integration and testing processes have fortified the system's functionality, reliability, and preparedness for real-world implementation, marking a significant milestone in the advancement of healthcare technology.

4   Discussion

The RETENTION platform marks a substantial leap forward in the realm of HF management through its innovative approach to remote patient monitoring. Below, the discussion delves into various pivotal points and implications stemming from the architectural design and conceptual framework of the RETENTION project [34].

The primary aim of the RETENTION initiative is to significantly enhance HF management by curbing mortality and hospitalisation rates while simultaneously elevating the overall quality of life for HF patients. Through the seamless integration of continuous data collection, cutting-edge data analytics, and machine learning, the platform endeavours to offer personalised interventions grounded in robust evidence. This paradigm shift holds the promise of revolutionising HF management and ushering in substantial improvements in patient outcomes. By capitalising on a meticulously structured IoT architecture, the RETENTION platform sets a groundbreaking standard for patient monitoring in the realm of chronic diseases [34].

The integration of big data analytics and artificial intelligence stands as a linchpin in HF management. ML models, encompassing Bayesian networks, ANNs, and SVMs, offer substantial potential for enhancing risk assessments and mortality predictions [35, 36]. However, it is imperative for these models to adhere to stringent ethical standards and data protection regulations, as underscored by GDPR. The unwavering commitment of the RETENTION project to uphold lawful, ethical, and robust decision-making processes is indispensable for establishing the platform's credibility and ensuring compliance.

The imperatives of interpretability and explainability in machine learning models cannot be overstated. The RETENTION project's exploration of model-agnostic methods for interpreting ML models signifies a significant stride towards fostering transparency in decision-making processes. This approach resonates with the broader trajectory in healthcare AI, where the ability to comprehend and validate model decisions holds paramount importance.

The integration of IoT devices into healthcare holds tremendous promise for revolutionising traditional healthcare systems into more streamlined and patient-centric environments. These cutting-edge technologies offer real-time monitoring capabilities and facilitate personalised interventions, thereby redefining the landscape of healthcare delivery [37]. RETENTION's adept utilisation of real-time sensor measurements and tailored treatment strategies underscores the transformative potential of IoT applications in enhancing HF management, with potential extensions to other chronic diseases.

Security and privacy emerge as non-negotiable priorities in healthcare systems, particularly when IoT applications are in play [38]. The RETENTION project's robust approach to security, encompassing privacy-preserving encryption and stringent access control policies, provides a comprehensive framework for addressing these challenges. Ensuring the sanctity of user privacy while facilitating secure data exchanges serves as a cornerstone for the success of any healthcare platform.

Additionally, it is imperative to acknowledge the ethical and societal implications of the RETENTION project. As healthcare systems increasingly rely on data-driven technologies, questions surrounding data ownership, consent, and equity come to the forefront [39]. The RETENTION project addresses these concerns by prioritising patient privacy, transparency, and equity in access to healthcare services. By adhering to strict data protection regulations and fostering open dialogue with stakeholders, the project endeavours to uphold the highest ethical standards while leveraging technology for the betterment of patient care [40].

The user-centric design ethos embraced by the RETENTION project underscores the significance of factoring in user needs and usability considerations. This approach assumes heightened relevance in healthcare settings, where diverse user groups, including patients, clinicians, and data scientists, engage with the system. The emphasis on adaptive visualisations and user interfaces aligns seamlessly with the overarching trend of democratising healthcare technologies and rendering them accessible to a broader spectrum of users.

The commitment of the RETENTION project to validation via a clinical study involving a sizable cohort of HF patients across multiple EU countries represents a pivotal milestone. This rigorous evaluation ensures that the platform's efficacy and benefits are rigorously assessed in real-world scenarios, encompassing diverse patient demographics and clinical contexts. Moreover, the forthcoming clinical study is not merely a validation exercise but a pivotal opportunity to assess the real-world impact of the RETENTION platform. By engaging a diverse cohort of HF patients across multiple EU countries, the study aims to capture nuanced variations in patient demographics, treatment modalities, and healthcare settings. This comprehensive approach ensures that the platform's efficacy and benefits are rigorously evaluated in diverse clinical contexts, thus enhancing its generalizability and potential for broader applications in healthcare data management and personalised interventions.

In summation, the RETENTION platform stands as a beacon of progress in HF management, leveraging state-of-the-art technologies and a holistic approach. By tackling challenges pertaining to data analytics, explainability, IoT, security, and user-centric design, the project lays the groundwork for the emergence of more efficacious, personalised, and secure healthcare solutions. The forthcoming clinical study holds the promise of furnishing invaluable insights into the platform's real-world impact, propelling its potential for broader applications in healthcare data management and personalised interventions.

5 Conclusions

Overall, this paper offers a thorough exploration of the RETENTION system, delving into its technical intricacies and constituent modules. Specifically, the architecture of the RETENTION Platform is elucidated, comprising the pivotal GIC, CSB, and PE components. The GIC serves as the nerve centre for data analysis and ML model training, facilitating evidence-based personalised interventions. Meanwhile, the CSB facilitates daily patient monitoring, data collection, and the implementation of ML-driven interventions. Complementing these, the PE ensures continuous patient surveillance and feedback acquisition. The infrastructure underpinning the RETENTION system is anchored in virtual machines (VMs) and Docker containers, bolstered by a cloud-based deployment. The rigorous integration and testing procedures employed were paramount in ensuring the system's reliability and efficacy. This paper lays a robust foundation for the continued evolution and implementation of the RETENTION system, poised to advance healthcare data management and personalised interventions.

Extending the discourse, the RETENTION Project epitomises a paradigm shift in healthcare, ushering in a new era of patient-centric remote monitoring for HF. The platform's architecture, encapsulating the GIC, CSB, and PE components, not only promises personalised interventions grounded in data-driven insights but also fosters a holistic approach to HF management. By harnessing the power of virtualization technologies and cloud infrastructure, the RETENTION system ensures scalability and accessibility, essential for widespread adoption and impact. Moreover, the rigorous integration and testing procedures undertaken underscore the project's commitment to reliability and effectiveness in real-world settings. As we look ahead, the RETENTION Project stands as a testament to the potential of technology to revolutionise healthcare, offering a beacon of hope for HF patients and clinicians alike.

Acknowledgments. The RETENTION project was financed by the European Union's Horizon 2020 Research and Innovation Programme, Grant Agreement Number 965343.

Disclosure of Interests. The authors have no competing interests to declare that are relevant to the content of this article.

References

1. Bernell, S., Howard, S.W.: Use your words carefully: what is a chronic disease? Front. Public Heal. **4** (2016). https://doi.org/10.3389/fpubh.2016.00159
2. Smith, S.C., et al.: Our time: a call to save preventable death from cardiovascular disease (heart disease and stroke). J. Am. Coll. Cardiol. **60**, 2343–2348 (2012). https://doi.org/10.1016/j.jacc.2012.08.962
3. The Global Cardiovascular Disease Pandemic, Current Status and Future Projections (2015)
4. Braunschweig, F., Cowie, M.R., Auricchio, A.: What are the costs of heart failure? Europace **13** (2011). https://doi.org/10.1093/europace/eur081
5. Ponikowski, P., et al.: 2016 ESC guidelines for the diagnosis and treatment of acute and chronic heart failure. Eur. Heart J. **37**, 2129–2200m (2016)
6. Calmette, L., Clauser, S.: Von willebrand disease. Rev. Med. Interne **39**, 918–924 (2018)
7. Reiss, N., et al.: Telemonitoring of left-ventricular assist device patients-current status and future challenges. J. Thorac. Dis. **10** (2018)
8. Ayyadurai, P., et al.: An update on the CardioMEMS pulmonary artery pressure sensor. Ther. Adv. Cardiovasc. Dis. **13** (2019)
9. Rosen, D., McCall, J.D., Primack, B.A.: Telehealth protocol to prevent readmission among high-risk patients with congestive heart failure. Am. J. Med. **130**, 1326–1330 (2017)
10. Black, J.T., et al.: A remote monitoring and telephone nurse coaching intervention to reduce readmissions among patients with heart failure: study protocol for the better effectiveness after transition - heart failure (BEAT-HF) randomized controlled trial. Trials **15** (2014). https://doi.org/10.1186/1745-6215-15-124
11. Koehler, F., et al.: Efficacy of telemedical interventional management in patients with heart failure (TIM-HF2): a randomised, controlled, parallel-group unmasked trial. Lancet **392**, 1047–1057 (2018). https://doi.org/10.1016/S0140-6736(18)31880-4
12. Bashi, N., Karunanithi, M., Fatehi, F., Ding, H., Walters, D.: Remote monitoring of patients with heart failure: an overview of systematic reviews. J. Med. Internet Res. **19** (2017)
13. Mielczarek, B.: Review of modelling approaches for healthcare simulation. Oper. Res. Decis. **26**, 55–72 (2016)
14. Weiss, E.S., et al.: Development of a quantitative donor risk index to predict short-term mortality in orthotopic heart transplantation. J. Hear. Lung Transplant. **31**, 266–273 (2012). https://doi.org/10.1016/j.healun.2011.10.004
15. Khodadadi, M., Shayanfar, H., Maghooli, K., Mazinan, A.H.: Fuzzy cognitive map based approach for determining the risk of ischemic stroke. IET Syst. Biol. **13**, 297–304 (2019). https://doi.org/10.1049/iet-syb.2018.5128

16. Tian, D., Shi, Z.: MPSO: modified particle swarm optimization and its applications. Swarm Evol. Comput. **41**, 49–68 (2018). https://doi.org/10.1016/J.SWEVO.2018.01.011
17. Danciu, G., Nicolae, I.E., Ilie, I., Septimiu Nechifor, C.: Advanced notebook: a tool for enhanced management of machine learning models and procedures in the healthcare domain. In: Proceedings of 2023 International Conference on Applied Mathematics & Computer Science ICAMCS 2023, pp. 36–41 (2023). https://doi.org/10.1109/ICAMCS59110.2023.00013
18. Sung, J.M., et al.: Development and verification of prediction models for preventing cardiovascular diseases. PLoS One (2019)
19. Quaglini, S., Sacchi, L., Lanzola, G., Viani, N.: Personalization and patient involvement in decision support systems: current trends. Yearb. Med. Inform. **10**, 106–118 (2015)
20. Bryan, M., Heagerty, P.J.: Multivariate analysis of longitudinal rates of change. PubMed Cent. **35** (2016)
21. Linkous, L., Zohrabi, N., Abdelwahed, S.: Health monitoring in smart homes utilizing Internet of Things. In: Proceedings of the Proceedings - 4th IEEE/ACM Conference on Connected Health: Applications, Systems and Engineering Technologies, CHASE 2019; Institute of Electrical and Electronics Engineers Inc., September 1 2019, pp. 29–34 (2019)
22. Akmandor, A.O., Jha, N.K.: Keep the stress away with SoDA: stress detection and alleviation system. IEEE Trans. Multi-Scale Comput. Syst. **3**, 269–282 (2017). https://doi.org/10.1109/TMSCS.2017.2703613
23. Crema, C., Depari, A., Flammini, A., Lavarini, M., Sisinni, E., Vezzoli, A.: A smartphone-enhanced pill-dispenser providing patient identification and in-take recognition. In: Proceedings of the 2015 IEEE International Symposium on Medical Measurements and Applications, MeMeA 2015 - Proceedings; Institute of Electrical and Electronics Engineers Inc., June 30 2015, pp. 484–489 (2015)
24. Tripoliti, E.E., et al.: A knowledge management system targeting the management of patients with heart failure. J. Biomed. Inform. **94** (2019). https://doi.org/10.1016/j.jbi.2019.103203
25. Assunção, M.D., Calheiros, R.N., Bianchi, S., Netto, M.A.S., Buyya, R.: Big data computing and clouds: trends and future directions. J. Parallel Distrib. Comput. **79–80**, 3–15 (2015). https://doi.org/10.1016/j.jpdc.2014.08.003
26. Sparks, E.R., Venkataraman, S., Kaftan, T., Franklin, M.J., Recht, B.: KeystoneML: Optimizing Pipelines for Large-Scale Advanced Analytics
27. Du, M., Liu, N., Hu, X.: Techniques for Interpretable Machine Learning (2018)
28. Blandford, A.: HCI for health and wellbeing: challenges and opportunities. Int. J. Hum. Comput. Stud. **131**, 41–51 (2019). https://doi.org/10.1016/j.ijhcs.2019.06.007
29. Patel, V., Kannampallil, T., Kaufman Editors, D.: Health Informatics Human Computer Interaction in Healthcare (2015)
30. Groenvold, M., et al.: Letter to the editor. Palliat. Med. **20**, 59–61 (2006). https://doi.org/10.1191/0269216306pm1133xx
31. Salah, K., Khan, M.: IoT security: review, blockchain solutions, and open challenges. Futur. Gener. Comput. Syst. (2017)
32. Hassija, V., Chamola, V., Saxena, V., Jain, D., Goyal, P., Sikdar, B.: A survey on IoT security: application areas, security threats, and solution architectures. IEEE Access **7**, 82721–82743 (2019)
33. Li, J., Zhang, Y., Chen, X., Xiang, Y.: Secure attribute-based data sharing for resource-limited users in cloud computing. Comput. Secur. **72**, 1–12 (2018). https://doi.org/10.1016/j.cose.2017.08.007
34. Manta, O., et al.: Architectural design for enhancing remote patient monitoring in heart failure: a case study of the RETENTION project. In: Proceedings of 17th International Joint Conference on Biomedical Engineering Systems and Technologies, pp. 708–715 (2024). https://doi.org/10.5220/0012458500003657

35. Tasnim, N., Tanvir, K., Bin, S., Sezan, K.: Machine learning for heart disease prediction a comparison analysis. J. Artif. Intell. Learn. Neural Netw. **3**, 28–35 (2023). https://doi.org/10.55529/JAIMLNN.35.28.35. ISSN 2799-1172

36. Moradi, R., Cofre-Martel, S., Lopez Droguett, E., Modarres, M., Groth, K.M.: Integration of deep learning and Bayesian networks for condition and operation risk monitoring of complex engineering systems. Reliab. Eng. Syst. Saf. **222**, 108433 (2022). https://doi.org/10.1016/J.RESS.2022.108433

37. Zhang, P., Kamel Boulos, M.N.: Generative AI in medicine and healthcare: promises, opportunities and challenges. Futur. Internet **15**, 286 (2023). https://doi.org/10.3390/FI15090286

38. Ibraheem, H.R., Zaki, N.D., Al-mashhadani, M.I.: Security and privacy in IoT-based healthcare systems: a review. Mesopotamian J. Comput. Sci. **2022**, 29–39 (2022). https://doi.org/10.58496/MJCSC/2022/005

39. Murdoch, B.: Privacy and artificial intelligence: challenges for protecting health information in a new era. BMC Med. Ethics **22** (2021). https://doi.org/10.1186/S12910-021-00687-3

40. Mohan, K., Kitsos, P., Williamson, S.M., Prybutok, V.: Balancing privacy and progress: a review of privacy challenges, systemic oversight, and patient perceptions in AI-driven healthcare. Appl. Sci. **14**, 675 (2024). https://doi.org/10.3390/APP14020675

Semantic Integration of Heterogeneous PGHD Sources in a Digital Health System

Rens Kievit[1]([⊠])(ID), Abdullahi Abubakar Kawu[2](ID), Harold Ekow Eshun[3](ID),
Samson Yohannes Amare[1,4](ID), Mirjam van Reisen[1](ID), Dympna O'Sullivan[2](ID),
and Lucy Hederman[5](ID)

[1] Leiden University Medical Centre (LUMC), Leiden University, Leiden, The Netherlands
r.kievit@lumc.nl
[2] School of Computer Science, Technological University Dublin, Dublin, Ireland
[3] Leiden Institute of Advanced Computer Science (LIACS), Leiden University,
Leiden, The Netherlands
[4] School of Public Health, Mekelle University, Mek'ele, Ethiopia
[5] School of Computer Science and Statistics, Trinity College Dublin, Dublin, Ireland

Abstract. Patient Generated Health Data (PGHD) can be communicated to a
health facility without the need for frequent hospital visits. This is very valuable
to patients with long-term health conditions that require regular monitoring of
vitals. The VODAN project, which deployed a digital health data system based
on the FAIR principles, commenced in 2020 and has increased the potential for
digital data curation and use in clinics in different countries in both Africa and
Asia, but currently no systems are in place for the integration of external data
from patients with long term health problems. In this paper, we combine two (2)
PGHD sources - a wearable device and a home digital monitor whose data is
communicated through an Interactive Voice Response (IVR) system - to increase
the connectivity of patients with long term health problems with the clinics using
the VODAN system, and propose a solution in the form of a data pipeline prototype based upon multiple PGHD sources. Additionally, we design a visualization
tool useful for the practitioner to interact with this data.

Keywords: PGHD · Wearable · Digital health system · IVR

1 Introduction

In most low resource settings like Africa, health information or data are mostly collected
in health settings (clinics or hospitals) and stored only in paper forms. In addition, there
is little opportunity to incorporate Patient Generated Health Data (PGHD) - health information that patient's collect themselves. By offering more information from different
settings about a patient health, data from PGHD sources can aid in predictive health
diagnosis [3]. The creation of VODAN [10] has improved the health data capabilities
of many African countries. VODAN is a novel healthcare framework that is entirely
based on the FAIR principles (Findable, Accessible (under well-defined conditions),
Interoperable, and Reusable) [13]. Within the VODAN project patient data is made

M. P. Guarino et al. (Eds.): BIOSTEC 2024, CCIS 2546, pp. 431–441, 2026.
https://doi.org/10.1007/978-3-031-96899-0_24

more useful for primary use (clinical) and secondary use (research and planning). As part of the secondary use, the platform enables the analysis of healthcare trends on large geographical scales while being able to maintain data ownership within the clinics. The former happens through the standardization of the data flow and creation of controlled vocabularies which allows interoperability between clinics in various countries, the latter is ensured by only storing data within the facilities. Insights are generated through knowledge graphs for which queries are run in a federated manner through a smart aggregating data visiting system [8]. The architecture of VODAN is currently based on decentralised mini-services of CEDAR (The Center for Expanded Data Annotation and Retrieval, a curation tool that provides digital forms backed by ontologies which is used to FAIRify data) [7] with data control (ownership) by the health facilities, and is defined as FAIR - based data Ownership in Locale under Regulatory Compliance (OLR) [9]. The controlled vocabularies were created using Bioportal which is integrated with the CEDAR derived templates to create semantic machine-actionable instances of the patient data [12].

Currently, the data collection and registration only happens during clinical encounters. Medical staff treat the patients and collect data, and trained data clerks insert this data into the system. Traveling to or communicating with these clinics is not always trivial. In poorer or more rural regions, proper access to infrastructure such as roads or the internet might be complicated. This can be especially difficult for patients with long term physical-conditions such as asthma, diabetes, epilepsy and high blood pressure. These are patients that do not need to be in a clinic at all times, but their vitals would ideally be tracked at short intervals over a long period of time to detect developments in their condition or predict deterioration in advance so that proper care can be administered.

To increase the connectivity of this type of patient, Kievit et al. [5] have developed a proof of concept using Interactive Voice Response (IVR) for a FAIR-based data pipeline that is capable of processing PGHD in a way that makes it interoperable with the existing VODAN technology without requiring access to the internet. Their work is based on the FAIR4PGHD framework [4] which uses CEDAR for the FAIRification of PGHD, making it a good candidate for integration with VODAN which is also based on CEDAR. The VODAN registers in their current form have limited information, purposefully chosen to meet public health surveillance purpose. PGHD can enrich the current data registries, and take a step towards enabling personalized care. For instance, there are many predictors of cardiovascular diseases (the main disease focus of [5]) that are not currently available as data points in the current registers, but which can be made available through some PGHD sources like wearables. Wearables could allow for the collection and communication of important information such as a patient's activity, sleep or stress levels outside of a clinical setting which could provide further insight when combined with the blood pressure data on a patient's cardiovascular health.

This paper builds upon the previous work on by Kievit et al. (2024) [5] on the three phase structure of the Patient Generated Health Data data flow, by including another PGHD source (wearable) in the workflow. The three phases are (1) *Collection & Communication*; (2) *Storage & Processing*; and (3) *Application & Access*. The aspects of each phase are presented in Fig. 1. The main contributions of this paper are two-fold.

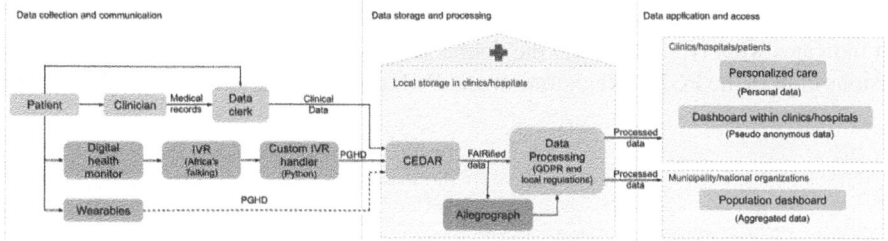

Fig. 1. Data pipeline of Patient Generated Health Data (PGHD) from point of collection up to and including visualization and analysis. Figure slightly adjusted from [5] to reflect the work done in this paper.

First we expand the Collection & Communication phase by introducing a patient registration template which allows for the storing of private information such as phone numbers or pass codes for authentication, and the inclusion of an extra template to connect various heterogeneous sources of PGHD to a single patient, which we present using data from a blood pressure monitor and a Fitbit. Second, we expand on the Application & Access phase by creating a dashboard that can be used for care by doctors.

2   Implementation

In this section we will describe each component in more detail, starting with the system for semantic integration of heterogeneous sources of PGHD to a single patient in Subsect. 2.1. We then introduce and describe the two sources of PGHD used in this paper: the Interactive Voice Response system designed in the previous work [5] in Subsect. 2.2; and the Fitbit wearable in Subsect. 2.3. Then we present the dashboard that integrates and visualizes all PGHD in Subsect. 2.4. All code for this project is publicly available at https://www.github.com/RenVit318/pghd.

2.1   PGHD Register and Connect

The overarching system we use to combine heterogeneous sources of PGHD to a single patient consists of two new CEDAR templates: the PGHD Registration and the PGHD Connector which are based on the PGHD_CONNECT ontology hosted on Bioportal[1]. The PGHD Registration template can be used to sign a patient up for PGHD by providing their VODAN Patient ID and any important information for the PGHD data pipeline. Right now the supported fields are the patient's phone number, an authentication code for the IVR system, the Fitbit device ID and authentication ID for the Fitbit system. Other information such as the International Mobile Equipment Identity number of a data collection device could be easily added at a later point.

The PGHD Connector template consists of three fields. The first two respectively contain the URI of the CEDAR instance of the patient to whom the PGHD pertains,

---

[1] https://bioportal.bioontology.org/ontologies/PGHD_CONNECT.

and the URI of the CEDAR instance of the data instance. The final field is a classifier that indicates what type of PGHD the connected instance is. In Fig. 2 we show filled in versions of both the PGHD Registration and PGHD Connector templates as an example.

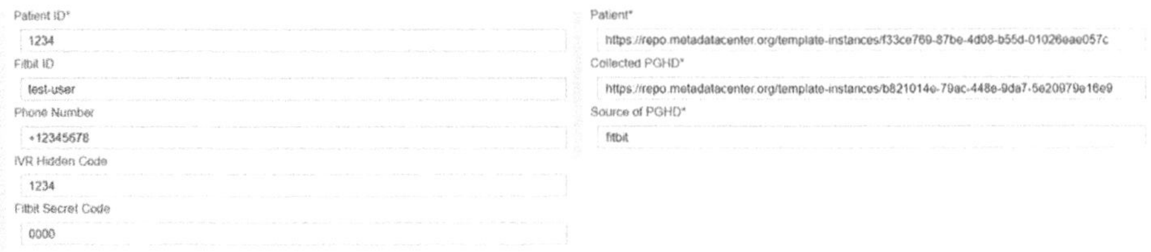

Fig. 2. The PGHD Registration (*left*) and -Connector (*right*) templates filled out on the CEDAR web interface with mock data. The URI under Patient corresponds to the unique instance ID of the form on the left.

Setting up the system in this way has two main benefits. First we set very little requirements on the storage format of the PGHD, as long as it has a resolvable URI. Second, we separate the patient information from the actual data meaning that if one only has access to the PGHD but not the PGHD Connector instances, the data would be fully anonymous by design. The schematic overview of this system is presented in Fig. 3. Here, it is clearly visible how multiple instances of PGHD collected through various devices are connected to a single patient through the connecting layer. The patient registration can be connected to the broader VODAN-Africa network through their Patient ID. This allows integrating the PGHD with data from other sources in the dashboard.

In the current implementation we store both the patient registration information and the PGHD on CEDAR. The registration instance is created in the health facility by the doctor or a data clerk, the PGHD instances are created dynamically through Python scripts which we describe in more detail in the next two sections. In both cases, this data is sent to CEDAR through HTTPS POST requests to the CEDAR REST API. When information from CEDAR is required, it is simply extracted from CEDAR through HTTPS GET request.

2.2 Interactive Voice Response

The Interactive Voice Response (IVR) tool deployed in this architecture was described in depth by Kievit et al. (2024) [5]. IVR is a technology that allows people to interact with an application through a phone call, where the application instructs an automated voice to talk to the user who can interact with the application either through speaking or by inserting numbers using their phone. This technology is used here to communicate simple types of PGHD. Specifically, the current implementation is based on a blood pressure monitor that is capable of recording the patients pulse rate, systolic blood pressure and diastolic blood pressure. Additionally the application allows the patient to provide simple information on the location, position and collector of the PGHD through

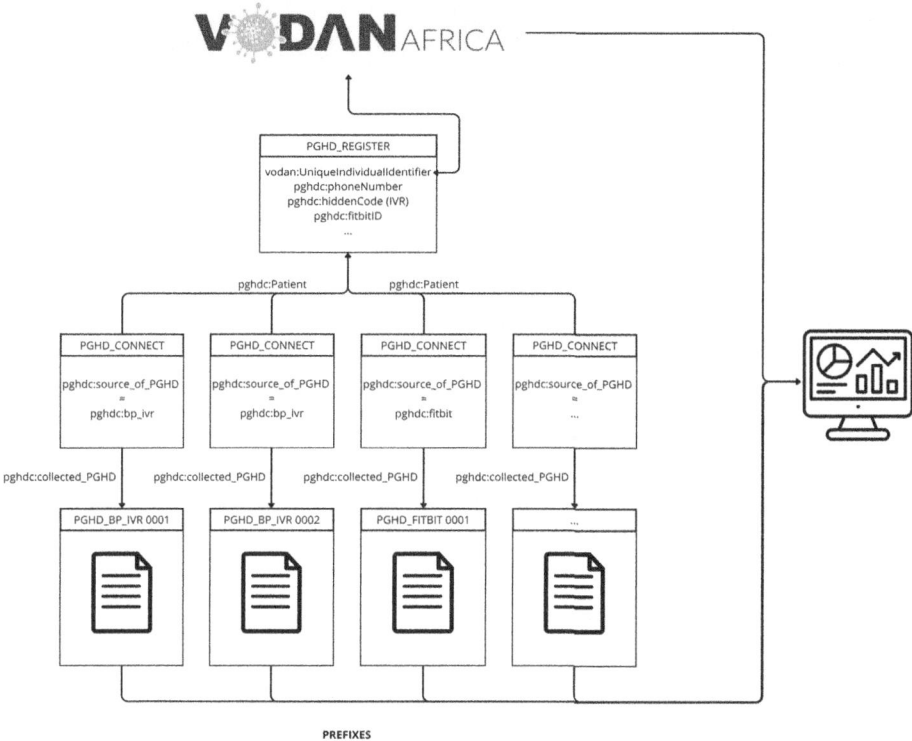

Fig. 3. The connections between a patient that is registered for the PGHD service in their clinic and the individual data instances collected through various devices. By connecting the PGHD to the rest of the VODAN-Africa network using the Patient ID we can combine the PGHD with all other information on that patient.

a drop-down like functionality (e.g. for position the patient should press 1 if they were laying down, 2 if they were sitting or 3 if they were standing).

The IVR system is implemented using the service provided by Africa's Talking (AT) which communicates with a script that is hosted on the website of one of the authors (only the application, the data is stored in CEDAR). If a patient calls the virtual phone number provided by AT, the AT service sends a POST request to our application which handles the incoming information and instructs the IVR service what to say through XML responses. Through multiple iterations we collect all the required information and then send the data as a template instance to CEDAR. Figure 4 shows a schematic overview of the flow of information from patient to CEDAR [5]. The call is initiated in steps 1–2, the data is collected iteratively in steps 3–7 and then sent to CEDAR in step 8.

The workflow is largely the same as was presented in [5], but with two main extensions. The first is of course the addition of the connector template to connect the BP IVR data to a patient registration, this is done in step 8. The second is that we have

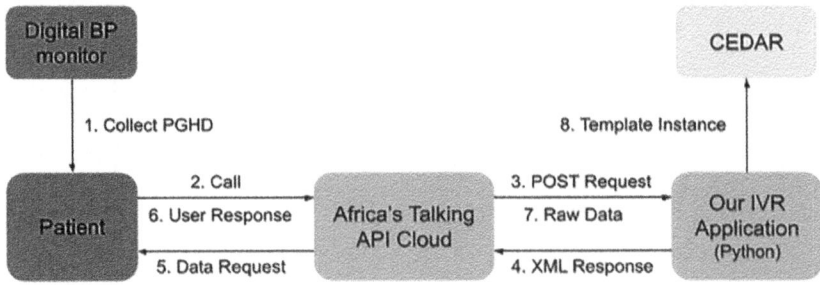

Fig. 4. Schematic overview of the Interactive Voice Response implementation using Africa's Talking for the collection of Patient Generated Health Data into CEDAR. It is discussed in more detail in [5].

incorporated a simple authentication system based on the phone number of the patient and a hidden code that is created at the time of registration in the PGHD Registration template. The authentication procedure occurs in the first data collection loop consisting of steps 3–7 plus a check to see if the combination of phone number and hidden code is correct in the form of a SPARQL query. In future work this could allow multiple types of PGHD to be easily supported by a single IVR service because patients could be routed to the specific services that are relevant to them. A downside of this implementation is that patients can only use a single phone to communicate their data to the clinic, which has to be determined at the time of registration. An alternative is to ask the patient for both their Patient ID and a hidden code for authentication in the call, however this does require the patient to remember two distinct sets of digits. Here we opt for the system that puts less mental load on the patient.

2.3 Fitbit

Fitbit[2] is a line of wireless-enabled wearable technology, physical fitness monitors and activity trackers such as smart watches, pedometers and monitors for heart rate, quality of sleep and other health features. Contrary to the blood pressure monitor described in the previous section the Fitbit can continuously collect data, as long as it is charged and worn by the patient, allowing greater insight into the vitals of the patient. The data collected by the device is periodically syncronized with the mobile application and then uploaded to the Fitbit cloud server when there is internet access. Our Python based application can then periodically send a request to the Fitbit Web API of the account belonging to the Fitbit device worn by the patient. From there it fetches the desired health data of the patient using the Fitbit Client ID and a secret code, which is stored in the PGHD Registration form. These values are obtained from each device and are used for solely for authorization and authentication. Upon collection of the information by the script, it is transformed into JSON-LD and sent to CEDAR as a template instance which is based on the Fitbit ontology which was created for this project, after which the Connector template is also uploaded similar to step 8 in the IVR system.

---

[2] https://www.fitbit.com.

2.4   Clinician PGHD Dashboard

To enable the use of the PGHD at point of care, we want to present the data in a fashion that is practical and actionable. According to a study conducted with service providers and patients, a dashboard to visualize PGHD is one of the best methods to assist clinicians [11]. To further ensure the usability of the dashboard and minimize the impact on clinician workload, PGHD should be incorporated with or easily accessible from the existing workflows [6]. In this work we take a first step towards this goal by emphasizing changes in values more than the absolute measurements, as they are easier to quickly analyse and may hold more benefit in the assessment of PGHD [1]. In future implementation work an investigation into factors impacting the usability in real life may be warranted.

The dashboard is set up using `rdflib` [2] for triple store and querying capabilities and `streamlit`[3] to create the dashboard itself. We start by importing all data directly from CEDAR through GET requests as JSON-LD and storing this into a single rdflib graph. This approach is not very scalable due to memory constraints in large implementations, however for this small proof-of-concept it is good enough. Once all data is imported into the graph we send a SPARQL query to the triple store to retrieve all required data for a single patient. An example mock query for the systolic blood pressure and observations dates for a single patient with UUI 1234 is given in Listing 1.1.

```
PREFIX pghdc: <https://github.com/RenVit318/pghd/tree/
               main/src/vocab/pghd_connect/>
PREFIX smash: <http://aimlab.cs.uoregon.edu/smash/
               ontologies/biomarker.owl#>
PREFIX vodan: <http://www.vodan-totafrica.info/
               vocs/vgt/>
PREFIX xsd: <http://www.w3.org/2001/XMLSchema#>
PREFIX dc: <http://purl.org/dc/elements/1.1/>
SELECT ?sys_bp ?date
WHERE {
        ?C pghdc:patient ?P ;
           pghdc:collected_PGHD ?D .
        ?P vodan:UniqueIndividualIdentifier
                                    "1234"^^xsd:int .
        ?D smash:hasSystolicBloodPressureValue ?sys_bp;
           dc:date ?date .
    }
```

Listing 1.1. SPARQL query to collect all systolic blood pressure information from PGHD sources pertaining to the patient with UUI "1234".

We do this in one query for all PGHD collected using both the IVR and Fitbit methods. This is then plotted as a trend graph showing the measured data as a function of time. The user can then hover over the corresponding data point to see the auxiliary

---

[3] https://www.streamlit.io.

information on that information which can potentially influence their analysis. This is in line with the desire of doctors to easily and quickly interpret the PGHD. We show an example of the implemented dashboard in Fig. 5. The data of different patients can be selected through the drop-down menu shown on the top left, and the different data types can be selected to be plotted through the buttons in the sidebar.

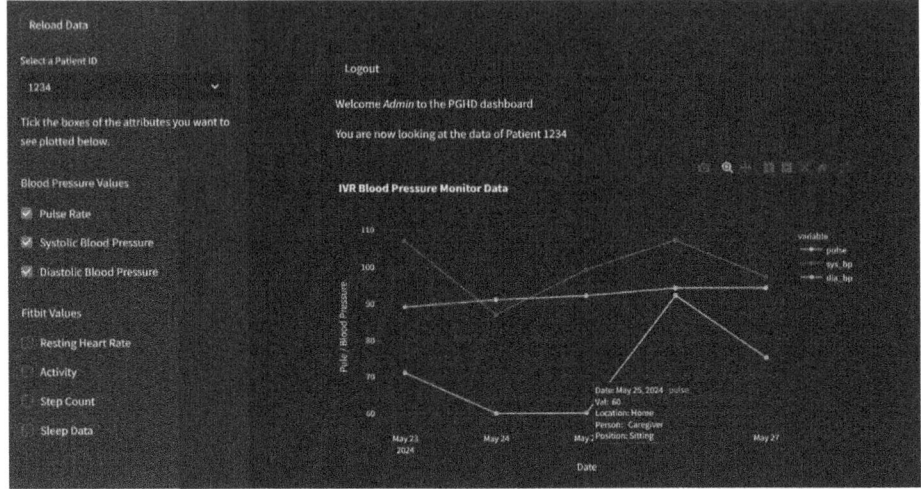

Fig. 5. Screenshot of the PGHD dashboard developed using Streamlit containing mock data. By hovering over a data point the clinician is able to both see the exact value of the measurement, and the auxiliary information communicated by the IVR pipeline.

3   Discussion

The architecture presented in this work is purely a proof-of-concept aligned with the current VODAN architecture based on, among others, the CEDAR microservice. In this proof-of-concept we have partially automated the data collection procedure, allowing for a new data stream to be included in the network without significantly increasing the workload of clinicians or data stewards in the facility. We have demonstrated the usability of the pipeline through a test setup based on the online version of CEDAR (hosted in Stanford, USA). In order to comply with the principles of ownership and localization the full pipeline needs to be under the control of the facility. For the CEDAR integration, it is relatively easy to do this as the current VODAN MVP already contains a local CEDAR service. In Fig. 6 we present what this in-clinic architecture could look like. Here the data storage is moved from CEDAR to AllegroGraph, the triple store currently in use in VODAN.

Through initial discussions with the VODAN technical team we have discovered two main technical obstacles in realizing the implementation of this architecture. Both

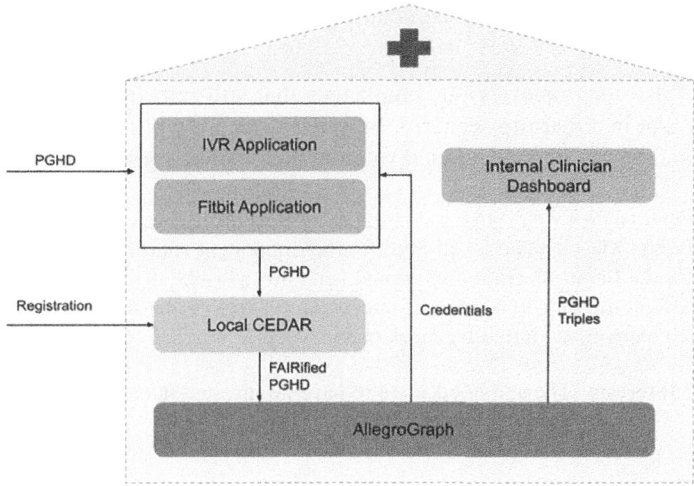

Fig. 6. In-clinic architecture for the PGHD pipeline compliant with the OLR principles.

issues are partially caused by the fact that the electricity network of the facilities in Nigeria where the VODAN MVP is deployed is unstable. On the one hand this leads to difficulty with deployment as computers can disconnect at unexpected times, however this issue has evidently been tackled previously as various aspects of the VODAN architecture are already deployed. The main problem caused by the unstable electricity lies in the PGHD collection step presented of our pipeline. Mainly for the IVR pipeline we require a continuous internet connection to allow patients to communicate their data to the facility at the moment of collection. A potential solution path is to outsource the data collection applications (the block of functions in the top left of Fig. 6) to a virtual machine hosted on a cloud server, under the control of the facility. PGHD could then periodically be collected by the facility. However this requires further investigation in terms of feasibility and security.

Despite these technological issues that are facing the potential of deployment of this pipeline, initial discussions with both clinicians and patients with long term health problems have shown that the potential of added value is present. In future work we also aim to verify this through experimentation with the deployed pipeline.

4   Conclusion

In this article we have expanded upon a proof-of-concept pipeline introduced by Kievit et al. (2024) [5] through three main contributions. We have

1. Designed a system based on CEDAR to connect various heterogeneous sources of Patient Generated Health Data (PGHD) with a single patient using a single Registration and multiple Connector templates.
2. Included a Fitbit into the pipeline that previously only consisted of the Interactive Voice Response (IVR) system.

3. Designed a dashboard aimed at clinicians to allow them to easily and quickly analyse PGHD.

We have also identified various challenges that still remain in implementing the proof-of-concept in a real-life scenario. In future work we will tackle these challenges and investigate the usability and added value of the pipeline presented in this work.

Acknowledgements. We would like to thank the MSc. students Jasper van Mosseveld, Esther van Dijk, Bidayatul Masulah and Swati Soni for their important contributions in developing the groundwork for the Fitbit integration presented here. We will like to also appreciate Abubakar Adamu - Data Steward with VODAN and our research partner - the Railway Clinic of Minna, Nigeria for their support and initial feedback on the work.

Disclosure of Interests. The authors declare to have no invested interests in the publication of this work.

References

1. Bendich, I., et al.: Changes in prospectively collected longitudinal patient-generated health data are associated with short-term patient-reported outcomes after total joint arthroplasty: a pilot study. Arthroplasty Today **5**(1), 61–63 (2019). https://doi.org/10.1016/j.artd.2019.01. 005. https://www.sciencedirect.com/science/article/pii/S235234411930007X
2. Boettiger, C.: rdflib: a high level wrapper around the redland package for common RDF applications (2018). https://doi.org/10.5281/zenodo.1098478
3. Kawu, A.A., Kievit, R., Abubakar, A., van Reisen, M., O'Sullivan, D., Hederman, L.: Exploring the integration of a patient generated health data in a fair digital health system in low-resourced settings: a user-centered approach. In: Proceedings of the 4th African Human Computer Interaction Conference, AfriCHI 2023, pp. 215–220. Association for Computing Machinery, New York (2024). https://doi.org/10.1145/3628096.3629059
4. Kawu, A.A., O'Sullivan, D., Hederman, L., Reisen, M.: FAIR4PGHD: a framework for fair implementation over PGHD. FAIR Connect **1**, 35–40 (2023). https://doi.org/10.3233/FC-230500
5. Kievit, R., Kawu, A.A., Reisen, M., O'Sullivan, D., Hederman, L.: Exploring the design of low-end technology to increase patient connectivity to electronic health records, pp. 194–200 (2024). https://doi.org/10.5220/0012460900003657
6. Lordon, R., et al.: How patient-generated health data and patient-reported outcomes affect patient-clinician relationships: a systematic review. Health Inform. J. **26**, 146045822092818 (2020). https://doi.org/10.1177/1460458220928184
7. Musen, M.A., et al.: The center for expanded data annotation and retrieval. J. Am. Med. Inform. Assoc. **22**(6), 1148–1152 (2015). https://doi.org/10.1093/jamia/ocv048
8. Plug, R., et al.: Fair and GDPR compliant population health data generation, processing and analytics (2022)
9. van Reisen, M., et al.: Federated fair principles: ownership, localisation and regulatory compliance (OLR). FAIR Connect **1**, 63–69 (2023). https://doi.org/10.3233/FC-230506
10. van Reisen, M., et al.: Design of a fair digital data health infrastructure in Africa for Covid-19 reporting and research. Adv. Genet. **2**(2), e10050 (2021). https://doi.org/10.1002/ggn2. 10050. https://onlinelibrary.wiley.com/doi/abs/10.1002/ggn2.10050
11. Sanger, P.C., et al.: A patient-centered system in a provider-centered world: challenges of incorporating post-discharge wound data into practice. J. Am. Med. Inform. Assoc. **23**(3), 514–525 (2016)

12. Van Reisen, M., et al.: Incomplete COVID-19 data: the curation of medical health data by the virus outbreak data network-Africa. Data Intell. **4**(4), 673–697 (2022). https://doi.org/10.1162/dint_e_00166
13. Wilkinson, M.D., et al.: The fair guiding principles for scientific data management and stewardship. Sci. Data **3**(1) (2016). https://doi.org/10.1038/sdata.2016.18

Classification of Augmented Motor Imagery Data Using Various Representations of Feature Vectors

Roman Mouček[1]([envelope]) [ORCID], Jakub Kodera[1] [ORCID], Pavel Mautner[1] [ORCID], and Jaroslav Průcha[2] [ORCID]

[1] Department of Computer Science and Engineering, Faculty of Applied Sciences, University of West Bohemia, Univerzitní 8, 301 00 Plzeň, Czech Republic
moucek@kiv.zcu.cz
[2] Department of Information and Communication Technologies in Medicine, Faculty of Biomedical Engineering, Czech Technical University, nám. Sítná 3105, 272 01 Kladno, Czech Republic

Abstract. Brain-controlled, robot-assisted rehabilitation is a promising approach in healthcare, with the potential to significantly enhance and partially automate the recovery of motor systems and the brain structures critical for movement. However, developing an effective rehabilitation system entails numerous challenges and limitations. A primary challenge is the limited data available from individuals recovering from motor function injuries, which is essential for training deep learning models to recognize motor imagery patterns. To address this issue, we present initial experiments using data augmentation and classification results on the collected and augmented dataset.

Three different representations of input feature vectors and three augmentation methods were employed. Binary classification involving hand movement and rest, as well as multiclass classification involving left-hand movement, right-hand movement, and rest, were performed. The highest accuracy, $76.00 \pm 0.80\%$, was achieved in binary classification with a CNN classifier without any dataset augmentation, using the time-series representation of the input feature vector.

Keywords: Brain-computer interface · Data augmentation · Deep learning · Electroencephalography · Feature vector representation · Motor imagery · Robot-assisted rehabilitation

1 Introduction

The advancement of robot-assisted rehabilitation holds great potential to enhance and partially automate rehabilitation processes, particularly for individuals recovering from motor function injuries. In these situations, a robot assists patients by guiding them through desired, usually pre-defined movements based on their current capabilities. Since motor rehabilitation ideally involves both the locomotor system and the brain areas responsible for movement, incorporating brain-controlled therapeutic robots into these procedures appears promising.

M. P. Guarino et al. (Eds.): BIOSTEC 2024, CCIS 2546, pp. 442–459, 2026.
https://doi.org/10.1007/978-3-031-96899-0_25

Brain-computer or brain-machine interface (BCI or BMI) enables direct communication between the human brain and external devices like computers. Non-invasive BCIs use electroencephalography (EEG) and event-related potential (ERP) techniques, where electrical activity recorded from the scalp is utilized to control applications or environments. Current BCI systems and applications are based on several key paradigms, including brain frequency detection, event-related or evoked components, Steady-State Visual Evoked Potentials (SSVEPs, VEPs), and Motor Imagery (MI).

Motor Imagery (MI), which involves mentally simulating a physical action without actually performing it, combined with monitoring the related EEG signals, is considered beneficial for retraining the neural pathways involved in movement. During the preparation and execution of a movement, the cortical EEG signal in the alpha and beta bands shows a decrease in amplitude, referred to as Event-Related Desynchronization (ERD). Conversely, Event-Related Synchronization (ERS) signifies an increase in the EEG amplitude in these bands during periods of rest or relaxation following a task. ERD is thus associated with cortical activation and is interpreted as the desynchronization of neuronal populations to facilitate information processing and motor execution. On the contrary, ERS reflects the brain's return to a more synchronized state associated with inhibitory processes. These two phenomena are essential for understanding the BCIs and MI paradigm since they indicate how the brain's electrical activity changes in response to different states and given tasks.

However, using the MI paradigm in BCI research and robot-assisted rehabilitation has numerous challenges and limitations, especially for practical, real-world applications. These challenges include the quality and interpretability of the EEG signals, the technology used for BCI data collection, the recognition of MI patterns, the use of appropriate signal processing methods, and the lack of adequate data from the target groups to train processing (especially deep learning) models. This paper specifically addresses the issue of insufficient data for training deep learning models; it follows up the authors' research presented in [9]. It subsequently explores options to augment existing MI datasets effectively when various representations of input feature vectors are used. Furthermore, the dimensionality of the feature vectors was reduced by shortening the period in which MI patterns are detected.

The paper is structured as follows: The state-of-the-art section reviews experiments, findings, and research on robot-assisted and brain-controlled rehabilitation, focusing on data augmentation methods and deep learning techniques for EEG signal analysis. The Materials and Methods section details the dataset and the data processing and augmentation techniques applied. The Results section presents the outcomes of applying augmentation techniques to a specific MI dataset and the classification results using various classifiers and representations of input feature vectors. Finally, the Discussion and Conclusions sections provide insights into the current results and suggest directions for future work.

2   State of the Art

A survey on robots controlled by motor imagery-based brain-computer interfaces (MI-BCIs) was conducted and detailed in [16] from several perspectives, including

EEG evocation/BCI paradigms, signal processing algorithms, and applications. The survey reviewed various brain-controlled robots through the lens of different BCI paradigms and introduced relevant EEG signal processing algorithms, such as feature extraction methods and classification algorithms. Additionally, the authors summarized experiences with MI brain-controlled robot applications. The study concluded that MI-BCI technology rapidly evolves and faces challenges in EEG signal processing and asynchronous control. Deep learning methods can then significantly enhance MI-BCI-controlled robotic systems' overall performance. Developing rehabilitation training robots is expected to be highly effective in helping patients recover from motor function injuries.

The augmentation techniques for MI-BCI data were used in several studies. The study by Yang et al. [15] aimed to detect four movements: left hand, right hand, tongue, and both feet. Their analysis showed that MI tasks caused ERD and ERS over the motor cortex's right and left hemispheres, mainly at the C4 and C3 electrodes. The Cz electrode was primarily affected by MI of the feet and tongue. The measured EEG signal used two-second-long time windows (epochs) for augmentation. They used Conditional Variational Autoencoder (CVAE) and Generative Adversarial Network (GAN) for data augmentation. Including the generated data in the dataset resulted in a several percent increase in cross-validation metric accuracy for all subjects.

A recurrent Generative Adversarial Network (GAN) for data augmentation to enhance the MI classification dataset using the publicly available PhysioNet dataset was used in [1]. Their findings highlighted the sensitivity of deep learning models to training dataset size, with all classifiers showing improved accuracy when the augmented dataset was employed.

Zhang et al. [17] experimented with various augmentation methods to enhance the classification performance of CNNs for MI detection. They evaluated the classifiers and augmentation methods using the freely available BCI Competition IV dataset 1 and BCI Competition IV dataset 2b. For analysis, a four-second-long EEG signal during MI was used. The Fréchet Inception Distance (FID) metric assessed each augmentation method's effectiveness. All methods, except the Gaussian Transform (GT), improved classification accuracy. The most significant improvement (12.6%) was achieved using the convolutional Generative Adversarial Network.

Alsaegh et al. [2] reviewed studies on EEG signal processing in MI tasks, examining 40 studies published between 2015 and 2020. Most of these studies (45.6%) focused solely on detecting two MI classes: left-hand and right-hand movements. The next most common classification task (31.6%) involved detecting left-hand, right-hand, tongue, and foot movements. CNNs were the most used classifier, appearing in 73% of the studies. Additionally, 14% of the studies utilized a hybrid architecture, typically combining CNN and LSTM.

Deep learning-based research for MI-EEG classification was systematically reviewed in [3]. It begins with an overview of the selection process for the studies reviewed and provides a summary of BCI, EEG, and MI systems. The review then analyzes DL-based techniques for MI classification from four perspectives: preprocessing, input formulation, deep learning architecture, and performance evaluation. Three significant questions about DL-based MI classification addressed include the necessity of preprocessing when using DL-based techniques, possible representations of input feature vectors, and current trends in DL-based techniques. Finally, the paper summarizes MI-EEG-based applications, explores public MI-EEG datasets, and visualizes the performance of each dataset based on the reviewed articles.

Tang et al. [13] utilized a deep Convolutional Neural Network (CNN) to classify single-trial left- and right-handed motor imagery (MI) already in 2017. They selected a three-second segment of the signal, divided into 50ms windows. The CNN outperformed the Support Vector Machine (SVM) classifier across various feature extraction methods, achieving an average classification accuracy of $86.41 \pm 0.77\%$. In comparison, the best result with the SVM classifier ($82.61 \pm 6.15\%$) was obtained using the Common Spatial Patterns (CSP) feature extraction method.

Another approach to classifying MI tasks using Deep Learning (DL) techniques is presented in [4]. The methodology used includes data preprocessing, feature extraction using Common Spatial Pattern (CSP), Wavelet Packet Decomposition (WPD), and the evaluation of four distinct classifiers that combine two, three, four, and five Convolutional Neural Networks (CNNs). Empirical evaluations show that employing five CNNs yields the best results, demonstrating promising performance metrics with score values of around 65%.

Regarding broader EEG analysis using deep learning, Roy et al. [10] conducted a systematic review covering studies published from 2010 to 2018. They found that a majority of studies (40%) employed Convolutional Neural Network (CNN) architectures for classification, followed by 13% using Recurrent Neural Networks (RNNs), another 13% using Autoencoders (AEs), and 7% utilizing a combination of CNN and RNN. Regarding the classification approach, 26% of studies focused on intra-subject classification, while 62% concentrated on inter-subject classification. Interestingly, only 8% of studies conducted both intra- and inter-subject classification.

Lashgari et al. [7] conducted a systematic review of studies on overall EEG data augmentation and deep learning methods applied to EEG datasets. Of 53 studies, only 29 provided classification results before and after dataset augmentation. The average improvement across all augmentation methods was $0.29 \pm 0.08\%$, with the most significant improvement seen using the Noise Injection (NI) method, which had an average improvement of 0.36%. The most commonly used classifier was the Convolutional Neural Network (CNN), appearing in 62% of the studies. The second most popular classifier used in 16% of the studies was a hybrid combination of Long Short-Term Memory (LSTM) and CNN. Multilayer Perceptron (MLP) was used in 8% of the studies, and LSTM alone was used in 6% of the studies.

Experiments on detecting motor MI patterns in EEG signals conducted in our neuroinformatics lab are broadly discussed in [8] and [11]. Various feature vectors as inputs to a multilayer perceptron (MLP) are introduced in [8]. The most effective feature vector, achieving a 90.05% average classification accuracy, was constructed by calculating ERD in the alpha band and ERS in the lower beta band. This inter-subject model classified movement versus resting state using MI from any limb. The detection of sensorimotor rhythms (SMR) by applying a band-pass filter in the alpha band to signal epochs was focused in [11]. The filtered epochs were used as inputs to either CSP methods or directly to SVM and linear discriminant analysis (LDA) classifiers. EEG signals from

C3, C4, and Cz electrodes were used to create intra-subject models, performing multi-class classification of left movement, right movement, and resting state.

In summary, various methods and techniques are employed for processing EEG signals and detecting MI patterns. During preprocessing, a band-pass filter is applied to the alpha and beta bands, and relevant channels, typically C3, Cz, and C4, are selected. Epochs, or segments of the EEG signal corresponding to specific events (such as hand movement), are identified, usually lasting between 2–4 s. Removing signal artifacts is also an essential but complex step, and many studies do not address it.

In the final preprocessing step, feature selection is crucial. Most studies use the time series of each epoch as classifier inputs without constructing feature vectors. Some studies, however, perform feature extraction by calculating signal properties or converting the spectrogram into an image. For example, directly calculated ERDs and ERSs, and each epoch's average power change as features were used in [8], while others used individual epochs.

Time series representation of the EEG signal is common, particularly with the rise of CNNs, due to its ease of implementation without needing feature extraction. Typically, preprocessing includes electrode selection, filtering, and artifact removal. Synchronization labels with the EEG signal are essential for MI detection, focusing on specific time intervals called epochs obtained by repeating MI tasks.

However, analyzing both time and frequency domains seems to be beneficial. MI is linked to desynchronization (ERD) and synchronization (ERS) in the alpha and beta bands, making frequency spectrum analysis important. Moreover, exclusive time or frequency domain feature extraction can omit valuable information. Therefore, methods like short-term Fourier transform (STFT), wavelet transform, and Hilbert filter, which combine time and frequency domain data, could be preferred to extract significant features.

In EEG signal processing, the large size of the original data poses a challenge. Classifiers may perform poorly if the training data is small relative to the feature vectors. It is recommended to have at least five to ten times more input vectors per class than the feature vector's dimensionality, which is often difficult due to typically small input data and high dimensionality [14]. With the growing use of DL for EEG signal processing, a large training set is essential for achieving robustness and generalization capability to DL-based classifiers [5,6]. However, obtaining extensive EEG datasets is challenging, and small datasets can lead to overfitting. Data augmentation is thus a promising solution to create a more complex dataset, reducing the distance between training and test data.

Data augmentation can be approached in two ways: directly manipulating collected feature vectors (e.g., geometric transformations or adding noise) or using generative models to learn and replicate the feature vector distribution. The former is simpler and requires fewer hyperparameters, though not all transformations are suitable for EEG as the augmented data may not resemble their original class. Generative models like Variational Autoencoders (VAEs) and GANs create new data samples from learned features, aiming to predict new vectors similar to the original set. However, their impact on classification accuracy has not been significantly proven.

There is no consensus on evaluation metrics for augmented data in EEG studies. Standard metrics include Frechet Inception Distance (FID), Signal-to-noise ratio (SNR), Root mean square error (RMSE), and Cross-correlation (CC), primarily used in machine vision [6].

According to the studies reviewed, CNNs are the most popular classifiers for MI detection, used in 73% of cases. This is followed by RNNs and combinations of both approaches, accounting for 14%. Traditional classifiers like MLP, LDA, and SVM are baselines for comparison with more advanced deep learning architectures. Additionally, some research has explored the use of transformers, as seen in [12].

3   Materials and Methods

This section presents the MI dataset created and utilized, detailing the fundamental parameters of EEG signal preprocessing and processing methods. It covers the representation of input feature vectors, augmentation techniques, classifiers, and evaluation metrics.

3.1   Dataset

The experiment protocol for acquiring EEG data using the rehabilitation robot was designed by Pavel Mochura [8]. Three experimenters utilized this protocol to generate the resulting dataset. A brief description is provided here, while a more detailed explanation can be found in [8].

During the experiment, the participant sits in a chair and holds the rehabilitation robot's arm with either their left or right hand. The measurement consists of alternating between resting and movement phases over a 10-min period. In the resting phase, the participant refrains from moving the robot arm for 10 s. In the movement phase, the participant moves the robot arm along a predefined trajectory for 20 s.

The EEG signal was recorded using a V-AMP 16 amplifier from BrainProducts, connected to a cap with electrodes. This amplifier was linked to a computer running BrainVision Recorder software. The EEG signal and stimuli generated by the rehabilitation robot serving as synchronization markers were recorded.

The final dataset includes data from 29 healthy subjects (men aged 21–26 and women aged 18–23). The data are anonymized and available for download at https://zenodo.org/record/7893847.

3.2   Data Preprocessing

In our previous work, we concentrated on detecting MI patterns using inter-subject models applied to a dataset introduced above, with input feature vectors represented directly by the measured time series. In this study, we aimed to enhance the classification performance of these models by implementing additional techniques. Although the data augmentation and classification processes remained largely unchanged, significant improvements were made in data preprocessing. We specifically expanded feature extraction methods and incorporated optional data dimensionality reduction.

First, each subject's raw signals from the electrodes Cz, C3, and C4 are epoched, selecting only the parts around the synchronization markers. Each epoch is originally four seconds long, spanning three and a half seconds before and half a second after the stimuli marker. However, upon further inspection, we found that using just two-second signals before the stimuli marker might suffice and yield similar classification results while reducing training time. A significant drop in signal power starts around two seconds before the stimuli marker in the movement epochs, as seen in Fig. 1. Time-frequency representation also supporting this observation is shown in Fig. 4.

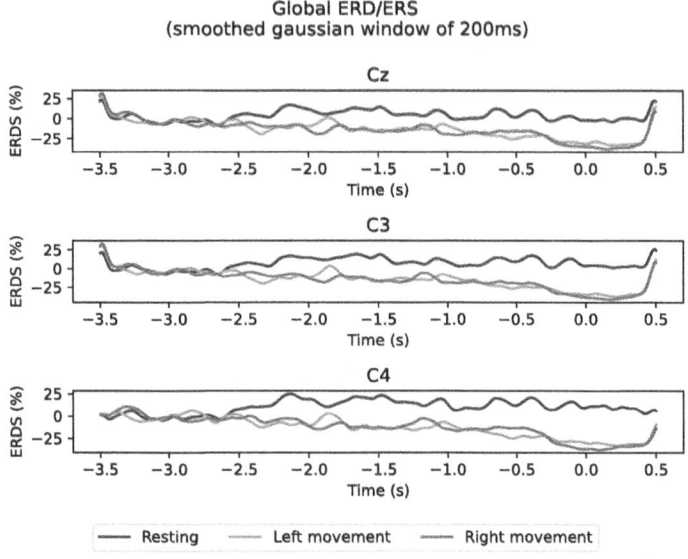

Fig. 1. Visualization of computed percentage values of ERD/ERS from epochs for each classification class. The visualization is smoothed with a Gaussian filter of length 200 ms.

In the subsequent phases of EEG signal preprocessing, baseline correction was applied, and the epochs were undersampled to 500 Hz. They were then filtered using a band-pass filter with a finite impulse response and 8–30 Hz cutoff frequencies. Artifacts exceeding 100 microvolts were rejected, and epochs were selected using an algorithm designed to maintain a balanced distribution of classification classes while adhering to the specified restrictions.

In our previous work, the feature vectors were represented by time series (as seen in Fig. 2) and preprocessed as described above. Using original four-second epochs sampled at 500 Hz resulted in input feature vectors with 2000 samples per electrode channel. This study expanded feature extraction by using two other input feature vector representations. First, we converted the time series to a frequency spectrum, explicitly calculating the power spectral density from the preprocessed time series. With the data band passed between 8–30 Hz, this produced feature vectors with 23 samples per channel. Figure 3 shows the filtered frequency spectrum. The third representation is created by transforming the preprocessed time series into the time-frequency domain; the continuous wavelet transform (CWT) was used. Figure 4 visualizes the resulting time-frequency spectrograms.

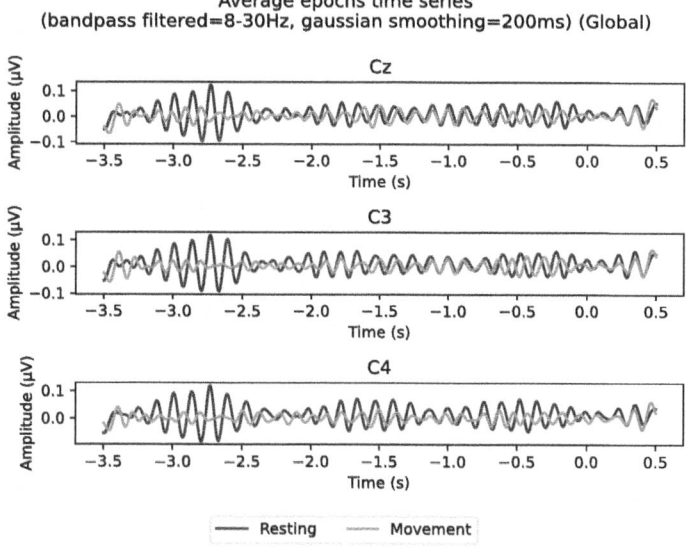

Fig. 2. Visualization of the preprocessed average time series data computed from epochs for the rest and movement classes.

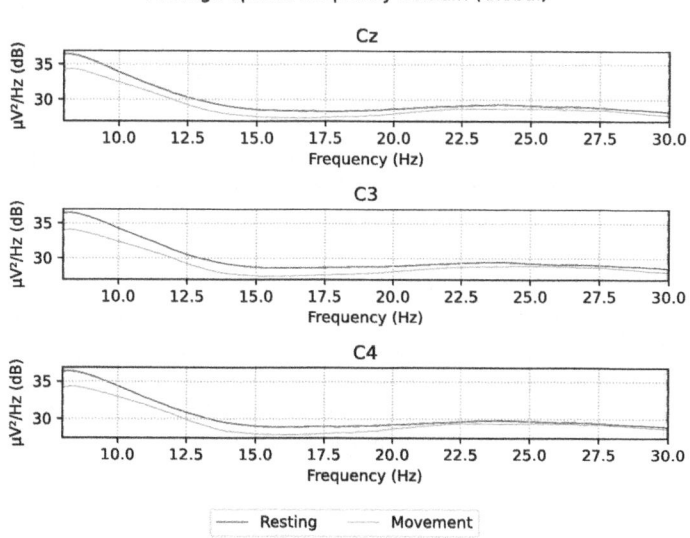

Fig. 3. Visualization of the preprocessed average frequency spectrum computed from epochs for the rest and movement classes.

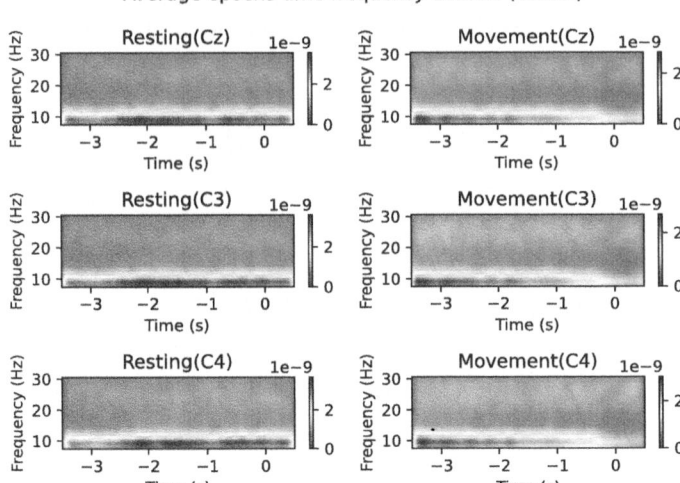

Fig. 4. Visualization of the preprocessed average spectrogram (time-frequency domain) computed from epochs for the rest and movement classes.

As an optional final preprocessing step, we applied a data dimensionality reduction method using PCA. Unless otherwise noted, this step was not used in the results presented. The preprocessed data from each subject was combined into a single dataset for input into the data augmentation methods and classifiers. The data was randomly shuffled and split, with 80% used for training and 20% for testing.

3.3   Data Augmentation

For data augmentation, we used noise injection (NI), conditional variational autoencoder (cVAE), and conditional generative adversarial network (GAN) with the Wasserstein loss function and gradient penalty (cWGAN-GP). We evaluated these augmentations using Fréchet Inception Distance (FID), Signal-to-Noise Ratio (SNR), Root Mean Square Error (RMSE), and Cross-Correlation (CC). Only the preprocessed training dataset was used to train the cVAE and cWGAN-GP models, and only the training data was augmented. The training dataset size was doubled, resulting in a final training set composed of half real measured preprocessed data and half generated data.

To improve the initial poor performance of the cWGAN-GP model, we conducted a grid search to find the optimal combination of hyperparameters instead of choosing them empirically. We evaluated the best model based on the calculated Fréchet inception distance (FID). The grid search included the following hyperparameters: generator learning rate, critic learning rate, and number of training epochs.

3.4   MI Patterns Classification

For MI patterns classification, we employed Linear Discriminant Analysis (LDA), Support Vector Machine (SVM), Multilayer Perceptron (MLP), Long Short-Term Memory

(LSTM), and Convolutional Neural Network (CNN). The classification results were assessed using traditional metrics: accuracy, precision, recall, and F1 score. Each classifier was trained using 10-fold cross-validation, employing early stopping based on monitoring the validation set training loss to prevent overfitting. Each fold's model was evaluated on the training dataset, and the classification metrics were averaged across the ten folds at the process conclusion.

4 Results

The classification results presented in the following tables are expressed as mean ± standard deviation. The best result for each classifier and augmentation method is highlighted in **bold**, while the overall best result for a classification metric across all used classifiers and augmentation methods is framed .

4.1 Input Feature Vectors as Time Series

Table 1 shows the metrics obtained when augmentation methods were applied to the input feature vectors represented as time series and when binary classification was performed. Table 2 presents classification metric results for different combinations of classifiers and augmentation methods used in binary classification when input feature vectors are represented as time series. Similarly, Tables 3 and 4 present similar results for multiclass classification.

Table 1. Resulting metrics for augmentation methods; input feature vectors are represented as time series and binary classification is performed.

Method	FID	SNR	RMSE	CC
NI	**3243.64**	4.207	1.41414	0.194
cVAE	9029.46	**15.772**	**1.41045**	0.489
cWGAN-GP	10900.1	2.953	1.41435	**0.492**

4.2 Input Feature Vectors as Frequency Spectra

Table 5 provides the resulting metrics for augmentation methods when input feature vectors were represented as frequency spectra and binary classification was performed. Table 6 presents classification metric results for different combinations of classifiers and augmentation methods used in binary classification when input feature vectors are represented as frequency spectra. Similarly, Tables 7 and 8 provide similar results for multiclass classification.

Table 2. Classification results; input feature vectors are represented as time series and binary classification is performed.

Method	Accuracy	Precision	Recall	F1 Score
SVM	57.28 ± 0.47	57.28 ± 0.47	57.26 ± 0.47	57.24 ± 0.47
NI SVM	**57.59 ± 0.71**	**57.85 ± 0.71**	**57.65 ± 0.70**	**57.34 ± 0.72**
cVAE SVM	53.58 ± 0.64	53.63 ± 0.66	53.52 ± 0.64	53.22 ± 0.66
cWGAN-GP SVM	57.47 ± 0.73	57.55 ± 0.75	57.42 ± 0.73	57.26 ± 0.73
LDA	50.51 ± 0.99	50.53 ± 0.99	50.52 ± 0.99	50.49 ± 0.98
NI LDA	51.00 ± 1.45	51.02 ± 1.46	51.02 ± 1.45	50.95 ± 1.45
cVAE LDA	50.66 ± 1.42	50.68 ± 1.43	50.68 ± 1.42	50.64 ± 1.43
cWGAN-GP LDA	**51.00 ± 1.02**	**51.02 ± 1.03**	**51.02 ± 1.03**	**50.96 ± 1.02**
MLP	51.12 ± 1.49	51.16 ± 1.55	51.13 ± 1.52	50.55 ± 1.90
NI MLP	51.45 ± 1.04	51.50 ± 1.05	51.47 ± 1.04	51.17 ± 1.18
cVAE MLP	49.82 ± 0.89	49.78 ± 0.92	49.77 ± 0.86	49.24 ± 0.65
cWGAN-GP MLP	**51.88 ± 0.99**	**51.98 ± 1.09**	**51.88 ± 0.97**	**51.38 ± 0.97**
CNN	**76.00 ± 0.80**	**76.73 ± 0.75**	**76.05 ± 0.79**	**75.86 ± 0.90**
NI CNN	75.34 ± 1.09	76.69 ± 0.67	75.41 ± 1.07	75.05 ± 1.30
cVAE CNN	75.39 ± 1.27	75.72 ± 1.31	75.42 ± 1.28	75.33 ± 1.28
cWGAN-GP CNN	74.29 ± 1.40	75.01 ± 1.13	74.30 ± 1.44	74.10 ± 1.56
LSTM	53.60 ± 1.64	53.62 ± 1.65	53.60 ± 1.64	53.55 ± 1.62
NI LSTM	**55.75 ± 1.13**	**55.79 ± 1.12**	**55.77 ± 1.12**	**55.71 ± 1.13**
cVAE LSTM	53.98 ± 1.21	54.00 ± 1.20	53.99 ± 1.21	53.95 ± 1.25
cWGAN-GP LSTM	55.41 ± 1.92	55.45 ± 1.89	55.43 ± 1.90	55.34 ± 1.96

4.3   Input Feature Vectors as Time-Frequency Spectra

The same method of results presentation is used in the time-frequency domain. Tables 9 and 10 provide the resulting metrics for augmentation methods and classification results when input feature data were represented as time-frequency spectra and binary classification was performed. Tables 11 and 12 then provide similar results for multiclass classification.

The training time (measured over ten-fold cross-validation) ranged from less than 1 s for the LDA method used for multiclass classification and using frequency spectrum representation of the input feature vector to over 40 min for the NI SVM used for binary classification and using time-frequency spectrum representation of the input feature vector. The classification time (for a single input sample) varied from 1 ms for LDA-based methods, binary and multiclass classification, and all representations of the feature vector to 1270 ms for the cWGAN-GP LSTM method, binary classification, and time-frequency representation of the feature vector. The classification time for CNNs ranged from 100 to 200 ms. A standard mid-range laptop was used for these calculations.

Table 3. Resulting metrics for augmentation methods; input feature vectors are represented as time series and multiclass classification is performed.

Method	FID	SNR	RMSE	CC
NI	**3303.68**	4.206	1.41461	0.202
cVAE	8869.08	**14.513**	1.41593	0.442
cWGAN-GP	10869.6	3.643	**1.4143**	**0.503**

Table 4. Classification results; input feature vectors are represented as time series and multiclass classification is performed.

Method	Accuracy	Precision	Recall	F1 Score
SVM	40.35 ± 0.82	**40.43 ± 0.82**	**39.82 ± 0.79**	**39.48 ± 0.80**
NI SVM	38.18 ± 1.09	39.56 ± 1.08	38.36 ± 1.10	38.21 ± 1.10
cVAE SVM	38.16 ± 0.51	36.88 ± 0.66	37.04 ± 0.50	36.15 ± 0.53
cWGAN-GP SVM	**40.48 ± 0.52**	39.30 ± 0.95	39.24 ± 0.56	37.97 ± 0.58
LDA	35.26 ± 1.46	35.34 ± 1.45	35.32 ± 1.47	35.20 ± 1.42
NI LDA	**35.88 ± 0.79**	**35.86 ± 0.79**	**35.91 ± 0.72**	**35.81 ± 0.77**
cVAE LDA	35.02 ± 1.11	35.04 ± 1.09	35.06 ± 1.06	34.96 ± 1.08
cWGAN-GP LDA	33.58 ± 1.27	33.68 ± 1.27	33.64 ± 1.33	33.53 ± 1.29
MLP	32.94 ± 1.13	33.03 ± 1.21	33.00 ± 1.21	32.49 ± 1.03
NI MLP	32.92 ± 1.55	33.05 ± 1.55	32.92 ± 1.52	32.85 ± 1.54
cVAE MLP	32.10 ± 0.99	32.01 ± 0.90	31.94 ± 1.07	31.70 ± 1.15
cWGAN-GP MLP	**34.65 ± 1.58**	**34.37 ± 0.91**	**34.30 ± 1.16**	**33.29 ± 1.74**
CNN	57.79 ± 1.69	59.36 ± 2.47	57.60 ± 1.84	57.17 ± 2.08
NI CNN	**58.57 ± 1.45**	**60.32 ± 1.48**	**58.43 ± 1.48**	**57.99 ± 1.72**
cVAE CNN	54.60 ± 1.83	55.39 ± 1.50	54.39 ± 1.66	53.98 ± 2.06
cWGAN-GP CNN	55.97 ± 2.71	58.28 ± 2.28	55.77 ± 2.60	54.87 ± 3.65
LSTM	36.54 ± 2.20	36.59 ± 2.25	36.47 ± 2.22	36.39 ± 2.22
NI LSTM	36.67 ± 0.84	36.76 ± 0.78	36.70 ± 0.79	36.50 ± 0.81
cVAE LSTM	35.44 ± 1.56	35.45 ± 1.52	35.37 ± 1.60	35.31 ± 1.58
cWGAN-GP LSTM	**37.22 ± 1.88**	**37.30 ± 1.96**	**37.12 ± 1.89**	**36.92 ± 1.93**

Table 5. Resulting metrics for augmentation methods; input feature vectors are represented as frequency spectra and binary classification is performed.

Method	FID	SNR	RMSE	CC
NI	146.959	3.234	1.41416	0.085
cVAE	**88.063**	**27.25**	1.41159	**0.194**
cWGAN-GP	151.276	11.651	**1.41107**	0.173

Table 6. Classification results; input feature vectors are represented as frequency spectra and binary classification is performed.

Method	Accuracy	Precision	Recall	F1 Score
SVM	64.79 ± 0.46	64.78 ± 0.46	64.77 ± 0.46	64.76 ± 0.46
NI SVM	**65.17 ± 0.50**	**65.18 ± 0.50**	**65.14 ± 0.51**	**65.13 ± 0.51**
cVAE SVM	64.55 ± 0.46	64.56 ± 0.46	64.56 ± 0.46	64.55 ± 0.46
cWGAN-GP SVM	64.92 ± 0.45	64.93 ± 0.44	64.93 ± 0.44	64.92 ± 0.44
LDA	59.56 ± 0.81	59.71 ± 0.81	59.43 ± 0.82	59.20 ± 0.86
NI LDA	**62.71 ± 0.53**	**63.25 ± 0.59**	**62.54 ± 0.52**	**62.13 ± 0.52**
cVAE LDA	58.87 ± 1.09	58.92 ± 1.10	58.77 ± 1.09	58.63 ± 1.11
cWGAN-GP LDA	59.47 ± 0.76	59.70 ± 0.81	59.33 ± 0.75	59.01 ± 0.75
MLP	63.85 ± 1.18	64.29 ± 1.00	63.89 ± 1.18	63.59 ± 1.38
NI MLP	64.00 ± 1.08	64.42 ± 1.14	64.04 ± 1.11	**63.77 ± 1.14**
cVAE MLP	62.60 ± 1.73	62.76 ± 1.73	62.54 ± 1.74	62.40 ± 1.81
cWGAN-GP MLP	**64.16 ± 0.77**	**64.94 ± 1.11**	**64.17 ± 0.75**	63.71 ± 0.79
CNN	63.54 ± 0.72	63.68 ± 0.72	63.56 ± 0.73	63.47 ± 0.75
NI CNN	**64.55 ± 0.65**	**64.64 ± 0.67**	**64.54 ± 0.67**	**64.47 ± 0.68**
cVAE CNN	61.29 ± 1.78	61.95 ± 1.76	61.29 ± 1.85	60.71 ± 2.12
cWGAN-GP CNN	63.53 ± 0.92	64.00 ± 1.00	63.62 ± 0.92	63.31 ± 0.99
LSTM	62.99 ± 0.84	63.12 ± 0.80	62.95 ± 0.88	62.84 ± 0.94
NI LSTM	**64.14 ± 0.49**	**64.40 ± 0.62**	**64.05 ± 0.48**	**63.88 ± 0.50**
cVAE LSTM	62.46 ± 0.85	62.56 ± 0.91	62.42 ± 0.81	62.34 ± 0.77
cWGAN-GP LSTM	63.15 ± 1.29	63.26 ± 1.26	63.18 ± 1.28	63.10 ± 1.31

5   Discussion

The best classification accuracy ($76.00 \pm 0.80\%$) was achieved using the CNN classifier without any augmentation for binary classification of time series input feature vectors. For binary classification of input feature vectors represented in the frequency spectrum, the highest accuracy ($65.17 \pm 0.50\%$) was obtained with the SVM classifier on data augmented using the NI method. When classifying data in which input feature vectors are represented in the time-frequency domain, the CNN classifier combined with the NI augmentation method achieved the best result ($74.36 \pm 0.66\%$). The results of other classification metrics closely matched the classification accuracy, indicating that the models performed well, which was expected given the balanced representation of the classes. We can thus state that the representation of the input feature vector in the frequency or time-frequency domain has not improved the classification results.

The CNN classifier produced the best results in 4 out of 6 combinations of input feature vector representations and classification tasks. Additionally, it significantly outperformed the other classifiers, as demonstrated by the McNemar test, with $p < 0.01$. These results also show an improvement over those reported in [8] and [11]. The differences

Table 7. Resulting metrics for augmentation methods; input feature vectors are represented as frequency spectra and multiclass classification is performed.

Method	FID	SNR	RMSE	CC
NI	148.893	3.248	1.41391	0.145
cVAE	**84.142**	**23.527**	**1.41121**	0.207
cWGAN-GP	153.797	18.413	1.4326	**0.265**

Table 8. Classification results; input feature vectors are represented as frequency spectra and multiclass classification is performed.

Method	Accuracy	Precision	Recall	F1 Score
SVM	49.45 ± 0.54	49.72 ± 0.62	49.11 ± 0.47	49.02 ± 0.45
NI SVM	49.01 ± 0.62	49.19 ± 0.64	48.61 ± 0.63	48.47 ± 0.66
cVAE SVM	**50.81 ± 0.57**	**51.01 ± 0.54**	**50.79 ± 0.55**	**50.76 ± 0.57**
cWGAN-GP SVM	47.30 ± 0.81	47.71 ± 1.07	46.78 ± 0.80	46.28 ± 0.85
LDA	45.62 ± 0.71	45.78 ± 0.78	45.63 ± 0.70	45.46 ± 0.72
NI LDA	**48.82 ± 0.66**	**48.93 ± 0.62**	**48.73 ± 0.64**	**48.75 ± 0.65**
cVAE LDA	43.51 ± 0.97	43.57 ± 0.97	43.52 ± 0.96	43.39 ± 0.97
cWGAN-GP LDA	45.22 ± 0.80	45.40 ± 0.75	45.21 ± 0.81	45.10 ± 0.79
MLP	49.08 ± 1.37	50.24 ± 1.23	48.93 ± 1.60	48.33 ± 2.13
NI MLP	48.12 ± 2.81	49.56 ± 1.73	48.18 ± 2.50	47.13 ± 3.65
cVAE MLP	48.38 ± 1.41	48.53 ± 1.40	48.23 ± 1.45	47.72 ± 1.81
cWGAN-GP MLP	**49.83 ± 0.97**	**51.25 ± 2.35**	**50.00 ± 1.31**	**49.06 ± 1.21**
CNN	**49.03 ± 1.22**	**49.70 ± 1.14**	48.59 ± 1.33	48.03 ± 1.73
NI CNN	48.92 ± 1.34	49.18 ± 1.35	**48.65 ± 1.28**	**48.40 ± 1.48**
cVAE CNN	43.47 ± 1.28	46.18 ± 1.74	43.05 ± 1.08	40.37 ± 1.38
cWGAN-GP CNN	46.36 ± 0.66	46.99 ± 1.39	46.25 ± 0.92	45.34 ± 1.03
LSTM	47.57 ± 0.43	47.96 ± 0.49	47.47 ± 0.59	47.06 ± 0.73
NI LSTM	48.25 ± 2.05	48.56 ± 1.94	48.09 ± 2.03	47.87 ± 2.03
cVAE LSTM	47.74 ± 1.39	47.78 ± 1.57	47.81 ± 1.48	47.60 ± 1.53
cWGAN-GP LSTM	**48.75 ± 1.06**	**48.88 ± 1.26**	**48.69 ± 1.18**	**48.47 ± 1.17**

Table 9. Resulting metrics for augmentation methods; input feature vectors are represented as time-frequency spectra and binary classification is performed.

Method	SNR	RMSE	CC
NI	3.739	1.41512	0.068
cVAE	**23.958**	1.40526	**0.211**
cWGAN-GP	7.895	**1.37666**	0.175

Table 10. Classification results; input feature vectors are represented as time-frequency spectra and binary classification is performed.

Method	Accuracy	Precision	Recall	F1 Score
SVM	67.91 ± 0.51	67.92 ± 0.51	67.90 ± 0.51	67.90 ± 0.51
NI SVM	$\mathbf{69.11 \pm 0.60}$	$\mathbf{69.20 \pm 0.59}$	$\mathbf{69.14 \pm 0.60}$	$\mathbf{69.09 \pm 0.60}$
cVAE SVM	67.40 ± 0.42	67.46 ± 0.42	67.38 ± 0.41	67.35 ± 0.42
cWGAN-GP SVM	67.26 ± 0.58	67.30 ± 0.59	67.24 ± 0.58	67.23 ± 0.58
LDA	55.27 ± 1.34	55.31 ± 1.35	55.29 ± 1.34	55.23 ± 1.34
NI LDA	54.38 ± 1.41	54.42 ± 1.42	54.40 ± 1.41	54.34 ± 1.41
cVAE LDA	$\mathbf{55.33 \pm 1.56}$	$\mathbf{55.33 \pm 1.56}$	$\mathbf{55.33 \pm 1.56}$	$\mathbf{55.31 \pm 1.56}$
cWGAN-GP LDA	52.57 ± 2.29	52.58 ± 2.29	52.57 ± 2.29	52.57 ± 2.29
MLP	66.93 ± 1.50	67.44 ± 1.44	66.93 ± 1.54	66.68 ± 1.70
NI MLP	66.28 ± 1.00	66.94 ± 1.16	66.33 ± 1.00	66.00 ± 1.06
cVAE MLP	67.46 ± 1.53	67.78 ± 1.36	67.46 ± 1.56	67.30 ± 1.71
cWGAN-GP MLP	$\mathbf{67.58 \pm 1.71}$	$\mathbf{68.08 \pm 1.56}$	$\mathbf{67.57 \pm 1.75}$	$\mathbf{67.33 \pm 1.92}$
CNN	74.02 ± 1.15	74.50 ± 1.09	74.07 ± 1.15	73.92 ± 1.19
NI CNN	$\mathbf{74.36 \pm 0.66}$	$\mathbf{74.85 \pm 0.72}$	$\mathbf{74.40 \pm 0.66}$	$\mathbf{74.25 \pm 0.69}$
cVAE CNN	73.43 ± 1.29	73.98 ± 0.81	$73.46 \pm \pm 1.26$	73.28 ± 1.46
cWGAN-GP CNN	73.58 ± 1.53	74.72 ± 1.60	73.64 ± 1.52	73.30 ± 1.65
LSTM	65.30 ± 1.08	65.43 ± 1.11	65.31 ± 1.08	65.24 ± 1.07
NI LSTM	65.49 ± 1.70	65.58 ± 1.71	65.51 ± 1.71	65.45 ± 1.71
cVAE LSTM	64.48 ± 1.08	64.61 ± 1.07	64.50 ± 1.08	64.42 ± 1.11
cWGAN-GP LSTM	$\mathbf{66.97 \pm 1.25}$	$\mathbf{67.21 \pm 1.19}$	$\mathbf{66.98 \pm 1.25}$	$\mathbf{66.86 \pm 1.30}$

in performance among the classifiers used are likely due to the high dimensionality of the input feature vectors.

It is interesting to compare the results of binary and multiclass classification. The best multiclass classification accuracy ($58.57 \pm 1.45\%$) was achieved by the CNN on data augmented with NI. Overall, the multiclass classification results are significantly worse than those of binary classification, with most classifiers failing to reach 50% accuracy in the multiclass task. This indicates that while the classifiers could distinguish between the subject's resting state and movement state, they struggled to differentiate between left-hand and right-hand movements.

The impact of augmentation methods on classification results is generally not encouraging. However, in most cases, at least one augmentation method led to some improvement in classification accuracy compared to classification without augmentation. These modest improvements are consistent with the findings reported in [7].

A key factor in the usability of a BCI system is the classification time. The longer the classification time, the longer the BCI system takes to respond to a request, such as assisting with a movement. If the response time is too long, it can be uncomfortable for the user. While the training time of the classifier is also important, it can be performed

Table 11. Resulting metrics for augmentation methods; input feature vectors are represented as time-frequency spectra and multiclass classification is performed.

Method	SNR	RMSE	CC
NI	3.711	1.41177	0.072
cVAE	**24.332**	1.40101	**0.263**
cWGAN-GP	5.704	**1.3565**	0.227

Table 12. Classification results; input feature vectors are represented as time-frequency spectra and multiclass classification is performed.

Method	Accuracy	Precision	Recall	F1 Score
SVM	50.46 ± 1.06	50.36 ± 1.08	49.95 ± 1.08	49.83 ± 1.16
NI SVM	**50.97 ± 0.82**	**51.22 ± 0.84**	**50.83 ± 0.83**	**50.85 ± 0.83**
cVAE SVM	49.47 ± 0.41	49.04 ± 0.41	48.91 ± 0.39	48.86 ± 0.39
cWGAN-GP SVM	47.94 ± 0.60	48.60 ± 0.68	47.20 ± 0.62	45.82 ± 1.04
LDA	**39.03 ± 1.67**	**38.92 ± 1.65**	**38.93 ± 1.72**	**38.86 ± 1.67**
NI LDA	38.12 ± 1.89	38.20 ± 1.96	38.14 ± 1.95	38.04 ± 1.91
cVAE LDA	34.76 ± 1.15	35.39 ± 1.20	35.00 ± 1.17	34.71 ± 1.16
cWGAN-GP LDA	34.03 ± 2.08	33.86 ± 2.14	33.82 ± 2.11	33.78 ± 2.10
MLP	48.49 ± 1.45	49.75 ± 1.39	48.33 ± 1.46	**47.01 ± 2.67**
NI MLP	46.21 ± 2.12	47.18 ± 2.38	46.06 ± 1.91	44.93 ± 1.89
cVAE MLP	45.61 ± 1.56	47.52 ± 2.93	45.62 ± 1.84	44.44 ± 2.12
cWGAN-GP MLP	**48.93 ± 1.95**	**50.59 ± 2.30**	**48.55 ± 1.85**	46.98 ± 2.94
CNN	56.05 ± 1.83	57.78 ± 1.46	56.18 ± 1.78	56.03 ± 1.88
NI CNN	**56.99 ± 0.91**	**58.17 ± 0.94**	**56.93 ± 0.91**	**56.92 ± 0.88**
cVAE CNN	55.02 ± 1.86	56.53 ± 1.80	55.12 ± 1.92	54.80 ± 2.10
cWGAN-GP CNN	55.46 ± 1.51	56.17 ± 1.48	55.21 ± 1.49	55.07 ± 1.58
LSTM	40.28 ± 1.64	40.46 ± 1.62	40.08 ± 1.58	39.28 ± 2.17
NI LSTM	40.44 ± 2.03	**40.72 ± 2.01**	**40.26 ± 2.04**	**40.10 ± 2.10**
cVAE LSTM	**40.61 ± 1.60**	40.29 ± 1.87	40.21 ± 1.55	39.28 ± 2.07
cWGAN-GP LSTM	39.72 ± 1.72	39.96 ± 1.74	39.53 ± 1.78	39.37 ± 1.83

offline and is, therefore, not as crucial as the classification time, which needs to occur in real time. It can be stated that the classification times achieved by most classifiers in these experiments are in acceptable time ranges.

It is important to note that although a reasonably good classification accuracy was achieved, the data were collected from a relatively small, non-representative sample of 29 healthy individuals aged 19 to 25 years. The target users of the BCI system are individuals recovering from motor function injuries, so it is uncertain whether the EEG signals of these individuals will be similar to those of healthy subjects.

Most hyperparameters for the classifiers and augmentation methods were set empirically or based on similar studies; a more comprehensive search of the hyperparameter space could potentially improve classification results. Additionally, it would be beneficial to investigate the impact of augmentation methods on classification results using a larger amount of generated data. Furthermore, intra-subject models may also yield better classification results.

6   Conclusion

This paper presents the results achieved by applying augmentation and classification methods on a dataset collected from motor imagery experiments when three different representations of input feature vectors are used. Overall, these experiments aim to verify whether the MI paradigm can be effectively used for real BCI-controlled and robot-assisted motor rehabilitation.

Data augmentation was performed using three different methods. A single-trial inter-subject model was trained, and MI patterns were detected using five classifiers. The highest accuracy ($76.00 \pm 0.80\%$) was achieved with the CNN classifier without any dataset augmentation using the time-series representation of the input feature vector. While the results of data augmentation and classification are not particularly encouraging, they are comparable to those reported in the literature and show some improvements over previous work described in [8] and [11].

Future work will focus on completing the experiments, increasing the size of real-world data by conducting experiments with the target population, generating more artificial data, and training and utilizing intra-subject models.

Acknowledgments. This work was supported by project FW03010025 Therapeutic rehabilitation robot controlled by brain signals, and the university-specific research project SGS-2022-016 Advanced Methods of Data Processing and Analysis (project SGS-2022-016).

Disclosure of Interests. The authors have no competing interests.

References

1. Abdelfattah, S.M., Abdelrahman, G.M., Wang, M.: Augmenting the size of EEG datasets using generative adversarial networks. In: 2018 International Joint Conference on Neural Networks (IJCNN), pp. 1–6 (2018). https://doi.org/10.1109/IJCNN.2018.8489727
2. Al-Saegh, A., Dawwd, S.A., Abdul-Jabbar, J.M.: Deep learning for motor imagery EEG-based classification: a review. Biomed. Signal Process. Control **63**, 102172 (2021). https://doi.org/10.1016/j.bspc.2020.102172. https://www.sciencedirect.com/science/article/pii/S1746809420303116
3. Altaheri, H., et al.: Deep learning techniques for classification of electroencephalogram (EEG) motor imagery (MI) signals: a review. Neural Comput. Appl. **35**(20), 14681–14722 (2023)
4. Echtioui, A., Zouch, W., Ghorbel, M.: Merged CNNs for the classification of EEG motor imagery signals. Multimed. Tools Appl. 1–23 (2024)

5. He, C., Liu, J., Zhu, Y., Du, W.: Data augmentation for deep neural networks model in EEG classification task: a review. Front. Hum. Neurosci. **15** (2021). https://doi.org/10.3389/fnhum.2021.765525. https://www.frontiersin.org/articles/10.3389/fnhum.2021.765525
6. Iglesias, G., Talavera, E., Gonzalez-Prieto, A., Mozo, A., Gómez-Canaval, S.: Data augmentation techniques in time series domain: a survey and taxonomy. Neural Comput. Appl. **35**(14), 10123–10145 (2023). https://doi.org/10.1007/s00521-023-08459-3
7. Lashgari, E., Liang, D., Maoz, U.: Data augmentation for deep-learning-based electroencephalography. J. Neurosci. Methods **346**, 108885 (2020). https://doi.org/10.1016/j.jneumeth.2020.108885. https://www.sciencedirect.com/science/article/pii/S0165027020303083
8. Mochura, P.: Detection of limb movement from EEG signal during exercise on a rehabilitation robot. Diploma thesis (2021). (in Czech)
9. Mouček, R., Kodera, J., Mautner, P., Průcha, J.: Augmentation of motor imagery data for brain-controlled robot-assisted rehabilitation. In: Proceedings of the 17th International Joint Conference on Biomedical Engineering Systems and Technologies - Volume 2: HEALTHINF, pp. 812–819. INSTICC, SciTePress (2024). https://doi.org/10.5220/0012575700003657
10. Roy, Y., Banville, H., Albuquerque, I., Gramfort, A., Falk, T.H., Faubert, J.: Deep learning-based electroencephalography analysis: a systematic review. J. Neural Eng. **16**(5), 051001 (2019). https://doi.org/10.1088/1741-2552/ab260c
11. Saleh, J.Y.: Design of movement detector of measured EEG data. Bachelor thesis (2022)
12. Tan, X., Wang, D., Chen, J., Xu, M.: Transformer-based network with optimization for cross-subject motor imagery identification. Bioengineering **10**(5), 609 (2023). https://doi.org/10.3390/bioengineering10050609. https://www.ncbi.nlm.nih.gov/pmc/articles/PMC10215191/
13. Tang, Z., Li, C., Sun, S.: Single-trial EEG classification of motor imagery using deep convolutional neural networks. Optik **130**, 11–18 (2017). https://doi.org/10.1016/j.ijleo.2016.10.117. https://www.sciencedirect.com/science/article/pii/S0030402616312980
14. Vařeka, L.: Methods for signal classification and their application to the design of brain-computer interfaces (2018). https://dspace5.zcu.cz/bitstream/11025/33651/1/PhdThesisVareka2018.pdf, disertační práce
15. Yang, J., Yu, H., Shen, T., Song, Y., Chen, Z.: 4-class MI-EEG signal generation and recognition with CVAE-GAN. Appl. Sci. **11**(4) (2021). https://doi.org/10.3390/app11041798. https://www.mdpi.com/2076-3417/11/4/1798
16. Zhang, J., Wang, M.: A survey on robots controlled by motor imagery brain-computer interfaces. Cogn. Robot. **1**, 12–24 (2021)
17. Zhang, K., et al.: Data augmentation for motor imagery signal classification based on a hybrid neural network. Sensors **20**(16) (2020). https://doi.org/10.3390/s20164485. https://www.mdpi.com/1424-8220/20/16/4485

Diagnosis of Resting Tremor in Parkinson's Disease Using Accelerometer and Gyroscope Sensors Built into a Smartwatch

Carlos Polvorinos-Fernández[1] , Luis Sigcha[2] , Luigi Borzì[4,5] ,
Paulo Cardoso[3] , Nelson Costa[3] , Susana Costa[3] , Juan Manuel López[6] ,
César Asensio[7] , Guillermo de Arcas[1] , and Ignacio Pavón[1(✉)]

[1] Department of Mechanical Engineering, Instrumentation and Applied Acoustics Research
Group, ETS Ingenieros Industriales, Universidad Politécnica de Madrid, Madrid, Spain
c.polvorinos@upm.es
[2] Department of Physical Education and Sports Science, Health Research Institute, &
Data-Driven Computer Engineering (D2iCE) Group, University of Limerick,
Limerick V94 T9PX, Ireland
[3] ALGORITMI Research Center, School of Engineering, University of Minho, Guimarães,
Portugal
[4] PolitoBIOMed Lab–Biomedical Engineering Lab, Politecnico Di Torino, 10129 Turin, Italy
[5] ANTHEA Lab–Data Analytics and Technologies for Health Lab, Department of Control and
Computer Engineering, Politecnico Di Torino, 10129 Turin, Italy
[6] Department of Physical Electronics, Electrical Engineering and Applied Physics,
Instrumentation and Applied Acoustics Research Group, ETS Ingeniería y Sistemas de
Comunicación, Universidad Politécnica de Madrid, Madrid, Spain
[7] Department of Audiovisual Engineering and Communications, Instrumentation and Applied
Acoustics Research Group, ETS Ingeniería y Sistemas de Comunicación, Universidad
Politécnica de Madrid, Madrid, Spain

Abstract. Monitoring resting tremor in Parkinson's disease (PD) can be performed using wearable technology and machine learning. Smartwatches offer a
cost-effective and non-intrusive way to track tremors remotely. However, to ensure
precise monitoring in free-living environments, optimized systems are needed.
This chapter discuss about the performance of inertial sensors to identify resting tremors and its classification according to MDS-UPDRS III. Six PD patients
wore a smartwatch on their wrists while performing different exercise based on
MDS-UPDRS. During eight weeks, data from triaxial accelerometers and gyroscopes were collected simultaneously and analyzed using machine learning techniques. In tremor presence detection, using binary classification, the use of only
accelerometer gives the best results in terms of accuracy (97%) and training time
(47 s) compared accelerometer and gyroscope combined (96.4% and 67 s) and only
gyroscope alone (93% and 59 s). In the MDS-UPDRS scale detection, using multiclass models, the best accuracy is offered by the combination of accelerometer and
gyroscope (96.5%) but offers the worst training times (77 s), while accelerometer
is slightly worse (96.1%) but require the less training time (57 s). These results
show the performance and training times of Machine Learning models for the
detection of resting tremor and prediction of the MDS-UPDRS assessment for the

© The Author(s), under exclusive license to Springer Nature Switzerland AG 2026
M. P. Guarino et al. (Eds.): BIOSTEC 2024, CCIS 2546, pp. 460–481, 2026.
https://doi.org/10.1007/978-3-031-96899-0_26

correct decision making of sensors and models to be used in future application developments. The results could be used to contribute to the development of reliable tremor monitoring systems using devices equipped with inertial sensors and Machine Learning algorithms.

Keywords: Motor symptoms · Wearables · Accelerometer · Gyroscope · Machine Learning

1 Introduction

Parkinson's disease (PD) is a neurodegenerative disorder that primarily affects the central nervous system, leading to both motor and non-motor symptoms. The disease is characterized by the death of dopamine-producing neurons in the brain, which results in a deficit of dopamine—a critical neurotransmitter responsible for regulating movement and coordination [1].

Globally, Parkinson's disease affects an estimated 7 to 10 million people, with the number of cases rising in recent years. The prevalence of PD shows a marked increase with advancing age, particularly affecting about 1% of individuals aged 60 and older [2]. While the disease can occur at younger ages, it is relatively rare before the age of 50. Additionally, epidemiological studies indicate that men are more likely to develop Parkinson's disease than women. The development of the disease varies significantly from person to person. Over time, patients go through different stages of the disease, which are directly related to the severity of the symptoms and the degree of physical disability they cause.

The symptoms of the disease can be classified into two main groups (Balestrino & Schapira, 2020). The non-motor or "premotor" symptoms can occur prior to the motor symptoms or coexist with the motor symptoms. These mainly consist of neuropsychiatric disorders, such as anxiety, depression or apathy, sleep disorders, digestive or sensory disorders, and may experience various types of pain or paresthesia (tingling sensation, cold or heat in a localized part of the body). The motor symptoms are bradykinesia (loss of speed and amplitude in voluntary mobility) together with muscle stiffness, tremor, freezing or instability of gait. Other motor symptoms may be decreased facial expression, decreased tone of voice or accumulation of saliva in the mouth [3].

Among the motor symptoms in PD, tremor is the most prevalent and diagnostically significant motor symptom [4]. Tremors are characterized by involuntary, rhythmic oscillations affecting various parts of the body, commonly the hands or feet. PD-associated tremors are categorized into two main types: resting tremors and action tremors. Resting tremors occur when the affected body part is relaxed and not engaged in purposeful movement, whereas action tremors manifest during voluntary movements or when maintaining a position against gravity [5].

The frequency of this type of tremor in PD is found around 3.5–7 Hz range [6], whereas normal human movements generally occur within the 0–20 Hz band [7].

Levodopa is the principal drug used to treat PD actively [8]. It acts by converting to dopamine in the brain and works vigorously on the tremors of patients, although as the disease progresses, the effect of levodopa diminishes and may even have negative effects due to its accumulation.

The diagnosis and monitoring of this disease is nowadays carried out by a medical specialist who observes a series of exercises carried out by the patients and subjectively classifies them into a stage of the disease [9]. One of the ways to assess the severity of PD is using standardized guidelines, composed of a series of items that relate to symptoms caused by PD quantitatively assessed. In this work, the Movement Disorders Society's review of the Unified Parkinson's Disease Rating Scale (MDS-UPDRS) [10] has been taken as a reference.

During these check-ups, medication is regulated based on a diagnosis provided by the patients themselves of their condition since the last appointment in a diary known as the patient's notebook. It should be noted that 70% of Parkinson's patients are over 65 years of age, and it is therefore often the case that memory loss occurs, sometimes caused by the disease itself, which means that the diagnosis provided by the specialist cannot fulfil its optimal purpose. For this reason, the need of tools to improve the diagnosis and continuous monitoring is still required.

Currently, smart technologies for use in diseases such as PD are increasing, in particular, wearable technologies, stand out for their low cost, battery life, non-invasiveness, and above all their accuracy in data collection, creating the perfect cocktail of attributes to monitor PD [11].

The use of inertial sensors such as accelerometers and gyroscopes in smart wearable watches, their low battery consumption, their light weight, and in combination with advances in communication systems are bringing new ways of diagnosing PD to the patient [12]. Therefore, the combination of data collection from inertial sensors included in wearable devices together with an appropriate processing of these data and a subsequent implementation of artificial intelligence algorithms can be a valid alternative for the monitoring of motor symptoms in PD in free-living conditions.

This study evaluated the performance of inertial sensors integrated into a smartwatch to determine which provides greater accuracy in classifying tremors in Parkinson's disease patients using machine learning models. In [13] has been explored in the comparative between accelerometer and gyroscope. This paper will study will discuss the comparison of using accelerometer and gyroscope data independently versus using accelerometer and gyroscope data in combination. In addition, the time required to each combination to train the Machine Learning models will be studied. The dataset [14] comprises weekly records from multiple Parkinson's disease patients who wore a smartwatch during various planned activities.

2 Background

Currently, the predominant standardized method for assessing PD is the MDS-UPDRS. In this guide, motor symptoms are assessed in part III, utilizing a scale from 0 to 4, where 0 indicates the absence of symptoms and 4 denotes the most severe manifestation. Item 3.17 is of special interest, where the object of study is the "Amplitude of tremor at rest", and which will be the criterion used in this work to compare it with the clinical assessment performed. In this task, the patient should sit quietly in a chair with hands resting on the armrest (not on the lap) and feet resting comfortably on the floor, for 10 s, without any other indication. Resting tremor is evaluated separately for each limb, lip and jaw.

However, this evaluation of tremor amplitude (and the rest of the sections of the guide) is subjective on the part of the physician and depends on his or her perception at the time, which may vary from one neurologist to another. This, together with the fact that patients make very occasional visits to the clinic, has led many authors to study the possibility of remote and objective symptom monitoring. This initiative has been enhanced by the situation during the COVID-19 pandemic emergency, when many patients, especially those living in remote areas, found it difficult to attend consultations [15].

Hence, in recent years, lot of studies have explored the potential of wearable devices in healthcare applications. Some studies have focused on the development of specific devices, while others have used commercial devices for the evaluation of PD pathologies [16].

Regardless of how the monitoring has been approached, MEMS (Micro Electronic Mechanical Systems) type sensors have been used due to their small size and low cost. Specifically, the most common sensors used in motor symptom monitoring are the accelerometer and the gyroscope. The combination of data from these sensors has allowed to understand better how a patient moves and to identify anomalous patterns.

A study conducted by [17] used the Axivity AX3 accelerometers to compare tremor detection in semi-free-living conditions and in the laboratory environment, achieving a 10% and 5% error. In [18], a comparison of peak frequencies of tremor measurements using a triaxial accelerometer versus data collected using different smartphones was made, showing a variability in measurements of 13.4%.

[12] performed a follow-up of parkinsonian tremor severity using a gyroscope placed on the wrist and ankle of the most affected side, achieving a correlation of $r = 0.93$ with the clinical evaluation. A study [19]conducted one year of monitoring using an Android app installed on a smartwatch that collected data from a gyroscope yielded a Spearman coefficient between the mean of the resting tremor (UPDRS-III) scores and smartwatch measurements for tremor intensity was 0.81.

The combination of accelerometer and gyroscope data for tremor detection was evaluated in [20], where a watch integrating both sensors was developed, achieving a tremor detection accuracy of over 94%. In [21], a correlation of $p = 0.8$ was obtained between the clinical assessment of tremor and the accelerometer and gyroscope signal from an Apple Watch.

Despite advancements in tremor monitoring, previous studies have overlooked the specific evaluation of which inertial sensor (accelerometer or gyroscope) can offer more information for assessing this symptom. If live monitoring of PD motor symptoms using these sensors is desired, it is of interest to perform the measurements with devices that have an optimal battery cost-computational cost-accuracy ratio. This study aims to explore the potential of inertial sensors embedded in commercial smartwatches for detecting resting tremor and their computational time cost.

3 Materials and Methods

3.1 Data Collection

The data used in this study were collected during the TECAPARK project [22], using a proprietary m-health application named Monipar [23]. A consumer-grade smartwatch and a smartphone were used to monitor motor symptoms in PD patients. Monipar application guides the user through exercises by showing the tasks to be performed on the mobile screen while collect data from the inertial sensors of the smartwatch.

The Monipar dataset comprises weekly records from individuals with Parkinson's disease engaged in planned activities, which included standardized exercises and resting periods for their upper limbs, all while wearing a smartwatch. This project was approved by the ethics committee of the Universidad Politécnica de Madrid and all study participants were informed prior to participation and signed an informed consent agreement.

Six PD patients (3 males/3 females, 64.2 ± 8.2 years) were recruited from a Parkinson's association in Guimaraes (Portugal) who were in the early stages of the disease according to the Hoehn and Yahr scale [24] (H&Y = 1).

Three participants did not present tremors while the other three presented tremors. Tremor amplitude was evaluated by a specialist neurologist according to MDS-UPDRS 3.17 between 0 (no tremor) and 2 (mild tremor).

The data collection process was carried out over 8 weeks. Patients were evaluated in their optimal ON state, characterized by the effective control of motor symptoms through medication, as determined through clinical assessments and patient-reported histories. Throughout the study, all patients maintained their usual medication regimen.

MATLAB software (R2017a) was utilized for tasks such as signal labeling, preprocessing, and feature extraction. For model evaluation and training, Python (3.6) was used, along with the Pandas and Scikit-learn libraries.

3.2 Acquisition Device (SmartWatch)

A consumer-grade smartwatch was used as the data acquisition device during the measurement sessions and was worn on the wrist of the most affected side. The wearable device used will collect all the vibration signals in the time domain thanks to the built-in inertial sensors (accelerometer and gyroscope). Both sensors collect the signals distributed in three axes, in the case of the accelerometer, acceleration in m/s2, and for the gyroscope, angular acceleration in rad/s.

In this study, the smartwatch used is a Mobvoi TicWatch S2 with WearOs® as the operating system. Its dimensions are 46.6 × 51.8 × 12.9 mm and it has a weight of 32.5 g. This smartwatch is equipped with an LSM6DS3 type package, which is comprised of 3-axial gyroscope (measurement range of ±2000 dps) and a 3-axial accelerometer (maximum measurement amplitude of ±2 g).

The smartwatch was configured to record data at a sampling rate of 50 Hz. This frequency is suitable for analyzing human movement, as typical movements occur in the 0–20 Hz range. It also allows for the recording of typical Parkinson's disease tremors, which fall within the 3.5–7 Hz range [6].

3.3 Experimental Protocol

In each measurement session, each participant performed the 8 tasks using Monipar application, supervised by a staff member. These 8 exercises were designed to evaluate their PD motor status. In specific, each exercise belongs to the MDS-UPDRS part III. The exercises proposed in this app are related to the amplitude of resting and postural tremor of the hands, movement of the hands towards the chest, finger tapping, hand movements, pronation-supination of the hands, getting up and gait.

Each exercise, which includes a short explanation, varies in duration in its execution; some last 15 s, while others may require more than 40 s. Additionally, there is a 30-s break between exercises, so the approximate duration of each measurement session about 7 min. Additionally, each patient's sessions were also video recorded for subsequent labeling.

For the development of this study, only the data associated with resting tremor amplitude was used. The resting tremor amplitude is evaluated by Sect. 3.17 of the MDS-UPDRS. During this evaluation, the patient sits calmly in a chair with their hands on the armrests (not on their lap) and their feet flat on the floor for a duration of 10 s, with no further instructions given. The interface for the resting tremor exercise is depicted in Fig. 1.

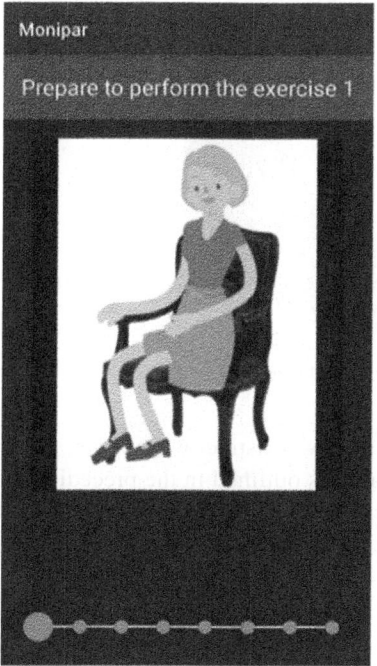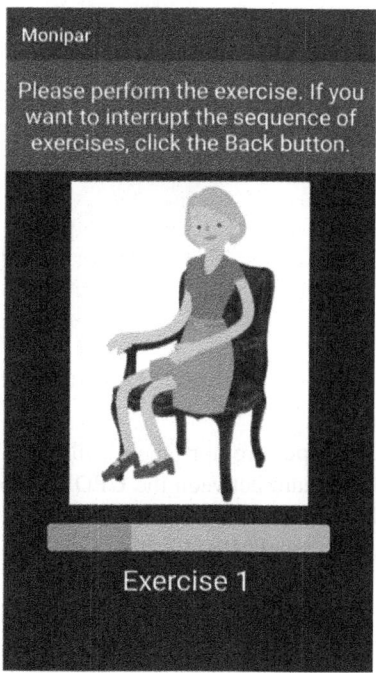

Fig. 1. Exercise related to resting tremor amplitude in mobile application (a) explanation (b) execution [23].

3.4 Data Labeling

For data labeling, the label generated automatically for each exercise from Monipar application were used. The exercises are numbered sequentially from 1 to 8, based on the order in which the participants performed it. The label for the resting tremor exercise is 1.

The data related to resting tremor were labeled according to the maximum amplitude of the movement according to MDS-UPDRS Sect. 3.17. In particular, the label 0 (Normal) corresponds if no tremor is observed, 1 (Minimal) if the maximum amplitude of the movement is less than 1 cm, 2 (Mild) if the maximum amplitude is between 1 and 3 cm, 3 (Moderate) if it is between 3 and 10 cm and 4 (Severe) if the amplitude is greater than 10 cm. These labels were verified and corrected using video recording for each of the measurement session.

Figure 2 illustrates the distribution of tremor labels according to UPDRS Sect. 3.17. For the dataset used, the available labels are 0, 1, and 2. Label 0 is the most prevalent, appearing in 78% of the data, while 1 represents the 15% and 2 the 7%.

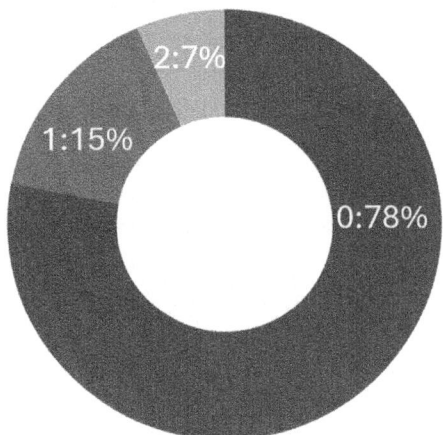

Fig. 2. Observations distributed by tremor label.

In this paper, tremor labels will be utilized in two distinct ways. First, the analysis will differentiate between the UPDRS categories as outlined in the preceding sections. Second, the focus will shift to a binary distinction between the presence and absence of tremor, with labels 1 and 2 combined into a single category.

3.5 Algorithmic Approach

This paper introduces machine learning models designed to predict tremor amplitude levels using data from accelerometers and gyroscopes. In this context, it will be evaluated which option, accelerometer or gyroscope alone, or the combination of both provides better results for the detection of resting tremor. Figure 3 shows the following steps followed in this work.

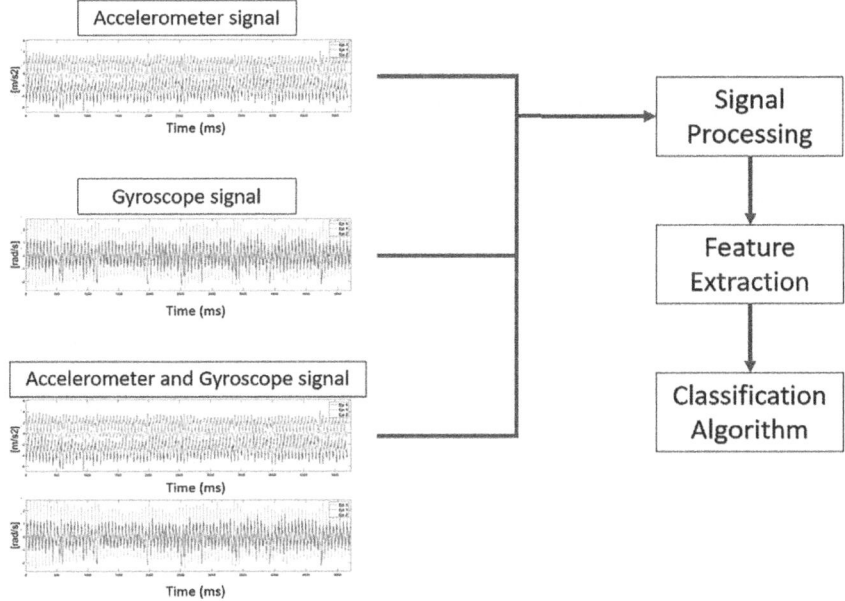

Fig. 3. Diagram of Algorithm Development.

For the training and evaluation of the proposed models, the smartwatch signals were processing. Initially, signals from each of the three sensor axes were merged into a single signal using the Euclidean Norm, as defined in Eqs. (1) and (2). This merging was necessary to account for the arbitrary orientation of the wearable device's inertial sensors, thus mitigating errors from potential data collection inconsistencies. Furthermore, this approach helps to reduce the computational complexity.

$$Accel = \sqrt{accel_x^2 + accel_y^2 + accel_z^2} \tag{1}$$

$$Gyro = \sqrt{gyro_x^2 + gyro_y^2 + gyro_z^2} \tag{2}$$

Subsequently, the signal obtained from the Euclidean norm was filtered with a third-order Butterworth band-pass filter to select the data between frequencies between 0.5 and 10 Hz. This range is ideal for recognizing human activities and is particularly relevant for detecting tremors in Parkinson's disease [25].

Following, the signal was segmented into windows of 128 samples each, equating to 2.56 s per window, with a 50% overlap between consecutive windows. In total, 8817 windows were defined. This method of segmentation and overlapping is recommended for analyzing Parkinson's disease tremors using inertial sensors [26], and will be employed to evaluate which sensor provides the most accurate results.

Finally, the signal was converted to the frequency domain using the Fast Fourier Transform (FFT). According to [27], signals in the frequency domain may offer a more accurate evaluation of tremors compared to those in the time domain.

Once this has been calculated, the feature extraction will be carried out. Features will be extracted from both the time domain and the frequency domain. Time domain variables are easy to obtain and computationally inexpensive; however, often yield less robust conclusions due to the complexity to interpret the tremors associated with human motion in this domain. On the other hand, frequency domain variables, although more computationally intensive due to the need to perform an FFT, improve the accuracy of tremor detection.

For both domains, the same types of features were extracted from the signal. Table 1 lists these calculated features along with brief descriptions of each. 18 features in total - 9 from the time domain and 9 from the frequency domain - will be calculated for training the Machine Learning models.

Table 1. Features extracted from the accelerometer and gyroscope signals in each domain [13].

Feature	Description
STD	Returns the standard deviation of the signals collected in the windows in each domain
MEAN	Calculates the median value of all the measurements provided in each domain
MEDIAN	Finds the median value of the filtered signals in each domain
PERCET25	The 25th percentile of the input data have been calculated for each domain signal slice
PERCET75	The 75th percentile of the input data have been calculated for each domain signal slice
SKEWNESS	Asymmetry of the filtered signals in each domain
MAX	Finds the maximum of the values for each window in each domain
MIN	Finds the minimum of the values for each window in each domain
ENTROPY	Returns the entropy of the filtered signals in each domain

In addition to the initial 18 characteristics, an additional characteristics derived from the FFT of the signal are included. These features correspond to the calculated spectral lines, so, as there are 128 samples per window, 65 features were calculated. This results in a total of 83 characteristics for developing the algorithmic models.

Given the complexity associated with such a high-dimensional dataset, 83 features for the 8817 windows defined for each data source, a reduction strategy has been devised through Principal Components Analysis (PCA). Before conducting PCA, normalization has been implemented to center the data around a mean of 0 and ensure an explained variance of 0.98.

For the development of machine learning models, the dataset was divided using Hold Out Validation. Specifically, 80% of the data was allocated for training the algorithm, while the remaining 20% was set aside for validation purposes. Despite all measurements being taken during the same task, the inherent variability in human movement, particularly in individuals with Parkinson's Disease (PD), necessitated randomizing the train-test split across the entire dataset.

A series of machine learning models have been proposed to predict resting tremor. As the target variable is categorical, the models proposed are classification models. In this study, the following models are proposed: Gradient Boosting (XGB), AdaBoost (ADAB), KNeighbours (KNN), Random Forest (RF), Logistic Regression (LR) and Decision Tree (TREE). The Table 2 shows the selected models and the parameters used. The models were evaluated using several metrics: accuracy, sensitivity, specificity, precision, and F1-score.

Table 2. Machine learning algorithm and parameters used.

ML algorithm	Parameters
Gradient Boosting (XGB)	n_estimators = 20
AdaBoost (ADAB)	n_estimators = 20
KNeighbors (KNN)	n_neighbors = 10
Random Forest (RF)	n_estimators = 20
MLP Classifier (MLPC)	Solver = 'lbfgs', alpha = 10^{-5}, hidden_layer_sizes = (10)
Logistic Regression (LR)	–
Decision Tree (TREE)	–
Support Vector Machine (SVM)	–

4   Experiments and Results

This section presents the results obtained in the present study. Multiple experiments were conducted to evaluate the suggested approaches and to determine which sensors provide the best performance. First, Sect. 4.1 shows the results obtained with the trained models using a binary classification of the presence or absence of tremor with the different combinations of data sources in terms of both the metrics evaluated and the time required to train the models. Then, in Sect. 4.2, the same study has been performed but training the models using a labelling according to the MDS-UPDRS scale.

4.1   Results of the Training of Binary Models

The classification models proposed in Sect. 3.5 were implemented and trained using features extracted from both the time and frequency domains for each data source. In specific, three datasets have been defined: one with only accelerometer data, one with only gyroscope data and one with both accelerometer and gyroscope data. Each dataset has the defined windows labelled as tremor or non-shudder, and the aim of the models will be to predict to which of these two categories each window fits.

Due to the unbalanced nature of the database, metrics such as accuracy and precision can be misleading. These metrics often yield a high percentage of correct predictions, which might predominantly reflect correct predictions of the "no tremor" class. Therefore, the study focuses on the F1-score, as it combines precision and recall through their harmonic mean. A high F1-score indicates that both precision and recall are being max-imized simultaneously. Figure 4 presents the first approach, showing the F1-scores for each proposed model using each data source.

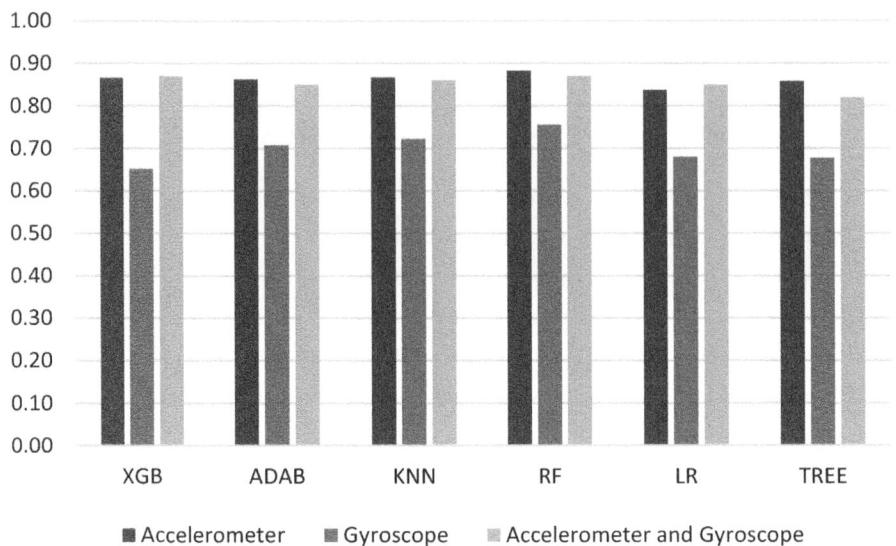

Fig. 4. F1-score comparison for each algorithm using only accelerometer training dataset, only gyroscope training dataset, and both accelerometer and gyroscope training dataset for binary classification.

From Fig. 4, it is significant relevant that using only the gyroscope data is the com-bination that gives the weakest performance in each of the proposed models, with a substantial difference in the F1-score values obtained in comparison to the rest of the dataset combinations. The average F1-score value of the models trained with only gyro-scope data is 0.70, while for only accelerometer and the combination of accelerometer and gyroscope is 0.86 and 0.85 respectively. A gap of 0.15 in the value of the F1-score is a considerable variation and indicates that the performance of the models is significantly worse.

However, the performance offered by the models trained with only accelerometer and the combination of accelerometer and gyroscope is quite similar as can be seen in the average F1-score, 0.86 vs 0.85. But in the case of the accelerometer models, the F1-score is between 0.84 and 0.88 (standard deviation of 0.013) while the combination models is between 0.82 and 0.87 (standard deviation of 0.017).

Therefore, it can be said that, of the three data source alternatives proposed, the one that offers the best performance in the trained models is the use of only accelerometer data, with an average F1-score of 0.86.

To reinforce these first findings, the study will be approached using a single model and comparing all the proposed metrics with the test data set. For this purpose, it has to be evaluated which is the best model of the six studied models, by comparing all the metrics for all the models using the training data. Tables 3, 4 and 5 show the accuracy, sensitivity, specificity, precision and f1-score for the six proposed models for the three training data sets.

Table 3. Metrics obtained for proposed models from accelerometer training data for binary classification [13].

	Accuracy	Sensitivity	Specificity	Precision	F1-score
XGB	0,94	0,86	0,96	0,87	0,87
ADAB	0,94	0,87	0,96	0,86	0,86
KNN	0,94	0,86	0,97	0,88	0,87
RF	0,95	0,87	0,97	0,90	0,88
LR	0,93	0,81	0,97	0,87	0,84
TREE	0,94	0,86	0,96	0,86	0,86

Table 4. Metrics obtained for proposed models from gyroscope training data for binary classification [13].

	Accuracy	Sensitivity	Specificity	Precision	F1-score
XGB	0,88	0,51	0,99	0,92	0,65
ADAB	0,89	0,61	0,97	0,84	0,71
KNN	0,90	0,61	0,98	0,89	0,72
RF	0,90	0,68	0,97	0,86	0,76
LR	0,88	0,57	0,97	0,85	0,68
TREE	0,86	0,68	0,90	0,67	0,68

Table 5. Metrics obtained for proposed models from combination of accelerometer and gyroscope training data for binary classification.

	Accuracy	Sensitivity	Specificity	Precision	F1-score
XGB	0,94	0,86	0,97	0,88	0,87
ADAB	0,93	0,86	0,96	0,85	0,85
KNN	0,94	0,83	0,97	0,90	0,86
RF	0,94	0,86	0,97	0,88	0,87
LR	0,94	0,81	0,97	0,89	0,85
TREE	0,92	0,82	0,95	0,82	0,82

For almost all metrics calculated on the three datasets, Randon Forest algorithm offers the best performance, with the best results for F1-score, accuracy, and sensitivity of all the models evaluated. Therefore, Random Forest algorithm will be used with test data set, corresponding to 20% of the total data, to identify whether the results previously identified in the training dataset are maintained in the test dataset or whether there is a change in behaviors of the models. The metrics obtained are shown in Table 6.

Table 6. Metrics associated with Random Forest algorithm for the three test dataset for binary classification.

[%]	Accelerometer	Gyroscope	Accelerometer and gyroscope
Accuracy	96.98	92.99	96.37
Sensitivity	91.06	75.07	89.95
Specificity	98.56	97.70	98.18
Precision	94.38	89.54	93.32
F1-score	92.69	81.67	91.60

It can be appreciated that the pattern observed with the training datasets is consistent with the test datasets, as all metrics obtained using only the gyroscope data are the lowest performance, while the other combinations offer superior performance. In terms of specificity, all three combinations provide a similar result, but it's in the other metrics where the gyroscope performs significantly worse.

For all the metrics evaluated, the accelerometer dataset shows better performance than the combination of accelerometer and gyroscope and far superior to gyroscope dataset. The major difference in the performance of accelerometer data compared to the combination of accelerometer and gyroscope is about 1%, while the difference compared with the performance of only gyroscope is about 16%.

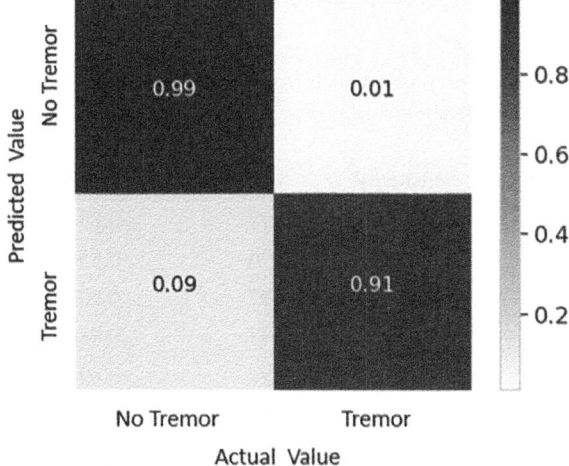

Fig. 5. Confusion matrix for Random Forest model with accelerometer test data for binary classification [13].

Figure 7 shows the normalized confusion matrix of the Random Forest algorithm evaluating the accelerometer test data. It predicts with a reliability of 99% the cases of no tremor and 91% when tremor is present. The most notable error is when, in 9% of cases, it predicts tremor in non-shaking situations, while the vice versa has a 1% error rate. This is due to 91.06% sensitivity and 98.56% specificity, indicating a very high accuracy rate in the prediction of resting tremor.

The standardized confusion matrix for the case of the Random Forest algorithm trained with the accelerometer data can be seen in Fig. 6. It can be appreciated that the gyroscope data has a 25% error rate in predicting no tremor when tremor is present, which brings the prediction rate of true tremor cases to 75%. In the prediction of non-tremor cases, the model has a higher accuracy, being correct in 98% of the cases, predicting only 2% of them as tremor.

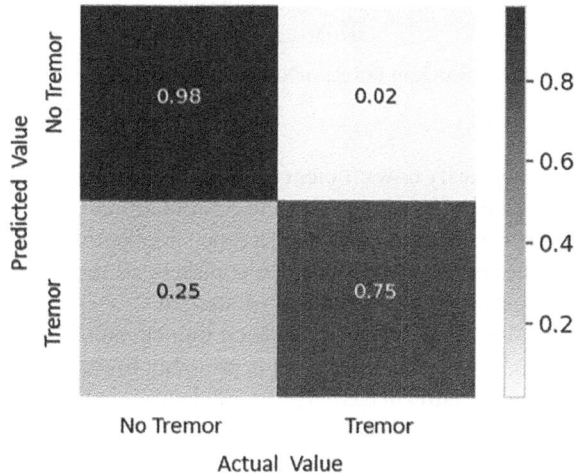

Fig. 6. Confusion matrix for Random Forest model with gyroscope test data for binary classification [13].

Figure 7 shows the normalized confusion matrix of the random forest models trained with the combined accelerometer and gyroscope data. The accuracy rates in the tremor and non-tremor cases are very similar to those of the models trained with the accelerometer, being 1% lower in both cases. This aligns with the previous findings, as for all metrics calculated, the combination of accelerometer and gyroscope data was similar but lower than the accelerometer-only data.

Although accelerometer data has been found to have the best performance, computational efficiency needs to be studied. A balance must be achieved between the performance of the models and the cost of training them. As the acquisition system is a watch and the aim is to perform measurements in free-living conditions, battery consumption is a very important fact to consider, so a very accurate but computationally very expensive model would not be as interesting as a slightly less accurate but computationally very cheap one.

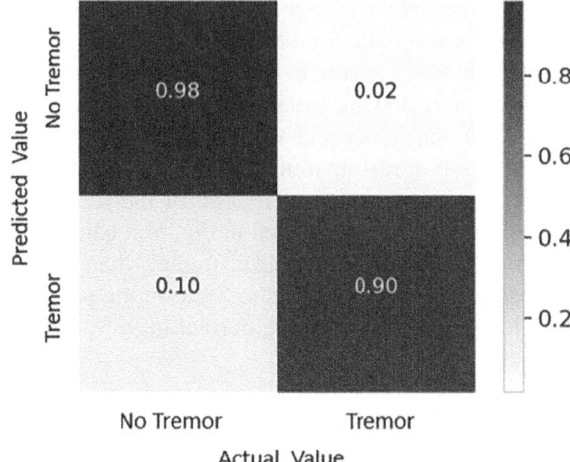

Fig. 7. Confusion matrix for Random Forest model with accelerometer and gyroscope test data for binary classification.

Therefore, in order to clarify how efficient are the algorithms implemented to improve the battery life of wearable devices, as well as the computational capacity required by the software used for the processing of these data, a time variable that indicates the seconds used to carry out all the iterations necessary to complete all the algorithms on 80% of the data used in the training of the model will be studied.

It should be noted that these models have been trained using the free version of the Google Colab platform, so the time measured is probably higher than that which could be obtained on a dedicated platform designed for model training. Table 7 shows the time collected in seconds for each combination.

Table 7. Time measured for training of all models for each data source for binary classification.

[s]	Accelerometer	Gyroscope	Accelerometer and gyroscope
Time	47.02	58.65	67.43

Once again, the data set that produces the best result is the one obtained from the accelerometer of the smartwatch. The time required for the training and validation of all the models tested with the accelerometer data is 11 s faster than the time required with the gyroscope data and 20 s faster than the combination of accelerometer and gyroscope data.

4.2 Results of the Training of Multiclass Models

This experiment will take a more qualitative approach to predicting resting tremor, moving away from binary classification. Instead, it aims to assess the algorithms' performance by accurately predicting the tremor labels assigned by the MDS-UPDRS scale through multi-class classification.

For this study, since the report of metrics in multiclass models is extensive, it has been simplified by considering that the best model for the binary classification is the same for the multiclass classification. Therefore, for this section, a Random Forest algorithm has been used.

Table 8 shows the metrics obtained from this model trained with the data labeled according to the MDS-UPDRS scale for each of the data sources combinations. These metrics have been obtained with the test dataset, 20% of the total data.

Table 8. Metrics associated with Random Forest algorithm for the three test dataset for multiclassification.

[%]	Accelerometer			Gyroscope			Accelerometer and gyroscope		
	0	1	2	0	1	2	0	1	2
Accuracy	96.1			88.6			96.5		
Sensitivity	92.6	97.7	99.6	73.5	94.5	99.1	90.7	98.4	99.9
Specificity	98.3	87.2	90.6	97.7	57.1	55.2	98.6	86.1	95.6
Precision	97.9	87.5	94.6	92.9	65.6	81.0	97.4	90.8	98.2
F1-score	98.1	87.3	92.7	95.2	91.1	65.6	98.0	88.4	97.9

The trend observed in the binary classification is maintained in the multi-class classification, as again it's the gyroscope data that gives the worst results. Although it should be noted that certain metrics are high for the gyroscope database, such as almost 98% specificity for MDS-UPDRS score 0 or 99% sensitivity for score 2, it can be observed that there are very low values, such as 65% precision for MDS-UPDRS score 1, 65% f1-score for score 2 and 55–57% specificity for scores 1 and 2, respectively.

So, as for the binary classification, the highest and most consistent values are those obtained from the accelerometer data and the combination of these with the gyroscope. The values of both combinations are quite similar, but, unlike the binary classification, the metrics obtained using the accelerometer and gyroscope data that are slightly higher in more metrics.

For the cases of no tremor (label 0), the values are practically the same, and it is in the cases where tremor is present (label 1 and 2) where the largest differences are observed, with the marked contrast being much more significant in the higher tremor score. In particular, the f1-score and specificity for label 2 show a maximum difference of around 5%.

These results correlate quite well with the data from the confusion matrices of the test data, which can be seen in the Fig. 8, Fig. 9 and Fig. 10 for accelerometer, gyroscope and the combination, respectively.

In the case of the accelerometer data, in Fig. 8, the model shows very low error rates. It is 98% correct for no tremor (score 0), 87% correct for mild tremor (score 1) and 91% correct for more severe tremor (score 2). In general, the errors occur because the model assumes that the data is located at a higher score than the real one, as can be seen, for example, that it makes an error of 11% when predicting as score 1 instead of score 0 and 2% in the opposite case.

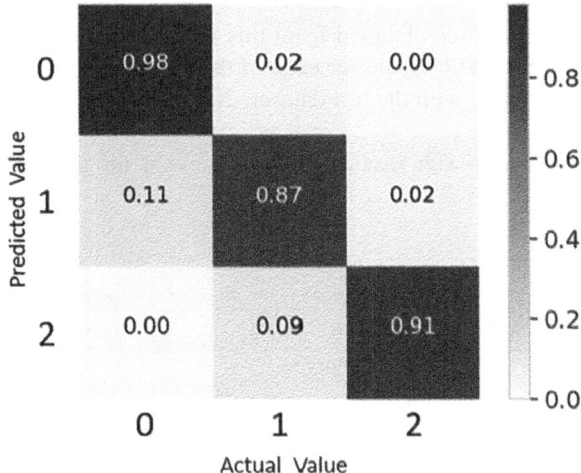

Fig. 8. Confusion matrix for Random Forest model with accelerometer test data for multiclassification.

Figure 9 shows the confusion matrix for the gyroscope data. As can be concluded from the presented metrics, the trained model has a higher error rate. The only exception is the score 0 data, with a 98% accuracy. The rest of the accuracy rates are quite low, as only 57% of the predicted score 1 and 55% of the predicted score 2 cases are correct.

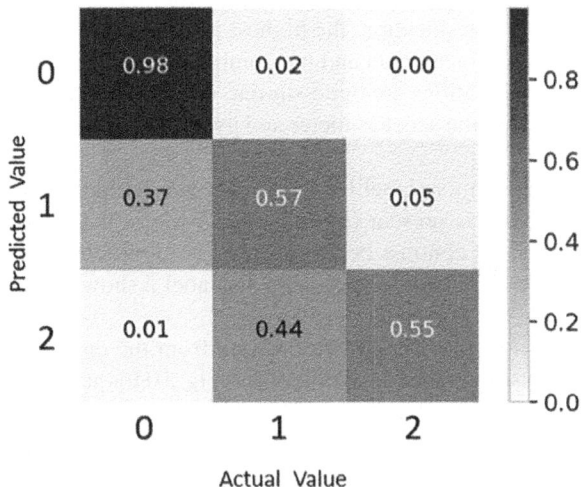

Fig. 9. Confusion matrix for Random Forest model with gyroscope test data for multiclassification.

However, it has the same kind of error as the accelerometer case, as it has to presume that the data are located in a higher score than the score. 37% of the cases predicted as score 1 are score 0 and 44% of those predicted as score 1 are score 2, while in the opposite case, only 2% of those predicted as score 0 are score 1 and 5% of those predicted as score 2 are score 1.

The confusion matrix for the combination of dataset is shown in Fig. 10. The results obtained are like those shown in the case of the accelerometer. This dataset is more accurate with score 2, which in this case is 96% vs. 91% for the accelerometer alone. Metric 0 (98% vs 99%) and score 1 (86% vs 87%) are practically identical. The trend to overestimate the present tremor of the previous cases is sustained in this model, as it produces an error of 4% predicting score 2 when it is 1 (1% otherwise) and 13% labelling it as 1 when it is 0 (1% otherwise).

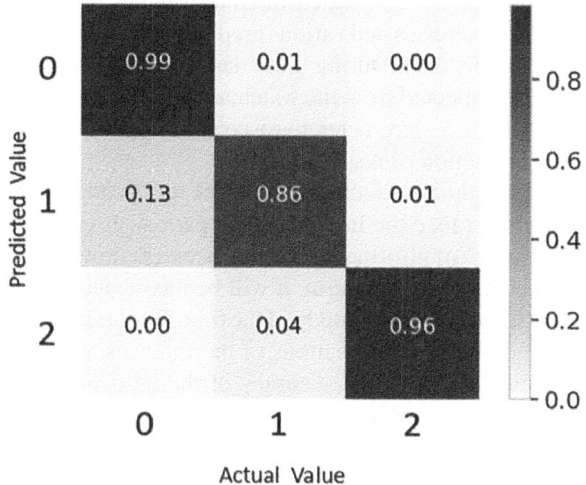

Fig. 10. Confusion matrix for Random Forest model with accelerometer and gyroscope test data for multiclassification.

As it has been seen in the metrics and in the confusion matrix calculated, the models trained with the accelerometer data and the combination of accelerometer and gyroscope are quite accurate and similar, being slightly above the second one. Therefore, the study of the time needed to train the models can be a very decisive factor in determining which of the two options is more interesting to perform measurements in free-living conditions where the computational cost due to battery consumption must be considered.

Table 9 shows the measured times needed to train the models using only the training data in the Google Colab platform. The results obtained show that the accelerometer data require the shortest time for model training, using 57 s for this purpose. The models trained with the gyroscope data need 8 s more, while the models that require more time are those trained with the data from both inertial sensors, as they need 77 s to do so. It can be seen that the change from binary to multiclassification has increased the time required by about 10 s.

Table 9. Time measured for training of all models for each data source for multiclassification.

[s]	Accelerometer	Gyroscope	Accelerometer and gyroscope
Time	57.36	65.53	77.28

5 Conclusions

Accurate tracking of disease progression and treatment efficacy in individuals with Parkinson's Disease (PD) is critical. This study focuses on improving this monitoring process through the implementation of efficient algorithms designed to streamline and enhance tracking capabilities.

By utilizing inertial sensors embedded in smartwatches, the study collected data during eight standardized exercises and various predictive models for resting tremor were then developed based on this data. During these data collection sessions, accelerometer and gyroscope data were collected from the watch, and this study has been carried out on which data source, whether accelerometer, gyroscope or a combination of both, provides the best results in the prediction of resting tremor.

Leveraging technological advancements over recent decades, the trend is towards free-living monitoring to reduce the burden on the patient. It is therefore necessary to assess not only which source of information is more accurate, but also which requires less computational cost, since, in the long term, it will be the devices themselves that make real-time predictions. So, in addition, a study of the time required to train several machine learning models using different combinations of inertial sensors has been proposed. A balance must be achieved between the accuracy of the models and the computational cost (time) required. A very accurate but computationally expensive model may not be as interesting as a slightly less accurate but computationally cheap one.

In this study, two different approaches have been proposed: one focused on a binary classification of the presence or absence of tremor, and the other based on a multiclassification focused on the assessment of tremor according to the MDS-UPDRS scale.

For binary classification between the presence or not of tremor, the use of only accelerometer data is the option that provides the best results, both in terms of the overall accuracy of the models and the time required to train them. Using this data, the best model, a Random Forest algorithm, achieves an accuracy, sensitivity, specificity, precision, and F1-score of 94%, 86%, 97%, 88%, 87%, respectively, in training data and 97%, 91%, 99%,94% and 93%, respectively, in test data. These impressive results demonstrate the model's effectiveness in automatically detecting resting tremor, comparable to the findings of [20] and [17]. In addition, the accelerometer is the source that requires the shortest time to train all the proposed algorithms, requiring 47 s for this task.

Alternatively, the combined data with the gyroscope provides much better results in terms of model accuracy than the only gyroscope data, but this trend turn around in the training time calculation, where the gyroscope data is faster than the combined data.

On the other hand, related to the multiclass classification according to the MDS-UPDRS scale, the results are not as robust as with the previous proposal in terms of performance of the models. The models trained with the combined accelerometer and gyroscope data and those trained with only accelerometer data provide much better performance than the models trained with only gyroscope. The models trained with the combination of inertial sensors that offer slightly better performance, as they have an accuracy of 99%, 86% and 96% for the 0,1,2 scores respectively versus 98%, 87% and 91% for the accelerometer models, as well as having a lower error in the misclassified data. But, as it can be seen, the results are very similar.

Regarding the time required for training, the results are more conclusive. The models trained with the accelerometer require the least time, 57 s, compared to 65 s for those trained with the gyroscope and 77 s for those trained with the combination of sensors. Models trained with the combination of sensors provide better accuracy but require much more training time compared to the time needed for accelerometer-only trained models, which have a slightly lower accuracy.

Although these results are quite promising, it is important to acknowledge certain limitations of this study that should be addressed in future research. The study was conducted with a relatively small sample size, involving only 6 PD patients over an 8-week period, 48 measurement sessions. This limited sample size may affect the generalizability of the findings. Additionally, as 75% of the samples corresponding to a single label (score 0, no tremor), this imbalance could potentially bias the results and reduce the robustness of the predictive models. To enhance the reliability and validity of the findings, increasing the number of measurement sessions and ensuring a more balanced dataset will help in obtaining more comprehensive and generalizable results.

The results indicate that, for detecting presence or not of tremor, using the accelerometer as the only inertial sensor yields excellent results in Parkinson's Disease (PD) patients. In the case of the classification according to the MDS-UPDRS scale, the use of only the accelerometer data also provides very encouraging results, although the combination of these data with the gyroscope shows a competitive alternative, as it has a slightly better performance despite having a higher computational cost. For this reason, a more detailed study would have to be carried out to study which combination could be the most interesting for a study and deployment in free-living conditions, in the case of multiclassification. It should be noted that these models have been developed a posteriori, but, in the future, if these algorithms are going to be used in real time on the edge, the computational cost will be a very important factor to consider.

Computing-wise, using a single inertial sensor in wearable devices offers several significant advantages. Firstly, it can enhance battery life and reduce power consumption, making the devices more practical for continuous, long-term use. Secondly, it lowers the computational demands required for data processing, model training and new data classification, which can lead to faster and more efficient real-time monitoring.

Overall, focusing on a single sensor without compromising the accuracy of tremor prediction paves the way for more accessible and user-friendly wearable solutions for PD management, as in a future real-world application, it would contribute to the clinician's understanding and tracking of patient data.

Acknowledgements. This study was funded by the Project BIOCLITE PID2021-123708OB-I00, funded by MCIN/AEI/10.13039/501100011033/FEDER, EU. The authors acknowledge to the Instrumentation and Applied Acoustics Research Group (I2A2) at Universidad Politécnica de

Madrid and the Physical Education and Sports Science (PESS) department, the Health Research Institute (HRI), and the Data-Driven Computer Engineering (D2iCE) Group at University of Limerick.

Disclosure of Interests. The authors have no competing interests to declare that are relevant to the content of this article.

References

1. Wirdefeldt, K., Adami, H., Cole, P., Trichopoulos, D., Mandel, J.: Epidemiology and etiology of Parkinson's disease: a review of the evidence. Eur. J. Epidemiol. **26**(Suppl 1), S1–58 (2011)
2. Rocca, W.: The burden of Parkinson's disease: a worldwide perspective. Lancet Neurol. **17**(11); 928–929 (2018)
3. Halli-Tierney, A.D., Luker, J., Carroll, D.G.: Parkinson disease. Am. Family Phys. **102**(11), 679–691 (2020)
4. Rodge, J.E.: Tremor. Springer International Publishing, Neuro-Geriatrics (2017)
5. Gironell, A., Pascual-Sedano, B., Aracil, I., Marín-Lahoz, J., Pagonabarraga, J., Kulisevsky, J.: Tremor types in Parkinson disease: a descriptive study using a new classification. Parkinson's Dis. **2018**, 4327597 (2018)
6. Salarian, A., et al.: An ambulatory system to quantify bradykinesia and tremor in Parkinson's disease. In: Proceedings of the 4th International IEEE EMBS Special Topic Conference on Information Technology Applications in Biomedicine, Birmingham, England (2003)
7. Mannini, A., Intille, S., Rosenberger, M., Sabatini, A., Haskell, W.: Activity recognition using a single accelerometer placed at the wrist or ankle. Med. Sci. Sports Exercise **45**(11), 2193–203 (2013)
8. LeWitt, P.A.: Levodopa for the treatment of Parkinson's disease. New Englad J. Med. **359**(23), 2468–76 (2008)
9. Bhidayasiri, R., Martinez-Martin, P.: Clinical assessments in Parkinson's disease: scales and monitoring. Int. Rev. Neurobiol. **132**, 129–182 (2017)
10. Goetz, C., et al.: Movement disorder society-sponsored revision of the unified Parkinson's disease rating scale (MDS-UPDRS): scale presentation and clinimetric testing results. Movement Disord. **23**(15), 2129–2170 (2008)
11. Rovini, E., Maremmani, C., Cavallo, F.: How wearable sensors can support Parkinson's disease diagnosis and treatment: a systematic review. Front. Neurosci. (2017)
12. Hssayeni, M., Jimenez-Shahed, J., Burack, M., Ghoraani, B.: Wearable sensors for estimation of parkinsonian tremor severity during free body movements. Sensors (2019)
13. Polvorinos-Fernández, C., et al.: Evaluation of the performance of wearables' inertial sensors for the diagnosis of resting tremor in Parkinson's disease. In: Proceedings of the 17th International Joint Conference on Biomedical Engineering Systems and Technologies - HEALTHINF, Rome, Italy (2024)
14. Sigcha, L., et al.: Monipar database: smartwatch movement data to monitor motor competency in subjects with Parkinson's disease (1.0) (2023). https://doi.org/10.5281/zenodo.8104853
15. Luis-Martínez, R., et al.: Impact of social and mobility restrictions in Parkinson's disease during COVID-19 lockdown. BMC Neurology (2021)
16. Sigcha, L., et al.: Automatic resting tremor assessment in parkinson's disease using smartwatches and multitask convolutional neural networks. Sensors (2021)
17. San-Segundo, R., et al.: Parkinson's Disease tremor detection in the wild using wearable accelerometers. Sensors **20**(20), 5817 (2020)

18. van Brummelen, E., et al.: Quantification of tremor using consumer product accelerometry is feasible in patients with essential tremor and Parkinson's disease: a comparative study. J. Clin. Movement Disord. (2020)
19. López-Blanco, R., et al.: Smartwatch for the analysis of rest tremor in patients with Parkinson's disease. J. Neurol. Sci. **401**, 37–42 (2019)
20. Sun, M., et al.: TremorSense: tremor detection for Parkinson's disease using convolutional neural network. In: IEEE/ACM Conference on Connected Health: Applications, Systems and Engineering Technologies (CHASE), Washington, DC, USA (2021)
21. Powers, R., et al.: Smartwatch inertial sensors continuously monitor real-world motor fluctuations in Parkinson's disease. Sci. Transl. Med. (2021)
22. TECAPARK. https://www.i2a2.upm.es/tecapark/. Accessed 29 May 2024
23. Sigcha, L., et al.: Monipar: Movement data collection tool to monitor motor symptoms in Parkinson's disease using smartwatches and smartphones. Front. Neurol. 14 (2023)
24. Hoehn, M., Yahr, M.: Parkinsonism: onset, progression, and mortality. Neurology **17**(5), 427–42 (1998)
25. Khan, A., Hammerla, N., Mellor, S., Plötz, T.: Optimising sampling rates for accelerometer-based human activity recognition. Pattern Recognit. **73**, 33–40 (2016)
26. Patel, S., et al.: Monitoring motor fluctuations in patients with Parkinson's disease using wearable sensors. IEEE Trans. Inf. Technol. Biomed. **13**(6), 864–73 (2009)
27. Ahlrichs, C., Samà, A.: Is "frequency distribution" enough to detect tremor in PD patients using a wrist worn accelerometer?. In: Proceedings of the 8th International Conference on Pervasive Computing Technologies for Healthcare, Oldenburg, Germany (2014)

Author Index

The manufacturer's authorised representative in the EU is Springer
Nature Customer Service Centre GmbH, Europaplatz 3, 69115 Heidelberg,
Germany. If you have any concerns regarding our products, please
contact ProductSafety@springernature.com

Printed and bound by CPI Group (UK) Ltd, Croydon, CR0 4YY
28/04/2026
02098524-0012